2015
The Year Book of SURGERY®

Editor-in-Chief
Kevin E. Behrns, MD
Chairman, Edward R. Woodward Professor, Department of Surgery, University of Florida, Gainesville, Florida

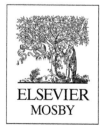

ELSEVIER
MOSBY

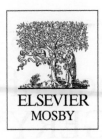

ELSEVIER
MOSBY

Vice President, Global Medical Reference: Mary E. Gatsch
Acquisitions Editor: John Vassallo
Developmental Editor: Susan Showalter
Production Supervisor, Electronic Year Books: Donna M. Skelton
Electronic Article Manager: Mike Sheets
Illustrations and Permissions Coordinator: Dawn Vohsen

2015 EDITION

Printed in the United States of America
Composition by TNQ Books and Journals Pvt Ltd, India

Editorial Office:
Elsevier
1600 John F. Kennedy Blvd.
Suite 1800
Philadelphia, PA 19103-2899

International Standard Serial Number: 0090-3671
International Standard Book Number: 978-0-323-35554-4

Editorial Board

Table of Contents

Journals Represented

Journals represented in this YEAR BOOK are listed below.

Academic Emergency Medicine
Acta Anaesthesiologica Scandinavica
Acta Paediatrica
Air Medical Journal
American Journal of Clinical Nutrition
American Journal of Rhinology & Allergy
American Journal of Surgery
American Journal of Transplantation
Annals of Surgery
Annals of Surgical Oncology
Annals of Thoracic Surgery
British Journal of Surgery
British Medical Journal
Burns
Cancer
Clinical Journal of the American Society of Nephrology
Clinical Orthopaedics and Related Research
Critical Care Medicine
Digestive Diseases and Sciences
European Journal of Surgical Oncology
Gut
Gynecologic Oncology
Health affairs
Injury
Intensive Care Medicine
International Journal of Obstetric Anesthesia
Journal of Adolescent Health
Journal of Burn Care & Research
Journal of Cardiothoracic and Vascular Anesthesia
Journal of Clinical Endocrinology & Metabolism
Journal of Clinical Oncology
Journal of Pediatric Gastroenterology and Nutrition
Journal of Pediatrics
Journal of Surgical Research
Journal of Thoracic and Cardiovascular Surgery
Journal of Trauma and Acute Care Surgery
Journal of Vascular and Interventional Radiology
Journal of Vascular Surgery
Journal of the American College of Surgeons
Journal of the American Medical Association
Journal of the American Medical Association Surgery
Journal of the American College of Cardiology
JPEN Journal of Parenteral and Enteral Nutrition
Lancet
Medicine
New England Journal of Medicine
Pediatrics

Proceedings of the National Academy of Sciences of the United States of America
Stroke
Surgery
Thyroid
Transplantation
Transplantation Proceedings
Wound Repair and Regeneration

STANDARD ABBREVIATIONS

The following terms are abbreviated in this edition: acquired immunodeficiency syndrome (AIDS), cardiopulmonary resuscitation (CPR), central nervous system (CNS), cerebrospinal fluid (CSF), computed tomography (CT), deoxyribonucleic acid (DNA), electrocardiography (ECG), health maintenance organization (HMO), human immunodeficiency virus (HIV), intensive care unit (ICU), intramuscular (IM), intravenous (IV), magnetic resonance (MR) imaging (MRI), ribonucleic acid (RNA), and ultrasound (US).

NOTE

The YEAR BOOK OF SURGERY is a literature survey service providing abstracts of articles published in the professional literature. Every effort is made to assure the accuracy of the information presented in these pages. Neither the editors nor the publisher of the YEAR BOOK OF SURGERY can be responsible for errors in the original materials. The editors' comments are their own opinions. Mention of specific products within this publication does not constitute endorsement.

To facilitate the use of the YEAR BOOK OF SURGERY as a reference tool, all illustrations and tables included in this publication are now identified as they appear in the original article. This change is meant to help the reader recognize that any illustration or table appearing in the YEAR BOOK OF SURGERY may be only one of many in the original article. For this reason, figure and table numbers appear to be out of sequence within the YEAR BOOK OF SURGERY.

1 General Considerations

Association of the 2011 ACGME Resident Duty Hour Reform With General Surgery Patient Outcomes and With Resident Examination Performance
Rajaram R, Chung JW, Jones AT, et al (American College of Surgeons, Chicago, IL; Northwestern Univ, Chicago, IL; American Board of Surgery, Philadelphia, PA; et al)
JAMA 312:2374-2384, 2014

Importance.—In 2011, the Accreditation Council for Graduate Medical Education (ACGME) restricted resident duty hour requirements beyond those established in 2003, leading to concerns about the effects on patient care and resident training.

Objective.—To determine if the 2011 ACGME duty hour reform was associated with a change in general surgery patient outcomes or in resident examination performance.

Design, Setting, and Participants.—Quasi-experimental study of general surgery patient outcomes 2 years before (academic years 2009-2010) and after (academic years 2012-2013) the 2011 duty hour reform. Teaching and nonteaching hospitals were compared using a difference-in-differences approach adjusted for procedural mix, patient comorbidities, and time trends. Teaching hospitals were defined based on the proportion of cases at which residents were present intraoperatively. Patients were those undergoing surgery at hospitals participating in the American College of Surgeons National Surgical Quality Improvement Program (ACS NSQIP). General surgery resident performance on the annual in-training, written board, and oral board examinations was assessed for this same period.

Exposures.—National implementation of revised resident duty hour requirements on July 1, 2011, in all ACGME accredited residency programs.

Main Outcomes and Measures.—Primary outcome was a composite of death or serious morbidity; secondary outcomes were other postoperative complications and resident examination performance.

Results.—In the main analysis, 204 641 patients were identified from 23 teaching (n = 102 525) and 31 nonteaching (n = 102 116) hospitals. The unadjusted rate of death or serious morbidity improved during the study period in both teaching (11.6% [95% CI, 11.3%-12.0%] to 9.4% [95% CI, 9.1%-9.8%], $P < .001$) and nonteaching hospitals (8.7% [95% CI, 8.3%-9.0%] to 7.1% [95% CI, 6.8%-7.5%], $P < .001$). In adjusted analyses, the 2011 ACGME duty hour reform was not associated with a significant change in death or serious morbidity in either postreform year 1 (OR, 1.12; 95% CI, 0.98-1.28) or postreform year 2 (OR, 1.00; 95% CI, 0.86-1.17) or when both postreform years were combined (OR, 1.06; 95% CI, 0.93-1.20). There was no association between duty hour reform and any other postoperative adverse outcome. Mean (SD) in-training examination scores did not significantly change from 2010 to 2013 for first-year residents (499.7 [85.2] to 500.5 [84.2], $P = .99$), for residents from other postgraduate years, or for first-time examinees taking the written or oral board examinations during this period.

Conclusions and Relevance.—Implementation of the 2011 ACGME duty hour reform was not associated with a change in general surgery patient outcomes or differences in resident examination performance. The implications of these findings should be considered when evaluating the merit of the 2011 ACGME duty hour reform and revising related policies in the future.

▶ Few topics have engendered as much discussion in the surgical world as resident duty-hour reform. After more than a decade, vigorous debate regarding the merit of duty hours persists. Since the introduction of the 2011 Accreditation Council for Graduate Medical Education revised duty-hour regulations, investigation of the effect of these work hour rules on patient outcomes has come in the form of single institutional studies that have largely found no improvement in patient outcomes. In this study, Rajaram et al used the National Surgical Quality Improvement Program database to assess outcomes in teaching ($n = 23$) and nonteaching ($n = 31$) hospitals in 204 641 patients. The primary end point was the composite of mortality and major complication. The results are crystal clear (Fig 2 in the original article). Further restriction in duty hours did not result in improved patient outcomes. Furthermore, American Board of Surgery test scores were not improved with duty-hour changes. Therefore, this study clearly demonstrates a lack of an association between duty hours and major outcome measurements. However, is this the real question we need to address? Although this information is clearly beneficial, the most important question is: are we producing trainees that can competently care for patients in an autonomous setting? Many senior surgeons opine that our surgical resident product is less well trained than in the past, and this has led to a large proportion of the residents securing additional training. This should not be surprising in that we have essentially eliminated 1 year of training through duty-hour restrictions. The ongoing prospective trial (FIRST—Flexibility in Duty Hour Requirements for Surgical Trainees) will provide us with helpful information, but we will still need to assess the competence of our residents to care for surgical patients independently.

K. E. Behrns, MD

Are We Paying Our Housestaff Fairly?
Morris JB, Burke SV, Berns JS (Univ of Pennsylvania, Philadelphia)
Ann Surg 260:1-2, 2014

Background.—Interns, residents, and fellows in US graduate medical education (GME) training programs are currently paid based on postgraduate year (PGY) of training rather than hours worked and without considering specialty or subspecialty. This method of housestaff compensation causes substantial discrepancies between hourly pay rates that have existed for at least 25 years. It is time to consider changing the approach in the interest of fairness.

Proposals.—Alternatives to the current system have been proposed. First, regional or national benchmarking data on usual hours worked per week in each different training program may be used to devise weekly salaries based on an effective hourly rate adjusted to each subsequent PGY level. With this system, a PGY-1 Dermatology resident and a PGY-1 General Surgery resident would each be paid the same effective hourly rate, but the General Surgery resident would receive a higher annual salary that reflects the greater number of hours required in that specialty.

Trainees could also be compensated at different levels based on benchmark data concerning approximate hours worked in each specialty or subspecialty area. Stepwise salary increases would then be assigned to each successive PGY level in the program.

Institutions could also identify a scale of hours worked. Programs whose trainees work well below an established threshold are paid less, then the saved money is used to increase compensation for trainees who work the most hours. The percentage of lower-hour employees who contribute to the increased salaries for the maximum-hour employees need not be at the same rate. For example, money from the bottom 20% of employees may be used to increase salaries for just the top 10% of the most-hours-worked employees. Home calls could be compensated with an additional hourly stipend.

Salary structure changes may be costly. Other salaries may need to be reduced, or new and innovative revenue sources may be sought. If these options are not feasible, the hospital and/or clinical program that benefits from the work of the housestaff may need to foot the bill. All training programs would have to be included in changes to avoid discrepancies among programs that use different compensation formulas. However, a new compensation system that considers hours worked as well as specialty or subspecialty and PGY would likely reduce the need for residents and fellows with longer working hours to seek opportunities to moonlight and earn more money.

Objections.—Several objections may arise. The argument that housestaff who choose programs that require long work hours know what they are getting into should not override the exercise of fundamental fairness. Considering future earning capability as offsetting a lower housestaff pay rate is also unfair. A tiered salary structure may be seen as a creating a hierarchy of value that undermines teamwork and morale, but in fact can be countered by pointing out the equitable hourly rates regardless of specialty or subspecialty. People are unlikely to select a training program based on housestaff salary, so the fear that remedying inequities in such compensation will diminish the appeal of certain specialties that are currently experiencing shortages is largely unfounded.

Conclusions.—Since 2005, federal law has viewed housestaff pay as the same as pay for other hospital employees and taxes it accordingly. To be fair, the considerations that guide other employee compensation should be followed for housestaff.

▶ Morris et al raise the interesting question of fair pay for housestaff, who, depending on the discipline, have markedly different jobs and hours worked yet receive the same pay. They suggest that resident pay is unfair and should be based on the number of hours worked. Their proposal suggests that trainees be compensated in 3 tiers based on the hours worked per week with the intervals of less than 50 hours, 50 to 65 hours, and greater than 65 hours with a predetermined hourly rate. In addition, home call would be compensated by an additional hourly stipend. Although this compensation plan levels the playing field and addresses inequities in pay for hours worked, several issues should be thoroughly examined because unintended consequences are sure to arise. First, pay for home call opens the door for presumed hourly compensation for other duties that may be deemed outside the usual duties of patient care and education. Would participation on a quality committee come with additional pay? In addition, would home study be a criterion for pay? Second, for young trainees, who are often debt-laden, an hourly rate would invite the perverse incentive of working longer hours merely for pay that is needed to pay the bills at home. Finally, and importantly, medicine and surgery are professions that have a long tradition of service and duty that supersede compensation. As surgeons, we are committed to our patients' well-being regardless of whether we are called in during off-hours, and compensation for this commitment is irrelevant.

K. E. Behrns, MD

Graded Autonomy in Medical Education — Managing Things That Go Bump in the Night
Halpern SD, Detsky AS (Perelman School of Medicine of the Univ of Pennsylvania, Philadelphia; Univ of Toronto, Ontario, Canada)
N Engl J Med 370:1086-1089, 2014

Background.—After the death of Libby Zion in a New York emergency department in 1984, measures were taken to improve patient safety by reducing medical errors related to fatigued residents and poor supervision. Resident fatigue was cited as less important than inadequate supervision in this case, but the first changes were to restrict work hours. After a decade of duty-hour reforms, evidence shows that most residents get a bit more sleep but patient care is not safer and outcomes have not improved. Changes in supervision are now proposed but before they are enacted, careful analysis of their value and the potential for increasing patient safety while maintaining the growth of medical trainees in terms of autonomy must be undertaken.

Proposed Changes.—Increasingly, residents must discuss all newly admitted patients with their attending physicians at night. Intensive care units (ICUs) are being staffed with more supervisors, including nighttime intensivists. Evidence supporting these changes is lacking, with some reports noting no change in outcomes. Newer resident-training approaches may not improve patient safety, and questions arise about how training models that reduce the opportunities for autonomous decision making will affect the quality of care of future patients. Organizations that regulate training programs should allow and promote assessments of various models of graded autonomy, especially at night, rather than set a single rigid standard without supporting evidence.

When physicians become independent practitioners, they are expected to function competently and without supervision. The term *core competencies* reflects a change in the curriculum from imparting and testing residents on a specific knowledge base to promoting expertise in the functions and attributes characteristic of independent physicians. Attending physicians assess "educational milestones" or the attainment of core competencies defined by accrediting bodies. Other terms used in regard to this new approach include *entrustable professional activities* and *statements of awarded responsibility*. These reflect the goal of translating theory into practice.

Another change seen in autonomous physicians is the expectation that they will simultaneously provide trainees with appropriate supervision and autonomy. Most residents resent close supervision and believe their autonomy is compromised by having an intensivist looking over their shoulders. Accrediting institutions and regulators should permit and encourage experimentation with various supervisory strategies to determine the most effective approach. Studies comparing the various approaches and the varying degrees of autonomy allowed would provide high-quality evidence to guide the development of more effective training programs. Both long-term and short-term studies are needed. Among the outcomes to be determined are accuracy of residents' initial diagnoses compared to those of the attending physician; physicians' evaluations of the likelihood residents will become excellent doctors; and number of independent, consequential decisions made by physicians during residency.

Issues.—The cost of increased supervision must be determined and compared to the effect on patient safety to determine the most efficient means of improving outcomes. Among the cost considerations should be the opportunity cost of using the attending physicians to supervise residents rather than provide more services to patients. Both quality of life and risk of burnout should also be assessed in relation to a heavier load of resident supervision.

Conclusions.—It is unsafe to require overly tired trainee physicians to make decisions independently for serious ill patients, but just getting more rest has not provided better outcomes. Studies of resident-training models are needed to determine the best way to train physicians without imposing supervision that will stifle their growth into mature, independent, successful physicians.

▶ More than a decade ago, surgical training underwent major restructuring with the implementation of duty-hour regulations. The changes in duty hours have been controversial and have generated robust discussion in the literature about the consequences, both intended and unintended. Now, 11 years later, it is clear that duty-hour restrictions have neither improved care nor have they generated a resident workforce that is substantially more rested. With accumulating evidence that duty-hour restrictions did not improve patient care, regulatory bodies have implemented new rules regarding resident supervision. These new regulations essentially mandate that a supervising faculty member be immediately available for consultation and review of clinical details. Not unexpectedly, these changes have dramatically reduced trainee autonomy. Neither the trainee nor the faculty accepts these changes as universally sound for the advancement of education and training. Importantly, increased supervision has the intended consequence of loss of autonomy, but too often an unintended consequence is the lack of engagement of the trainee. If residents must review all the clinical data with a supervisor, they may not fully interpret the clinical data and make an informed decision for which they are responsible. The abdication of responsibility to the attending physician is associated with a high cost to the trainee and, more important, to future patients. When will the trainees learn to make the difficult decisions if they experience loss of autonomy during their training? Is it advantageous to have them make these potentially life-altering decisions when they have no supervision? We should rethink resident training such that we have structured independent decision making and the trainees receive important feedback on autonomous care of patients.

K. E. Behrns, MD

Interventions to address challenges associated with the transition from residency training to independent surgical practice
Sachdeva AK, Flynn TC, Brigham TP, et al (American College of Surgeons, Chicago, IL; Accreditation Council for Graduate Med Education, Chicago, IL; Washington Univ School of Medicine, St Louis, MO; et al)
Surgery 155:867-882, 2014

Background.—Concerns regarding preparation of residents for independent surgical practice are widespread and support for junior surgeons entering practice is variable across institutions and practices. The American College of Surgeons (ACS) Division of Education partnered with the Accreditation Council for Graduate Medical Education (ACGME) to convene a National Invitational Conference to define key issues relating to the transition to practice and develop recommendations to address various challenges.

Outcomes of the National Invitational Conference.—Leaders from ACS, ACGME, certifying boards, residency review committees, program director organizations, and professional societies representing the breadth of surgical specialties, along with other key stakeholders, were invited to participate in the 1.5-day conference in July 2012. Key recommendations generated during the conference included the need to focus on the transition to practice within the context of the continuum of professional development; definition of specific levels of knowledge and skills expected of graduating surgery residents; development and adoption of competency-based methods for training, assessment, and advancement of residents; implementation of special interventions during the chief resident year to prepare residents for practice; robust evaluations of residents before graduation; intake assessments of junior surgeons during the onboarding processes; and effective mentorship for junior surgeons as they enter practice. Recommendations also highlighted major regulatory, legal, and financial issues. The key role of ACS and other national organizations in implementing the recommendations was underscored.

Conclusion.—The recommendations from the conference should be of great help in addressing various challenges associated with the transition from surgery residency to independent practice.

▶ Since the inception of duty-hours regulations, the loss of resident autonomy caused by billing criteria from payers, and decreased reimbursement that necessitated increased clinical productivity by supervising faculty, a widespread observation that surgical trainees are less prepared to practice independently has been promulgated. The broadcast of this observation has been so loud that numerous constituencies of surgical training have taken notice and responded with a call to action. A major response to this supposition was the National Invitational Conference organized by the American College of Surgeons and the Accreditation Council on Graduate Medical Education. Here, Sachdeva et al report the findings of this conference in which education thought leaders gathered for 1.5 days to exchange ideas about theoretic and operational ways to enhance the autonomy and function of graduating surgical residents. This masterful, comprehensive publication details many approaches to improving surgical education, and this work is a must read for all surgical educators. However, this work must be placed in temporal context. The report was written in the framework of a fee-for-service surgical business model that drives patient care delivery. How will we train surgical residents in a new model of care that emphasizes surgery as a valuable resource that is to be used nearly exclusively when its benefits clearly outdistance other treatments? This article offers numerous strategies for improving surgical training, and it certainly addresses necessary competencies. Three major factors that need to be placed in the context of new models of surgical care delivery are (1) the necessity for patient-centered care and quality outcomes, (2) the mandate that health care delivery occurs through teamwork, (3) and the obligation for lifelong learning. These 3 factors must take center stage in the education of surgical trainees. All actions must be geared toward patient outcomes, and surgeons not only must be integrated in teams, but they must lead health care units that put the patient outcome as the top priority. Finally, all surgeons must commit to lifelong training, and it is the responsibility of our certifying bodies to ensure the public that we, as a surgical community, are committed to lifelong betterment of surgical care.

K. E. Behrns, MD

Surgical Coaching for Individual Performance Improvement

Greenberg CC, for the Wisconsin Surgical Coaching Program (Univ of Wisconsin, Madison; et al)

Ann Surg 261:32-34, 2015

Background.—Surgical outcomes can be altered by the surgeon's skill. Unfortunately skill levels can vary significantly between surgeons. Among the possible new approaches to improving individual performance is one-on-one coaching. The definition of coaching and characteristics of an effective coach and coaching program were outlined.

Definitions.—Coaching is defined as a cooperative process involving a coach and coachee in which the coach provides objective, constructive instruction to help the coachee expand and apply specific skills, knowledge, and abilities. In surgery, coaching focuses on improving and refining the surgeon's existing skills, empowering the surgeon to become an agent of change, and applying the results throughout the surgeon's career.

Characteristics.—Effective coaches should demonstrate strong interpersonal skills such as effective communication that emphasizes active and engaged listening, encouragement, and challenges for the coachee. Coaches should also be highly respected in their field, which is useful in building rapport with and gaining the appreciation of the coachee. The coach should be able to recognize the individual surgeon's ability and experience, build rapport and trust, and work with him or her to define the appropriate goals and develop strategies for working toward them.

The coaching program begins with setting goals, then it provides encouragement and motivation and guides the surgeon toward enhancements of the appropriate skills. Some programs may be focused on transitioning the surgeon to independent practice but often they will involve peer coaching. The three domains targeted for performance improvement are technical skill, cognitive skill, and nontechnical skill. These interrelated domains are addressed as appropriate to optimize components that are controllable, such as whether the coaching should be done by a video review or live interaoperative instruction, peer versus expert coaching, and the setting from which coaches and surgeons are identified. The advantages and disadvantages of each must be considered. Other components of the program that can be of importance are the coachee's experience, skill level, disposition, and interpersonal skills and the types of operations, practice settings, and system characteristics in which the surgeon works.

Conclusions.—Increasingly the focus in health care is on improving the quality and safety of care and developing practical continuing education offerings. The American Board of Surgery has included lifelong learning and self-assessment and the evaluation of performance in practice in its requirements for the Maintenance of Certification. Surgeons who want to improve their performance may benefit from the use of a coach to meet these requirements.

▶ Lifelong learning is a basic tenet of high-quality surgical care. Surgeons must continue to evolve their knowledge, psychomotor skill set, and decision-making ability throughout their career. In decades past, it was assumed that practitioners would accomplish these tasks independently, but as the availability of information rapidly proliferated, the need for clinical productivity increased, technological advances burgeoned, and the demands of nonclinical activities increased, career development became overwhelming and perhaps burdensome. This is true generally, not only for surgical specialties, and thus, academic centers experienced the creation of faculty development programs as guides to orderly and carefully planned career progression. Although these faculty development programs are useful, they were developed for faculty of diverse disciplines and therefore offer general advice and guidelines. Out of the need for specific development and instruction arose coaching. For the surgeon, coaching may be related to technical skills, cognitive development, or possibly enhanced communication skills. Greenberg et al nicely describe an approach to coaching and carefully discuss the benefits of such a program. Even though their approach is clearly appropriate, one wonders why a coach is necessary when a surgical chairman or division or section chief should already be leading these efforts. The description of a coach lists the attributes of a good surgical chief or mentor. In addition, although individual coaching may be necessary, surgery is now clearly a "team sport," so should coaching not occur in the context of a team? The benefits of coaching are undeniable, but likely a coaching program should be developed within the organizational matrix of a surgical department, division or unit, and the program should be address the needs of all, including the coach. As a surgical community, we are only at the basecamp of ensuring the public of our continued professional development and investment in improved outcomes.

K. E. Behrns, MD

Underlying Reasons Associated With Hospital Readmission Following Surgery in the United States
Merkow RP, Ju MH, Chung JW, et al (American College of Surgeons, Chicago, IL; Northwestern Univ, Chicago, IL; et al)
JAMA 313:483-495, 2015

Importance.—Financial penalties for readmission have been expanded beyond medical conditions to include surgical procedures. Hospitals are working to reduce readmissions; however, little is known about the reasons for surgical readmission.

Objective.—To characterize the reasons, timing, and factors associated with unplanned postoperative readmissions.

Design, Setting, and Participants.—Patients undergoing surgery at one of 346 continuously enrolled US hospitals participating in the American College of Surgeons National Surgical Quality Improvement Program (ACS NSQIP) between January 1, 2012, and December 31, 2012, had clinically abstracted information examined. Readmission rates and reasons (ascertained by clinical data abstractors at each hospital) were assessed for all surgical procedures and for 6 representative operations: bariatric procedures, colectomy or proctectomy, hysterectomy, total hip or knee arthroplasty, ventral hernia repair, and lower extremity vascular bypass.

Main Outcomes and Measures.—Unplanned 30-day readmission and reason for readmission.

Results.—The unplanned readmission rate for the 498 875 operations was 5.7%. For the individual procedures, the readmission rate ranged from 3.8% for hysterectomy to 14.9% for lower extremity vascular bypass. The most common reason for unplanned readmission was surgical site infection (SSI) overall (19.5%) and also after colectomy or proctectomy (25.8%), ventral hernia repair (26.5%), hysterectomy (28.8%), arthroplasty (18.8%), and lower extremity vascular bypass (36.4%). Obstruction or ileus was the most common reason for readmission after bariatric surgery (24.5%) and the second most common reason overall (10.3%), after colectomy or proctectomy (18.1%), ventral hernia repair (16.7%), and hysterectomy (13.4%). Only 2.3% of patients were readmitted for the same complication they had experienced during their index hospitalization. Only 3.3% of patients readmitted for SSIs had experienced an SSI during their index hospitalization. There was no time pattern for readmission, and early (≤7 days postdischarge) and late (>7 days postdischarge) readmissions were associated with the same 3 most common reasons: SSI, ileus or obstruction, and bleeding. Patient comorbidities, index surgical admission complications, non-home discharge (hazard ratio [HR], 1.40 [95% CI, 1.35-1.46]), teaching hospital status (HR, 1.14 [95% CI 1.07-1.21]), and higher surgical volume (HR, 1.15 [95% CI, 1.07-1.25]) were associated with a higher risk of hospital readmission.

Conclusions and Relevance.—Readmissions after surgery were associated with new postdischarge complications related to the procedure and not exacerbation of prior index hospitalization complications, suggesting that readmissions after surgery are a measure of postdischarge complications. These data should be considered when developing quality indicators and any policies penalizing hospitals for surgical readmission.

▶ The Centers for Medicare and Medicaid Services has recently included readmission of surgical patients as a metric that may lead to a financial penalty in the assessment of quality and cost containment. The introduction of readmission as a metric has spurred numerous articles on readmission rates for a number of surgical conditions and operations. Most of these articles define the scope of the problem and provide an assessment of readmission risks. However, the question that should be answered is whether these readmissions were preventable. If, indeed, these readmissions can be prevented by treatment during the hospitalization, then readmission would be a valid metric of quality. However, if the readmissions cannot be prevented, then the readmission measure loses value. Merkow et al addressed this question in an investigation with nearly 500 000 patients that underwent surgery and were followed through the American College of Surgeons National Surgical Quality Improvement Program. They conducted a careful and thorough analysis, which determined that the unplanned readmission rate was 5.7% with surgical site infection the most common reason for readmission followed by bowel obstruction or ileus. Because neither of these complications was the result of an in-hospital event and the time of occurrence was unpredictable, the authors concluded that these readmissions were not preventable and the unplanned readmission rate was not a quality measure that could be readily altered. This study demonstrates the power of a collective database that can address pertinent outcome questions. Moreover, the investigation demonstrates that studies conducted by active surgeons can provide a foundation for policy making. This work is a superb demonstration of the ability of surgeons to select appropriate outcome measures that help shape meaningful policy.

K. E. Behrns, MD

The Medical Liability Climate and Prospects for Reform
Mello MM, Studdert DM, Kachalia A (Stanford Law School, CA; Brigham and Women's Hosp, Boston, MA)
JAMA 312:2146-2155, 2014

For many physicians, the prospect of being sued for medical malpractice is a singularly disturbing aspect of modern clinical practice. State legislatures have enacted tort reforms, such as caps on damages, in an effort to reduce the volume and costs of malpractice litigation. Attempts to introduce similar traditional reform measures at the federal level have so far failed. Much less prominent, but potentially more important, are proposed alternative approaches for resolving medical injuries; a number of these efforts are currently being tested in federally sponsored demonstration projects. These nontraditional reforms have considerable promise for addressing some of the system's most challenging issues, including high costs and barriers to accessing compensation. In this Special Communication, we review recent national trends in medical liability claims and costs, which indicate a sharp reduction in the rate of paid claims and flat or declining levels in compensation payments and liability insurance costs over the last 7 to 10 years. We discuss a number of nontraditional reform approaches—communication-and-resolution programs, presuit notification and apology laws, safe harbor legislation, judge-directed negotiation, and administrative compensation systems—and we conclude by describing

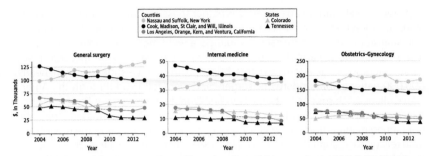

FIGURE 3.—Liability Insurance Rates Charged to General Surgeons, Internal Medicine Physicians, and Obstetrician-Gynecologists in 5 Locations, 2004-2013. Medical Liability Monitor Annual Rate Survey data. Rates shown are in 2013 dollars and indicate those charged by the dominant insurer in the local market. Dashed line between 2009 and 2010 in California indicates the shift from Los Angeles and Orange counties (2004-2009) to Los Angeles, Orange, Kern, and Ventura counties (2010-2013). Blue segment on each y-axis corresponds to the range $0 to $50 000. For interpretation of the references to color in this figure legend, the reader is referred to web version of this article. (Reprinted from Mello MM, Studdert DM, Kachalia A. The medical liability climate and prospects for reform. *JAMA.* 2014;312:2146-2155, Copyright 2014, American Medical Association. All rights reserved.)

several forces likely to shape change in the medical liability environment over the next decade (Fig 3).

▶ Surgeons' daily patient care activities are high risk and require complex decision making and sound judgment. Surgical training cultivates these behaviors, and the vast majority of the time, most surgeons exercise sound judgment with creditable results. On occasion, however, the surgeon may have a lapse in judgment, a technical error occurs, or perhaps the patient outcome is not what was anticipated despite delivery of sound care. All of these situations may result in a dissatisfied patient and potential litigation. Surgeons live with the prospect of a lawsuit on a regular basis, and when it occurs, they are often consumed by efforts to address the litigation. These efforts are not only time-consuming but also emotionally exhausting for the busy surgeon. Over the years, surgical organizations have attempted to improve the legal landscape with medical liability reform, but with little significant progress. However, Mello et al report that the number of claims has decreased substantially over time while the average indemnity is $195 000. Malpractice premium costs have held relatively steady over time but vary somewhat based on geographic practices (Fig 3). Notably, the proportion of claims paid out of a jury trial was only 3.4%, suggesting that nearly all claims are paid out of settlements. Importantly, the authors thoroughly discuss new approaches to medical liability. One approach, which has been in practice primarily in academic institutions, is communication-and-resolution programs. These programs identify adverse outcomes and approach resolution through open, transparent discussion and explanation of the case along with apology with the patient and family. In cases in which the standard of care was not met, compensation is offered. This approach has been practiced at the University of Michigan Health System and resulted in a 36% decrease in the number of claims and a 59% decrease in patient compensation. This refreshing approach should become the norm because it engenders trust among the medical center, physician, and the patient and family. When we meet patients preoperatively, we engage their trust; reciprocally, when outcomes are less desirable, we owe them a complete, heart-felt explanation and compensation when warranted.

K. E. Behrns, MD

Big Data And New Knowledge In Medicine: The Thinking, Training, And Tools Needed For A Learning Health System
Krumholz HM (Yale Univ School of Medicine, in New Haven, CT)
Health Aff 33:1163-1170, 2014

Big data in medicine—massive quantities of health care data accumulating from patients and populations and the advanced analytics that can give those data meaning—hold the prospect of becoming an engine for the knowledge generation that is necessary to address the extensive unmet information needs of patients, clinicians, administrators, researchers, and health policy makers. This article explores the ways in which big data can be harnessed to advance prediction, performance, discovery, and comparative effectiveness research to address the complexity of patients, populations, and organizations. Incorporating big data and next-generation analytics into clinical and population health research and practice will require not only new data sources but also new thinking, training, and tools. Adequately utilized, these reservoirs of data can be a practically inexhaustible source of knowledge to fuel a learning health care system.

▶ Medicine has firmly entered the era of big data, which has the potential to vastly change how we care for patients, assess our outcomes, ask research questions, and educate the next generation of trainees. In this work, Krumholz reflects on the likely opportunities that big data hold for the future with specific attention to clinical research. However, these concepts are not limited to clinical research but will likely guide clinical surgical practice because we will be able to mine the electronic health record for data that will allow predictive analytics. How this might change clinical practice? It is the hope that analyses of large data sets will direct more personalized approaches to medicine. Much like genomic assessment promises personalized medicine based on a genetic signature, personalized surgery could evolve from a big data signature that predicts surgical outcomes for patients exhibiting a pattern of characteristics. Employment of such a system will require a marked shift in research culture in that we will be required to embrace inductive reasoning and data pattern recognition rather than proving hypotheses through standard experimental clinical trial design. In addition to adopting changing approaches to clinical practice and research, incorporation of big data will mandate a learning culture across the health system. A new learning system and knowledge disbursement must permeate our approaches to education so that we can rapidly take advantage of big data. These unique opportunities will require dramatic shifts in the culture of clinical care, research, and education, but the opportunities to provide more accurate assessment in these missions are too great to delay implementation. We should ready ourselves for an exciting shift in data-directed surgical practice.

K. E. Behrns, MD

Introduction of Surgical Safety Checklists in Ontario, Canada

Urbach DR, Govindarajan A, Saskin R, et al (Univ of Toronto, Ontario, Canada; et al)

N Engl J Med 370:1029-1038, 2014

Background.—Evidence from observational studies that the use of surgical safety checklists results in striking improvements in surgical outcomes led to the rapid adoption of such checklists worldwide. However, the effect of mandatory adoption of surgical safety checklists is unclear. A policy encouraging the universal adoption of checklists by hospitals in Ontario, Canada, provided a natural experiment to assess the effectiveness of checklists in typical practice settings.

Methods.—We surveyed all acute care hospitals in Ontario to determine when surgical safety checklists were adopted. Using administrative health data, we compared operative mortality, rate of surgical complications, length of hospital stay, and rates of hospital readmission and emergency department visits within 30 days after discharge among patients undergoing a variety of surgical procedures before and after adoption of a checklist.

Results.—During 3-month periods before and after adoption of a surgical safety checklist, a total of 101 hospitals performed 109,341 and 106,370 procedures, respectively. The adjusted risk of death during a hospital stay or within 30 days after surgery was 0.71% (95% confidence interval [CI], 0.66 to 0.76) before implementation of a surgical checklist and 0.65% (95% CI, 0.60 to 0.70) afterward (odds ratio, 0.91; 95% CI, 0.80 to 1.03; $P = 0.13$). The adjusted risk of surgical complications was 3.86% (95% CI, 3.76 to 3.96) before implementation and 3.82% (95% CI, 3.71 to 3.92) afterward (odds ratio, 0.97; 95% CI, 0.90 to 1.03; $P = 0.29$).

Conclusions.—Implementation of surgical safety checklists in Ontario, Canada, was not associated with significant reductions in operative mortality or complications. (Funded by the Canadian Institutes of Health Research.)

▶ In 2009, the effectiveness of checklists was documented by a study demonstrating improved mortality and morbidity with the implementation of a standardized approach to surgical safety.[1] Because of the dramatic improvement in mortality and morbidity with the introduction of a simple, inexpensive safety tool, checklists were readily adopted with significant rapidity. Implementation of checklists was assumed to result in similar reductions in mortality and morbidity regardless of the site of employment. However, the study by Urbach et al challenges the concept that implementation of checklists results in marked improvement. In this Canadian study, the authors show that in 101 hospitals in the Ontario province 3 months before checklist implementation and 3 months after introduction of the checklist failed to produce the previously documented improvement. What are the potential reasons that the implementation was not associated with expected improvements? Likely, in many sites, the checklists were introduced with too little education, and the checklist became a rote exercise of checking off standardized approaches to improve surgical care. A checklist was never intended as a mechanical exercise but as a document to engender discussion about potential safety issues with each unique patient. Checklists should be adapted to the clinical situation and may differ significantly in a pediatric surgery patient compared with an adult cardiac patient. The purpose of a checklist is to ensure a thorough and direct discussion of the unique safety issues for each patient. Furthermore, the communication among the care team should permit early identification and management of any safety issue that may arise. As the leader in the operating room, the surgeon should lead the efforts with checklists to ensure the safety of our patients.

K. E. Behrns, MD

Reference

1. Haynes AB, Weiser TG, Berry WR, et al. A surgical safety checklist to reduce morbidity and mortality in a global population. *N Engl J Med*. 2009;360:491-499.

Aligning Private Sector Incentives With Health Care Quality: Need for Quality-Adjusted Hospital Bond Ratings

Chang DC (Univ of California San Diego)
Ann Surg 260:3-4, 2014

Background.—Efforts to improve the quality of health care in the United States have primarily been led by public sector insurers, but if the goal is to transform the system, the involvement of the private sector is needed. Social change in the United States tends to be driven by the engagement of the private sector. Private insurance companies have tried to participate by linking the contracting process with quality and outcome data, but these efforts are undermined because for every dollar insurers withhold, they reap an additional dollar in profit. The goal must be to align the profit motives of the private sector with health care quality.

Approaches.—The private sector is the source of capital for most US health care organizations. Nearly all these organizations raise startup and expansion capital from private sector sources, which offers a unique opportunity to engage the private sector by engaging capital markets that provide money through the issuance of bonds. Most health care organizations are not-for-profit and therefore cannot raise equity financing or sell ownership shares through stock offerings. To engage these capital markets, health care quality must be connected to the debt financing process.

If quality is linked to financial performance, more favorable bond ratings may become available for hospitals offering higher quality care. As with auto insurance discounts for good driving, high-quality hospitals would be offered lower interest rates and save money over the course of the bond life. Bond investors would support such an approach because they could benefit from an organization that produces higher revenue and has lower expenses. Hospital quality could affect not only the revenue but also the expense side of profitability. Default risk is also lowered because high health care quality will make debt default less likely. Bond investors would profit only when a health care organization profits. Financial incentives would be aligned with public good.

Industry Perspective.—The financial industry would support this type of investment based on the growing interest in "social impact investing." Financial leaders can choose to view outcomes and quality data as marketing incentives for the debt instrument and sell it to socially conscious investors. No government backing would be required. This does require a change from the current practice of basing bond ratings solely on financial assessments, primarily generated by volume projections. It seems reasonable, however, to base bond ratings for health care organizations also on the health care outcomes achieved and quality data relating to the care delivered.

Conclusions.—Engaging Wall Street in the health care quality movement offers an opportunity to make changes that will benefit not only the investor but also the entire health care system.

▶ For nearly 15 years much of the focus of health care has been quality improvement, and numerous government programs (mainly Centers for Medicare and Medicaid Services) have been initiated to improve the quality of patient care. Several of these programs started as incentive programs and then, over a few years, transitioned to programs that result in a penalty if a benchmark is not achieved. Overall, the results of these programs have been modest at best. For these reasons, substantial skepticism has emerged about these programs and significant proportions of patient populations, those without Medicare or Medicaid, are not included in the assessment of the quality mission. Therefore, Chang introduced a novel approach to engage the private sector by including quality metrics in hospital bond ratings. This innovative approach has several unique and attractive features, including a long duration of assessment because mortgages are held for years, it also incorporates the expense side of the ledger because quality outcomes affect costs, and, finally, this goal emphasizes the public mission of most hospitals and is socially conscious. However, several questions should be addressed with this approach. First, would tying hospital bond ratings to quality outcomes reach most hospitals? Likely, small hospitals would be affected little, whereas larger health care systems would have several mortgages within a short period of time. Second, would all private sector groups participate equally? Third, quality metrics will likely change over time, and given the long duration of mortgages, how would evolving metrics be incorporated into mortgage rates? This interesting concept, and others like it, deserves further investigation, but ultimately surgeons should have a primary role in driving quality forward.

K. E. Behrns, MD

Quantifying Innovation in Surgery
Hughes-Hallett A, Mayer EK, Marcus HJ, et al (Imperial College London, UK)
Ann Surg 260:205-211, 2014

Objectives.—The objectives of this study were to assess the applicability of patents and publications as metrics of surgical technology and innovation; evaluate the historical relationship between patents and publications; develop a methodology that can be used to determine the rate of innovation growth in any given health care technology.

Background.—The study of health care innovation represents an emerging academic field, yet it is limited by a lack of valid scientific methods for quantitative analysis. This article explores and cross-validates 2 innovation metrics using surgical technology as an exemplar.

Methods.—Electronic patenting databases and the MEDLINE database were searched between 1980 and 2010 for "surgeon" OR "surgical" OR "surgery." Resulting patent codes were grouped into technology clusters. Growth curves were plotted for these technology clusters to establish the rate and characteristics of growth.

Results.—The initial search retrieved 52,046 patents and 1,801,075 publications. The top performing technology cluster of the last 30 years was minimally invasive surgery. Robotic surgery, surgical staplers, and image guidance were the most emergent technology clusters. When examining the growth curves for these clusters they were found to follow an S-shaped pattern of growth, with the emergent technologies lying on the exponential phases of their respective growth curves. In addition, publication and patent counts were closely correlated in areas of technology expansion.

Conclusions.—This article demonstrates the utility of publically available patent and publication data to quantify innovations within surgical technology and proposes a novel methodology for assessing and forecasting areas of technological innovation.

▶ Out of necessity, surgeons have always been innovators. They have had to design the tools with which they perform their craft. Consider for a moment the development of the surgical stapler, the heart-lung machine, energy devices, ventricular assist devices, endovascular grafts, the laparoscope, adaptation of the robot—the impressive list goes on. Over the years, the tools have become increasingly sophisticated and the design and production of these tools have become big businesses. In addition, implementation of these tools may be used in marketing strategies as methods to attract patients. Thus, the development of these tools is big business for the surgeon inventor, the business, and the health care marketplace. Surprisingly, quantifying the development of these innovations has lagged significantly. However, Hughes-Hallett et al performed an interesting analysis that looked at a 30-year period, and then a more recent 10-year period, of development and attempted to quantify innovation in surgery with a combination of patent data and publication data or bibliometrics. Over the 30-year period, the search identified more than 50 000 patents and 1.8 million publications. When clusters of technology were analyzed for the longer time period, developments in minimally invasive surgery topped the list. In the more recent 10-year assessment, emerging technologies included image-guided surgery, robotic surgery, and, surprisingly, the development of new surgical staplers remains in the forefront of innovation. Patent counts and bibliometrics were closely correlated as reflective measures of technologic expansion. This intriguing article applies straightforward measurements to the assessment of innovation and affords inventors, businesspeople, and health care executives an avenue to assess trends in technology and the application of these new inventions. The information is also likely to be useful to investors!

K. E. Behrns, MD

Comparison of Treatment Effect Estimates From Prospective Nonrandomized Studies With Propensity Score Analysis and Randomized Controlled Trials of Surgical Procedures
Lonjon G, Boutron I, Trinquart L, et al (Assistance Publique-Hôpitaux de Paris, France)
Ann Surg 259:18-25, 2014

Objective.—We aimed to compare treatment effect estimates from NRSs with PS analysis and RCTs of surgery.

Background.—Evaluating a surgical procedure in randomized controlled trials (RCTs) is challenging. Nonrandomized studies (NRSs) involving use of propensity score (PS) analysis to limit bias are of increasing interest.

Design.—Meta-epidemiological study.

Methods.—We systematically searched MEDLINE via PubMed for all prospective NRSs with PS analysis evaluating a surgical procedure. Related RCTs, addressing the same clinical questions, were systematically retrieved. Our primary outcome of interest was all-cause mortality. We also selected 1 subjective outcome. We calculated the summary odds ratios (OR) for each study design, the ratio of OR (ROR) between the designs and the summary ROR across clinical questions. An ROR < 1 indicated that the experimental intervention is more favorable in NRSs with PS analysis than RCTs.

Results.—We retrieved 70 reports of NRSs with PS analysis and 94 related RCTs evaluating 31 clinical questions, of which 22 assessed all-cause mortality and 26 a subjective outcome. The combined ROR for all-cause mortality was 0.83 (95% confidence interval: 0.65−1.04). For subjective outcomes, the combined ROR was 1.07 (0.87−1.33).

Conclusions.—There was no statistically significant difference in treatment effect between NRSs with PS analysis and RCTs. Prospective NRSs

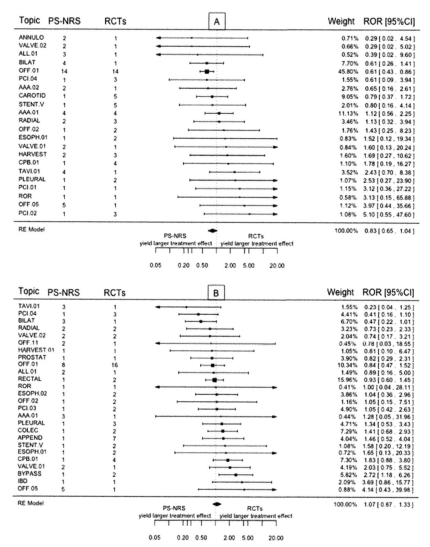

FIGURE 3.—Forest plot of ratio of ORs and 95% CIs between PS-based NRSs and RCTs for all-cause mortality (A) and subjective outcomes (B). RE indicates random effect. (Reprinted from Lonjon G, Boutron I, Trinquart L, et al. Comparison of treatment effect estimates from prospective nonrandomized studies with propensity score analysis and randomized controlled trials of surgical procedures. *Ann Surg.* 2014;259:18-25, © 2014, Southeastern Surgical Congress.)

with suitable and careful PS analysis can be relied upon as evidence when RCTs are not possible (Fig 3).

▶ For several decades, the randomized controlled clinical trial has been the method of comparison for clinical treatment effects. Although the use of this experimental design is certainly advantageous, the method has several limitations, especially for surgeons. First, the nature of the design of the randomized trial is that the application of techniques and the standardization of care are rigid, and thus, the total care of the patient likely does not represent real-world surgical care. That is, how applicable are the findings to the surgical community at large? Second, these trials are costly, often prohibitively so, such that they cannot be conducted at many institutions. Third, single institutions may not have sufficient volume to address a clinical question in a randomized fashion, and therefore, a multi-institutional approach is required. Although alternative methods of experimental design may not alleviate this limitation, the regulatory burden for alternative clinical experimental designs may be substantially decreased, and the trials may be more readily conducted from a logistics standpoint. An alternative to conducting a randomized controlled trial is a nonrandomized study with propensity score analysis. In the manuscript by Lonjon et al, this experimental design is compared to a randomized control trial, and the results demonstrate equivalency (Fig 3). This publication may open the door for surgeons to be more heavily engaged in comparative effective studies, and, hence be a game-changer for the conduct of clinical trials. It behooves the surgical community to engage in the propensity score methodology and to determine if this scientific approach is a suitable alternative to a randomized trial.

K. E. Behrns, MD

Patient expectations and patient-reported outcomes in surgery: A systematic review

Waljee J, McGlinn EP, Sears ED, et al (The Univ of Michigan Health System, Ann Arbor)
Surgery 155:799-808, 2014

Background.—Recent events in health care reform have brought national attention to integrating patient experiences and expectations into quality metrics. Few studies have comprehensively evaluated the effect of patient expectations on patient-reported outcomes (PROs) after surgery. The purpose of this study is to systematically review the available literature describing the relationship between patient expectations and postoperative PROs.

Methods.—We performed a search of the literature published before November 1, 2012. Articles were included in the review if (1) primary data were presented, (2) patient expectations regarding a surgical procedure were measured, (3) PROs were measured, and (4) the relationship between patient expectations and PROs was specifically examined. PROs were categorized into 5 subgroups: Satisfaction, quality of life (QOL), disability, mood disorder, and pain. We examined each study to determine the relationship between patient expectations and PROs as well as study quality.

Results.—From the initial literature search yielding 1,708 studies, 60 articles were included. Fulfillment of expectations was associated with improved PROs among 24 studies. Positive expectations were correlated with improved PROs for 28 studies (47%), and poorer PROs for 9 studies (15%). Eighteen studies reported that fulfillment of expectations was correlated with improved patient satisfaction, and 10 studies identified that positive expectations were correlated with improved postoperative. Finally, patients with positive preoperative expectations reported less pain (8 studies) and disability (15 studies) compared with patients with negative preoperative expectations.

Conclusion.—Patient expectations are inconsistently correlated with PROs after surgery, and there is no accepted method to capture perioperative expectations. Future efforts to rigorously measure expectations and explore their influence on postoperative outcomes can inform clinicians and policymakers seeking to integrate PROs into measures of surgical quality.

▶ Quality in health care, especially in surgery, is a water cooler topic that creates much consternation among practicing clinicians. Universally, surgeons desire excellent outcomes for their patients, yet the surgical literature clearly tells us that complications are a part of surgery. Part of the art of surgery is choosing patients wisely and applying an appropriate operation that will alleviate symptoms or risks with as little harm as possible. Sometimes, however, the measurement of harm is difficult to determine. In major operations with an anticipated risk of death or major morbidity, measuring these outcomes, such as death or deep venous thrombosis, is straightforward. However, in some practices, the measurement of mortality or major complications is meaningless, as the rate of occurrence is so low. In these circumstances, we often measure patient satisfaction. But, what is patient satisfaction and how do we measure it? Waljee et al offer insight into our ability to satisfy patients by aligning patient expectations with patient-reported outcomes. Unfortunately, the alignment is poor. Too often the outcomes do not achieve expectations. This could result because the outcomes are poor, or, alternatively, the expectations may not be realistic. We should pause to assess whether our preoperative description of outcomes will match the patient expectations. When a cosmetic procedure is performed, the outcome may not match the perceived expectations. Thus, we need to ensure that our preoperative assessment provides exquisite detail and, possibly, video confirmation of results. Furthermore, having a patient discuss the potential outcome with a previous patient is an excellent approach to setting expectations. We need to ensure that we go the extra mile to align patient expectations with realistic results.

K. E. Behrns, MD

Surgeon-Family Perioperative Communication: Surgeons' Self-Reported Approaches to the "Surgeon-Family Relationship"
Jordan AL, Rojnica M, Siegler M, et al (Univ of Chicago Pritzker School of Medicine, IL; Univ of Chicago Medicine, IL)
J Am Coll Surg 219:958-967, 2014

Background.—Family members are important in the perioperative care of surgical patients. During the perioperative period, communication about the patient occurs between surgeons and family members. To date, however, surgeon-family perioperative communication remains unexplored in the literature.

Study Design.—Surgeons were recruited from the surgical faculty of an academic hospital to participate in an interview regarding their approach to speaking with family members during and immediately after an operative procedure. An iterative process of transcription and theme development among 3 researchers was used to compile a well-defined set of qualitative themes.

Results.—Thirteen surgeons were interviewed and described what informs their communication, how they practice surgeon-family perioperative communication, and how the skills integral to perioperative communication are taught. Surgeons saw perioperative communication with family members as having a special role of providing support and anxiety alleviation that is distinct from the role of communication during clinic or postoperative visits. Wide variability exists in how interviewed surgeons practice perioperative communication, including who communicates with the family, and the frequency and content of the communication. Surgeons universally reported that residents' instruction in perioperative communication with families was lacking.

Conclusions.—Surgeons recognize perioperative communication with family members to be a part of their role and responsibility to the patient. However, during the perioperative period, they also acknowledge an independent responsibility to alleviate family members' anxieties. This independent responsibility supports the existence of a distinct "surgeon-family relationship."

▶ The patient-physician relationship has recently received much deserved attention largely in the form of patient satisfaction metrics. However, the patient-physician relationship is rapidly evolving to include not only discussion between the patient and physician but also informed, shared decision making. The patient generally makes health care decisions with the support of family or loved ones. Therefore, family engagement is an important component of shared decision making in the perioperative period. Jordan et al have examined surgeon-family communication in the perioperative period by admittedly investigating the surgeons' role in this dynamic interplay. By interviewing 13 surgeons with varied practices, they found that surgeons view the immediate perioperative period as distinct from the preoperative assessment and postoperative care. Furthermore, a major thematic finding was that surgeon-family communication should allay the anxiety of the family. The mechanisms through which surgeon-family communication occurred, however, were varied, and resident instruction in perioperative communication was lacking. These findings provide insights that should allow each of us to reflect on our approach to surgeon-patient/family communication. What are the goals of these communications? Undoubtedly, patients and families not only want to know how the procedure proceeded, but they want to know what will transpire next. In effect, the surgeon needs to manage the expectations of the patient and family by laying out the anticipated plan for the operation and the recovery. Managing expectations is a routine behavior of surgeons, and thus, communicating with patients and families should be well within our skill set. However, patient and family cultural expectations, level of education, family dynamics, and a host of other personal factors may complicate these conversations. Thus, establishing effective communication between a surgeon and family is not a "one size fits all" proposition, and improved communication will require education for all health care providers. Kudos to Jordan et al for bringing this important topic forward.

K. E. Behrns, MD

Being a Surgeon—The Myth and the Reality: A Meta-Synthesis of Surgeons' Perspectives About Factors Affecting Their Practice and Well-being
Orri M, Farges O, Clavien P-A, et al (INSERM-U669, Paris, France; Hôpital Beaujon, Clichy, France; Univ Hosp Zurich, Switzerland; et al)
Ann Surg 260:721-729, 2014

Objectives.—Synthesize the findings from individual qualitative studies about surgeons' account of their practice.

Background.—Social and contextual factors of practice influence doctors' well-being and therapeutic relationships. Little is known about surgery, but it is generally assumed that surgeons are not affected by them.

Methods.—We searched international publications (2000–2012) to identify relevant qualitative research exploring how surgeons talk about their practice. Meta-ethnography (a systematic analysis of qualitative literature that compensates for the potential lack of generalizability of the primary studies and provides new insight by their conjoint interpretation) was used to identify key themes and synthesize them.

Results.—We identified 51 articles (>1000 surgeons) from different specialties and countries. Two main themes emerged. (i) The patient-surgeon relationship, described surgeons' characterizations of their relationships with patients. We identified factors influencing surgical decision making, communication, and personal involvement in the process of care; these were surgeon-related, patient-related, and contextual. (ii) Group relations and culture described perceived issues related to surgical culture (image and education, teamwork, rules, and guidelines); it highlighted the influence of a social dimension on surgical practice. In both themes, we uncovered an emotional dimension of surgeons' practice.

Conclusions.—Surgeons' emphasis on technical aspects, individuality, and performance seems to impede a modern patient-centered approach to care and to act as a barrier to well being. Our findings suggest that taking into account the relational and emotional dimensions of surgical practice (both with patients and within the institution) might improve surgical innovation, surgeons' well-being, and the attractiveness of this specialty.

▶ Surgical practice is a high-risk discipline that involves several complex relationships between the patient and the surgeon and the surgeon and his or her coworkers. These relationships have largely remained unexplored, although recently, emphasis on the surgeon-patient relationship and shared decision making has received attention in the literature. Orri et al bring these complex relationships to light using a meta-synthesis approach that assesses qualitative information. Their review of 51 evaluable manuscripts suggests 2 major themes: the patient-surgeon relationship and surgical culture. The findings related to the patient-surgeon relationship highlight the necessity of thorough communication and the contextual factors that influence good communication. The findings related to surgical culture are steeped in surgical tradition and how surgeons should behave and interact. Many of the findings highlight the individualism of the surgeon, which is often disguised as being the "art" of surgery. Are surgical operations and the care of the postoperative patient so unique that we cannot apply evidence-based guidelines? We know that this is, indeed, not true. Most importantly, medicine is on a direct path to be a team sport, and surgeons must embrace the team concept that will deliver care to a patient along a continuum. This should not diminish our role, and, alternatively, we should be leaders in the team concept because we have been doing this for years in the operating room.

K. E. Behrns, MD

2 Trauma

Patterns of Injury, Outcomes, and Predictors of In-Hospital and 1-Year Mortality in Nonagenarian and Centenarian Trauma Patients

Hwabejire JO, Kaafarani HMA, Lee J, et al (Massachusetts General Hosp, Boston; et al)
JAMA Surg 149:1054-1059, 2014

Importance.—With the dramatic growth in the very old population and their concomitant heightened exposure to traumatic injury, the trauma burden among this patient population is estimated to be exponentially increasing.

Objective.—To determine the clinical outcomes and predictors of in-hospital and 1-year mortality in nonagenarian and centenarian trauma patients (NCTPs).

Design, Setting, and Participants.—All patients 90 years or older admitted to a level 1 academic trauma center between January 1, 2006, and December 31, 2010, with a primary diagnosis of trauma were included. Standard trauma registry data variables were supplemented by systematic medical record review. Cumulative mortality rates at 1, 3, 6, and 12 months after discharge were investigated using the Social Security Death Index. Univariate and multivariable analyses were performed to identify the predictors of in-hospital and 1-year postdischarge cumulative mortalities.

Main Outcomes and Measures.—Length of hospital stay, in-hospital mortality, and cumulative mortalities at 1, 3, 6, and 12 months after discharge.

Results.—Four hundred seventy-four NCTPs were included; 71.7% were female, and a fall was the predominant mechanism of injury (96.4%). The mean patient age was 93 years, the mean Injury Severity Score was 12, and the mean number of comorbidities per patient was 4.4. The in-hospital mortality was 9.5% but cumulatively escalated at 1, 3, 6, and 12 months after discharge to 18.5%, 26.4%, 31.3%, and 40.5%, respectively. Independent predictors of in-hospital mortality were the Injury Severity Score (odds ratio [OR], 1.09; 95% CI, 1.02-1.16; $P = .01$), mechanical ventilation (OR, 6.23; 95% CI, 1.42-27.27; $P = .02$), and cervical spine injury (OR, 4.37; 95% CI, 1.41-13.50; $P = .01$). Independent predictors of cumulative 1-year mortality were head injury (OR, 2.65; 95% CI, 1.24-5.67; $P = .03$) and length of hospital stay (OR, 1.06; 95% CI, 1.02-1.11; $P = .005$). Cumulative 1-year mortality in NCTPs with a head injury was 51.1% and increased to 73.2% if the Injury Severity Score was 25 or higher and to 78.7% if mechanical ventilation was required. Most NCTPs required rehabilitation; only 8.9% were discharged to home.

Conclusions and Relevance.—Despite low in-hospital mortality, the cumulative mortality rate among NCTPs at 1 year after discharge is significant, particularly in the presence of head injury, spine injury, mechanical ventilation, high injury severity, or prolonged length of hospital stay. These considerations can help guide clinical decisions and family discussions.

▶ This selection was chosen to show the dilemma encountered in caring for aging patient populations. In this study, examining the outcomes of trauma patients 90 years of age or greater, a misleadingly low in-hospital mortality rate was seen. The mortality rate increased by more than 4-fold by the end of the first year after discharge. Cervical spine injury, head injury, intensive care unit admission, need for mechanical ventilation, high injury severity score, and prolonged length of hospital stay were correlated with a high risk of in-hospital or postdischarge death within the first year. This risk is depicted in Fig 1 from the original article. Discharge to home is uncommon. Mortality was worse among patients discharged to skilled nursing facilities than those discharged to rehabilitation centers. These findings portray a realistic picture of the outcomes after injury in the extremes of age. This information may help trauma care providers set appropriate goals and facilitate discussions with families about their ultimate expectations. This study is somewhat limited by being retrospective and from a single institution; however, it would be easily validated using existing large data sets. It would also be interesting to explore the concept of frailty indices in this population.

D. W. Mozingo, MD

Increased Trauma Center Volume Is Associated With Improved Survival After Severe Injury: Results of a Resuscitation Outcomes Consortium Study
Minei JP, Fabian TC, Guffey DM, et al (Univ of Texas Southwestern Med Ctr, Dallas; Univ of Tennessee Health Science Ctr, Memphis. TN; Univ of Washington, Seattle; et al)
Ann Surg 260:456-465, 2014

Objective.—To investigate the relationship between trauma center volume and outcome.

Background.—The Resuscitation Outcomes Consortium is a network of 11 centers and 60 hospitals conducting emergency care research. For many procedures, high-volume centers demonstrate superior outcomes versus low-volume centers. This remains controversial for trauma center outcomes.

Methods.—This study was a secondary analysis of prospectively collected data from the Resuscitation Outcomes Consortium multicenter out-of-hospital Hypertonic Saline Trial in patients with Glasgow Coma Scale score of 8 or less (traumatic brain injury) or systolic blood pressure of 90 or less and pulse of 110 or more (shock). Regression analyses evaluated associations between trauma volume and the following outcomes: 24-hour mortality, 28-day mortality, ventilator-free days, Multiple Organ Dysfunction Scale incidence, worst Multiple Organ Dysfunction Scale score, and poor 6-month Glasgow Outcome Scale—Extended score.

Results.—A total of 2070 patients were evaluated: 1251 in the traumatic brain injury cohort and 819 in the shock cohort. Overall, 24-hour and 28-day mortality was 16% and 25%, respectively. For every increase of 500 trauma center admissions, there was a 7% decreased odds of 24-hour and 28-day mortality for all patients. As trauma center volume increased, nonorgan dysfunction complications increased, ventilator-free days increased, and worst Multiple Organ Dysfunction Scale score decreased. The associations with higher trauma center volume were similar for the traumatic brain injury cohort, including better neurologic outcomes at 6 months, but not for the shock cohort.

Conclusions.—Increased trauma center volume was associated with increased survival, more ventilator-free days, and less severe organ failure. Trauma system planning and implementation should avoid unnecessary duplication of services.

▶ The role of patient volume has been a source of debate regarding whether level I centers have higher survival rates than level II trauma centers. There are studies that both support and refute this debate. The results of this selection show that severely injured patients admitted to high-volume trauma centers have lower odds of mortality than if they are brought to low-volume trauma centers. This finding was associated with additional complications, but high-volume centers were able to deal with the consequences of these complications. This finding may have been related, in part, to improved processes and protocols that led to fewer ventilator days and less severe organ failure. High-volume trauma centers likely have systems in place to deliver the highest quality efficient trauma care to the most severely injured patients brought to their centers. Therefore, prehospital triage guidelines should bring the most severely injured patients to the highest-volume centers. Trauma center proliferation should be approached with caution because of the volume reduction effect resulting from a wider distribution of the same number of patients to a greater number of trauma centers. This study is limited somewhat by sample size, and further study is warranted to define those factors that lead to improved outcomes at high-volume trauma centers.

D. W. Mozingo, MD

A Crew Resource Management Program Tailored to Trauma Resuscitation Improves Team Behavior and Communication
Hughes KM, Benenson RS, Krichten AE, et al (York Hosp, PA)
J Am Coll Surg 219:545-551, 2014

Background.—Crew Resource Management (CRM) is a team-building communication process first implemented in the aviation industry to improve safety. It has been used in health care, particularly in surgical and intensive care settings, to improve team dynamics and reduce errors. We adapted a CRM process for implementation in the trauma resuscitation area.

Study Design.—An interdisciplinary steering committee developed our CRM process to include a didactic classroom program based on a preimplementation survey of our trauma team members. Implementation with new cultural and process expectations followed. The Human Factors Attitude Survey and Communication and Teamwork Skills assessment tool were used to design, evaluate, and validate our CRM program.

Results.—The initial trauma communication survey was completed by 160 team members (49% response). Twenty-five trauma resuscitations were observed and scored using Communication and Teamwork Skills. Areas of concern were identified and 324 staff completed our 3-hour CRM course during a 3-month period. After CRM training, 132 communication surveys and 38 Communication and Teamwork Skills observations were completed. In the post-CRM survey, respondents indicated improvement in accuracy of field to medical command information ($p = 0.029$); accuracy of emergency department medical command information to the resuscitation area ($p = 0.002$); and team leader identity, communication of plan, and role assignment ($p = 0.001$). After CRM training, staff were more likely to speak up when patient safety was a concern ($p = 0.002$).

Conclusions.—Crew Resource Management in the trauma resuscitation area enhances team dynamics, communication, and, ostensibly, patient safety. Philosophy and culture of CRM should be compulsory components of trauma programs and in resuscitation of injured patients (Table 2).

▶ Crew Resource Management is a communication tool developed in the aviation industry. Review of airline disasters determined safety information was

TABLE 2.—Communication and Teamwork Skills Metrics: Improved Post Implementation

Observation Metric	Pre-CRM (n = 25), %*	Post-CRM (n = 38), %*	p Value
Briefing	40	89	<0.0001
Verbalize plan of care	44	89	<0.0001
Establish team leader	12	82	<0.0001
Assign roles	4	89	<0.0001
ED gives patient summary to trauma personnel	48	84	0.0021
Request external resources if needed	12	87	<0.0001
Ask for help from team as needed	28	68	0.0016
Cross monitoring	16	87	<0.0001
Closed loop	8	76	<0.0001
Verbal updates-think aloud	8	71	0.0007
Use names	8	84	<0.0001

CRM, Crew Resource Management; ED, emergency department.
*Percentage of observations.

often known to individual crew members but not to all crew members. Inadequate interpersonal communication, poor decision making, and lack of leadership resulted in ineffective information sharing, which inspired Crew Resource Management to improve safety through improved communication between all team members. This is particularly applicable to those teams in which there is a perceived power inequality. By flattening the hierarchy, communication is encouraged, leading to improved team interactions.

A growing number of health care disciplines now use Crew Resource Management techniques. Such initiatives have been described as transformative and culturally sustainable in improving patient safety. Crew Resource Management in the authors' facility was initially implemented in the operating rooms. The Crew Resource Management Model, which has been endorsed by the Joint Commission for Accreditation for Healthcare Organizations, and methods of improving communication, leadership, team effectiveness, and safety, have been used in high-risk hospital environments, such as operating rooms and intensive care settings; however, conclusive evidence about Crew Resource Management effectiveness has yet to emerge, as implementation has not been adequately studied. In this selection, the authors report their evaluation of this system relative to training the multidisciplinary trauma team. Table 2 is included and shows the results of this training. Crew Resource Management enhances team dynamics and communication and likely improves patient safety. The authors suggest that the philosophy and culture of Crew Resource Management should be compulsory components in organization of trauma programs and in resuscitation of injured patients.

D. W. Mozingo, MD

Changing Patterns of In-Hospital Deaths Following Implementation of Damage Control Resuscitation Practices in US Forward Military Treatment Facilities
Langan NR, Eckert M, Martin MJ (Madigan Army Med Ctr, Tacoma, WA)
JAMA Surg 149:904-912, 2014

Importance.—Analysis of combat deaths provides invaluable epidemiologic and quality-improvement data for trauma centers and is particularly important under rapidly evolving battlefield conditions.

Objective.—To analyze the evolution of injury patterns, early care, and resuscitation among patients who subsequently died in the hospital, before and after implementation of damage control resuscitation (DCR) policies.

Design, Setting, and Participants.—In a review of the Joint Theater Trauma Registry (2002-2011) of US forward combat hospitals, cohorts of patients with vital signs at presentation and subsequent in-hospital death were grouped into 2 time periods: pre-DCR (before 2006) and DCR (2006-2011).

Main Outcomes and Measures.—Injury types and Injury Severity Scores (ISSs), timing and location of death, and initial (24-hour) and total volume of blood products and fluid administered.

Results.—Of 57 179 soldiers admitted to a forward combat hospital, 2565 (4.5%) subsequently died in the hospital. The majority of patients (74%) were severely injured (ISS >15), and 80% died within 24 hours of admission. Damage control resuscitation policies were widely implemented by 2006 and resulted in a decrease in mean 24-hour crystalloid infusion volume (6.1-3.2 L) and increased fresh frozen plasma use (3.2-10.1 U) (both $P < .05$) in this population. The mean packed red blood cells to fresh frozen plasma ratio changed from 2.6:1 during the pre-DCR period to 1.4:1 during the DCR period ($P < .01$). There was a significant increase in mean ISS between cohorts (pre-DCR ISS = 23 vs DCR ISS = 27; $P < .05$) and a marked shift in injury patterns favoring more severe head trauma in the DCR cohort.

Conclusions and Relevance.—There has been a significant shift in resuscitation practices in forward combat hospitals indicating widespread military adoption of DCR. Patients who died in a hospital during the DCR period were more likely to be severely injured and have a severe brain injury, consistent with a decrease in deaths among potentially salvageable patients.

▶ The most important advancement in combat trauma care has been the widespread adoption of damage control resuscitation (DCR). The basic principles of DCR include the early administration of blood products in a balanced ratio, aggressive correction of coagulopathy, and limiting the infusion of crystalloid fluids to a minimum. Ever since these resuscitation strategies have been adopted widely in civilian trauma centers, there has been a noticeable shift toward reducing the volume of both crystalloid and blood products administered and associated improvements in survival. In the combat setting, the use of DCR has been credited with improvements in survival among severely injured patients, particularly for those requiring a massive transfusion. Data for this study were obtained from the Joint Theater Trauma Registry (JTTR), which is maintained by the Joint Theater Trauma System under the US Army Institute of Surgical Research, Fort Sam Houston, Texas. Established in 2003, the JTTR is the largest and most comprehensive database of wartime wounded and injured patients ever recorded.

This study provides a valuable addition to the currently available DCR literature in that it removes survivor bias and confirms that severely injured patients who die of wounds are receiving more balanced transfusion ratios and less crystalloid. Fig 3 in the original article, included in this selection, depicts a dramatic downward trend in mortality after adoption of the DCR protocol.

D. W. Mozingo, MD

Attribution: Whose complication is it?

Murry J, Hambright G, Patel N, et al (Methodist Dallas Med Ctr, TX)
J Trauma Acute Care Surg 77:974-977, 2014

Background.—To improve quality, programs such as accountable care organizations need to determine the part of the health care system most "responsible" for a complication. This is referred to as attribution. This provides a framework to compare physicians for patients and third-party payers. Traditionally, the attribution of complications has been to the admitting physician. This may misidentify the physician "responsible" for the complication. This is especially difficult in trauma patients who have multiple providers. We hypothesized that the current mechanism for attributing complications in trauma patients is inadequate and will need to be modernized.

Methods.—All trauma admissions during a 12-month period were reviewed. Patients with single-system trauma were excluded. We reviewed our trauma database for mechanism of injury, complications, and readmissions. The trauma director and the medical director of our accountable care organizations reviewed all complications and attributed them to the appropriate health care provider. These were compared with the hospital decisions using the traditional definition.

Results.—The trauma service had 1,526 admissions. After exclusions, 1,019 patients were reviewed. One hundred twenty-five complications occurred in 73 patients. Using the traditional definition, the acute care surgery service was assigned all 125 complications. Using the trauma director and medical director method, the neurosurgical attending accounted for 36% (45 of 125) of complications. The acute care surgery attending was responsible for 34% (43 of 125) of complications, and orthopedic surgery was identified as the causative factor in 22% (27 of 125). The remaining 8% (10 of 125) were attributed to various other services. Seven patients had unexpected readmissions. Most (6 of 7) of these were related to orthopedics.

Conclusion.—Hospital complications are now being assigned to individual surgeons. Which physician is responsible for each complication will be a controversial matter. Without a critical review process with physician input, up to two thirds of complications could be attributed incorrectly. The attribution process needs to be refined.

Level of Evidence.—Epidemiologic study, level IV.

▶ Surgeons have been leaders in performance improvement for many years, and the attribution of complications to individual practitioners is not new to them. What is new is the potential effect on physicians in the future when it comes to professional viability, reimbursement, and public reporting. In this study, two-thirds of all complications were potentially misattributed to the acute care surgeons under the existing model. This can have deleterious effects on a practicing physician for several reasons. For a surgeon planning to relocate, there may be difficulty obtaining privileges because a high rate of complications could be seen as an unacceptable risk to the new hospital. Additionally, hospitals may be in a position to restrict a physician's privileges if certain procedures are considered too high risk. The authors conclude that the policy of assigning all trauma complications to the admitting acute care surgery attending resulted in misattribution 66% of the time. The fallout of incorrectly assigning complications is significant. This could have severe unintended consequences to the health care system. They submit that a physician-led, multidisciplinary solution is necessary and should be applied uniformly across the country.

D. W. Mozingo, MD

Superiority of Frailty Over Age in Predicting Outcomes Among Geriatric Trauma Patients: A Prospective Analysis
Joseph B, Pandit V, Zangbar B, et al (Univ of Arizona Med Ctr, Tucson)
JAMA Surg 149:766-772, 2014

Importance.—The Frailty Index (FI) is a known predictor of adverse outcomes in geriatric patients. The usefulness of the FI as an outcome measure in geriatric trauma patients is unknown.

Objective.—To assess the usefulness of the FI as an effective assessment tool in predicting adverse outcomes in geriatric trauma patients.

Design, Setting, and Participants.—A 2-year (June 2011 to February 2013) prospective cohort study at a level I trauma center at the University of Arizona. We prospectively measured frailty in all geriatric trauma patients. Geriatric patients were defined as those 65 years or older. The FI was calculated using 50 preadmission frailty variables. Frailty in patients was defined by an FI of 0.25 or higher.

Main Outcomes and Measures.—The primary outcome measure was in-hospital complications. The secondary outcome measure was adverse discharge disposition. In-hospital complications were defined as cardiac, pulmonary, infectious, hematologic, renal, and reoperation. Adverse discharge disposition was defined as discharge to a skilled nursing facility or in-hospital mortality. Multivariate logistic regression was used to assess the relationship between the FI and outcomes.

Results.—In total, 250 patients were enrolled, with a mean (SD) age of 77.9 (8.1) years, median Injury Severity Score of 15 (range, 9-18), median Glasgow Coma Scale score of 15 (range, 12-15), and mean (SD) FI of 0.21 (0.10). Forty-four percent (n = 110) of patients had frailty. Patients with frailty were more likely to have in-hospital complications (odds ratio, 2.5; 95% CI, 1.5-6.0; $P = .001$) and adverse discharge disposition (odds ratio, 1.6; 95% CI, 1.1-2.4; $P = .001$). The mortality rate was 2.0% (n = 5), and all patients who died had frailty.

Conclusions and Relevance.—The FI is an independent predictor of in-hospital complications and adverse discharge disposition in geriatric trauma patients. This index should be used as a clinical tool for risk stratification in this patient group.

▶ Frailty is defined as a syndrome of decreased physiologic reserve and resistance to stressors that results in increased vulnerability to poor health outcomes, worsening mobility and disability, hospitalizations, and death. Frailty has been used to predict in-hospital complications, discharge to institutional care, and mortality among geriatric surgical patients. However, the role of frailty evaluation in trauma patients remains unclear and has only recently been studied. Current guidelines defining the management of geriatric trauma patients usually do not take into account the low physiologic reserve and the altered response to injury in these patients. In addition, there is a lack of an effective assessment tool for evaluating outcomes in geriatric trauma patients. The aim of this study was to assess the usefulness of the Frailty Index as an assessment tool in predicting outcomes in geriatric trauma patients.

Such early assessment and identification of vulnerable patients is critical in optimizing outcomes in an aging trauma patient population. This study shows that the Frailty Index is an effective tool to predict outcomes in this patient group. Trauma patients with frailty are more likely to have in-hospital complications and adverse discharge disposition than patients without frailty. The Frailty Index is superior to age and other routinely used assessment tools for determining outcomes among geriatric trauma patients. This index could be used as a clinical tool for risk stratification across trauma centers to standardize geriatric trauma patient management. Geriatric patients represent a growing trauma patient population without well-defined guidelines for their management.

D. W. Mozingo, MD

Isolated Free Fluid on Abdominal Computed Tomography in Blunt Trauma: Watch and Wait or Operate?
Gonser-Hafertepen LN, Davis JW, Bilello JF, et al (Univ of California San Francisco, Fresno)
J Am Coll Surg 219:599-605, 2014

Background.—Isolated free fluid (FF) on abdominal CT in stable blunt trauma patients can indicate the presence of hollow viscus injury. No criteria exist to differentiate treatment by operative exploration vs observation. The goals of this study were to determine the incidence of isolated FF and to identify factors that discriminate between patients who should undergo operative exploration vs observation.

Study Design.—A review of blunt trauma patients at a Level I trauma center from July 2009 to March 2012 was performed. Patients with a CT showing isolated FF after blunt trauma were included. Data collected included demographics, injury severity, physical examination, CT, and operative findings.

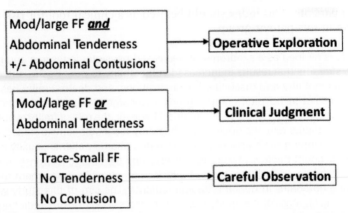

FIGURE 2.—Recommendations for stable blunt trauma patients with isolated free fluid (FF) on CT scan. Mod/Large, moderate to large. (Reprinted from the Journal of the American College of Surgeons. Gonser-Hafertepen LN, Davis JW, Bilello JF, et al. Isolated free fluid on abdominal computed tomography in blunt trauma: watch and wait or operate? *J Am Coll Surg.* 2014;219:599-605, Copyright 2014, with permission from the American College of Surgeons.)

Results.—Two thousand eight hundred and ninety-nine patients had CT scans, 156 (5.4%) of whom had isolated FF. The therapeutic operative group included 13 patients; 9 had immediate operation and 4 failed non-operative management. The nonoperative/nontherapeutic operation group consisted of 142 patients with successful nonoperative management and 1 patient with a nontherapeutic operation. Abdominal tenderness was documented in 69% of the therapeutic operative group and 23% of the nonoperative/nontherapeutic group (odds ratio = 7.5; $p < 0.001$). The presence of a moderate to large amount of FF was increased in the therapeutic operative group (85% vs 8%; odds ratio = 66; $p < 0.001$).

Conclusions.—Isolated FF was noted in 5.4% of stable blunt trauma patients. Blunt trauma patients with moderate to large amounts of FF without solid organ injury on CT and abdominal tenderness should undergo immediate operative exploration. Patients with neither of these findings can be safely observed (Fig 2).

▶ The detection of isolated free fluid on abdominal and pelvic CT scan in the stable adult blunt trauma patient presents a management dilemma. Free fluid in the absence of solid organ injury might be a clue to the presence of hollow viscus or mesenteric injury, which is associated with an increased risk of morbidity and mortality if diagnosis is delayed. Consensus has still not been reached regarding the detection of isolated free fluid. A survey of the members of the American Association for the Surgery of Trauma showed significant variation with regard to diagnostic approach and treatment for patients with this finding.[1] Based on the findings from this study, the authors of this selection recommend the following guidelines for treatment of the stable blunt trauma patient with isolated free fluid on CT scan. Patients with a moderate to large amount of free fluid on CT and abdominal tenderness (with or without abdominal wall contusion) should undergo operative exploration. Patients with a trace to small amount of free fluid and no abdominal tenderness are unlikely to require operative intervention and should be observed carefully with serial abdominal examinations and laboratory studies. For those patients with either a moderate to large amount of isolated free fluid or abdominal tenderness, the decision for operative exploration should be made based on careful clinical judgment. Fig 2 from this article is included summarizing these recommendations.

D. W. Mozingo, MD

Reference

1. Brownstein MR, Bunting T, Meyer AA, Fakhry SM. Diagnosis and management of blunt small bowel injury; a survey of the membership of the American association for the surgery of trauma. *J Trauma*. 2000;48:403-407.

Whole-body computed tomographic scanning leads to better survival as opposed to selective scanning in trauma patients: A systematic review and meta-analysis
Caputo ND, Stahmer C, Lim G, et al (Lincoln Medical and Mental Health Center, Bronx, NY; Mount Sinai Hosp, NY)
J Trauma Acute Care Surg 77:534-539, 2014

Background.—Traumatic injury in the United States is the Number 1 cause of mortality for patients 1 year to 44 years of age. Studies suggest that early identification of major injury leads to better outcomes for patients. Imaging, such as computed tomography (CT), is routinely used to help determine the presence of major underlying injuries. We review the literature to determine whether whole-body CT (WBCT), a protocol including a noncontrast scan of the brain and neck and a contrast-enhanced scan of the chest, abdomen, and pelvis, detects more clinically significant injuries as opposed to selective scanning as determined by mortality rates.

Methods.—Scientific publications from 1980 to 2013 involving the study of the difference between pan scan and selective scan after trauma were identified. The Preferred Reporting Items for Systematic Reviews and Meta-analyses was used. Publications were categorized by level of evidence. Injury Severity Score (ISS) and pooled odds for mortality rate of patients who received WBCT scan versus those who received selective scans were compared.

Results.—Of the 465 publications identified, 7 were included, composing of 25,782 trauma patients who received CT scan following trauma. Of the patients, 52% (n − 13,477) received pan scan and 48% (n − 12,305) received selective scanning. Overall ISS was significantly higher for patients receiving WBCT versus those receiving selective scan (29.7 vs. 26.4, $p < 0.001$, respectively). Overall mortality rate was significantly lower for WBCT versus selective scanning (16.9; 95% confidence interval [CI],

16.3–17.6 vs. 20.3; 95% CI, 19.6–21.1, $p < 0.0002$, respectively). Pooled odds ratio for mortality rate was 0.75 (95% CI, 0.7–0.79), favoring WBCT.

Conclusion.—Despite the WBCT group having significantly higher ISS at baseline compared with the group who received selective scanning, the WBCT group had a lower overall mortality rate and a more favorable pooled odds ratio for trauma patients. This suggests that in terms of overall mortality, WBCT scan is preferable to selective scanning in trauma patients.

Level of Evidence.—Systematic review and meta-analysis, level III.

▶ The authors of this selection present the largest systematic review and meta-analysis determining the odds of mortality in trauma patients when comparing the use of whole-body CT scan vs selective scanning in the initial diagnostic evaluation of these patients. Fig 3 in the original article is included and supports their literature review meta-analysis. The analysis suggests that in severely injured trauma patients, those who receive whole-body CT scan are less likely to have a fatal outcome. They, therefore, recommend its use until current randomized controlled trials are reported. The finding of lower mortality among the whole-body CT scan group could be interpreted as an underestimation of the overall benefit associated with the whole-body CT scan, as these patients were more seriously injured as indicated by higher injury severity scores. We await the outcome of a prospective, randomized, controlled trial, the REACT-2 trial, which is currently underway. The results of this trial will help better define the answer to this dilemma in the initial treatment of seriously injured patients.

D. W. Mozingo, MD

Computed tomography scans with intravenous contrast: Low incidence of contrast-induced nephropathy in blunt trauma patients
Colling KP, Irwin ED, Byrnes MC, et al (Univ of Minnesota Med Ctr, Minneapolis; North Memorial Med Ctr, Robbinsdale, MN)
J Trauma Acute Care Surg 77:226-230, 2014

Background.—Computed tomography (CT) with intravenous (IV) contrast is an important step in the evaluation of the blunt trauma patient; however, the risk for contrast-induced nephropathy (CIN) in these patients still remains unclear. The goal of this study was to describe the rate of CIN in blunt trauma patients at a Level 1 trauma center and identify the risk factors of developing CIN.

Methods.—After internal review board approval, we reviewed our Level 1 trauma registry to identify blunt trauma patients admitted during a 1-year period. Chart review was used to identify patient demographics, creatinine levels, and vital signs. CIN was defined as an increase in creatinine by 0.5 mg/dL from admission after undergoing CT with IV contrast.

TABLE 4.—Multivariate Analysis of Risk Factors of Development of Acute Kidney Injury in Blunt Trauma Patients

Variable	Adjusted Odds Ratio	95% Confidence Interval	p
Sex (male)	1.72	0.62–4.78	0.295
Age >55 y	5.48	1.86–16.11	0.002
ISS ≥16	3.17	1.02–9.83	0.046
Admission SBP <90 mm Hg	1.27	0.25–6.41	0.775
DM	6.08	1.09–34.05	0.040
IV contrast	0.507	0.12–2.91	0.579

Hosmer-Lemeshow test, $p = 0.943$.
SBP, systolic blood pressure; ISS, Injury Severity Score; DM, Diabetes Mellitus.
Reprinted from Colling KP, Irwin ED, Byrnes MC, et al. Computed tomography scans with intravenous contrast: Low incidence of contrast-induced nephropathy in blunt trauma patients. *J Trauma Acute Care Surg.* 2014;77:226-230.

Results.—Four percent of patients developed CIN during their admission following receipt of IV contrast for CT; 1% had continued renal impairment on discharge. No patients required dialysis during their admission. Diabetic patients had an increased rate of CIN, with 10% rate of CIN during admission and 4% at discharge. In multivariate analysis, only preexisting diabetes and Injury Severity Score (ISS) of greater than 25 were independently associated with risk for CIN.

Conclusion.—The rate of CIN in trauma patients following CT scan with IV contrast is low. Diabetes and ISS were independent risk factors of development of CIN in trauma patients.

Level of Evidence.—Epidemiologic/prognostic study, level III (Table 4).

▶ Computed tomography with iodinated intravenous contrast media is common in the evaluation of hemodynamically stable patients with blunt traumatic injuries. Computed tomography imaging allows quick and accurate identification of injuries, leading to faster final treatment and improved patient care. However, this modality is not without risk, and the association between the administration of intravenous (IV) iodinated contrast and the subsequent development of acute kidney injury or contrast-induced nephropathy is well known. The incidence of renal injury after IV contrast administration is highly dependent on the risk profile of the patient, ranging from negligible rates in patients with no risk factors to rates of 5% to 50% reported in patients with diabetes or preexisting renal insufficiency. The goal of this study was to assess the risk for contrast-induced nephropathy in blunt trauma patients, to identify patient risk factors that may contribute to its development, and to evaluate the rate of contrast-induced nephropathy in high-risk subgroups. The authors concluded that the rate of contrast-induced nephropathy in their patient population was low, with 4% developing contrast-induced nephropathy transiently and 1% having residual renal impairment at discharge. Diabetes and Injury Severity Score were the only independent risk factors associated with contrast-induced nephropathy shown by multivariate analysis as seen in Table 4.

D. W. Mozingo, MD

The public health burden of emergency general surgery in the United States: A 10-year analysis of the Nationwide Inpatient Sample—2001 to 2010

Gale SC, Shafi S, Dombrovskiy VY, et al (East Texas Med Ctr, Tyler, TX; Baylor Inst for Health Care Res and Improvement, Dallas, TX; Rutgers-Robert Wood Johnson Med School, New Brunswick, NJ)
J Trauma Acute Care Surg 77:202-208, 2014

Background.—Emergency general surgery (EGS) represents illnesses of very diverse pathology related only by their urgent nature. The growth of acute care surgery has emphasized this public health problem, yet the true "burden of disease" remains unknown. Building on efforts by the American Association for the Surgery of Trauma to standardize an EGS definition, we sought to describe the burden of disease for EGS in the United States. We hypothesize that EGS patients represent a large, diverse, and challenging cohort and that the burden is increasing.

Methods.—The study population was selected from the Nationwide Inpatient Sample, 2001 to 2010, using the AAST EGS DRG International Classification of Diseases—9th Rev. codes, selecting all EGS patients 18 years or older with urgent/emergent admission status. Rates for operations, mortality, and sepsis were compiled along with hospital type, length of stay, insurance, and demographic data. The χ^2 test, the t test, and the Cochran-Armitage trend test were used; $p < 0.05$ was significant.

Results.—From 2001 to 2010, there were 27,668,807 EGS admissions, 7.1% of all hospitalizations. The population-adjusted case rate for 2010 was 1,290 admissions per 100,000 people (95% confidence interval, 1,288.9-1,291.8). The mean age was 58.7 years; most had comorbidities. A total of 7,979,578 patients (28.8%) required surgery. During 10 years, admissions increased by 27.5%; operations, by 32.3%; and sepsis cases, by 15% ($p < 0.0001$). Mortality and length of stay both decreased ($p < 0.0001$). Medicaid and uninsured rates increased by a combined 38.1% ($p < 0.0001$). Nearly 85% were treated in urban hospitals, and nearly 40% were treated in teaching hospitals; both increased over time ($p < 0.0001$).

Conclusion.—The EGS burden of disease is substantial and is increasing. The annual case rate (1,290 of 100,000) is higher than the sum of all new cancer diagnoses (all ages/types): 650 per 100,000 (95% confidence interval, 370.1−371.7), yet the public health implications remain largely unstudied. These data can be used to guide future research into improved access to care, resource allocation, and quality improvement efforts.

Level of Evidence.—Epidemiologic study, level III (Fig 1).

► Although not a study of the trauma population, this selection is included as more emergency general surgery is performed by trauma surgeons in the practice setting of acute care surgery.

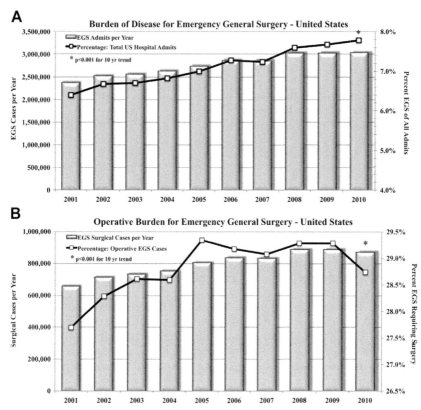

FIGURE 1.—(*A*), Annual burden of disease for EGS: hospital admissions per year and percentage of total US admissions for that year. (*B*), Surgical burden of disease for EGS: number of EGS admissions with surgical intervention during the same admission and annual percentage of EGS admissions requiring surgery. (Reprinted from Gale SC, Shafi S, Dombrovskiy VY, et al. The public health burden of emergency general surgery in the United States: a 10-year analysis of the Nationwide Inpatient Sample—2001 to 2010. *J Trauma Acute Care Surg.* 2014;77:202-208, with permission from Lippincott Williams & Wilkins.)

Emergency general surgery conditions represent a large and complex patient population that is growing annually. This escalation in patients presenting annually is included as Fig 1. These are also complex patients, with half of them being older than 60 years and most having significant comorbidities. They showed that sepsis rates remained relatively stable during the study period but documented a 40% reduction in mortality. In this study, the authors evaluated, for the first time, the public health implications of this massive disease burden and suggest that a crisis is at hand. There is a growing need for emergency surgical care at a time of progressively declining surgeon availability. Although large urban centers are better equipped to care for many of these complex patients and may serve as centers for regionalization, the sheer volume of patients requiring treatment for emergency general surgery conditions may be prohibitive. Further efforts, using similar approaches, should be directed at studying processes of care and quality improvement and ensuring adequate organizational planning and resource allocation for the growth of acute care surgery programs.

D. W. Mozingo, MD

Disparities in trauma: the impact of socioeconomic factors on outcomes following traumatic hollow viscus injury

Hazlitt M, Hill JB, Gunter OL, et al (Meharry Med College, Nashville, TN; Vanderbilt Univ School of Medicine, Nashville, TN; Vanderbilt Univ Med Ctr, Nashville, TN)
J Surg Res 191:6-11, 2014

Background.—This piece aims to examine the relationships between hollow viscus injury (HVI) and socioeconomic factors in determining outcomes. HVI has well-defined injury patterns with complex postoperative convalescence and morbidity, representing an ideal focus for identifying potential disparities among a homogeneous injury population.

Materials and Methods.—A retrospective review included patients admitted to a level I trauma center with HVI from 2000–2009, as identified in the Trauma Registry of the American College of Surgeons. Patients with concomitant significant solid organ or vasculature injury were excluded. US Census (2000) median household income by zip code was used as socioeconomic proxy. Demographic and injury-related variables were also included. Endpoints were mortality and outcomes associated with HVI morbidity.

Results.—A total of 933 patients with HVI were identified and 256 met inclusion criteria. There were 23 deaths (9.0%), and mortality was not associated with race, gender, income, or payer source. However, lower median household income was significantly associated with longer intervals to ostomy takedown ($P = 0.032$). Additionally, private payers had significantly lower rates of anastomotic leak (0% [0/73] versus 7.1% [13/183], $P = 0.019$) and fascial dehiscence (5.5% [4/73] versus 16.9% [31/183], $P = 0.016$), while self-payers had significantly higher rates of abscess formation, both overall (24% [24/100] versus 10.2% [16/156], $P = 0.004$) and among penetrating injuries (27.4% [23/84] versus 13.6% [12/88], $P = 0.036$).

Conclusions.—Socioeconomic status may not impact overall mortality among trauma patients with hollow viscus injuries, but private insurance appears to be protective of morbidity related to anastomotic leak, fascial dehiscence, and abscess formation. This supports that socioeconomic disparity may exist within long-term outcomes, particularly regarding payer source (Fig 2).

▶ There is a growing body of evidence that nonclinical factors such as socioeconomic status and health insurance status impact health outcomes. Such disparity has been described in a wide array of conditions, including cardiac revascularization, prevention and early detection of colorectal cancer, and rejection after renal

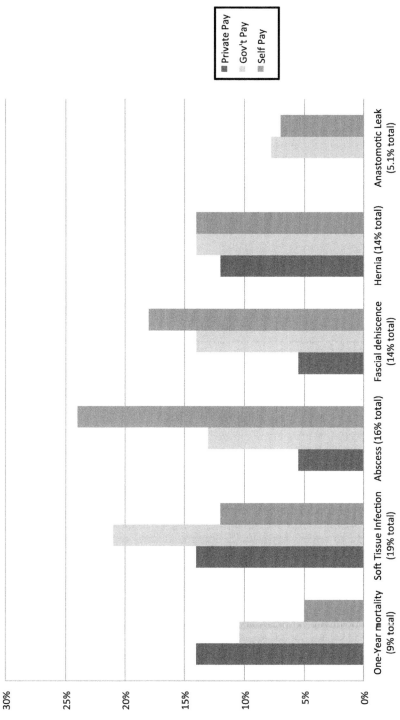

FIGURE 2.—Incidence of 1-y complications following HVI surgical intervention among different payer groups. (Reprinted from The Journal of Surgical Research. Hazlitt M, Hill JB, Gunter OL, et al. Disparities in trauma: the impact of socioeconomic factors on outcomes following traumatic hollow viscus injury. *J Surg Res.* 2014;191:6-11, Copyright 2014, with permission from Elsevier.)

transplant. Socioeconomic factors and insurance status have been described to affect outcomes across many medical conditions, perhaps more profoundly than race or income. One might infer that these factors would have a diminished effect on traumatic injury outcomes in the short term because of the emergent and protocolled nature of acute care. Also, the behavior of surgeons and allied health professionals may not be affected by variations in socioeconomic status indicators within the limited timeline of standardized care that defines trauma care. In this study, the authors sought to characterize the relationships among the homogenous population of abdominal hollow viscus injuries. Hollow viscus injuries represent an injury pattern characterized by early intervention and complex, yet well-defined, recovery and predictable morbidity. It is therefore an ideal focus for independently examining the impact of socioeconomic and nonclinical factors on both mortality and morbidity. The authors hypothesize that there is no difference between outcomes in trauma with isolated hollow viscus injuries based on demographic or socioeconomic variables. Fig 2, included in this selection, describes the authors' main findings in this study, namely, that private insurance appears to be protective of morbidity related to anastomotic leak, fascial dehiscence, and abscess formation. The major limitation of this study is that it is retrospective and from a single institution. Thus, these findings may not be generalizable, and additional investigation is warranted.

D. W. Mozingo, MD

A Human Factors Subsystems Approach to Trauma Care

Catchpole K, Ley E, Wiegmann D, et al (Cedars-Sinai Med Ctr, Los Angeles, CA; Univ of Wisconsin, Madison; et al)
JAMA Surg 149:962-968, 2014

Importance.—A physician-centered approach to systems design is fundamental to ameliorating the causes of many errors, inefficiencies, and reliability problems.

Objective.—To use human factors engineering to redesign the trauma process based on previously identified impediments to care related to coordination problems, communication failures, and equipment issues.

Design, Setting, and Participants.—This study used an interrupted time series design to collect historically controlled data via prospective direct observation by trained observers. We studied patients from a level I trauma center from August 1 through October 31, 2011, and August 1 through October 31, 2012.

Interventions.—A range of potential solutions based on previous observations, trauma team engagement, and iterative cycles identified the most promising subsystem interventions (headsets, equipment storage, medication packs, whiteboard, prebriefing, and teamwork training). Five of the 6 subsystem interventions were successfully deployed. Communication headsets were found to be unsuitable in simulation.

Main Outcomes and Measures.—The primary outcome measure was flow disruptions, with treatment time and length of stay as secondary outcome measures.

Results.—A total of 86 patients were observed before the intervention and 120 after the intervention. Flow disruptions increased if the patient had undergone computed tomography (CT) ($F_{1200} = 20.0$, $P < .001$) and had been to the operating room ($F_{1200} = 63.1$, $P < .001$), with an interaction among the intervention, trauma level, and CT ($F_{1200} = 6.50$, $P = .01$). For total treatment time, there was an effect of the intervention ($F_{1200} = 21.7$, $P < .001$), whether the patient had undergone CT ($F_{1200} = 43.0$, $P < .001$), and whether the patient had been to the operating room ($F_{1200} = 85.8$, $P < .001$), with an interaction among the intervention, trauma level, and CT ($F_{1200} = 15.1$, $P < .001$), reflecting a 20- to 30-minute reduction in time in the emergency department. Length of stay was reduced significantly for patients with major mortality risk ($P = .01$) from a median of 8 to 5 days.

Conclusions and Relevance.—Deployment of complex subsystem interventions based on detailed human factors engineering and a systems analysis of the provision of trauma care resulted in reduced flow disruptions, treatment time, and length of stay.

▶ In this selection, the authors describe the human factors engineering process as based on the principle that system performance and human well-being can be improved through an integrated approach to individual skills, teamwork, equipment, task, environment, and organizational design. The authors apply this process to a performance improvement initiative to improve the care of their trauma patients. Evidence supports improving work systems through such interventions as checklists, briefings, standardized care pathways, formal protocols, team resource management training, and technological development to improve teamwork, shared knowledge, workflow, and outcomes. The greatest success is usually achieved by involving physicians, nurses, and other team members in the process of developing improvements and by designing systems around human needs. This person-centered approach to systems design is fundamental to diminishing the causes of many errors, inefficiencies, and reliability problems. Fig 1 in the original article, included in this selection, illustrates the general process by which the interventions were developed. This novel study objectively examined the effects of multiple subsystem interventions in trauma care. The detailed study of the trauma system and the collection of data prospectively were central in guiding the authors toward the largest improvement opportunities. By reviewing hospital policy documentation, they were able to map the process and conducted interviews and focus groups with a broad range of physicians to discover their impressions of the problems. Through a combination of statistical analysis and multidisciplinary consensus, the authors were able to identify key aspects of process, workplace modification, teamwork, technology, and information management that would benefit from re-engineering. By piecing together all the collected data elements, they were able to target the interventions that had the greatest positive effect on the process.

D. W. Mozingo, MD

Association Between Race and Age in Survival After Trauma
Hicks CW, Hashmi ZG, Velopulos C, et al (Johns Hopkins School of Medicine, Baltimore, MD)
JAMA Surg 149:642-647, 2014

Importance.—Racial disparities in survival after trauma are well described for patients younger than 65 years. Similar information among older patients is lacking because existing trauma databases do not include important patient comorbidity information.

Objective.—To determine whether racial disparities in trauma survival persist in patients 65 years or older.

Design, Setting, and Participants.—Trauma patients were identified from the Nationwide Inpatient Sample (January 1, 2003, through December 30, 2010) using International Classification of Diseases, Ninth Revision, Clinical Modification diagnosis codes. Injury severity was ascertained by applying the Trauma Mortality Prediction Model, and patient comorbidities were quantified using the Charlson Comorbidity Index.

Main Outcomes and Measures.—In-hospital mortality after trauma for blacks vs whites for younger (16-64 years of age) and older ($\geq$65 years of age) patients was compared using 3 different statistical methods: univariable logistic regression, multivariable logistic regression with and without clustering for hospital effects, and coarsened exact matching. Model covariates included age, sex, insurance status, type and intent of injury, injury severity, head injury severity, and Charlson Comorbidity Index.

Results.—A total of 1 073 195 patients were included (502 167 patients 16-64 years of age and 571 028 patients $\geq$65 years of age). Most older patients were white (547 325 [95.8%]), female (406 158 [71.1%]), and insured (567 361 [99.4%]) and had Charlson Comorbidity Index scores of 1 or higher (323 741 [56.7%]). The unadjusted odds ratios (ORs) for death in blacks vs whites were 1.35 (95% CI, 1.28-1.42) for patients 16 to 64 years of age and 1.00 (95% CI, 0.93-1.08) for patients 65 years or older. After risk adjustment, racial disparities in survival persisted in the younger black group (OR, 1.21; 95% CI, 1.13-1.30) but were reversed in the older group (OR, 0.83; 95% CI, 0.76-0.90). This finding was consistent across all 3 statistical methods.

Conclusions and Relevance.—Different racial disparities in survival after trauma exist between white and black patients depending on their age group. Although younger white patients have better outcomes after trauma than younger black patients, older black patients have better outcomes than older white patients. Exploration of this paradoxical finding may lead to a better understanding of the mechanisms that cause disparities in trauma outcomes.

▶ Disparities in survival after trauma among minority and uninsured patients have been well described for those younger than 65 years. Despite recent demonstration of racial disparities after trauma among younger patients, information regarding the effect of race on trauma outcomes in older patients is lacking. The objective of this study was to determine whether the previously described racial disparities in outcomes after trauma continue to persist among older trauma patients. Using an approach that allows for the incorporation of patient comorbidity information with traumatic injury severity information, the authors of this selection assessed in-hospital mortality in white vs black patients after traumatic injury. The authors queried the Nationwide Inpatient Sample data set for their analysis. In this study, which risk-adjusts for both patient-specific comorbidity data and injury severity information, differential racial disparities in survival after traumatic injury exist between black and white patients depending on their age. For patients younger than 65 years, white patients have better outcomes after trauma than black patients. Conversely, among older patients, black patients have better outcomes than similarly injured, matched white patient cohorts. This finding is depicted in Fig 1 from the original article and included with this selection. This finding has not been described previously in the trauma patient population. Further study of this racial disparity within different populations, including analysis of the effect of insurance status, may help explain these findings in the population 65 years or older. Also, future studies that incorporate the use of frailty indexes might shed additional light on these outcomes.

D. W. Mozingo, MD

A Review of the First 10 Years of Critical Care Aeromedical Transport During Operation Iraqi Freedom and Operation Enduring Freedom: The Importance of Evacuation Timing

Ingalls N, Zonies D, Bailey JA, et al (Univ of Nevada, Las Vegas; Landsthul Regional Med Ctr, Kaiserlautern, Germany; US Army Inst of Surgical Res, Ft Sam Houston, TX; et al)
JAMA Surg 149:807-813, 2014

Importance.—Advances in the care of the injured patient are perhaps the only benefit of military conflict. One of the unique aspects of the military medical care system that emerged during Operation Iraqi Freedom and Operation Enduring Freedom has been the opportunity to apply existing civilian trauma system standards to the provision of combat casualty care across an evolving theater of operations.

Objectives.—To identify differences in mortality for soldiers undergoing early and rapid evacuation from the combat theater and to evaluate the capabilities of the Critical Care Air Transport Team (CCATT) and Joint

Theater Trauma Registry databases to provide adequate data to support future initiatives for improvement of performance.

Design, Setting, and Participants.—Retrospective review of CCATT records and the Joint Theater Trauma Registry from September 11, 2001, to December 31, 2010, for the in-theater military medicine health system, including centers in Iraq, Afghanistan, and Germany. Of 2899 CCATT transport records, those for 975 individuals had all the required data elements.

Exposure.—Rapid evacuation by the CCATT.

Main Outcomes and Measures.—Survival as a function of time from injury to arrival at the role IV facility at Landstuhl Regional Medical Center.

Results.—The patient cohort demonstrated a mean Injury Severity Score of 23.7 and an overall 30-day mortality of 2.1%. Mortality en route was less than 0.02%. Statistically significant differences between survivors and decedents with respect to the Injury Severity Score (mean [SD], 23.4 [12.4] vs 37.7 [16.5]; $P < .001$), cumulative volume of blood transfused among the patients in each group who received a transfusion ($P < .001$), worst base deficit (mean [SD], -3.4 [5.0] vs -7.8 [6.9]; $P = .02$), and worst international normalized ratio (median [interquartile range], 1.2 [1.0-1.4] vs 1.4 [1.1-2.2]; $P = .03$) were observed. We found no statistically significant difference between survivors and decedents with respect to time from injury to arrival at definitive care.

Conclusions and Relevance.—Rapid movement of critically injured casualties within hours of wounding appears to be effective, with a minimal mortality incurred during movement and overall 30-day mortality. We found no association between the duration of time from wounding to arrival at Landstuhl Regional Medical Center with respect to mortality.

▶ Since September 11, 2001, we have seen dramatic changes undertaken by US military medicine. One of the unique aspects of the military medical care system emerging from and during Operation Iraqi Freedom and Operation Enduring Freedom has been the opportunity to apply existing civilian trauma system standards to the provision of combat casualty care across an evolving theater of operations. Medical operations in support of these conflicts represent the first large-scale opportunity for the US military to adapt and incorporate lessons from the civilian trauma system to the combat casualty care arena. This transformation was accelerated in part by the presence of a generation of military surgeons who went to war after fellowship training in large, civilian, urban-based trauma centers and systems. Tools such as trauma registries, performance improvement processes, and clinical practice guidelines were familiar to this group of fellowship-trained surgeons. These same tools had yet to be incorporated to any great extent into the US military medical system. Fellowship-trained trauma surgeons successfully advocated and partnered with military medical corps leadership to implement change and incorporate important trauma system principles as advocated by the American College of Surgeons Committee on Trauma and the optimal resources guidelines. The results of this study suggest that the critical care air transport teams process has proved itself to be an important component of the continuum of combat casualty care. The process of rapid movement of critically injured casualties within hours of their wounding appears to be effective, with minimal mortality incurred during movement (<0.02%) and an overall 30-day mortality of 2.1%. This study is yet another in a long series of excellent publications documenting the improvements in care of our wounded soldiers in recent years, and the military surgeons and their patient care teams should be congratulated for their success.

D. W. Mozingo, MD

A 6-year retrospective review of pediatric firearm injuries: Do patients < 14 years of age differ from those 15–18 years of age?

Hendry PL, Suen A, Kalynych CJ, et al (Univ of Florida College of Medicine, Jacksonville; et al)
J Trauma Acute Care Surg 77:S41-S45, 2014

Background.—Pediatric firearm injuries are an increasing source of morbidity. Firearm injuries in adolescents are common but not well studied in younger children. The aims were to describe the epidemiology of firearm injuries in patients 0 year to 18 years old, with a case study of patients 14 years or younger for determining shooting characteristics and epidemiologic trends.

Methods.—Part 1 obtained data from hospital trauma registry. Inclusion criteria were patients 0 year to 18 years of age presenting from 2005 to 2010 with firearm injury and registry inclusion. Demographic and injury data were extracted. Part 2 included a retrospective review of patients 14 years or younger including hospital and emergency medical services records. Data from the group 0 year to 14 years included shooting and treatment details. Categorical variables were described using counts and percentages. Differences between the groups were assessed using odds ratios (ORs), along with 95% confidence intervals (CIs), extracted from logistic regression models.

Results.—Registry query resulted in 456 patients (0–18 years), including 78 patients who are 14 years or younger. In the group of 0 to 18 years, 86% were male; 83% were black in the group of 15 to 18 years and 64% in the group 0 to 14 years. Overall death rate was 7%. Patients in the group of 15 years to 18 years were twice more likely (23% vs. 11%) to arrive via car or walk-in compared with the patients in the group of 0 year to 14 years (OR, 2.32; 95% CI, 1.07–5.03). Patients in the group of 0 year to 14 years were almost four times more likely to be shot at home compared with those who are 15 years to 18 years (OR, 3.76, 95% CI, 2.29–6.19). Patients in the group of 5 years to 9 years were six times more likely to have multiple injury sites compared with those who are 10 years to 14 years (OR, 6.26; 95% CI, 1.26–31.09). Only 13% had documented child protective services notification.

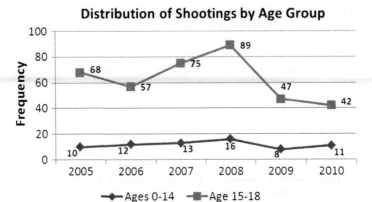

FIGURE 1.—Distribution of firearm injuries by age group. (Reprinted from Hendry PL, Suen A, Kaly-nych CJ, et al. A 6-year retrospective review of pediatric firearm injuries: do patients < 14 years of age differ from those 15-18 years of age? *J Trauma Acute Care Surg.* 2014;77:S41-S45, with permission from Lippincott Williams & Wilkins.)

Conclusion.—Results from this study suggest that firearm injuries differ in younger patients compared with adolescents. The younger subset was more likely to be shot at home versus public settings. Hospital and emergency medical services records lacked important shooting details often found in crime scene reports, which are necessary for the development of effective crime and prevention strategies.

Level of Evidence.—Epidemiologic study, level III (Fig 1).

▶ In light of recent national firearm tragedies involving young children, there is renewed interest in firearm safety and prevention. In this selection, the authors attempted to further define the differences between firearm injuries in children younger than 14 years and firearm injuries in the adolescent population. Results suggest that firearm injuries differ in younger patients compared with adolescents. The younger subset was more likely to arrive by emergency medical services compared with adolescents. The mode of arrival in the group 15 years to 18 years old was 23% by private car or walk in compared with 11% in the group of 0 to 14 years. A possible explanation for this finding is that adolescents are more likely to be involved in a gang or criminal activity at the time of the firearm injury. The mode of arrival was often by private car or walk in vs emergency medical services to avoid contact with law enforcement. The younger subset of our study was 4 times more likely to be shot at home versus public settings compared with the group of 15 years to 18 years, indicating that future prevention strategies should be aimed at the home setting. Unintentional shootings may occur when children are unsupervised in a home and find a loaded firearm. This study suggests that firearm injuries differ in the circumstances and type of injury in younger children compared with adolescents. Future research funding for pediatric firearm injury prevention is currently being addressed as the epidemic of gun violence continues to escalate. Successful linkage of emergency medical services, hospital, law enforcement, and primary care records is a priority for improved epidemiologic study and development of prevention strategies targeted at this population.

D. W. Mozingo, MD

Association Between the Seat Belt Sign and Intra-abdominal Injuries in Children With Blunt Torso Trauma in Motor Vehicle Collisions

Borgialli DA, for the Pediatric Emergency Care Applied Research Network (Hurley Med Ctr, Flint, MI; et al)
Acad Emerg Med 21:1240-1248, 2014

Objectives.—The objective was to determine the association between the abdominal seat belt sign and intra-abdominal injuries (IAIs) in children presenting to emergency departments with blunt torso trauma after motor vehicle collisions (MVCs).

Methods.—This was a planned subgroup analysis of prospective data from a multicenter cohort study of children with blunt torso trauma after MVCs. Patient history and physical examination findings were documented before abdominal computed tomography (CT) or laparotomy. Seat belt sign was defined as a continuous area of erythema, ecchymosis, or abrasion across the abdomen secondary to a seat belt restraint. The relative risk (RR) of IAI with 95% confidence intervals (CIs) was calculated for children with seat belt signs compared to those without. The risk of IAI in those patients with seat belt sign who were without abdominal pain or tenderness, and with Glasgow Coma Scale (GCS) scores of 14 or 15, was also calculated.

Results.—A total of 3,740 children with seat belt sign documentation after blunt torso trauma in MVCs were enrolled; 585 (16%) had seat belt signs. Among the 1,864 children undergoing definitive abdominal testing (CT, laparotomy/laparoscopy, or autopsy), IAIs were more common in patients with seat belt signs than those without (19% vs. 12%; RR = 1.6, 95% CI = 1.3 to 2.1). This difference was primarily due to a greater risk of gastrointestinal injuries (hollow viscous or associated mesentery) in those with seat belt signs (11% vs. 1%; RR = 9.4, 95% CI = 5.4 to 16.4). IAI was diagnosed in 11 of 194 patients (5.7%; 95% CI = 2.9% to 9.9%) with seat belt signs who did not have initial complaints of abdominal pain or tenderness and had GCS scores of 14 or 15.

Conclusions.—Patients with seat belt signs after MVCs are at greater risk of IAI than those without seat belt signs, predominately due to gastrointestinal injuries. Although IAIs are less common in alert patients with seat belt signs who do not have initial complaints of abdominal pain or tenderness, the risk of IAI is sufficient that additional evaluation such as observation, laboratory studies, and potentially abdominal CT scanning is generally necessary.

▶ The objective of this study was to determine the association between the presence of seat belt sign and intra-abdominal injuries in children presenting to emergency departments after motor vehicle crashes. The authors also sought to determine the rate of intra-abdominal injury among the subset of children with seat belt signs who do not have abdominal pain or tenderness and have Glasgow Coma Scale scores of 14 or 15 on initial examination. This was a planned subanalysis of a large prospective observational multicenter study of children with blunt torso trauma. The study was conducted at 20 pediatric emergency departments in the Pediatric Emergency Care Applied Research Network as part of a larger study to derive clinical prediction rules for identifying children at low risk of intra-abdominal injuries undergoing acute intervention. In this study, the authors included patients younger than 18 years of age with histories of blunt abdominal trauma after motor vehicle crashes who were evaluated in the emergency department and had the presence or absence of seat belt sign documented during the initial evaluation. Pediatric patients with seat belt signs after motor vehicle crashes are at a greater risk of intra-abdominal injuries than those without seat belt signs, primarily due to a greater risk of gastrointestinal injuries. In addition, the authors found that these patients had more interventions than those without seat belt signs. The authors conclude that although intra-abdominal injuries are uncommon in patients with seat belt signs and no initial complaints of abdominal pain or abdominal tenderness, the risk of intra-abdominal injury is such that additional evaluation with observation, laboratory studies, and potentially abdominal computed tomography is generally necessary.

D. W. Mozingo, MD

3 Burns

Costs of burn care: A systematic review
Hop MJ, Polinder S, van der Vlies CH, et al (Maasstad Hosp, Rotterdam, The
Netherlands; Erasmus Med Ctr, Rotterdam, The Netherlands; et al)
Wound Repair Regen 22:436-450, 2014

Burn care is traditionally considered expensive care. However, detailed information about the costs of burn care is scarce despite the increased need for this information and the enhanced focus on healthcare cost control. In this study, economic literature on burn care was systematically reviewed to examine the problem of burn-related costs. Cost or economic evaluation studies on burn care that had been published in international peer-reviewed journals from 1950 to 2012 were identified. The methodology of these articles was critically appraised by two reviewers, and cost results were extracted. A total of 156 studies met the inclusion criteria. Nearly all of the studies were cost studies ($n = 153$) with a healthcare perspective ($n = 139$) from high-income countries ($n = 127$). Hospital charges were often used as a proxy for costs ($n = 44$). Three studies were cost-effectiveness analyses. The mean total healthcare cost per burn patient in high-income countries was \$88,218 (range \$704–\$717,306; median \$44,024). A wide variety of methodological approaches and cost prices was found. We recommend that cost studies and economic evaluations employ a standard approach to improve the quality and harmonization of economic evaluation studies, optimize comparability, and improve insight into burn care costs and efficiency (Table 4).

▶ The objectives of this study were 3-fold: (1) to assess the methodologic quality of economic studies on burn care, (2) to present the range of medical costs and nonmedical costs of burn care, and (3) to present economic evaluation studies of burn care. Costs per treatment and per day compared with nonburn care costs were also included in the analyses. A summary of the findings appears as Table 4. The most expensive burn care component in this review was hospital stay. The included studies, however, often focused on medication or dressings. This finding suggests that future research on cost-effective burn care should focus on reducing length of hospital stay without compromising the quality of care.

Furthermore, more studies on medical and nonmedical costs in the rehabilitation phase are lacking and need to be performed to gain better insight into the total cost of burn care. Additionally, because this study surveyed the international literature on the cost of burn care, the authors stated that data from

TABLE 4.—Healthcare Costs of Burn Patients in High-Income Countries (Converted to US Dollars, 2012)

	Mean ($)	Range ($)	Median ($)	References
Costs per burn center day	2,705	111–11,607	2,060	25,26,29,31,38,41,42,47,49–51,55,57,60,64, 72,75,83,87,99,103,122,135,140,141,146,148
Costs per burn center ICU day	3,164	1,590–4,657	2,969	26,41,42,87,140,141
Costs per general hospital day	1,959	585–4,314	1,468	25,45,59,84
Costs per general ICU day	4,356	4,356	4,356	45
Total healthcare costs/pt	88,218	704–717,306	44,024	1,8,25–69,71,72,76,78,80,81,83–85,87–89, 91,93,94,96,98,99,101–103
Flame	87,140	50,508–109,469	94,291	49,59,62,71
Scald	33,960	15,882–32,526	33,981	49,59,62,71
Electric	55,281	26,076–70,311	69,457	49,62,71
Costs per 1% TBSA	4,159	162–20,663	2,633	1,8,25,26,28–30,32,34–36,38–43,45,50,52,54 –58,60, 63–67,70,72–74,78,83,85,87,89,93,96,99,102

ICU, intensive care unit; pt, patient; TBSA, total body surface area.
Editor's Note: Please refer to original journal article for full references.
Reprinted from Hop MJ, Polinder S, van der Vlies CH, et al. Costs of burn care: A systematic review. *Wound Repair Regen.* 2014;22:436-450, with permission from Wound Repair and Regeneration and John Wiley and Sons, www. interscience.wiley.com.

mid- and low-income countries was limited, and additional studies are needed to gain better insight into costs and cost effectiveness in these regions.

D. W. Mozingo, MD

Burn Disaster-Management Planning: A Preparedness Tool Kit
Joho BS, Lozano D, Pagella P, et al (Regional Burn Ctr, Allentown, PA)
J Burn Care Res 35:e205-e216, 2014

It is vital that preburn center emergency providers have the knowledge and equipment needed to treat burn-injured patients should there be an extended delay in transporting the patients to a burn center as may be the case during a mass-casualty incident or weather-related emergency. Since 2007 a collaborative effort has been underway to build an emergency-response tool kit that provides to and draws from local, state, and federal resources. This tool kit is designed to fill knowledge deficits regarding burn treatment as well as address gaps in stockpiled treatment materials. This tool kit was implemented in four modules: provide equipment, provide guidance, provide education, and provide drill. Module one ensures that equipment needed for treating burn injuries is available to emergency providers. Module two ensures that policies and procedures congruent with the practice of the regional burn center are in place. Module three ensures that preburn center providers are provided education on modern burn care. Module four is to drill. The sum of the effort by the authors is the

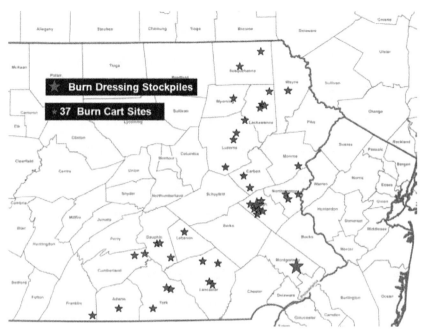

FIGURE 9.—Burn cart locations. (Reprinted from Joho BS, Lozano D, Pagella P, et al. Burn disaster-management planning: a preparedness tool kit. *J Burn Care Res*. 2014;35:e205-e216, with permission from American Burn Association.)

establishment of a tool kit that enhances the capabilities of preburn center emergency providers. Implementation has led to improved collaborative relationships, increased the awareness of available resources, and reduced knowledge deficit regarding burn care among preburn center providers. This tool kit provides greater continuity of care for all burn patients affected by a delay in transport to a burn center, and its modular structure makes it adaptable to other regions as a whole or in part (Fig 9).

▶ Since 2007, the authors' institution has been implementing a collaborative plan to ensure that all burn patients of a mass casualty incident or weather-related emergency in eastern Pennsylvania receive appropriate treatment. The ultimate goal of this plan is to create a network of resources that non-burn center providers can rely on to assist them in successfully treating burn patients for up to 72 hours after injury. To achieve these goals, they focused on filling gaps in both emergency provider burn triage and treatment knowledge and availability of burn treatment supplies. Their tool kit was implemented in 4 stages: provide equipment, provide guidance, provide education, and provide opportunities to drill. Fig 9 is included and shows the location of burn supply carts relative to the regional burn center. The sum of this effort is the establishment of a comprehensive, modular program designed to enhance the capabilities of preburn center emergency responders in the event they are required to care for a burn patient because of a delay in transfer to the regional burn center.

D. W. Mozingo, MD

Cost-Effectiveness Comparison Between Topical Silver Sulfadiazine and Enclosed Silver Dressing for Partial-Thickness Burn Treatment

Sheckter CC, Van Vliet MM, Krishnan NM, et al (Univ of Southern California, Los Angeles; Geisel School of Medicine, Dartmouth, Hanover, NH)
J Burn Care Res 35:284-290, 2014

The standard treatment of partial-thickness burns includes topical silver products such as silver sulfadiazine (SSD) cream and enclosed dressings including silver-impregnated foam (Mepilex Ag; Molnlycke Health Care, Gothenburg, Sweden) and silver-laden sheets (Aquacel Ag; ConvaTec, Skillman, NJ). The current state of health care is limited by resources, with an emphasis on evidence-based outcomes and cost-effective treatments. This study includes a decision analysis with an incremental cost-utility ratio comparing enclosed silver dressings with SSD in partial-thickness burn patients with TBSA less than 20%. A comprehensive literature review was conducted to identify clinically relevant health states in partial-thickness burn patients. These health states include successful healing, infection, and noninfected delayed healing requiring either surgery or conservative management. The probabilities of these health states were combined with Medicare CPT reimbursement codes (cost) and patient-derived utilities to fit into the decision model. Utilities were obtained using a visual analog scale during patient interviews. Expected cost and quality-adjusted life years (QALYs) were calculated using the roll-back method. The incremental cost-utility ratio for enclosed silver dressing relative to SSD was $40,167.99/QALY. One-way sensitivity analysis of complication rates confirmed robustness of the model. Assuming a maximum willingness to pay $50,000/QALY, the complication rate for SSD must be 22% or higher for enclosed silver dressing to be cost effective. By varying complication rates for SSD and enclosed silver dressings, the two-way sensitivity analysis demonstrated the cost effectiveness of using enclosed silver dressing at the majority of complication rates for both treatment modalities. Enclosed silver dressings are a cost-effective means of treating partial thickness burns (Fig 1).

▶ For nearly 50 years, topical silver delivered from silver sulfadiazine has been the standard treatment for partial-thickness burns. Owing to its formulation as a cream, silver sulfadiazine is easily applied topically and has few side effects, although transient pancytopenia sometimes occurs. It is affordable and can be used with little cost to cover large burns. In the last 10 years, alternatives to silver sulfadiazine have been developed that deliver therapeutic silver to the burn in a way that does not require daily dressing changes and has minimal time investment by the practitioner. Therapeutic levels of silver are present in

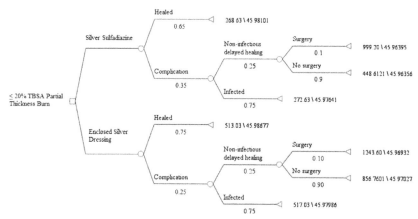

FIGURE 1.—Decision model used in our analysis for partial-thickness burn treatment with silver sulfadiazine and enclosed silver dressing (Mepilex/Aquacel). Probabilities are displayed below terminal branches whereas cost and quality-adjusted life years (QALYs) are displayed to the right of the terminal branches. Expected values were calculated for both cost and QALYs, based on the probability of each health state and were summed across both the silver sulfadiazine and enclosed silver dressing (Mepilex/Aquacel) arms for comparison. (Reprinted from Sheckter CC, Van Vliet MM, Krishnan NM, et al. Cost-effectiveness comparison between topical silver sulfadiazine and enclosed silver dressing for partial-thickness burn treatment. *J Burn Care Res.* 2014;35:284-290, with permission from American Burn Association.)

these dressings up to 2 weeks after application. The study in this selection describes a decision analysis comparing silver sulfadiazine with closed silver dressings for partial-thickness burns in patients with burns less than 20% of the total body surface area. The decision analysis used appears as Fig 1. Decision analysis is a technique that compares the cost effectiveness of competing management strategies by evaluating the cost and clinical efficacy for each treatment option. This type of analysis is often used when comparing a more expensive treatment option thought to provide greater clinical efficacy relative to the current standard treatment. The authors conclude that enclosed silver dressings offer a cost-effective means of treating partial-thickness burns. They also suggest that the enclosed silver dressings have a higher utility than silver sulfadiazine, which offers patients a better quality of life in burn treatment.

D. W. Mozingo, MD

Effect of Platelet-rich Plasma Therapy Associated With Exercise Training in Musculoskeletal Healing in Rats

Cunha RC, Francisco JC, Cardoso MA, et al (Instituto de Pesquisa Pelé Pequeno Príncipe, Curitiba, Paraná, Brazil; et al)
Transplant Proc 46:1879-1881, 2014

Background.—Muscle healing is a time-dependent process associated with an increase in the total amount of local collagen fibers. Platelet-rich plasma therapy (PRPT) associated with exercise may improve this healing process. The aim of this study was to demonstrate the regenerative effect of PRPT in association with exercise training on musculoskeletal healing.

Methods.—Male Wistar rats were submitted to an injury in the vastus lateralis muscle and randomly divided into 4 groups ($n = 5$/group): sedentary sham-operated (SSO); sedentary group submitted to PRPT (SPR); swim-trained (SWT); and swim-trained group submitted to PRPT (SWP). Serum lactate level was used to confirm the training protocol effectiveness to increase aerobic fitness. The collagen fiber concentration was measured by the polarization colors in picrosirius red-stained tissue sections.

Results.—Lactate levels decreased in both training groups (SWT and SWP; $P < .05$) after training (SWT: from 6.2 ± 0.44 to 4.7 ± 0.22 mmol/L; SWP: from 5.5 ± 0.99 to 4.0 ± 0.78 mmol/L). There were less type 1 collagen fibers in SWP group compared with other groups (SSO = 31.8 ± 10.3, SSP = 32.3 ± 13.5, SWT = 14.6 ± 13.4, SWP = 5.7 ± 4.7, $P < .05$), while there were more type 3 collagen fibers on SWP (SSO = 68.7 ± 9.8, SSP = 71.2 ± 12.2, SWT = 85.4 ± 13.4, SWP = 94.4 ± 4.6, $P < .05$) in the injured region.

Conclusion.—Exercise in association with PRPT enhances the skeletal muscle-healing process.

▶ Healing of tissue after trauma is often thought of as progressing in a stepwise fashion and, in normal individuals, is determined by the degree of trauma. Meanwhile, a number of agents have shown efficacy in certain conditions such as malnutrition, steroid use, radiated wounds, and diabetes. However, the holy grail of wound management is to improve the healing process in healthy people. In addition, resting the affected area was often espoused to allow for maximum healing to occur. This experimental study in animals reverses these previous dictums. Exercise (swimming) and platelet-rich plasma accelerated the healing of rat muscle wounds compared with results in other control groups.

It would be of great interest if this experimental method were to be studied in Phases 1, 2, and 3 human trials after determining the safety and dosages required for muscle healing.

J. M. Daly, MD

Major wound complication risk factors following soft tissue sarcoma resection

Moore J, Isler M, Barry J, et al (Maisonneuve-Rosemont Hosp, Montreal, Canada)
Eur J Surg Oncol 40:1671-1676, 2014

Background and Objectives.—Wound-healing complications represent an important source of morbidity in patients treated surgically for soft tissue sarcomas (STS). The purpose of this study was to determine which factors are predictive of major wound complication rates following STS resection, including tumor site, size, grade, and depth, as well as radiotherapy and chemotherapy.

Methods.—We reviewed 256 cases of STS treated surgically between 2000 and 2011. The primary outcome was occurrence of major wound complications post STS resection.

Results.—Major wound complications were more likely to occur post STS resection with larger tumor diameters ($p = 0.001$), high grade tumors ($p = 0.04$), location in the proximal lower extremity ($p = 0.01$), and use of preoperative radiotherapy ($p = 0.01$). Tumors located in the adductor compartment were at highest risk of complications. We did not demonstrate a significant difference in complications rates based on method of closure. Diabetes, smoking, obesity, tumor diameter, tumor location in the proximal lower extremity, and preoperative radiotherapy were independent predictors on multivariate analysis.

Conclusions.—There are multiple predictors for major wound complications post STS resection. A more aggressive resection irradiated soft tissues, combined with primary reconstruction, should be considered in cases with multiple risk factors.

▶ This retrospective review evaluated a variety of clinical and patient personal factors associated with wound complications in 256 patients undergoing resection of soft tissue sarcomas. As predicted and reported previously by other authors, the risk of wound complications increased as the size of the tumor increased (particularly > 20 cm). In addition, the use of preoperative radiotherapy was significantly associated with increased wound complications. Location in the adductor compartment and proximal lower leg was associated with poorer wound healing but was not significant on multivariate analysis.

Studies such as these do provide insight into the preoperative management of patients with soft tissue sarcomas in that under certain circumstances, one should plan for plastic reconstruction perhaps with use of muscle flaps to obviate wound breakdown.

J. M. Daly, MD

Hyaluronan enhances wound repair and increases collagen III in aged dermal wounds
Damodarasamy M, Johnson RS, Bentov I, et al (Univ of Washington, Seattle; et al)
Wound Repair Regen 22:521-526, 2014

Age-related changes in the extracellular matrix contribute to delayed wound repair in aging. Hyaluronan, a linear nonsulfated glycosaminoglycan, promotes synthesis and assembly of key extracellular matrix components, such as the interstitial collagens, during wound healing. The biological effects of hyaluronan are mediated, in part, by hyaluronan size. We have previously determined that dermal wounds in aged mice, relative to young mice, have deficits in the generation of lower molecular weight hyaluronan (defined as <300 kDa). Here, we tested the effect of exogenous hyaluronan of 2, 250, or 1,000 kDa sizes on full-thickness excisional wounds in aged mice. Only wounds treated with 250 kDa hyaluronan (HA250) were significantly improved over wounds that received carrier (water) alone. Treatment with HA250 was associated with increased expression of transcripts for the hyaluronan receptors CD44 and RHAMM, as well as collagens III and I. Analyses of dermal protein content by mass spectrometry and Western blotting confirmed significantly increased expression of collagen III in wounds treated with HA250 relative to control wounds. In summary, we find that HA250 improves wound repair and increases the synthesis of collagen III in aged dermal wounds.

▶ It is well known that in older subjects, wound healing does not progress as well as in young individuals. In fact, fetal wound healing has been described as "scarless," which is thought to be influenced by hyaluronan (HA). In this animal experiment, the investigators sought to understand whether the exogenous local supplementation with various kD sizes of HA would positively influence wound healing in aged mice. They demonstrated that over a 5-day period, aged mice showed improvement in wound closure when they received HA2, HA250, or HA1000 compared with control mice that received carrier (water) only. However, improvement in wound closure achieved statistical significance only in mice treated with HA250. Wounds of control mice (injected with water only) healed in a manner nearly identical to wounds in aged mice that received no fluid injections suggesting that the carrier for HA (water) did not influence wound healing in the control mice of the present study.

It would be valuable to understand the deficits in HA in older subjects and to conduct early clinical trials to determine the safety and efficacy of HA supplementation on open wounds, decubiti, venous stasis ulcers, and other lesions in aged patients.

J. M. Daly, MD

A modified collagen gel dressing promotes angiogenesis in a preclinical swine model of chronic ischemic wounds

Elgharably H, Ganesh K, Dickerson J, et al (The Ohio State Univ Wexner Med Ctr, Columbus)
Wound Repair Regen 22:720-729, 2014

We recently performed proteomic characterization of a modified collagen gel (MCG) dressing and reported promising effects of the gel in healing full-thickness excisional wounds. In this work, we test the translational relevance of our aforesaid findings by testing the dressing in a swine model of chronic ischemic wounds recently reported by our laboratory. Full-thickness excisional wounds were established in the center of bipedicle ischemic skin flaps on the backs of animals. Ischemia was verified by laser Doppler imaging, and MCG was applied to the test group of wounds. Seven days post wounding, macrophage recruitment to the wound was significantly higher in MCG-treated ischemic wounds. In vitro, MCG up-regulated expression of Mrc-1 (a reparative M2 macrophage marker) and induced the expression of anti-inflammatory cytokine interleukin (IL)-10 and of fibroblast growth factor-basic (β-FGF). An increased expression of CCR2, an M2 macrophage marker, was noted in the macrophages from MCG treated wounds. Furthermore, analyses of wound tissues 7 days post wounding showed up-regulation of transforming growth factor-β, vascular endothelial growth factor, von Willebrand's factor, and collagen type I expression in MCG-treated ischemic wounds. At 21 days post wounding, MCG-treated ischemic wounds displayed higher abundance of proliferating endothelial cells that formed mature vascular structures and increased blood flow to the wound. Fibroblast count was markedly higher in MCG-treated ischemic wound-edge tissue. In addition, MCG-treated wound-edge tissues displayed higher abundance of mature collagen with increased collagen type I: III deposition. Taken together, MCG helped mount a more robust inflammatory response that resolved in a timely manner, followed by an enhanced proliferative phase, angiogenic outcome, and postwound tissue remodeling. Findings of the current study warrant clinical testing of MCG in a setting of ischemic chronic wounds.

▶ Chronic ischemic wounds are a major clinical problem. The ischemia may come from the arterial side or the venous side of the equation but results in a chronic wound that is difficult to heal. Many studies have attempted to provide growth factors locally in an attempt to initiate robust recruitment of wound macrophages and other cells to the wound to sustain the healing process. According to the manufacturer, the unique formulation of the modified collagen gel (MCG) represents a mixture of 52% collagen of long and short polypeptides, along with glycerine, water, and fragrance. The MCG is a highly concentrated modified collagen (mainly type I) in a gel form.

The authors applied this gel on 1 side of ischemic flaps using the same animals as their own controls (Tegaderm alone on the control side). The treated side had far greater recruitment of wound macrophages along with growth factors associated with healing.

Importantly, however, the authors did not describe the entire process but only the biochemical and cellular changes taking place in the wounds. Although they wish to proceed to clinical trials, they should conduct additional safety experiments and also determine that earlier healing does indeed take place using the MCG dressing.

J. M. Daly, MD

Prospective, randomized, multi-institutional clinical trial of a silver alginate dressing to reduce lower extremity vascular surgery wound complications

Ozaki CK, Hamdan AD, Barshes NR, et al (Brigham and Women's Hosp, Boston, MA; Beth Israel Deaconess Med Ctr, Boston, MA; Baylor College of Medicine, Houston, TX)

J Vasc Surg 61:419-427, 2015

Objective.—Wound complications negatively affect outcomes of lower extremity arterial reconstruction. By way of an investigator initiated clinical trial, we tested the hypothesis that a silver-eluting alginate topical surgical dressing would lower wound complication rates in patients undergoing open arterial procedures in the lower extremity.

Methods.—The study block-randomized 500 patients at three institutions to standard gauze or silver alginate dressings placed over incisions after leg arterial surgery. This original operating room dressing remained until gross soiling, clinical need to remove, or postoperative day 3, whichever was first. Subsequent care was at the provider's discretion. The primary end point was 30-day wound complication incidence generally based on National Surgical Quality Improvement Program guidelines. Demographic, clinical, quality of life, and economic end points were also collected. Wound closure was at the surgeon's discretion.

Results.—Participants (72% male) were 84% white, 45% were diabetic, 41% had critical limb ischemia, and 32% had claudication (with aneurysm, bypass revision, other). The overall 30-day wound complication incidence was 30%, with superficial surgical site infection as the most common. In intent-to-treat analysis, silver alginate had no effect on wound complications. Multivariable analysis showed that Coumadin (Bristol-Myers Squibb, Princeton, NJ; odds ratio [OR], 1.72; 95% confidence interval [CI], 1.03-2.87; $P = .03$), higher body mass index (OR, 1.05; 95% CI, 1.01-1.09; $P = .01$), and the use of no conduit/material (OR, 0.12; 95% CI, 0.82-3.59; $P < .001$) were independently associated with wound complications.

Conclusions.—The incidence of wound complications remains high in contemporary open lower extremity arterial surgery. Under the study conditions, a silver-eluting alginate dressing showed no effect on the incidence of wound complications.

▶ Previous reports have suggested that silver-eluting dressings have significant antibacterial effects not only for burn victims but also for others suffering open wounds. This prospective, randomized trial was conducted in 3 major hospitals and accrued 500 patients comparing a silver alginate dressing with a control dressing after open incisions for vascular reconstruction of the lower extremities. No significant differences were noted between the groups in terms of wound infections and other complications. There was a significant association of complications with patient body mass index, use of Coumadin, and use of no conduit or material. The dressing was left in place for only a maximum of 3 days, presumably because after that point, there was sealing of the wound. These results suggest that patient phenotype, medications, and the operation itself play a more major role in wound complications compared with an antibacterial dressing.

J. M. Daly, MD

A novel immune competent murine hypertrophic scar contracture model: A tool to elucidate disease mechanism and develop new therapies
Ibrahim MM, Bond J, Bergeron A, et al (Duke Univ, Durham)
Wound Repair Regen 22:755-764, 2014

Hypertrophic scar (HSc) contraction following burn injury causes contractures. Contractures are painful and disfiguring. Current therapies are marginally effective. To study pathogenesis and develop new therapies, a murine model is needed. We have created a validated immune-competent murine HSc model. A third-degree burn was created on dorsum of C57BL/6 mice. Three days postburn, tissue was excised and grafted with ear skin. Graft contraction was analyzed and tissue harvested on different time points. Outcomes were compared with human condition to validate the model. To confirm graft survival, green fluorescent protein (GFP) mice were used, and histologic analysis was performed to differentiate between ear and back skin. Role of panniculus carnosus in contraction was analyzed. Cellularity was assessed with 4',6-diamidino-2-phenylindole. Collagen maturation was assessed with Picrosirius red. Mast cells were stained with Toluidine blue. Macrophages were detected with F4/80 immune. Vascularity was assessed with CD31 immune. RNA for contractile proteins was detected by quantitative real-time polymerase chain reaction (qRT-PCR). Elastic moduli of skin and scar tissue were analyzed using a microstrain analyzer. Grafts contracted to ~45% of their original size by day 14 and maintained their size. Grafting of GFP mouse skin onto wild-type mice, and analysis of dermal thickness and hair follicle density, confirmed graft survival. Interestingly, hair follicles disappeared after grafting and regenerated in ear skin configuration by day 30. Radiological analysis revealed that panniculus carnosus doesn't contribute to contraction. Microscopic analyses showed that grafts show increase in cellularity. Granulation tissue formed after day 3. Collagen analysis revealed increases in collagen maturation over time. CD31 stain revealed increased vascularity. Macrophages and mast cells were increased. qRT-PCR showed up-regulation of transforming growth factor beta, alpha smooth muscle actin, and rho-associated protein kinase 2 in HSc. Tensile testing revealed that human skin and scar tissues are tougher than mouse skin and scar tissues (Table 1).

▶ Hypertrophic burn scars remain a formidable clinical problem for which no effective therapy has yet been developed. Despite the significance of hypertrophic scar contractures, preclinical investigations into the pathogenesis of hypertrophic scar contraction and development of new therapies to prevent hypertrophic scar contraction are lacking. One of the major hurdles to developing an effective hypertrophic scar therapy is the lack of an animal model that

TABLE 1.—Characteristics of Human and Murine Hypertrophic Scars

Parameter		Human HSc	Murine HSc
Initial injury	Burn	Third-degree burn	Third-degree burn
Management	Surgical	Excision and skin graft	Excision and skin graft
Gross appearance	Scar contraction	Increased	Increased
Matrix	Collagen maturation/type I	Increased	Increased
Cellularity	Vascularity	Increased	Increased
	Macrophage density	Increased	Increased
	Mast cell density	Increased	Increased
	Proliferation	Increased	Increased
Cytokines	TGF-β	Increased	Increased
Cytoskeletal changes	ASMA	Increased	Increased
	NMMIIA	Increased	Increased
	ROCK2	Increased	Increased
Elasticity	Elastic modulus	Increased compared with uninjured human skin	Increased compared with uninjured mouse skin

ASMA, alpha smooth muscle actin; HSc, hypertrophic scar contraction; NMMIIA, nonmuscle myosin II A; ROCK2, rho-associated protein kinase; TGF-β, transforming growth factor beta.

Reprinted from Ibrahim MM, Bond J, Bergeron A, et al. A novel immune competent murine hypertrophic scar contracture model: A tool to elucidate disease mechanism and develop new therapies. *Wound Repair Regen.* 2014;22:755-764, with permission from Wound Repair and Regeneration and John Wiley and Sons, www.interscience.wiley.com.

mimics the human skin scarring response, particularly an immune-competent murine model. Human hypertrophic scar has typically been studied in immune-compromised mouse models, which have their limitations. Although this murine hypertrophic model shares many characteristics with the human condition as evidenced in Table 1, there are still some differences between mice and human hypertrophic scar lacking in this model. According to the authors, this model does not use a true split-thickness skin graft because harvesting of mouse skin with a dermatome is unreliable. Additionally, the scars observed in this model were initially flat and red, eventually becoming pale. Hypertrophic scar in humans are classically described as red, raised, and itchy. This may be due to a diminished level of mechanical tension in the murine skin graft bed. Despite these limitations, this novel model of hypertrophic burn scar will likely facilitate preclinical screening of new interventions aimed at reducing the hypertrophic scarring response.

D. W. Mozingo, MD

A systematic review of the management and outcome of toxic epidermal necrolysis treated in burns centres

Mahar PD, Wasiak J, Hii B, et al (The Alfred Hosp, Melbourne, Victoria, Australia; et al)
Burns 40:1245-1254, 2014

Introduction.—Toxic epidermal necrolysis (TEN) is a rare condition characterised by mucocutaneous exfoliation of greater than 30% total body surface area (%TBSA), increasingly being treated in burns centres.

The rate of mortality varies significantly in the literature, with recent prospective studies in non-burns centres reporting percentage mortality of approximately 45%. We undertook a systematic review of published studies that included TEN patients treated specifically in burns centres to determine a cumulative mortality rate.

Methods.—Electronic searches of MEDLINE, EMBASE and The Cochrane Library (Issue 4, 2010) databases from 1966 onwards were used to identify English articles related to the treatment of TEN in burns centres.

Results.—The systematic literature search identified 20 studies which specifically described patients with TEN grater than 30% %TBSA. Treatment regimens varied amongst studies, as did mortality. The overall percentage mortality of the combined populations was 30%. Risk factors commonly described as associated with mortality included age, %TBSA and delay to definitive treatment.

Conclusion.—The review highlights the variation between principles of treatment and mor-tality amongst burns centres. It offers a standard that burns centre can use to internationally compare their mortality rates. The review supports the ongoing reporting of outcomes in TEN patients with epidermal detachment greater than 30%.

▶ Toxic epidermal necrolysis (TEN) is a rare condition characterized by areas of mucocutaneous exfoliation, usually as a result of an adverse drug reaction. It exists on the same spectrum of disease as Stevens-Johnson syndrome (SJS), with the 2 conditions differing based primarily on the degree of total body surface area (%TBSA) involved. The extensive degree of epidermal loss that occurs during the disease progression has led to TEN being described as a burnlike condition, despite there being significant differences in the etiology, pathophysiology, and outcomes associated with the 2 conditions. As such, a number of studies have suggested that management of TEN patients in burns centers may improve survival. One of the challenges when reviewing the mortality of TEN is the rarity of the disease and the difficulty in establishing an evidence base delineating a standard with respect to mortality as a measure of quality of care. Most reported case series tend to have small sample sizes, and the factors associated with mortality often differ substantially between studies. Also, to diagnose TEN accurately, patients must present with a minimum of 30% TBSA epidermal detachment. Many reported studies include patients with less than 30% TBSA in their data reporting and analyses; therefore, patients with a diagnosis of SJS (%TBSA <10%) and SJS/TEN overlap (%TBSA 10%–30%) are included. A recent multinational prospective study of 114 TEN patients with >30% epidermal detachment reported a 45 percent mortality.[1] This review was limited by a number of factors, perhaps the most significant being that patients treated outside of burns centers were not included in study selection. The authors made this decision only to use data from burn centers because multiple studies have reported a survival benefit from early referral to a burn center, and the search strategy was purposefully narrowed to this context assuming this paradigm to be correct. Even if this were not case, it may still be appropriate to transfer TEN patients to burns centers so that they can obtain experienced wound care and pain management.

D. W. Mozingo, MD

Reference

1. Auquier-Dunant A, Mockenhaupt M, Naldi L, et al. Correlations between clinical patterns and causes of erythema multiforme majus, Stevens-Johnson syndrome, and toxic epidermal necrolysis: results of an international prospective study. *Arch Dermatol.* 2002;138:1019-1024.

A clinician's guide to the treatment of foot burns occurring in diabetic patients
Jones LM, Coffey R, Khandelwal S, et al (The Ohio State Univ Wexner Med Ctr, Columbus)
Burns 40:1696-1701, 2014

Introduction.—Diabetes mellitus affects 25.8 million Americans and is predicted to almost double by 2050. The presence of diabetes complicates hospital courses because of the microvascular complications associated with disease progression. Patients with diabetes represent 18.3% of annual burn admissions to our unit and 27% have burns to the feet. The purpose of this project was to develop an evidence-based guideline for care of the patient with diabetes and foot burns.

Methods.—A multidisciplinary group was charged with developing an evidence-based guideline for the treatment of foot burns in patients with diabetes. Evidence was evaluated in the areas of diabetes, burn care, hyperbaric medicine, care of diabetic foot wounds and physical therapy. After guideline development and approval, key aspects were incorporated into order sets.

Results.—Key aspects of this guideline are the ability to identify patients with undiagnosed diabetes, assess diabetic control, optimize glycemic and metabolic control, optimize burn wound management, treat microvascular disease, and provide education and a discharge plan. Evaluated outcomes are glycemic control, length of stay, complication rates, amputation rates, infection rates and the use of hyperbaric oxygen.

Conclusions.—Best outcomes for this high risk population will be attainable with an evidence based guideline.

▶ In this selection, a multidisciplinary group of physicians, nurses, and allied health personnel from The Ohio State University Wexner Medical Center were assembled and charged with the task of producing an evidence-based guideline for the treatment of burns of the feet occurring in patients with diabetes. The published literature lacks studies specific to burns of the feet of patients with diabetes. Problems encountered in healing burns on the feet of patients with diabetes are caused by the same process as that causing diabetic foot ulcers—namely, tissue hypoxia due to small vessel disease, leading to both neuropathy and poor wound healing. The authors of this guideline apply the diabetic foot ulcer treatment recommendations to the management of diabetic foot burns because of this common pathology. The publication contains the guideline explaining the management of foot burns occurring in patients with diabetes. Burn patients with diabetes comprise 18.3% of their institution's acute burn admissions. Using this systematic evidence-based approach will likely improve care for these patients, including managing glycemic control, optimizing wound care, decreasing the length of stay, ensuring follow-up diabetes treatment, and decreasing amputation rates. Research to evaluate the outcomes associated with the use of this evidence-based guideline would be applicable to other burn centers to improve the care of burn patients with diabetes and burns of the feet.

D. W. Mozingo, MD

A pilot review of gradual versus goal re-initiation of enteral nutrition after burn surgery in the hemodynamically stable patient
Shields BA, Brown JN, Aden JK, et al (San Antonio Military Med Ctr, Ft Sam Houston, TX; United States Army Inst of Surgical Res, Ft Sam Houston, TX)
Burns 40:1587-1592, 2014

Severe weight loss resulting from inadequate nutritional intake along with the hypermetabolism after thermal injury can result in impaired immune function and delayed wound healing. This observational study was conducted on adults admitted between October 2007 and April 2012 with at least 20% total body surface area burn requiring excision who previously tolerated gastric enteral nutrition at calorie goal and who returned from surgery hemodynamically stable (no new pressor requirement) and compared the effect of goal rate re-initiation versus slow re-initiation after the first excision and grafting. Demographic, intake, and tolerance data were collected during the 36 h following surgery and were analyzed with descriptive and comparative statistics. Data were collected on 14 subjects who met the inclusion criteria. Subjects in the goal rate re-initiation group ($n = 7$) met a significantly greater percentage of caloric goals ($99 \pm 12\%$ versus $58 \pm 21\%$, $p = 0.003$) during the 36 h following surgery than subjects in the slow re-initiation group ($n = 7$). There were no incidences of emesis, aspiration, or ischemic bowel in either group. The goal rate reinitiation group had a 29% incidence of either stool output >1 L ($n = 1$) or gastric residual volumes >500 mL ($n = 1$), whereas these were not present in the slow re-initiation group ($p = 0.462$). In conclusion, in this small pilot study, we found that enteral nutrition could be re-initiated after the first excision and grafting in those patients who previously tolerated gastric enteral nutrition meeting caloric goals who return from surgery hemodynamically stable without a significant difference in intolerance and with a significantly higher percentage of calorie goals achieved, but larger studies are required.

▶ Thermal injuries result in increased energy expenditure, catabolism, and loss of lean body mass. Basal metabolic rates may double, and severe weight loss resulting from inadequate nutritional intake along with this hypermetabolic, catabolic state can exacerbate the already impaired host defenses and delayed wound healing. Multiple studies have shown that early postburn feeding results in increased provision of protein and calories. Improved outcomes associated with adequate provision of nutrition include increased wound healing rates, decreased wasting, reduced length of stay, and reduced mortality. A retrospective review associated with the Glue Grant published in the *Journal of Burn Care and Research* in 2011 found that burn patients who had enteral nutrition initiated within 24 hours of admission had a shorter intensive care unit (ICU) length of stay (LOS) and decreased incidences of wound infections ($P = .030$ and $P = .010$).[1] In the subjects who achieved a caloric goal with enteral nutrition before the first surgery, the authors of this selection found significant differences in the caloric achievement in the goal rate re-initiation group compared to the slow re-initiation group. There were no negative clinical outcomes of emesis or aspiration or ischemic bowel in either group. There was no significant difference in ventilator days, ICU LOS, hospital LOS, or mortality. Future studies with larger sample sizes are needed with the prospective measurement of weight loss, preservation of lean body mass, and evaluation of wound healing. Further investigation of subsequent episodes of surgery other than the initial excision and grafting, other surgical procedures, and subjects who tolerated less than goal enteral nutrition would enhance the interpretation the results from this pilot study.

D. W. Mozingo, MD

Reference

1. Mosier MJ, Pham TN, Klein MB, et al. Early enteral nutrition in burns: compliance with guidelines and associated outcomes in a multicenter study. *J Burn Care Res.* 2011;32:104-109.

A simple method for the treatment of cicatricial ectropion and eyelid contraction in patients with periocular burn: Vertical V-Y advancement of the eyelid
Yeşiloğlu N, Şirinoğlu H, Sarıcı M, et al (Dr. Lütfi Kırdar Kartal Training and Res Hosp, Turkey)
Burns 40:1820-1821, 2014

Lagophthalmos is a critical problem in patients with severe periocular burn causing corneal exposure which may result in corneal ulcers and even loss of vision. Many surgical techniques were described to overcome this problem with different rates of success. This article presents a simple

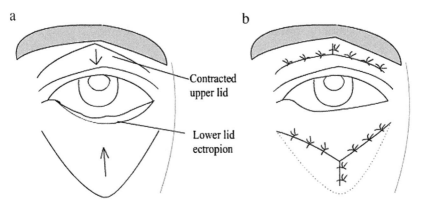

FIGURE 1.—The schematic appearance of the vertical V-Y advancement technique: (a) preoperative planning of the incisions and (b) the appearance of the V-Y advancement at the end of the operation. (Reprinted from Burns. Yeşiloğlu N, Şirinoğlu H, Sarıcı M, et al. A simple method for the treatment of cicatricial ectropion and eyelid contraction in patients with periocular burn: vertical V-Y advancement of the eyelid. *Burns.* 2014;40:1820-1821, Copyright 2014, with permission from International Society for Burn Injuries.)

but useful technique involving the V-Y advancement of the eyelid or eyelids in vertical direction for the prevention of cicatricial ectropion and eyelid contraction (Fig 1).

▶ Cicatricial ectropion and eyelid contracture seen in patients with severe periocular burns may cause lagophthalmos resulting in corneal exposure. Long-term corneal exposure may result in corneal ulcers and eventually loss of vision. The most commonly performed operation for the prevention of lagophthalmos is tarsorrhaphy in the acute setting. However, tarsorrhaphy is a morbid procedure with many long-term drawbacks and is also usually unsuccessful for the long-term prevention of cicatricial ectropion and eyelid contracture. Many surgical techniques have been described to overcome this problem with different rates of success. Releasing the contracture and closing the defect with a split- or full-thickness skin graft is usually successful in resolving the ectropion, but a good cosmetic result is often lacking. This article presents a simple but useful technique that involves one of the most basic plastic surgical maneuvers to solve this problem. The surgical technique is based on V-Y advancement of the contracted eyelid or if necessary both upper and lower eyelids and is included as Fig 1. After drawing the vertically oriented V-Y advancement flap or flaps and injection of local anesthetics, temporary sutures are placed to close the eyelids, which are helpful for determining the amount of advancement. The V-flap is harvested in musculocutaneous fashion by including the eyelid skin and the orbicularis oculi muscle to the flap and leaving the underlying orbital septum intact and advanced to the resultant defect until facilitating tension-free closure. This selection is included because it represents an alternative technique to the conventional skin graft correction of symptomatic ectropion caused by facial burns.

D. W. Mozingo, MD

Continuous wound infiltration with ropivacaine for analgesia after caesarean section: a randomised, placebo-controlled trial

Reinikainen M, Syväoja S, Hara K (North Karelia Central Hosp, Joensuu, Finland)
Acta Anaesthesiol Scand 58:973-979, 2014

Background.—We evaluated the analgesic effect of ropivacaine infiltration into the surgical wound after caesarean section.

Methods.—In a double-blind trial, 67 patients who were scheduled for caesarean section under spinal anaesthesia were randomly assigned to receive either 0.75% ropivacaine or placebo (NaCl 0.9%) through a multi-orifice catheter that was placed into the surgical wound, between the muscle fascia and the subcutaneous tissue. The study drug was administered as a bolus of 10 ml at the end of the operation, followed by an infusion at 2 ml/h for 48 h. All patients were also given paracetamol and ibuprofen. The primary outcome was the total amount of rescue oxycodone needed during the first 48 h post-operatively. Secondary outcomes included pain and patient satisfaction scores. Analyses were according to intention to treat.

Results.—The mean (± standard deviation) amount of oxycodone administered during the first 48 h was 47.5 ± 20.9 mg in the ropivacaine group and 57.8 ± 29.4 mg in the placebo group (95% confidence interval for the difference between means, −22.8−2.2 mg; $P = 0.10$). There were no differences between the groups in pain scores or in patient satisfaction scores.

Conclusion.—Continuous wound infiltration with ropivacaine did not decrease the need for opioids and had no impact on pain scores or patient satisfaction after caesarean section.

▶ The use of local wound instillation of Bupivicaine and other analgesics after surgery has had variable effects. Using Bupivicaine injected as a subcutaneous gel has resulted in significant benefit in terms of pain control. In this study, the wound catheter (above the fascia) instillation of the study drug (0.75% ropivacaine) was administered by continuous infusion at 2 mL/h during the first 48 hours after surgery. No major benefit was noted in terms of pain control, and no wound complications were different from those in the control group.

Certainly, the local instillation of analgesics is attractive as a means to control pain, particularly because there does not appear to be any difference in wound complications. But why are there such differences in study results? Are they due to dosage, placement of catheters (subfascial vs suprafascial spaces), duration of analgesic administration, or observer bias? Or is it simply that the differences in pain control are so small that variable results ensue under different conditions? Perhaps it is time for a large, multi-institutional study to lay the matter at rest.

J. M. Daly, MD

Commercially Available Topical Platelet-Derived Growth Factor as a Novel Agent to Accelerate Burn-Related Wound Healing

Travis TE, Mauskar NA, Mino MJ, et al (MedStar Washington Hosp Ctr, DC)
J Burn Care Res 35:e321-e329, 2014

The authors investigated whether the application of platelet-derived growth factor (PDGF) to donor site wounds would speed healing in a porcine model. In a red duroc pig model, three wounds that were 3 inches × 3 inches were created with a dermatome (0.06-inch depth) on one side of two different animals. These wounds were digitally and laser Doppler (LDI) imaged and biopsied immediately pre- and postwound creation and every 2 days for 2 weeks. A set of identical wounds were subsequently created on the opposite side of the same animals and treated with topical PDGF (becaplermin gel 0.01%, 4 g/wound) immediately on wounding. PDGF-treated wounds were imaged and biopsied as above. Digital images of wounds were assessed for epithelialization by clinicians using an ordinal scale. Perfusion units (PU) were evaluated by LDI. Wound healing was evaluated by hematoxylin and eosin histological visualization of an epithelium and intact basement membrane. First evidence of partial epithelialization was seen in control and PDGF-treated wounds within 7.7 ± 1.4 and 6.4 ± 1.1 days postwounding, respectively ($P = .03$). Completely epithelialized biopsies were seen in control and PDGF-treated wounds at 11.7 ± 2.6 and 9.6 ± 1.5 days, respectively ($P = .02$). Clinician evaluation of digital images showed that on day 9, control wounds were, on average, 48.3 ± 18.5% epithelialized vs 57.2 ± 20.2% epithelialized for PDGF-treated wounds. At day 16, control wounds showed an average of 72.9 ± 14.6% epithelialization and PDGF-treated wounds showed an average of 90 ± 11.8% epithelialization. Overall, PDGF-treated wounds had statistically significantly higher scores across all timepoints ($P = .02$). Average perfusion units as measured by LDI were similar for control and PDGF-treated wounds at time of excision (225 ± 81 and 257 ± 100, respectively). On day 2 postwounding, average PU for control wounds were 803 and were 764 for PDGF-treated wounds. Control wounds maintained higher PU values compared with PDGF-treated wounds at all time points and returned to excision PU values by day 12.2 ± 1.1 postwounding. PDGF-treated wounds reached the same values by day 9.7 ± 2.3 ($P = .03$). The authors conclude that topical PDGF speeds time to epithelialization of partial thickness wounds in a porcine model as evidenced by histology, clinical appearance, and time to return to prewounding vascularity.

▶ Many studies have attempted to use wound growth factors to heal wounds factor. Often, models such as radiated wounds and infected or ischemic wounds are used because control wounds heal very slowly. In most of the experiments, treated wounds heal faster and more completely. In patients with large, deep, second- and third-degree burns, it is important to be able to harvest their donor sites frequently to completely cover their wounds.

In this study, the use of a single application of platelet-derived growth factor (PDGF) improved the healing of experimental donor sites. As the authors noted "Prior researchers have postulated that PDGF does not actually alter the sequence of wound repair, rather it augments the amount and rate of the processes occurring. Perhaps the addition of exogenous PDGF just after injury is enough to ignite and accelerate the accessory cells and feedback loops that participate in synchrony with endogenous PDGF in wound healing."

It is interesting that greater differences in the 2 groups were noted at and beyond 7 days after treatment.

This type of approach certainly has merit and should be subjected to a proper clinical trial with safety and efficacy determinations.

J. M. Daly, MD

A phase II trial of a surgical protocol to decrease the incidence of wound complications in obese gynecologic oncology patients
Novetsky AP, Zighelboim I, Guntupalli SR, et al (Washington Univ School of Medicine and Siteman Cancer Ctr, St Louis, MO; St. Luke's Cancer Care Associates, Bethlehem, PA; Univ of Colorado, Denver; et al)
Gynecol Oncol 134:233-237, 2014

Objectives.—Obese women have a high incidence of wound separation after gynecologic surgery. We explored the effect of a prospective care pathway on the incidence of wound complications.

Methods.—Women with a body mass index (BMI) ≥ 30 kg/m^2 undergoing a gynecologic procedure by a gynecologic oncologist via a vertical abdominal incision were eligible. The surgical protocol required: skin and subcutaneous tissues to be incised using a scalpel or cutting electrocautery, fascial closure using #1 polydioxanone suture, placement of a 7 mm Jackson-Pratt drain below Camper's fascia, closure of Camper's fascia with 3-0 plain catgut suture and skin closure with staples.

Wound complication was defined as the presence of either a wound infection or any separation. Demographic and perioperative data were analyzed using contingency tables. Univariable and multivariable regression models were used to identify predictors of wound complications. Patients were compared using a multivariable model to a historical group of obese patients to assess the efficacy of the care pathway.

Results.—105 women were enrolled with a median BMI of 38.1. Overall, 39 (37%) had a wound complication. Women with a BMI of 30–39.9 kg/m^2 had a significantly lower risk of wound complication as compared to those with a BMI > 40 kg/m^2 (23% vs 59%, p < 0.001). After controlling for factors associated with wound complications the prospective care pathway was associated with a significantly decreased wound complication rate in women with BMI < 40 kg/m^2 (OR 0.40, 95% C.I.: 0.18–0.89).

Conclusion.—This surgical protocol leads to a decreased rate of wound complications among women with a BMI of 30–39.9 kg/m^2.

▶ The authors performed a phase II prospective trial using a clinical pathway protocol in an effort to reduce wound complications in obese women undergoing gynecologic procedures. They used historical controls from a study published in 2010 that evaluated preincisional skin preparation. They found that women with a body mass index (BMI) < 40 kg/m^2 had a lower rate of wound complication after treatment with our new surgical protocol compared with historical controls (23% vs 39%, $P = .038$). No benefit to the new surgical protocol was seen in women with BMI ≥40 kg/m^2 (59% vs 56%, $P = 0.76$).

It is important to realize that phase II studies primarily evaluate the role of a particular treatment for different disease states or situations to determine the most efficacious therapy in these states. For this study, the authors should conclude that there may be an improvement in wound complication rates using their protocol for women < 40 kg/m. However, because of the 4- to 6-year difference in the historical controls compared with the new experimental group, a prospective, randomized, controlled trial is necessary to compare their new protocol with standard treatment before solid conclusions can be determined.

J. M. Daly, MD

Effect of aerosolized fibrin sealant on hemostasis and wound healing after endoscopic sinus surgery: A prospective randomized study
Yu MS, Kang S-H, Kim B-H, et al (Konkuk Univ School of Medicine, Chungju, Korea)
Am J Rhinol Allergy 28:335-340, 2014

Background.—The purpose of this study was to investigate the effect of aerosolized fibrin sealant (FS) compared with that of polyvinyl acetal sponge packing on hemostasis and wound healing after functional endoscopic sinus surgery (FESS).

Methods.—We conducted a prospective randomized controlled trial of the use of aerosolized FS in 41 consecutive patients who underwent bilateral FESS between February 2011 and March 2012. The patients were randomized to receive FS applied via an aerosol spray in one nasal cavity and polyvinyl acetal sponge packing in the opposite cavity. The patients were followed up at 1, 2, 4, 8, and 12 weeks postoperatively. Crusting, adhesion, bleeding, granulation tissue formation, infection, and frontal sinus ostium stenosis after endoscopic surgery were assessed using a grading scale. Subjective symptoms related to nasal packing were evaluated using questionnaires quantified by visual analog scales.

Results.—The degree of granulation and crusting was significantly reduced in the side treated with FS compared with the polyvinyl acetal sponge side, as were bleeding and pain during nasal packing removal ($p < 0.05$). In addition, general satisfaction and willingness to reuse the material were significantly higher for the FS-treated side than for the polyvinyl acetal sponge-packed side ($p < 0.001$).

Conclusions.—Compared with polyvinyl acetal sponge, aerosolized FS shows beneficial effects on hemostasis and wound healing after FESS. The application of FS resulted in a high degree of patient satisfaction without additional morbidity.

▶ Functional endoscopic sinus surgery has become the standard therapy for patients with chronic sinusitis and nasal polyposis. However, the best method to obviate postoperative bleeding is unclear. In this prospective, randomized trial, fibrin sealant spray was compared with packing using 2 sides of the nose for comparison in the same patient. On the removal of the Merocel packing material, grade 1 bleeding was observed in 22 patients (53.6%), grade 2 bleeding was observed in 8 patients (19.5%), grade 3 bleeding was observed in 3 patients (7.3%), and no (grade 0) bleeding was observed in 8 patients (19.5%). In contrast, on the removal of fibrin sealant, no bleeding (grade 0) was observed in 18 patients (43.9%), grade 1 bleeding was observed in 16 patients (39.0%), grade 2 bleeding was observed in 5 patients (12.2%), and grade 3 bleeding requiring repacking was observed in 2 patients (4.8%). Pain felt during packing removal and nasal obstruction were significantly different between the 2 sides. Patients showed a significant preference for fibrin sealant compared with Merocel packing. The general satisfaction score for fibrin sealant was 8 compared with 2 for Merocel. Studies such as these are important because they answer real-world questions that have tremendous relevance to current day practice. Clearly, fibrin sealant is an improvement over Merocel packing after functional endoscopic sinus surgery.

J. M. Daly, MD

Bupivacaine-soaked absorbable gelatin sponges in caesarean section wounds: effect on postoperative pain, analgesic requirement and haemodynamic profile
Simavli S, Kaygusuz I, Kinay T, et al (Izzet Baysal State Hosp, Bolu, Turkey; Turgut Ozal Univ School of Medicine, Ankara, Turkey)
Int J Obstet Anesth 23:302-308, 2014

Background.—Pain is a common distressing adverse effect in the early postoperative period following caesarean section. The aim of this study was to investigate the effect on postoperative pain, analgesic requirement and haemodynamic profile of placing a suprafacial bupivacaine-soaked absorbable gelatin sponge in the caesarean section wound.

Methods.—A total of 164 healthy patients scheduled to undergo general anaesthesia for elective caesarean section were randomised to a study group ($n = 81$) or a control group ($n = 83$). In the study group, a bupivacaine-soaked absorbable gelatin sponge was placed subcutaneously in the caesarean section wound. Intramuscular diclofenac 75 mg was given to all patients at 8-h intervals during the first 24 h. Postoperatively, visual analogue scale pain scores, requirement for pethidine and diclofenac and changes in blood pressure and heart rate were compared between groups.

Results.—Pain scores were lower in the study group compared to the control group at all assessments ($P < 0.001$). During the first eight hours after surgery, fewer patients in the study group required rescue pethidine compared with the control group (4 vs. 33, $P < 0.001$). In the study group, total opioid and diclofenac consumption was lower ($P < 0.001$), and blood pressure and heart rate were lower ($P < 0.001$) compared to the control group.

Conclusion.—Suprafascial wound placement of a bupivacaine-soaked absorbable gelatin sponge improved postoperative analgesia and decreased opioid consumption following caesarean section.

▶ Pain control after surgery requires a multimodal approach, and no one method is ideal for all patients. In obstetrics practices, epidural analgesia is common, but as the authors noted, more than 90% of their patients do not wish spinal analgesia. It would be common to use patient-controlled analgesia, but again, in their hospital setting, it is not used for economic reasons. In that setting, bupivacaine injection into the wound seems ideal. The use of a sponge to absorb the bupivacaine presumably results in slower absorption and longer-lasting effects (but this remains to be proven). Mean pain scores were lower in the study group than the control group at all time points ($P < .001$). There were significant differences in group effect ($F = 1013.9$, $P < .001$), time effect ($F = 2.35$, $P < .001$), and the group by time interaction effect ($F = 194.4$, $P < .001$).

Cumulative analgesic consumption was lower in the study group compared with the control group.

The frequency of postoperative nausea, vomiting, antiemetic drug requirement, and sedation were lower in the study group compared with the control group at both 4 hours and 8 hours postoperatively ($P < .001$).

It is important to note that patients and nurses involved in data collection were blinded to group allocation. Thus, both patient and observer bias were eliminated.

This interesting study demonstrated the effectiveness of local anesthesia administered in a local wound sponge postoperatively to reduce pain and associated symptoms. It would be interesting to determine the effects of this approach alone or with minimal system analgesics in future studies.

J. M. Daly, MD

Trends in Bacterial Wound Isolates and Antimicrobial Susceptibility in a Pediatric Burn Hospital
DiMuzio EE, Healy DP, Durkee P, et al (Univ of Cincinnati, OH; Shriners Hosps for Children, Cincinnati, OH)
J Burn Care Res 35:e304-e311, 2014

The purpose of this retrospective study was to collate data dealing with organisms cultured from the burn patients and evaluate trends in antimicrobial susceptibility. All cultures collected from each acute admission patient between 2004 and 2011 in the 30-bed pediatric burn hospital were evaluated for their annual frequency and antimicrobial susceptibility. Duplicate cultures were excluded. *Staphylococcus aureus* was isolated most frequently (25% of total isolates; range, 69—408 isolates/yr), followed by *Pseudomonas aeruginosa* (13%; range, 40—202 isolates/yr), coagulase-negative staphylococci (9%; range, 2—188 isolates/yr), Enterobacter cloacae (8%; range, 22—128 isolates/yr), and *Escherichia coli* (6%; range, 19—91 isolates/yr). This rank order remained relatively consistent during the period of study. The emergence of methicillin-resistant *S. aureus* increased from 20% in 2004 to about 45% in 2009 to 2011. Susceptibility to vancomycin was still 100%. In comparing periods 2004 to 2007 and 2008 to 2011, *P. aeruginosa* showed increased susceptibility to cefepime (from 76% to 84%) and the aminoglycosides (from 68% to 81%), whereas susceptibility to piperacillin-tazobactam remained high (from 91% to 93%). *E. cloacae* demonstrated 90 to 100% susceptibility to aminoglycosides, cefepime, and imipenem. *E. coli* showed an increased rate of resistance to ceftazidime but was still susceptible to imipenem and amikacin. *S. aureus* and *P. aeruginosa* continue to be the most prevalent organisms cultured from our pediatric burn population. Almost half of the staphylococcal isolates were methicillin-resistant *S. aureus*. Despite widespread use of piperacillin-tazobactam, *P. aeruginosa* susceptibility remained high. Several classes of antimicrobials continued to demonstrate good to excellent activity against the majority of organisms cultured from the burn patients (Fig 2).

▶ Studying temporal changes in bacteria isolated from burn wounds and their susceptibility patterns can provide guidance for empiric antimicrobial therapy and monitor for the emergence of resistant organisms. The most convenient and widely available measure of organism susceptibility is the hospital antibiogram, which tabulates the proportion of organisms that are susceptible to an institution's formulary antibiotics during a given period. The purpose of this

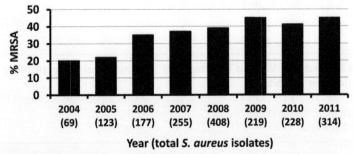

FIGURE 2.—Percentage of methicillin-resistant *Staphylococcus aureus* (MRSA) among total *S. aureus* isolates. (Reprinted from DiMuzio EE, Healy DP, Durkee P, et al. Trends in bacterial wound isolates and antimicrobial susceptibility in a pediatric burn hospital. *J Burn Care Res.* 2014;35:e304-e311, the American Burn Association.)

study was to collate and analyze data dealing with organisms cultured from our pediatric burn patients and evaluate trends in antimicrobial susceptibility using the institution's annual antibiogram during an 8-year period. This study confirms that there are significant shifts in microbial colonization and antibiotic sensitivities of burn wounds over time, with *Staphylococcus aureus* and *Pseudomonas aeruginosa* remaining the top pathogens. Fortunately, the incidence of methicillin-resistant *S. aureus* has remained steady during the last 4 years of the study despite an earlier increase in incidence as depicted in Fig 2. The patterns of antimicrobial resistance should be frequently reassessed by the institution to ensure that those factors affecting the proliferation of resistant organisms are controlled and that the most appropriate empiric drug regimen can be initiated.

D. W. Mozingo, MD

A New Marker of Sepsis Post Burn Injury?
Paratz JD, Lipman J, Boots RJ, et al (Univ of Queensland, Brisbane, Australia; et al)
Crit Care Med 42:2029-2036, 2014

Objectives.—Accurate diagnosis of sepsis is difficult in patients post burn due to the large inflammatory response produced by the major insult. We aimed to estimate the values of serum N-terminal pro-B-type natriuretic peptide and procalcitonin and the changes in hemodynamic variables as markers of sepsis in critically ill burn patients.

Design.—Prospective, observational study.

Setting.—A quaternary-level university-affiliated ICU.

Patients.—Fifty-four patients with burns to total body surface area of greater than or equal to 15%, intubated with no previous cardiovascular comorbidities, were enrolled.

Interventions.—At admission, a FloTrac/Vigileo system was attached and daily blood samples taken from the arterial catheter. Infection surveillance was carried out daily with patients classified as septic/nonseptic according to American Burns Consensus criteria.

Measurements and Main Results.—N-terminal pro-B-type natriuretic peptide, procalcitonin, and waveform analysis of changes in stroke volume index and systemic vascular resistance index were measured within the first 24 hours after burn and daily thereafter for the length of the ICU stay or until their first episode of sepsis. Prevalences of stroke volume variation less than 12% (normovolemia) with hypotension (systolic blood pressure <90 mm Hg) were recorded. Patients with sepsis differed significantly from "no sepsis" for N-terminal pro B-type natriuretic peptide, systemic vascular resistance index, and stroke volume index on days 3-7. Procalcitonin did not differ between sepsis and "no sepsis" except for day 3. Area under the receiver operating characteristic curves showed

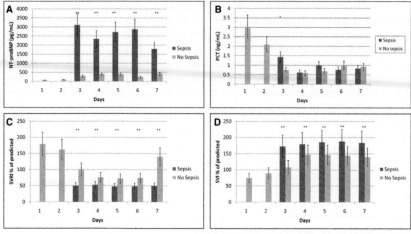

FIGURE 3.—N-terminal pro-B-type natriuretic peptide (NT-proBNP) % of predicted for days 1—7 (A), procalcitonin (PCT) over days 1—7 (B), systemic vascular resistance index (SVRI) % of predicted for days 1—7 (C), and stroke volume index (SVI) % of predicted for days 1—7 (D). Number of patients with sepsis (S) and those not reaching the criteria for sepsis (NS) differed each day, apart from days 1 and 2 on which no subjects had sepsis. Number of patients was as follows: day 1 (NS) $n = 54$, day 2 (NS) $n = 54$, day 3 (S) $n = 4$ and (NS) $n = 50$, day 4 (S) $n = 11$ and (NS) $n = 43$, day 5 (S) $n = 16$ and (NS) $n = 37$, day 6 (S) $n = 12$ and (NS) $n = 31$, and day 7 (S) $n = 5$ and (NS) $n = 28$. * indicates that on that particular day patients reaching sepsis criteria were significantly different from those not reaching sepsis criteria: $*p < 0.05$, $** p < 0.01$. (Reprinted from Paratz JD, Lipman J, Boots RJ, et al. A new marker of sepsis post burn injury? *Crit Care Med.* 2014;42:2029-2036, with permission from Society of Critical Care Medicine and Lippincott Williams & Wilkins.)

excellent discriminative power for B-type natriuretic peptide ($p = 0.001$; 95% CI, 0.99-1.00), systemic vascular resistance index ($p < 0.001$; 95% CI, 0.97-0.99), and stroke volume index ($p < 0.01$; 95% CI, 0.96-0.99) in predicting sepsis but not for procalcitonin (not significant; 95% CI, 0.29-0.46). A chi-square crosstab found that there was no relationship between hypotension with normovolemia (stroke volume variation <12%) and sepsis.

Conclusions.—Serum N-terminal pro-B-type natriuretic peptide levels and certain hemodynamic changes can be used as an early indicator of sepsis in patients with burn injury. Procalcitonin did not assist in the early diagnosis of sepsis (Fig 3).

▶ Despite an increased overall survival rate, severe infection remains the main cause of mortality in burn injury. Prompt antimicrobial therapy for septic shock shows a mortality benefit in general critical care patients; therefore, early diagnosis is important for beneficial outcomes. Diagnosing sepsis in burn patients has been associated with several difficulties. The hyperdynamic response to burn injury, elevated body temperature set point, and the severe systemic inflammatory response in thermally injured patients confound the diagnosis of sepsis in these patients. Early, accurate diagnosis of sepsis is vital in thermal injury both for a mortality advantage potentially achieved by timely initiation of empiric antibiotics and to decrease inappropriate antibiotic use, which increases the risk of antimicrobial resistance. The authors of this study found a high degree of both positive and negative predictive ability for B-type natriuretic peptide (BNP) and the hemodynamic values of stroke volume index (SVI) and systemic vascular resistance index (SVRI) but not for procalcitonin or hypotension with normovolemia. BNP is a well-known biomarker of cardiac failure, and high levels have been well documented and accepted to differentiate dyspnea in the emergency setting. However, increases in BNP have been well documented in other clinical conditions including sepsis. At first, this finding was attributed to cardiac failure in conjunction with sepsis and then later to the accompanying myocardial depression that occurs in 50% of patients with septic shock. It has also been found that high levels of BNP in sepsis are related to an alteration in the BNP clearance pathway. It can be seen in Fig 3 that BNP levels are highly predictive of the presence of sepsis in the burn patients studied by the authors of this selection. Limitations of this study included the fact that only the first episode of sepsis and the early stage of intensive care admission were recorded. Further work will be required to elucidate normal values for BNP and hemodynamics for the entire duration of the burn intensive care stay. Diagnosing sepsis in patients after burn injury remains a major problem, and this study indicates that the variables of N-terminal pro-B-type natriuretic peptide and the hemodynamic values of SVRI and SVI may assist in providing a high suspicion of sepsis prior to results of the blood culture. Further work is required to confirm these findings.

D. W. Mozingo, MD

Histomorphometric Analysis of Early Epithelialization and Dermal Changes in Mid—Partial-Thickness Burn Wounds in Humans Treated With Porcine Small Intestinal Submucosa and Silver-Containing Hydrofiber
Salgado RM, Bravo L, García M, et al (Instituto Nacional de Rehabilitación, Mexico City; Hosp Rubén Leñero, Mexico City; Hosp Darío Fernández Fierro, Mexico City; et al)
J Burn Care Res 35:e330-e337, 2014

The objective of this study was to determine the healing rates of mid—partial-thickness burns treated with a porcine intestinal submucosa (SIS) vs silver-containing cellulose hydrofiber (AgH) dressings. This was done by comparing healing response of burn wounds treated with SIS vs that of burns treated with AgH dressings. Five patients with mid—partial-thickness burns ≤10% of body surface were treated simultaneously, but in different areas, with SIS and AgH dressings; full-thickness biopsies were taken at days 0 and 7. Tissues treated with SIS presented higher epithelial maturation index (6.2 ± 0.84 vs 3.2 ± 3.28, [mean ± standard deviation], $P = .029$), better orientation and differentiation of epithelial cells, as well as an appropriate basal lamina structure, collagen deposition, and higher transforming growth factor—$\beta3$ expression (7.4 ± 8.1 vs

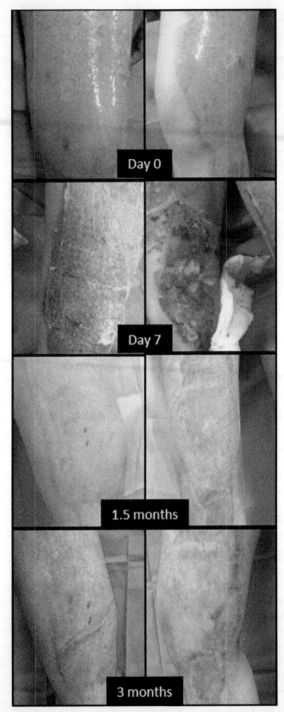

FIGURE 3.—Clinical photographs of patient treated with porcine intestinal submucosa (left-side panels) or silver-containing cellulose hydrofiber dressings (right-side panels). The lesion evolution observed with each treatment is shown from pretreatment, to 7 days, 1.5 months, and 3 months. Note that at 7 days the dressings were still adhered to most of wound. (Reprinted from Salgado RM, Bravo L, García M, et al. Histomorphometric analysis of early epithelialization and dermal changes in mid-partial-thickness burn wounds in humans treated with porcine small intestinal submucosa and silver-containing hydrofiber. *J Burn Care Res.* 2014;35:e330-e337, with permission from American Burn Association.)

2.1 ± 2.6; $P = .055$) than tissues treated with AgH dressings. Importantly, after the treatment SIS was not integrated in healed tissues. After 3 months of treatment, SIS produced a lower score according to Vancouver Scar Scale (3.6 ± 2.6 vs 7.2 ± 2.5, $P = .025$). The submucosa dressing does not simply act as scaffolding for the wound, it provides stimulation in the healing area, probably via growth factors initially present in SIS or matrikines derived from its digestion in the wound site. In conclusion, the present study demonstrated that biological matrices favor the wound-healing process (Fig 3).

▶ Vancouver Scar Scale analysis of the resulting scars showed that after 3 months the areas treated with small intestinal submucosa dressings differed significantly from the areas treated with silver-containing hydrofiber dressings. As shown in Fig 3, the cosmetic effect of each treatment group was different. The most important differences within the Vancouver Scar Scale score were observed in vascularity, pigmentation, and pliability. In this study, the authors found that, although in epithelialization was clinically evident in practically all patients after 7 days of treatment, there were differences in the rate of wound maturation and cosmetic appearance by the end of the study. Even with this small sample size, the results of this study suggest that biological and synthetic dressings evaluated can stimulate early epithelialization, although with varying degrees of effectiveness. The data presented here, related to the quality of epithelial repair, may lead to a therapeutic choice based not only on cost of the material but on the additional treatment benefits.

D. W. Mozingo, MD

A new, bioactive, antibacterial-eluting, composite graft for infection-free wound healing
Mittal A, Kumar N (Natl Inst of Pharmaceutical Education and Res (NIPER), SAS Nagar, India)
Wound Repair Regen 22:527-536, 2014

The current work focuses on the in vivo performance of a newly developed injectable composite graft in infected full-thickness wounds. The composite graft was composed of bioactive porous Poly dl-lactide-co-glycolide scaffolds, antibiotic gentamicin, and crosslinked gelatin as carrier gel. Treated infected wounds exhibited a faster wound closure, rapid weight gain, lower neutrophil count, higher breaking strength, and 100 times lesser microbial count (10^2 colony forming units/g in infected treated vs. 10^4 colony forming units/g in infected control group) in comparison with infected control group 28 days post treatment. During healing, collagen production was more in the treated groups at day 7 than controls and thereafter gradually reduced to normal levels. Histology revealed a mature scar tissue formation, fibroblast proliferation, epidermal resurfacing, and collagen deposition in reticular alignment similar to normal healthy skin in treated wounds. Further, the plasma concentration of gentamicin was 35–45 µg/mL during the initial 12 hours and reduced to 1 µg/mL in 24 hours, which indicated safe levels of the antibiotic drug during healing. These results clearly indicate a faster, infection-free, and safe after treatment with the developed graft.

▶ The use of biomaterials in full-thickness wounds has proliferated as new materials become available to act as a matrix for the healing wound. Most of the developed materials are used in noninfected wounds for many reasons. Thus, the patient with a chronically infected wound has great difficulty with healing. Because of this, the authors developed a composite graft in such a way that it could support wound healing by incorporating a bioactive scaffold material to support the cell proliferation/tissue formation along with an antibiotic drug to suppress the infection locally and for a prolonged period of time. They selected components such as cytomodulin functionalized porous poly dl-lactide-co-glycolide microspheres to be used as scaffold material. Gelatin was selected as a hydrogel-based carrier system to ensure that both the components—namely, bioactive scaffolds and antibiotic drug gentamicin—would remain at the wound site during the healing process. Being a hydrogel, it provides a moist environment and good fluid absorbance needed for wound healing. Gelatin is also biocompatible, completely bioresorbable, and nonimmunogenic. The authors noted significantly improved wound healing and wound closure, increased breaking strength, and lower microbial counts in the treated wounds compared with controls.

This is an important study because if reproduced in other animal models, it should undergo safety and then efficacy trials in humans with infected wounds.

J. M. Daly, MD

Effect of Wound Classification on Risk Adjustment in American College of Surgeons NSQIP
Ju MH, Cohen ME, Bilimoria KY, et al (American College of Surgeons; Chicago, IL)
J Am Coll Surg 219:371-381, 2014

Background.—Surgical wound classification has been used in risk-adjustment models. However, it can be subjective and could potentially improperly bias hospital quality comparisons. The objective is to examine the effect of wound classification on hospital performance risk-adjustment models.

Study Design.—Retrospective review of the 2011 American College of Surgeons NSQIP database was conducted for the following wound classification categories: clean, clean-contaminated, contaminated, and dirty-infected. To assess the influence of wound classification on risk adjustment, 2 models were developed for all outcomes: 1 including and 1 excluding wound classification. For each model, hospital postoperative complications were estimated using hierarchical multivariable regression methods. Absolute changes in hospital rank, correlations of odds ratios, and outlier status agreement between models were examined.

Results.—Of the 442,149 cases performed in 315 hospitals: 53.6% were classified as clean; 34.2% as clean-contaminated; 6.7% as contaminated; and 5.5% as dirty-infected. The surgical site infection rate was highest in dirty-infected (8.5%) and lowest in clean (1.8%) cases. For overall surgical site infection, the absolute change in risk-adjusted hospital performance rank between models, including vs excluding wound classification, was minimal (mean 4.5 of 315 positions). The correlations between odds ratios of the 2 performance models were nearly perfect ($R = 0.9976$, $p < 0.0001$), and outlier status agreement was excellent ($\kappa = 0.95$ss08, $p < 0.0001$). Similar findings were observed in models of subgroups of surgical site infections and other postoperative outcomes.

Conclusions.—In circumstances where alternate information is available for risk adjustment, there appear to be minimal differences in performance models that include vs exclude wound classification. Therefore, the American College of Surgeons NSQIP is critically evaluating the continued use of wound classification in hospital performance risk-adjustment models.

▶ Wound classification systems have been used as a predictor of surgical site infection (SSI; superficial or deep) for many years. However, more recent data sets such as National Surgical Quality Improvement Program (NSQIP) use so many variables that entry of wound classification may not be critical for risk adjustment. The authors examined more than 400 000 patients, and their procedures with wound classifications characterized as clean to dirty-infected. Overall, the incidence of any SSI (superficial incisional, deep incisional, or organ space) was 3.4%, with 1.9% as superficial incisional SSI, 0.6% as deep incisional SSI, and 1.1% as organ space SSI (as a case can have 2 types of SSI: superficial and organ space, or deep and organ space, but not superficial and deep). The rate of any SSI was highest among cases that had wound classification of dirty-infected (8.5%) and lowest in cases that were clean (1.8%). Interestingly, the use of wound classification did not add to the specificity of the risk adjustment model for NSQIP. However, I believe that within a hospital, it is still of value for the surgeon to classify the wound according to Centers for Disease Control and Prevention guidelines when describing a wound at the time of surgery to predict, in general, the risk of subsequent infection and the need for ancillary procedures, such as wound closure techniques or open wound techniques to ameliorate wound infections postoperatively.

J. M. Daly, MD

Impact of a novel, antimicrobial dressing on in vivo, *Pseudomonas aeruginosa* wound biofilm: Quantitative comparative analysis using a rabbit ear model

Seth AK, Zhong A, Nguyen KT, et al (Northwestern Univ, Chicago, IL; et al)
Wound Repair Regen 22:712-719, 2014

The importance of bacterial biofilms to chronic wound pathogenesis is well established. Different treatment modalities, including topical dressings, have yet to show consistent efficacy against wound biofilm. This study evaluates the impact of a novel, antimicrobial Test Dressing on *Pseudomonas aeruginosa* biofilm-infected wounds. Six-mm dermal punch wounds in rabbit ears were inoculated with 10^6 colony-forming units of *P. aeruginosa*. Biofilm was established in vivo using our published model. Dressing changes were performed every other day with either Active Control or Test Dressings. Treated and untreated wounds were harvested for several quantitative endpoints. Confirmatory studies were performed to measure treatment impact on in vitro *P. aeruginosa* and in vivo polybacterial wounds containing *P. aeruginosa* and *Staphylococcus aureus*. The Test Dressing consistently decreased *P. aeruginosa* bacterial counts, and improved wound healing relative to Inactive Vehicle and Active Control wounds ($p < 0.05$). In vitro bacterial counts were also significantly reduced following Test Dressing therapy ($p < 0.05$). Similarly, improvements in bacterial burden and wound healing were also achieved in polybacterial wounds ($p < 0.05$). This study represents the first quantifiable and consistent in vivo evidence of a topical antimicrobial dressing's impact against established wound biofilm. The development of clinically applicable therapies against biofilm such as this is critical to improving chronic wound care.

▶ This interesting article investigates the concept of bacterial boils that protect certain bacteria against antimicrobials and result in chronically infected wounds difficult to heal. In this experimental study, wounds were subject to 1 of 3 dressings: Telfa AMD was designated as the active control dressing. This dressing allows for consistent formation of intact and viable *Pseudomonas aeruginosa* wound biofilm, thus representing an appropriate control. The product AQUACEL Hydrofiber was used as the inactive vehicle dressing, representing a nonwoven gauze pad often used for dressing changes in the clinical setting. The inactive vehicle dressing also serves as the base dressing for the novel, antimicrobial dressing, AQUACEL Ag + Technology Hydrofiber or "Test Dressing," used in this study. This dressing is impregnated with 3 compounds, ionic silver, ethylenediaminetetra-acetic acid, and benzethonium chloride, which in combination function to clear wound biofilm. Ionic silver is known as an effective antimicrobial that functions to kill viable bacteria. The results showed that the experimental dressing dramatically reduced bacterial counts and improved the rate of wound healing.

If the safety and efficacy of this type of dressing could be proven in humans, it would be a major boon to help heal chronic wounds such as chronic venous ulcers, decubiti, and open, infected wounds. Further study in other animal models is warranted before bring to Phase I trails in humans.

J. M. Daly, MD

Do silver-based wound dressings reduce pain? A prospective study and review of the literature
Abboud EC, Legare TB, Settle JC, et al (Morsani College of Medicine, Tampa, FL; LLC, Mount Pleasant, SC)
Burns 40:s40-s47, 2014

Silver-containing dressings are a mainstay in the management of burn injury and acute and chronic wounds. In addition to antimicrobial activity, there is anecdotal evidence that silver dressings may modulate or reduce wound pain. Pain is subjective and difficult to quantify, and most studies of silver-containing dressings evaluate pain as a secondary rather than a primary outcome. Nevertheless, a dressing with a proven ability to reduce pain independent of systemic analgesics would have great utility.

In this study, we compared patient-reported pain levels in patients previously randomized to receiving silver-nylon dressings vs. conventional gauze dressings in a study of surgical site infection. Compared to gauze dressings, patients in the silver dressing group reported less pain between postoperative days 0 and 9 ($p < 0.02$). Post hoc analysis of analgesic use did not reach statistical significance between the groups. The study was completed with a literature review of the effect of silver on pain.

Silver-based dressings may reduce wound pain by providing an occlusive barrier or by other as-yet undefined mechanisms. The role of silver in pain relief, however, cannot be definitively stated until well-designed prospective randomized studies evaluating pain as a primary endpoint are carried out.

▶ Postoperative pain is a major issue for patients, affecting their recovery. In burn patients, silver-impregnated dressings are used for anti-infective properties, but there is also evidence to suggest that they diminish pain after burn injury compared with other dressing types. The authors sought to evaluate the use of silver-impregnated dressings in patients undergoing open abdominal colectomy and skin closure in a prospective study. They have previously reported the effects of these silver-impregnated dressings on wound infections. One hundred and ten patients were included in the final randomization. In the group of patients receiving the silver-nylon dressing, there was a statistically significant decrease in the self-reported pain scores from postoperative days 0 to 9. This reduction in self-reported pain was independent of surgical site infection status. The mean pain scores in the silver-nylon group continued to show a trend of decreased pain beyond postoperative day 9. There was little difference in opioid use between groups.

This is an interesting approach to evaluate pain control in a specific group of surgical patients and deserves further evaluation in other subsets of patients.

J. M. Daly, MD

Airborne bacterial dispersal during and after dressing and bed changes on burns patients

Bache SE, Maclean M, Gettinby G, et al (Glasgow Royal Infirmary, UK; Univ of Strathclyde, Glasgow, UK)
Burns 41:39-48, 2015

Background.—It is acknowledged that activities such as dressing changes and bed sheet changes are high-risk events; creating surges in levels of airborne bacteria. Burns patients are particularly high dispersers of pathogens; due to their large, often contaminated, wound areas. Prevention of nosocomial cross-contamination is therefore one of the major challenges faced by the burns team. In order to assess the contribution of airborne spread of bacteria, air samples were taken repeatedly throughout and following these events, to quantify levels of airborne bacteria.

Methods.—Air samples were taken at 3-min intervals before, during and after a dressing and bed change on a burns patient using a sieve impaction method. Following incubation, bacterial colonies were enumerated to calculate bacterial colony forming units per m^3 (cfu/m^3) at each time point. Statistical analysis was performed, whereby the period before the high-risk event took place acted as a control period. The periods during and after the dressing and bed sheet changes were examined for significant differences in airborne bacterial levels relative to the control period. The study was carried out four times, on three patients with burns between 35% total burn surface area (TBSA) and 51% TBSA.

Results.—There were significant increases in airborne bacteria levels, regardless of whether the dressing change or bed sheet change took place first. Of particular note, is the finding that significantly high levels (up to 2614 cfu/m^3) of airborne bacteria were shown to persist for up to approximately 1 h after these activities ended.

Discussion.—This is the most accurate picture to date of the rapidly changing levels of airborne bacteria within the room of a burns patient undergoing a dressing change and bed change. The novel demonstration of a significant increase in the airborne bacterial load during these events has implications for infection control on burns units. Furthermore, as these increased levels remained for approximately 1 h afterwards, persons entering the room both during and after such events may act as vectors of transmission of infection. It is suggested that appropriate personal protective equipment should be worn by anyone entering the room, and that rooms should be quarantined for a period of time following these events.

▶ Patients suffering from major burns are hypermetabolic because of their injury, and this increase in metabolic rate persists until the wound is covered.

Wound infection leads to significant sepsis, nonhealing of the burn wound, and death. Cross-contamination of burn patients as well as the spread of dangerous bacterial infections can lead to devastating events in an intensive care unit. The authors designed these studies for only a few patients, so the patients acted as their own controls. A minimal activity period at the start of each study established "control" airborne bacterial counts for the patient in that room at that time in his or her burn treatment. These baseline airborne bacterial levels were seen to significantly increase during dressing and bed sheet changes, regardless of which took place first. Furthermore, the effects lasted for approximately 45 to 60 minutes after the dressing and bed change was completed.

The importance of these studies in that hospital caregivers should continue to wear protective clothing for an hour after changing the patients' dressings or their beds. Typically, this is not done, and the yellow paper gowns are removed as soon as the dressing or sheet change is completed. In addition, because the airborne bacterial counts remain significantly raised for a period of up to 1 hour or longer after a dressing change, this cleaning should be delayed until the maximum number of bacteria has precipitated onto surfaces. This may be regarded as a high-risk time, during which anyone entering the room should wear adequate personal protective equipment.

J. M. Daly, MD

Airborne bacterial dispersal during and after dressing and bed changes on burns patients
Bache SE, Maclean M, Gettinby G, et al (Glasgow Royal Infirmary, UK; Univ of Strathclyde, Glasgow, UK)
Burns 41:39-48, 2015

Background.—It is acknowledged that activities such as dressing changes and bed sheet changes are high-risk events; creating surges in levels of airborne bacteria. Burns patients are particularly high dispersers of pathogens; due to their large, often contaminated, wound areas. Prevention of nosocomial cross-contamination is therefore one of the major chal-lenges faced by the burns team. In order to assess the contribution of airborne spread of bacteria, air samples were taken repeatedly throughout and following these events, to quantify levels of airborne bacteria.

Methods.—Air samples were taken at 3-min intervals before, during and after a dressing and bed change on a burns patient using a sieve impaction method. Following incubation, bacterial colonies were enumerated to calculate bacterial colony forming units per m^3 (cfu/m^3) at each time point. Statistical analysis was performed, whereby the period before the high-risk event took place acted as a control period. The periods during and after the dressing and bed sheet changes were examined for significant differences in airborne bacterial levels relative to the control period. The study was carried out four times, on three patients with burns between 35% total burn surface area (TBSA) and 51% TBSA.

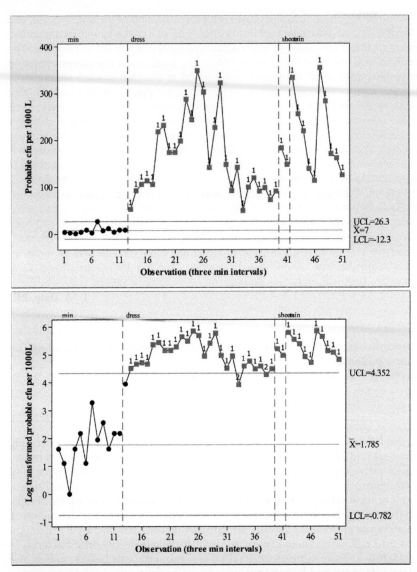

FIGURE 3.—Control Charts 3 (Minitab v16) based on raw data (top) and log-transformed data (bottom), demonstrating levels of airborne bacteria during events involving Patient C with 51%TBSA burns at an early point of care. Probable cfu per 1000 L (i.e. cfu/m^3) from air samples taken at 3 min intervals are given. The event has been divided into stages according to the activities taking place (min, minimal activity; dress, dressing change; sheet, bed sheet change). 'out of control' data points are flagged in red (online version only). They are marked with a number according to the failed test and appear as squares rather than circles (print version). (For interpretation of the references to color in this figure legend, the reader is referred to the web version of this article.) (Reprinted from Burns. Bache SE, Maclean M, Gettinby G. Airborne bacterial dispersal during and after dressing and bed changes on burns patients. *Burns.* 2015;41:39-48, Copyright 2015, with permission from International Society for Burn Injuries.)

Results.—There were significant increases in airborne bacteria levels, regardless of whether the dressing change or bed sheet change took place first. Of particular note, is the finding that significantly high levels (up to 2614 cfu/m^3) of airborne bacteria were shown to persist for up to approximately 1 h after these activities ended.

Discussion.—This is the most accurate picture to date of the rapidly changing levels of airborne bacteria within the room of a burns patient undergoing a dressing change and bed change. The novel demonstration of a significant increase in the airborne bacterial load during these events has implications for infection control on burns units. Furthermore, as these increased levels remained for approximately 1 h afterwards, persons entering the room both during and after such events may act as vectors of transmission of infection. It is suggested that appropriate personal protective equipment should be worn by anyone entering the room, and that rooms should be quarantined for a period of time following these events.

Conclusion.—Airborne bacteria significantly increase during dressing and sheet changes on moderate size burns, and remain elevated for up to an hour following their cessation (Fig 3).

▶ The primary modes of cross-contamination of pathogens between burn patients are believed to be direct and indirect contact either from the hospital environment and equipment or via health care providers. The contribution of the airborne route is less well defined. The authors of this selection studied 4 patients and quantified the dispersal of microorganisms during patient care activities. When a burn patient is at rest in bed, the dispersal of bacteria from their wounds is likely to be negligible. On the instigation of activity, however, a proliferation of bacteria are released into the air and onto surrounding surfaces, after traveling a distance of up to 2 meters. Certain events have been identified as high-risk periods of bacterial liberation. Bed sheet changes are 1 such event creating enhanced bacterial dispersion. This article has provided evidence of a substantial increase in the levels of airborne bacteria produced in the room of patients with moderate-size burns undergoing a dressing and bed sheet change. An example of 1 patient is included as Fig 3. The authors have created a detailed picture of the large surges and falls in bacteria suspended in the air that are produced during these events. It raises questions about whether the personal protective equipment worn by staff in the room should be increased. Finally, it highlights the length of time following a dressing and sheet change during which the airborne bacterial levels are still above baseline levels, suggesting a quarantine period may be observed in the room for up to an hour after the event takes place. These findings suggest that the airborne route of cross-contamination should not be ignored in the fight against nosocomial infection and further investigation is indicated.

D. W. Mozingo, MD

Efficacy of Silver-Loaded Nanofiber Dressings in *Candida albicans*–Contaminated Full-Skin Thickness Rat Burn Wounds

Ciloglu NS, Mert AI, Doğan Z, et al (Haydarpasa Numune Training and Research Hosp, Istanbul; Istanbul Technical Univ)
J Burn Care Res 35:e317-e320, 2014

In this experimental study, the effects of nanofiber dressings containing different forms of silver on full-thickness rat burn contaminated with *Candida albicans* was analyzed. A full-thickness skin burn was formed on a total of 32 Sprague-Dawley rats. After the burn wound was seeded with a 10^8 colony-forming units/ml standard strain of *Candida albicans* ATCC90028, the animals were divided into four groups. The effects of topical silver sulfadiazine and two recently designed nanofiber dressings containing nanosilver and silversulfadiazine as active materials were compared with the control group. There was a significant difference in the Candida growth on the burn eschar tissue among the groups. The difference for Candida growth in the burn eschar between the control group and the 1% silver sulfadiazine—containing nanofiber dressing group was statistically significant ($P < 0.01$). Silver sulfadiazine—containing nanofiber dressing was the most effective agent in the treatment of *Candida albicans*—contaminated burn wounds. Because of their regenerative potential, silver-loaded nanofiber dressings could be a good alternative for infected burn wounds.

▶ Burn wound colonization is ubiquitous and can lead to conversion of superficial second-degree burns ultimately to third-degree burns with attendant morbidity. Use of surface anti-infective agents such as silver nitrate and silver sulfadiazine has markedly reduced colonization and sepsis in burn patients. Newer technologies attempt to enhance the anti-infective properties of silver in unique ways. As the authors noted in their article, "nanofibers are used in the medical field as wound dressings and artificial vessels because of their high porosity, specific surface area, ability to mimic the extracellular matrix, effective use as a drug carrier, and ability to provide a convenient environment for cell proliferation and replication. Nanotechnology and the ability to deliver silver from a nanocrystalline structure markedly improve the biologic value of silver. There is a marked increase in surface area for water to react with silver in nanocrystalline form." Their experimental animal study used silver-impregnated nanofiber dressings and determined that they were much more effective against *Candida albicans* colonization of the burn eschar compared with controls. The safety and efficacy of these new compound dressings need to be tested in humans, for they may be useful in a wide variety of clinical situations.

J. M. Daly, MD

Laser Resurfacing and Remodeling of Hypertrophic Burn Scars: The Results of A Large, Prospective, Before-After Cohort Study, With Long-term Follow-up

Hultman CS, Friedstat JS, Edkins RE, et al (Univ of North Carolina Health Care System, Chapel Hill)

Ann Surg 260:519-532, 2014

Objectives.—Hypertrophic burn scars produce significant morbidity, including itching, pain, stiffness, and contracture, but best management practices remain unclear. We present the largest study to date that examines long-term impact of laser therapies, a potentially transformative technology, on scar remodeling.

Methods.—We conducted a prospective, before-after cohort study in burn patients with hypertrophic scars. Pulsed-dye laser was used for pruritus and erythema; fractional CO_2 laser was used for stiffness and abnormal texture. Outcomes included (1) Vancouver Scar Scale (VSS), which documents pigmentation, erythema, pliability, and height, and (2) University of North Carolina "4P" Scar Scale (UNC4P), which rates pain, pruritus, paresthesias, and pliability.

Results.—A total of 147 burn patients (mean age, 26.9 years; total body surface area, 16.1%) received 415 laser sessions (2.8 sessions/patient), 16 months (median) after injury, including pulsed dye laser (n = 327) and CO_2 (n = 139). Laser treatments produced rapid, significant, and lasting improvements in hypertrophic scar. Provider-rated VSS dropped from 10.43 [standard deviation (SD) 2.37] to 5.16 (SD 1.92), by the end of

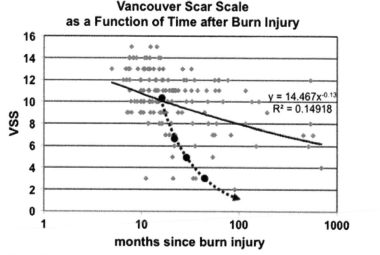

FIGURE 1.—Effect of laser treatment on VSS decay curve. (Reprinted from Hultman CS, Friedstat JS, Edkins RE, et al. Laser resurfacing and remodeling of hypertrophic burn scars: the results of a large, prospective, before-After cohort study, with long-term follow-up. *Ann Surg.* 2014;260:519-532, © 2014, Southeastern Surgical Congress.)

treatments, and subsequently decreased to 3.29 (SD 1.24), at a follow-up of 25 months. Patient-reported UNC4P fell from 5.40 (SD 2.54) to 2.05 (SD 1.67), after the first year, and further decreased to 1.74 (SD 1.72), by the end of the study period.

Conclusions.—For the first time, ever, in a large prospective study, laser therapies have been shown to dramatically improve both the signs and symptoms of hypertrophic burn scars, as measured by objective and subjective instruments. Laser treatment of burn scars represents a disruptive innovation that can yield results not previously possible and may displace traditional methods of operative intervention (Fig 1).

▶ Over the last 50 years, we have seen major advances in the resuscitation and rehabilitation of patients with thermal injury; however, reconstructive efforts are sometimes limited by the development and persistence of hypertrophic scar formation. Abnormal healing that results in hypertrophic scars may produce significant morbidity and impair quality of life because of intense pruritus, pain, stiffness, and contracture. Treatment of hypertrophic scars uses different approaches, depending on the severity of the scarring response. Usual management includes observation, massage, moisturizing agents, compression garments, silicone sheeting, steroid injection, and surgical excision. However, laser therapies have recently emerged as an attractive new modality to treat hypertrophic burn scars. Several publications have reported good short-term results, but none until now have provided long-term follow-up and comparison to the natural history of conventionally treated scars over time. Fig 1 from this selection is included, which depicts the decay over time in the Vancouver Scar Score with and without laser treatment. The authors concluded that laser- based and light-based therapies could be combined safely to treat hypertrophic burn scars, accelerate the maturation and remodeling of symptomatic burn scars, and improve quality of life.

D. W. Mozingo, MD

Ablative Fractional Photothermolysis for the Treatment of Hypertrophic Burn Scars in Adult and Pediatric Patients: A Single Surgeon's Experience
Khandelwal A, Yelvington M, Tang X, et al (MetroHealth Med Ctr, Cleveland, OH; Arkansas Children's Hosp Burn Ctr, Little Rock; Arkansas Children's Hosp Research Inst, Little Rock)
J Burn Care Res 35:455-463, 2014

Many patients develop hypertrophic scarring after a burn injury. Numerous treatment modalities have been described and are currently in practice. Photothermolysis or laser therapy has been recently described as an adjunct for management of hypertrophic burn scars. This study is a retrospective chart review of adult and pediatric patients undergoing fractional photothermolysis at a verified burn center examining treatment parameters as well as pre— and post—Vancouver Scar Scale scores. Forty-four patients underwent fractional photothermolysis during the

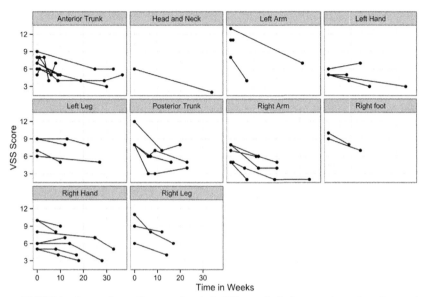

FIGURE 2.—Pre— and post—Vancouver Scar Scale (VSS) score by body area and over time. (Reprinted from Khandelwal A, Yelvington M, Tang X, et al. Ablative fractional photothermolysis for the treatment of hypertrophic burn scars in adult and pediatric patients: a single surgeon's experience. *J Burn Care Res.* 2014;35:455-463, with permission from American Burn Association.)

study period of 8 months. Mean pretreatment score was 7.6, and mean posttreatment score was 5.4. The mean decrease in score was 2.2, which was found to be statistically significant. There were no complications. Fractional photothermolysis is a safe and efficacious adjunct therapy for hypertrophic burn scars. Prospective trials would be beneficial to determine optimal therapeutic strategies (Fig 2).

▶ Despite timely intervention, many thermally injured patients have hypertrophic scarring (HTS). Numerous therapies have been used for the management of HTS, the most common being compression therapy, silicone or hydrogel sheeting, ultrasound scan, excision, and intralesional steroid injection. Photothermolysis or laser therapy has been used recently as an adjunct to traditional methods for the management of hypertrophic scars in burn patients, of which ablative fractional photothermolysis (FP) may be the most promising. This study evaluates an initial cohort of adult and pediatric patients treated with FP. Treatment strategies and subsequent pathways are presented. Relatively short-term follow-up is presented; however, a significant improvement occurred in the subjects treated as depicted in Fig 2. Laser therapy for hypertrophic burn scars is still in its infancy. Clinical and histologic studies need to be performed to assess the type of lasers that should be used, optimal treatment parameters, duration of treatment, and efficacy according to settings and body part treated. Multi-institutional studies to enroll appropriate patient volume and conduction of blinded studies should be entertained. In addition, novel methods for determining scar depth may help surgeons provide accurate treatment. The results of this study show that ablative FP is a safe and efficacious adjunct for the management of hypertrophic burn scars in adult and pediatric patients.

D. W. Mozingo, MD

Prophylactic synthetic mesh can be safely used to close emergency laparotomies, even in peritonitis
Argudo N, Pereira JA, Sancho JJ, et al (Hosp Universitari del Mar, Barcelona, Spain; et al)
Surgery 156:1238-1244, 2014

Background.—This study was conducted to determine the efficacy and safety of the use of a partially absorbable large pore synthetic prophylactic mesh in emergent midline laparotomies for the prevention of evisceration and incisional hernia.

Methods.—Retrospective analysis of all patients who underwent an emergency midline laparotomy between January of 2009 and July of 2010 was performed. Patients with complicated ventral hernia repair, postoperative death, and lack of follow-up were excluded.

Results.—A total of 266 patients were included. Laparotomies were closed with a running suture of slow reabsorbable material in 190 patients (Group S), and 50 patients within this group (26.3%) received additional retention sutures. In 76 patients (Group M), an additional partially absorbable lightweight mesh was placed in the Supra-aponeurotic space. Both groups presented similar complication rates (71.1% Group S vs 80.3% Group M, $P = .97$). There were no differences regarding surgical-site infection rates (17.9% Group S vs 26.3% Group M; $P = .13$) or postoperative mortality (13.7% Group S vs 18.3% Group M; $P = .346$). A total of 150 patients completed the follow-up (99 Group S; 51 Group M) at a mean time of 16.7 months. During follow-up, 36 cases of incisional hernia (24%) were diagnosed: 33 (33%) in Group S, whereas there were only three cases (5.9%) in Group M ($P = .0001$). Mesh removal for chronic infection was not required in any case.

Conclusion.—The use of a partially absorbable, lightweight large pore prophylactic mesh in the closure of emergency midline laparotomies is feasible for the prevention of incisional hernia without adding a substantial rate of morbidity to the procedure, even if high contamination or infections are present.

▶ There are multiple risk factors for incisional hernia after surgery, including smoking, comorbidities such as obesity, male sex, and previous abdominal surgery. Emergency midline operations are predisposing in the authors' experience. A correlation with the blood loss during operation and wound infection also has been found. In this retrospective study, the sutured alone patients, the linea alba was closed with a running suture of double loop number 1 polydioxanone. In some patients within this group, 3 or 4 retention sutures with polypropylene number 1 were added to prevent postoperative evisceration. In mesh patients, the same technique was performed with the addition of a partially absorbable lightweight large pore mesh. Of the 266 midline laparotomies performed during the study period, a prophylactic mesh was placed in 76 cases. In the remaining 190 patients, the midline closure consisted of a running suture in 140 cases (73.7%), with added reinforcement with retention sutures in 50 cases (26.3%).

Follow-up for 1 year was completed in 150 patients. Incisional hernia was identified in 36 patients (24%): 33 in the sutured group and only 3 in the mesh group. The subgroup treated with retaining sutures (n = 30) displayed the greatest incidence of incisional hernia among the series with 11 cases (36.7%). Most of the incisional hernias detected were clinically significant, and 15 (41.5%) required surgery.

This interesting study clearly requires an additional prospective, randomized trial. Different demographics occurred among groups. Some sutured patients had retention sutures presumably because the surgeon believed they were at higher risk for wound problems. In addition, follow-up was short, and longer-term follow-up (5 years) is necessary for definitive outcomes to be defined.

J. M. Daly, MD

Safety and efficacy of excision and direct closure in acute burns surgery: Outcome analysis in a prospective series of 100 patients and a survey of UK burns surgeons' attitudes
Bain CJ, Wang T, McArthur G, et al (Chelsea and Westminster NHS Foundation Trust, London, UK)
Burns 40:1635-1641, 2014

Many burns surgeons avoid excision and direct closure of acute burns owing to concerns over wound dehiscence, scarring and infection. There is no evidence in the literature to support this practice. We present outcomes of a prospective series of 100 patients who underwent excision and direct closure of 138 burns over a 2-year period, along with results from a survey sent to 33 senior burns surgeons to gauge attitudes towards direct closure in burns surgery. 47% of survey respondents never perform direct closure. Dehiscence was cited as the most common concern, followed by hypertrophic scarring (HTS). In our cohort, the superficial dehiscence rate was 12% and the HTS rate was 16%, with no scarring contractures. Patients with healing time greater than 14 days were more likely to develop HTS ($p = 0.008$), as were those with wound dehiscence ($p = 0.014$). Patients undergoing part-grafting in addition to direct closure took significantly longer to heal than those undergoing direct closure alone ($p = 0.0002$), with the donor site or graft delaying healing in the majority. Excision and direct closure of acute burn wounds avoids donor site morbidity and has an acceptable complication rate. It is a safe and effective treatment for full thickness burns in selected cases.

▶ There are many methods used to treat burn victims, including excision and direct closure, but little evidence documents the benefit of this approach. Data were collected prospectively on 138 consecutive excisions and direct closures of burn wounds in 100 patients between July 2010 and September 2012. Minor complications were recorded in 33 burns. There were 16 superficial dehiscences (12%), which were all managed successfully with dressings. Many of these wound problems were due to a reaction to buried suture material or extrusion of suture material. Healing was delayed in these cases, but all patients who attended follow-up had healed within 2 months.

The authors believe strongly in their techniques. It now remains for others to help them perform a prospective, randomized trial with adequate power to evaluate their hypothesis.

J. M. Daly, MD

Stress—Relaxation and Tension Relief System for Immediate Primary Closure of Large and Huge Soft Tissue Defects: An Old—New Concept: New Concept for Direct Closure of Large Defects
Topaz M, Carmel NN, Topaz G, et al (Hillel Yaffe Med Ctr, Hadera, Israel; Bar Ilan Univ, Ramat Gan, Israel; et al)
Medicine 93:e234, 2014

Stress—relaxation is a well-established mechanism for laboratory skin stretching, with limited clinical application in conventional suturing techniques due to the inherent, concomitant induction of ischemia, necrosis and subsequent suture failure. Skin defects that cannot be primarily closed are a common difficulty during reconstructive surgery. The TopClosure® tension-relief system (TRS) is a novel device for wound closure, providing secured attachment to the skin through a wide area of attachment, in an adjustable manner, enabling primary closure of medium to large skin defects.

The aim of this study was to evaluate the efficiency of the TopClosure® TRS as a substitute for skin grafting and flaps for primary closure of large soft tissue defects by stress—relaxation.

We present three demonstrative cases requiring resection of large to huge tumors customarily requiring closure by skin graft or flaps. TRS was applied during surgery serving as a tension-relief platform for tension sutures, to enable primary skin-defect closure by cycling of stress—relaxation, and following surgery as skin-secure system until complete wound closure.

All skin defects ranging from 7 to 26 cm in width were manipulated by the TRS through stress—relaxation, without undermining of skin, enabling primary skin closure and eliminating the need for skin grafts and flaps. Immediate wound closure ranged 26 to 135 min. TRS was applied for 3 to 4 weeks. Complications were minimal and donor site morbidity was eliminated. Surgical time, hospital stay and costs were reduced and wound aesthetics were improved.

In this case series we present a novel technology that enables the utilization of the viscoelastic properties of the skin to an extreme level, extending the limits of primary wound closure by the stress—relaxation principle. This is achieved via a simple device application that may aid immediate primary wound closure and downgrade the complexity of surgical procedures for a wide range of applications on a global scale.

▶ Closure of large skin defects is typically done using skin grafting with rotational or free flaps. However, it would be advantageous if it were possible to avoid these methods through other mechanical means. The system described by the authors in this article comprises 2 malleable polymer attachment plates (APs) that are fixed to the skin by adhesive or regular skin staples or sutures through a large area of adherence. The APs are placed a distance from the wound margins and are pulled together manually by an interconnecting flexible approximation strap for incremental advancement of wound edges through a lock/release ratchet mechanism.

The authors presented 3 cases in which the device was applied to close major skin defects with what appear to be good cosmetic results. Clearly, they should, after institutional review board approval, conduct Phase 2 and 3 trials to demonstrate effectiveness of this technique over other current, standard methods

J. M. Daly, MD

Management of Pediatric Skin-Graft Donor Sites: A Randomized Controlled Trial of Three Wound Care Products
Brenner M, Hilliard C, Peel G, et al (Univ College Dublin, Ireland; Our Lady's Children's Hosp, Crumlin, Ireland; et al)
J Burn Care Res 36:159-166, 2015

Skin grafts are used to treat many types of skin defects in children, including burns, traumatic wounds, and revision of scars. The objective of this prospective randomized controlled trial was to compare the effectiveness of three dressing types for pediatric donor sites: foam, hydrofiber, and calcium alginate. Children attending a pediatric Burns & Plastics Service from October 2010 to March 2013, who required a split-skin graft, were recruited to the trial. Patients were randomly assigned to the two experimental groups, foam or hydrofiber, and to the control group, calcium alginate. Data were gathered on the management of exudate, assessment of pain, time to healing, and infection. Fifty-seven children aged 1 to 16 years (mean – 4.9 years) were recruited to the trial. Fifty-six patients had evaluable data and one participant from the control group was lost to follow-up. Most children required skin grafting for a burn injury (78%). The median size of the donor site was 63.50 cm^2 (8—600 cm^2).

There was a statistically significant difference in time to healing across the three dressing groups (x^2 [2, n = 56] = 6.59, $P = .037$). The calcium alginate group recorded a lower median value of days to healing (median = 7.5 days) compared to the other two groups, which recorded median values of 8 days (hydrofiber) and 9.5 days (foam). The greatest leakage of exudate, regardless of dressing type, occurred on day 2 after grafting. No statistically significant difference was found in leakage of exudate, pain scores, or infection rates across the three groups. Calcium alginate emerged as the optimum dressing for pediatric donor site healing in this trial.

▶ The treatment of patients with major burn wounds is skin grafting, but in children, the management of donor sites is critically important. Many burn centers use a variety of donor-site dressings that help to accelerate healing, decrease wound exudate, and decrease pain. Exudate can be a major problem, and therefore the investigators performed a prospective, randomized trial to prospectively assess 3 donor-site dressings. Their results showed that when leakage was compared across each of the 3 dressing groups, 8 (42%) of the wounds dressed with Allevyn had a moderate to heavy amount of leakage, compared with 4 (21%) of wounds in the Aquacel group and 3 (16%) of the wounds in the Kaltostat group. The Kaltostat group had a faster time to healing (7.5 days), which was statistically significant when compared to Aquacel (8 days) and Allevyn (9.5 days). Time to healing was defined as the day on which epithelialization was achieved and a dressing was no longer required.

Studies such as these are useful; however, there were not huge differences among the groups, and clinically relevant differences may not have been apparent.

J. M. Daly, MD

Comparison of Barbed versus Conventional Sutures for Wound Closure of Radiologically Implanted Chest Ports

Ahmed O, Jilani D, Funaki B, et al (Univ of Chicago Medicine, IL; Wright State Univ Boonshoft School of Medicine, Dayton, OH)
J Vasc Interv Radiol 25:1433-1438, 2014

Purpose.—To retrospectively compare the incidences of complications with barbed suture versus conventional interrupted suture for incision closure in implantable chest ports.

Materials and Methods.—A total of 715 power-injectable dual-lumen chest ports placed between 2011 and 2013 were studied. Primary outcomes included wound dehiscence, local port infection, local infections treated by wound packing, early infections within 30 days, and total infections. A multivariate analysis of independent risk factors for port infection was also performed.

Results.—A total of 442 ports were closed with nonbarbed suture, versus 273 closed with barbed suture. Mean catheter-days in the traditional and barbed groups were 257.9 (range, 3—722) and 189.1 (range, 13—747), respectively ($P < .01$). The rate of dehiscence with traditional suture (1.6%; seven of 442) was significantly higher than that with barbed suture (zero of 273; $P = .04$). Percentage of total infections was also significantly higher with traditional suture (9.5% vs 5.1%; $P = .03$). No difference in rate of infection per 1,000 catheter-days was seen between traditional and barbed suture groups (0.0035 vs 0.0026; $P = .17$). The rate of local infection with traditional suture was significantly higher (2.7% vs 0.4%; $P = .02$). Additionally, multivariate analysis identified the use of traditional suture as the only independent risk factor for infection (39% vs 25%; $P = .03$).

Conclusions.—Barbed suture for incision closure in implantable dual-lumen chest ports was associated with lower rates of dehiscence and potentially lower rates of local infectious complications compared with traditional nonbarbed suture.

▶ There continues to be controversy regarding the best methods of skin closure that enhance healing, reduce infectious complications, and provide the maximum tensile strength over time. In this retrospective study, the authors sought to review the incidence of wound complications (infections) with 2 forms of suture closure. Using the barbed sutures, the percentage of total infections was significantly lower compared with the traditional suture group (9.5% vs 5.1%; $P < .03$). However, there was no difference in the rate of infection per 1000 catheter days in the traditional suture group versus the barbed suture group. The study had a large number of patients (> 700), and the methods of skin preparation, catheter insertion, and skin closure seemed to be the same during the study, but the retrospective nature of the trial certainly can introduce bias and provide "associations" but not definitive conclusions.

The authors should be commended for evaluation these new sutures but should also conduct a prospective, randomized trial to fully determine the efficacy of barbed sutures in this clinical situation.

J. M. Daly, MD

4 Critical Care

A Health System-Based Critical Care Program with a Novel Tele-ICU: Implementation, Cost, and Structure Details
Fortis S, Weinert C, Bushinski R, et al (Univ of Minnesota, Minneapolis)
J Am Coll Surg 219:676-683, 2014

Background.—Improving the efficiency of critical care service is needed as the shortfall of intensivists is increasing. Standardizing clinical practice, telemedicine, and organizing critical care service at a health system level improves outcomes. We developed a health system Critical Care Program based at an academic medical center. The main feature of our program is an intensivist who shares on-site and telemedicine clinical responsibilities. Tele-ICU facilitates the standardization of high-quality critical care across the system. A common electronic medical record made the communications among the ICUs feasible. Combining faculty from medical and surgical critical care divisions increased the productivity of intensivists.

Study Design.—We retrospectively reviewed the administrative database data from 2011 and 2012, including mean census, number of transfers, age, sex, case mix index, mortality, readmissions, and financial data.

Results.—The Critical Care program has 106 adult ICU beds; 54 of those beds can be managed remotely using tele-ICU based at the main University hospital. The mean midnight census of the system for 2012 was 69.44 and total patient-days were 34,406. The capital cost of the tele-ICU was $1,186,220. The annual operational cost is $1,250,112 or $23,150 per monitored ICU-bed. Unadjusted mortality was 6.5% before and 4.9% after implementation ($p < 0.0002$).

Conclusions.—We describe a novel health system level ICU program built using "off the shelf" technology based on a large University medical center and a tele-ICU with a full degree of treatment authority across the system.

▶ This study describes the development and operational details of a health care system-level intensive care unit (ICU) program patterned off the much larger Military Joint Theater Trauma System. This is 1 of few studies that provide details about the structure and the operation of ICUs at a health system level. The system-wide ICU program described in this selection led to standardization of some aspects of critical care in the system. Traditionally, decisions at a system level affect financial and organization issues and critical care service are organized at a unit level by the ICU directors. In this model, leadership participates in strategic decisions about the entire critical care service of the system. This kind of multidisciplinary approach to critical care is known to be beneficial at a hospital level. In addition, because all of the intensivists are in the same physician practice group and medical school, there is greater ability to adopt common critical care protocols and order sets, in turn decreasing unnecessary variation. Payment for professional work by the intensivist staff in their system is reimbursed only when provided directly at the bedside; therefore, the tele-ICU work is not reimbursed. Indirect financial benefits, such as improved efficiency outcomes from 24-hour intensivist availability and ability to keep ICU patients in their local hospital helps compensate for lack of reimbursement. The authors describe building a health system-level ICU program using "off-the-shelf" technology based at a university medical center and implementing a tele-ICU program with full treatment authority in all monitored ICUs. They describe the tele-ICU as the "eyes on the ground" for the system that facilitates the critical care program's efforts to standardize critical care practices across 7 ICUs. The tele-ICU business model is based on an intensivist who shares on-site and telemedicine clinical responsibilities, thereby subsidizing the operational cost to the remote ICUs. Combining the faculty clinical effort of academically distinct departments into 1 critical care program reduces nighttime work and creates new education and research opportunities.

D. W. Mozingo, MD

The Importance of the First Complication: Understanding Failure to Rescue after Emergent Surgery in the Elderly
Sheetz KH, Krell RW, Englesbe MJ, et al (Univ of Michigan, Ann Arbor)
J Am Coll Surg 219:365-370, 2014

Background.—Perioperative mortality in the elderly is high after emergency surgery and varies considerably among hospitals—an observation partially explained by differences in failure to rescue. We hypothesize that failure to rescue after certain types of complications underlies the disproportionately poor outcomes observed in elderly patients.

Study Design.—We identified 23,217 patients undergoing emergent general or vascular surgery procedures at 41 hospitals within the Michigan Surgical Quality Collaborative between 2007 and 2012. Patients' first complications were identified and categorized by type. We compared failure to rescue rates at the patient-level between patients younger than 75 and 75 years of age and older. We then compared failure to rescue rates after specific complications across hospitals grouped in tertiles by risk-adjusted 30-day mortality.

Results.—Risk-adjusted failure to rescue rates were significantly higher in the elderly after a first infectious (21.7% vs 10.3%; $p < 0.01$) or pulmonary (38.2% vs 20.4%; $p < 0.01$) complication when compared with younger patients. At the hospital level, high-mortality centers failed to rescue elderly patients more frequently than low-mortality centers after a first infectious (35.6% vs 22.2%; $p < 0.01$) and pulmonary (24.3 vs 14.3; $p < 0.01$) complication. Failure to rescue rates after cardiovascular

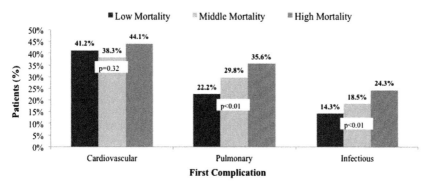

FIGURE 2.—Failure to rescue rates for elderly patients treated at low-, middle-, and high-mortality hospitals. Patients are stratified by the type of first documented complication. The *p* values represent the comparison between low- and high-mortality hospitals. (Reprinted from the Journal of the American College of Surgeons. Sheetz KH, Krell RW, Englesbe MJ, et al. The importance of the first complication: Understanding failure to rescue after emergent surgery in the elderly. *J Am Coll Surg.* 2014;219:365-370, Copyright 2014, with permission from the American College of Surgeons.)

complications did not differ significantly across patient ages or tertiles of hospital mortality.

Conclusions.—Hospitals fail to rescue elderly patients at higher rates than younger patients after infectious and pulmonary complications. Efforts to recognize and manage these specific complications have the potential to improve emergency surgical care of the elderly in Michigan (Fig 2).

▶ In this selection, the authors report on the differences in failure to rescue after specific complications in an elderly emergency surgery population. They discovered that failure-to-rescue rates were markedly different between elderly and nonelderly patients after an initial pulmonary or infectious complication.

However, there were no significant differences seen after cardiovascular complications. This observation persisted at the hospital level, at which high mortality centers failed to rescue elderly patients from pulmonary or infectious complications at significantly higher rates than low mortality centers. These findings, from a statewide database, offer more specific data for hospitals, as they address failure to rescue in elderly surgical patients. Fig 2 included in this review shows the effect of failure to rescue rates on hospital mortality rates. Managing the risks of surgical care in elderly patients is complex, and opportunities to improve outcomes may exist, not just before, but after the operation as well. This study substantiates growing sentiment that appropriate surgical care is age specific and that those efforts to improve the care for pulmonary and infectious complications could attenuate the large mortality differences between elderly and nonelderly patients.

D. W. Mozingo, MD

Predictors of mortality and morbidity for acute care surgery patients

Sudarshan M, Feldman LS, St. Louis E, et al (Montreal General Hosp, Québec, Canada)
J Surg Res 193:868-873, 2015

Background.—As the implementation of exclusive acute care surgery (ACS) services thrives, prognostication for mortality and morbidity will be important to complement clinical management of these diverse and complex patients. Our objective is to investigate prognostic risk factors from patient level characteristics and clinical presentation to predict outcomes including mortality, postoperative complications, intensive care unit (ICU) admission and prolonged duration of hospital stay.

Methods.—Retrospective review of all emergency general surgery admissions over a 1-year period at a large teaching hospital was conducted. Factors collected included history of present illness, physical exam and laboratory parameters at presentation. Univariate analysis was performed to examine the relationship between each variable and our outcomes with chi-square for categorical variables and the Wilcoxon rank-sum statistic for continuous variables. Multivariate analysis was performed using backward stepwise logistic regression to evaluate for independent predictors.

Results.—A total of 527 ACS admissions were identified with 8.1% requiring ICU stay and an overall crude mortality rate of 3.04%. Operative management was required in 258 patients with 22% having postoperative complications. Use of anti-coagulants, systolic blood pressure <90, hypothermia and leukopenia were independent predictors of in-hospital mortality. Leukopenia, smoking and tachycardia at presentation were also prognostic for the development of postoperative complications. For ICU admission, use of anti-coagulants, leukopenia, leukocytosis and tachypnea at presentation were all independent predictive factors. A prolonged length of stay was associated with increasing age, higher American Society of Anesthesiologists class, tachycardia and presence of complications on multivariate analysis.

Conclusions.—Factors present at initial presentation can be used to predict morbidity and mortality in ACS patients.

▶ The emergency general surgery cohort forms a challenging subgroup within the general surgery patient population. These patients can present with acute intra-abdominal crises with major underlying physiologic derangements caused by their illness. In addition to initial resuscitation, the decision for operative management needs to be made. Preoperative optimization of underlying medical comorbidities may be limited because of the need for urgent operative intervention. Outcomes in emergency general surgery are typically worse than their nonemergent counterparts. Performance variability among hospitals for common emergency procedures such as appendectomy, cholecystectomy, and colorectal resection could be compared with regard to quality improvement. The major prediction tools and estimates of risk often used in elective surgical cases to evaluate outcomes are not frequently used for acute care surgery patients. This study is one of the few series to investigate prognostication factors for the acute care surgery population. Use of anticoagulants, blood pressure less than 90 mm Hg, hypothermia, and leukopenia were independent predictors of in-hospital mortality after correction for age and comorbidities. Leukopenia, smoking, and tachycardia at presentation were also prognostic for the development of postoperative complications. The identification of such variables from factors known at presentation represents a potential to prognosticate patients' outcomes and course of stay in acute care surgery. Moreover, it may help identify those patients needing early intervention for morbidity reduction.

D. W. Mozingo, MD

The Opportunity Cost of Futile Treatment in the ICU
Huynh TN, Kleerup EC, Raj PP, et al (Univ of California, Los Angeles; Ronald Reagan-UCLA Med Ctr; et al)
Crit Care Med 42:1977-1982, 2014

Objective.—When used to prolong life without achieving a benefit meaningful to the patient, critical care is often considered "futile." Although futile treatment is acknowledged as a misuse of resources by many, no study has evaluated its opportunity cost, that is, how it affects care for others. Our objective was to evaluate delays in care when futile treatment is provided.

Design.—For 3 months, we surveyed critical care physicians in five ICUs to identify patients that clinicians identified as receiving futile treatment. We identified days when an ICU was full and contained at least one patient who was receiving futile treatment. For those days, we evaluated the number of patients waiting for ICU admission more than 4 hours in the emergency department or more than 1 day at an outside hospital.

Setting.—One health system that included a quaternary care medical center and an affiliated community hospital.

Patients.—Critically ill patients.

Interventions.—None.

Measurements and Main Results.—Boarding time in the emergency department and waiting time on the transfer list. Thirty-six critical care specialists made 6,916 assessments on 1,136 patients of whom 123 were assessed to receive futile treatment. A full ICU was less likely to contain a patient receiving futile treatment compared with an ICU with available beds (38% vs 68%, $p < 0.001$). On 72 (16%) days, an ICU was full and contained at least one patient receiving futile treatment. During these days, 33 patients boarded in the emergency department for more than 4 hours after admitted to the ICU team, nine patients waited more than 1 day to be transferred from an outside hospital, and 15 patients canceled the transfer request after waiting more than 1 day. Two patients died while waiting to be transferred.

Conclusions.—Futile critical care was associated with delays in care to other patients.

▶ There is no recognized objective method of prospectively defining futile treatment, and the assessments by critical care physicians participating in this study were entirely subjective. Nevertheless, the questions asked in this study are extremely important, and the issue of intensive care support when care is futile should continue to be examined. Because futile treatment was defined by the critical care physician, it is likely that many patients' families would not agree with the assessment. Lastly, patients delayed while waiting on the transfer list may not have benefited from transfer to the academic intensive care unit, as they may have been too ill to benefit from critical care, or perhaps another waiting patient may have filled the slot vacated by the patient receiving futile treatment. It is unfortunate when a patient is unable to access intensive care because intensive care unit beds are occupied by patients who may not benefit from such care. In the context of health care reform, which aims to more justly distribute medical care, opportunity cost is a significant reason that futile treatment should be brought under reins.

D. W. Mozingo, MD

Alcohol withdrawal syndrome in admitted trauma patients
Jawa RS, Stothert JC, Shostrom VK, et al (Stony Brook Univ School of Medicine, NY; Univ of Nebraska Med Ctr, Omaha; et al)
Am J Surg 208:781-787, 2014

Background.—As alcohol use is highly prevalent in trauma patients, we hypothesized that a significant proportion of hospitalized trauma patients would demonstrate alcohol withdrawal (AW).

Methods.—The trauma registries at a joint trauma center system from 1999 to 2008 were evaluated for patients aged at least 16 years.

Results.—Of 19,369 trauma admissions, 159 patients had AW. Blood alcohol concentration (BAC) testing was performed in 31.5% of the patients. BAC was significantly higher in AW patients versus other traumas (205.7 ± 130.1 vs 102.9 ± 121.7 mg/dL). BAC was 0 in 14.4% of AW patients. As compared with other trauma patients, patients with AW had a significantly greater age (50.2 vs 42.1 years), hospital length of stay (10 vs 3 days), intensive care unit length of stay (2 vs 0 days), need for mechanical ventilation (34% vs 12.7%), and pneumonia (12% vs 2.3%). AW patients were less frequently discharged to home (59.8% vs 69.9%). Mortality was not different.

Conclusions.—AW was diagnosed in few patients. Of note, it occurred in patients with an initial BAC of 0. AW is associated with adverse outcomes.

▶ Despite the reported prevalence of alcohol use in trauma patients, physicians diagnosed alcohol withdrawal in very few patients. As suggested by the literature, the low prevalence of alcohol withdrawal may be related in part to underdiagnosis and thereby indicates the need for education in its recognition for physicians and other health care providers. Additional factors may include low provider awareness or interest and societal beliefs about alcohol use. Since completion of the study, trauma patients at both medical centers involved in the study routinely undergo brief psychological screening by nursing and social work.

In this study, the authors demonstrated that alcohol withdrawal is associated with greater hospital and intensive care unit length of stay and need for mechanical ventilation. It is also associated with decreased likelihood of discharge to home. The development of pneumonia in alcohol withdrawal should be expeditiously treated, given the 22-fold increase odds of death. Although older age and higher blood alcohol content are progressively associated with increased risk of alcohol withdrawal syndrome development, a key finding of this study was that alcohol withdrawal can occur even in patients who are sober at admission. These findings argue for a careful assessment for chronic alcoholism in all trauma patients, using validated instruments, with subsequent intervention.

D. W. Mozingo, MD

Definition, prevalence, and outcome of feeding intolerance in intensive care: a systematic review and meta-analysis
Blaser AR, Starkopf J, Kirsimägi Ü, et al (Univ of Tartu, Estonia; Tartu Univ Hosp, Estonia; et al)
Acta Anaesthesiol Scand 58:914-922, 2014

Clinicians and researchers frequently use the phrase 'feeding intolerance' (FI) as a descriptive term in enterally fed critically ill patients. We aimed to: (1) determine what is the most accepted definition of FI; (2) estimate the prevalence of FI; and (3) evaluate whether FI is associated with important outcomes. Systematic searches of peer-reviewed publications using PubMed, MEDLINE, and Web of Science were performed with studies reporting FI extracted. We identified 72 studies defining FI. In 33 studies, the definition was based on large gastric residual volumes (GRVs) together with other gastrointestinal symptoms, while 30 studies relied solely on large GRVs, six studies used inadequate delivery of enteral nutrition (EN) as a threshold, and three studies gastrointestinal symptoms without reference to GRV. The median volume used to define a 'large' GRV was 250 ml (ranges from 75 to 500 ml). The pooled proportion ($n = 31$ studies) of FI was 38.3% (95% CI 30.7—46.2). Five studies reported outcomes, all of them observed adverse outcome in FI patients. In three studies, respectively, FI was associated with increased mortality and ICU length-of-stay. In summary, FI is inconsistently defined but appears to occur frequently. There are preliminary data indicating that FI is associated with adverse outcomes. A standard definition of FI is required to determine the accuracy of these preliminary data.

▶ Nutritional support is an accepted component of caring for the critically ill, with the enteral route favored in patients who have an intact gastrointestinal tract but who are unable to ingest food. The predominant method for administering nutrient in this group is via a nasogastric or orogastric tube. Clinicians frequently use the term "feeding intolerance" to describe the situation in which they cannot deliver satisfactory caloric and protein loads because of varied physiological responses of the patient. Researchers also use this term frequently in the scientific literature to describe numerous physiological responses. For a relatively commonly used term, it is surprising that there does not appear to be an agreed-on definition. Recognizing this lack of definition of feeding intolerance, the authors of this study undertook this systematic review to (1) evaluate the breadth of definitions used and determine what is the most frequently described term, (2) estimate the prevalence of feeding intolerance in intensive care patients, and (3) evaluate whether feeding intolerance is associated with important patient-centered outcomes. Because of its prevalence and association with outcome, the need for standardization of the definition of feeding intolerance in future research seems obvious. A standardized definition is required to accurately determine the incidence and associated outcomes. The need for definition is further supported by the fact that inability to feed the patients enterally is a common problem that clinicians confront every day.

D. W. Mozingo, MD

Flat or fat? Inferior vena cava ratio is a marker for occult shock in trauma patients
Nguyen A, Plurad DS, Bricker S, et al (Harbor-UCLA Med Ctr, Torrance, CA)
J Surg Res 192:263-267, 2014

Background.—Identification of occult shock (OS) or hypoperfusion is critical in the initial management of trauma patients. Analysis of inferior vena cava (IVC) ratio on computed tomography (CT) scan has shown promise in predicting intravascular volume. We hypothesized that a flat IVC is a predictor of OS and associated with worse outcomes in major trauma patients.

Materials and Methods.—We performed a 1-y retrospective analysis of our level 1 trauma center database to identify all major trauma activations that underwent evaluation with a CT scan of the torso, arterial blood gas, and serum lactate. A flat IVC was defined as a transverse-to-anteroposterior ratio ≥2.5 at the level of the suprarenal IVC. OS was defined as a base deficit ≥4.0 in the absence of hypotension (systolic blood pressure ≤90 mm Hg).

Results.—Two hundred sixty-four patients were included, of which 52 had a flat IVC. Patients with a flat IVC were found to have a higher injury severity score, lactate, and base deficit compared with patients with a fat IVC. Flat IVC patients also required greater amounts of fluids ($P < 0.04$) and blood ($P < 0.01$). On multivariate analysis, a flat IVC was independently associated with an increased risk for OS (odds ratio $= 2.87$, $P < 0.007$) and overall complications (odds ratio $= 2.26$, $P = 0.05$). The area under the receiver operating characteristic curve for a flat IVC to predict OS was 0.74.

Conclusions.—A flat IVC on CT is an accurate marker for OS in major trauma victims and may help stratify patients who require more aggressive resuscitation, monitoring, and support.

▶ Identification of occult shock is critical, as failure to recognize and reverse this pathologic state is associated with an increase in morbidity and mortality. The typical indicators of shock, namely blood pressure, heart rate, and urine output, may be unreliable in detecting the imbalance between cellular oxygen delivery and demand seen in occult shock. This common clinical entity may be present in up to 70% of severely injured, hemodynamically stable trauma patients. The authors of this selection sought to determine whether the dimensions of the suprarenal vena cava could help identify those patients at risk for occult shock. CT scan images were reviewed by 3 independent assessors who were blinded to patient outcome. Inferior vena cava (IVC) transverse and anteroposterior diameters were measured 2.5 to 5 mm above the left renal vein on axial views. A flat IVC was defined as a transverse-to-anteroposterior ratio ≥2.5 at the level of the suprarenal IVC. A fat IVC was defined as a transverse-to-anteroposterior ratio of less than 2.5. The authors found that patients with a flat IVC were more severely injured and critically ill than their fat IVC counterparts. The presence of a flat IVC on CT may, therefore, alert emergency and trauma personnel to the potential for both occult shock and severity of injury in the absence of other markers of occult shock. This may be most relevant in situations in which other indicators of shock were not ordered either by protocol or in undertriaged trauma patients. The results of this retrospective study are intriguing, and the authors should consider continuing this study prospectively.

D. W. Mozingo, MD

X Chromosome-Linked IRAK-1 Polymorphism Is a Strong Predictor of Multiple Organ Failure and Mortality Postinjury
Sperry JL, Zolin S, Zuckerbraun BS, et al (Univ of Pittsburgh, PA)
Ann Surg 260:698-705, 2014

Objective(s).—Clinical research characterizing the mechanisms responsible for sex-based outcome differences postinjury remain conflicting. We sought to characterize an X chromosome-linked IRAK-1 (IL-1 receptor-associated kinase) polymorphism as an alternative mechanism responsible for sex differences postinjury. IRAK-1 is key intermediate in the toll-like receptor (TLR) pathway thought to drive inflammation postinjury.

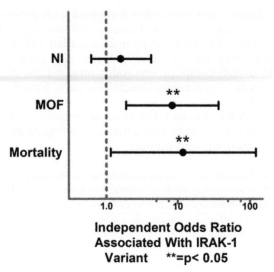

**Independent Odds Ratio
Associated With IRAK-1
Variant **=p< 0.05**

FIGURE 1.—Forest plot depicting the independent Odds Ratio for the development of NI, MOF, and mortality associated with the IRAK-1 variant. (Reprinted from Sperry JL, Zolin S, Zuckerbraun BS, et al. X chromosome-linked IRAK-1 polymorphism is a strong predictor of multiple organ failure and mortality postinjury. *Ann Surg.* 2014;260:698-705, © 2014, Southeastern Surgical Congress.)

Methods.—A prospective cohort study was performed over a 24-month period. Bluntly injured patients requiring intensive care unit admission were enrolled, whereas patients with isolated brain and spinal cord injuries were excluded. Outcomes of interest included multiple organ failure (MOF, Marshall MOD score > 5) and mortality. Logistic regression was utilized to determine the independent risk of poor outcome associated with the IRAK-1 variant after controlling for important differences.

Results.—In an enrolled cohort of 321 patients, the IRAK-1 variant was common (12.5%). Patients with and without the variant were similar in age, injury severity, and 24hr blood transfusion. After controlling for important confounders, the IRAK1 variant was independently associated with more than eightfold (OR = 8.4, $P = 0.005$, 95% CI: 1.9–37.1) and 11-fold (OR = 11.8, $P = 0.037$, 95% CI: 1.1–121) greater risk of MOF and mortality, respectively. These differences were most prominent in men, whereas women heterozygous for the variant demonstrated worse outcome in a dose-dependent fashion.

Conclusions.—The IRAK1 polymorphism is a strong independent predictor of MOF and mortality postinjury and represents a common variant with prognostic potential. These data demonstrate the importance of TLR signaling postinjury and supports that a genetic mechanism may drive sex outcome differences postinjury (Fig 1).

▶ Sex-based differences in outcome have been described for many years in trauma patients, with females having an improved survival advantage. The authors of this selection sought to characterize an X chromosome-linked interleukin-1 receptor-associated kinase (IRAK-1) polymorphism as an alternative mechanism responsible for sex differences postinjury. IRAK-1 is a protein constituent member of the toll-like receptor (TLR) signaling cascade, which resides on the X chromosome and has been shown to have 2 haplotypes. The IRAK-1 variant haplotype has been shown to be relatively common and associated with worse outcome in septic patients. The odds ratio plots for outcome observation associated with the IRAK-1 haplotype are included as Fig 1. IRAK-1 is a key intermediate in the TLR pathway thought to drive inflammation postinjury. TLRs are an evolutionarily conserved family of protein receptors, which are central to NF-κ B cellular signaling and the initiation of the innate immune response to infection. Accumulating evidence suggests that TLRs also recognize endogenous ligands that arise from cellular damage. Additional evidence has shown that the TLR receptor, specifically TLR4, is required and plays a critical role in the early activation and upregulation of the innate immune response, producing a systemic inflammatory response and secondary organ dysfunction. The results of this study show the importance of TLR signaling postinjury and support that an X chromosome-linked genetic mechanism may drive sex-based outcome differences after trauma.

D. W. Mozingo, MD

A Multicenter, Randomized Clinical Trial of IV Iron Supplementation for Anemia of Traumatic Critical Illness
Pieracci FM, Stovall RT, Jaouen B, et al (Univ of Colorado School of Medicine, Denver; et al)
Crit Care Med 42:2048-2057, 2014

Objective.—To evaluate the efficacy of IV iron supplementation of anemic, critically ill trauma patients.

Design.—Multicenter, randomized, single-blind, placebo-controlled trial.

Setting.—Four trauma ICUs.

Patients.—Anemic (hemoglobin <12 g/dL) trauma patients enrolled within 72 hours of ICU admission and with an expected ICU length of stay of more than or equal to 5 days.

Interventions.—Randomization to iron sucrose 100 mg IV or placebo thrice weekly for up to 2 weeks.

Measurements and Main Results.—A total of 150 patients were enrolled. Baseline iron markers were consistent with functional iron deficiency: 134 patients (89.3%) were hypoferremic, 51 (34.0%) were hyperferritinemic, and 64 (42.7%) demonstrated iron-deficient erythropoiesis as evidenced by an elevated erythrocyte zinc protoporphyrin concentration. The median baseline transferrin saturation was 8% (range, 2–58%). In the subgroup of patients who received all six doses of study drug ($n = 57$), the serum ferritin concentration increased significantly for the iron as compared with placebo group on both day 7 (808.0 ng/mL vs 457.0 ng/mL, respectively, $p < 0.01$) and day 14 (1,046.0 ng/mL vs

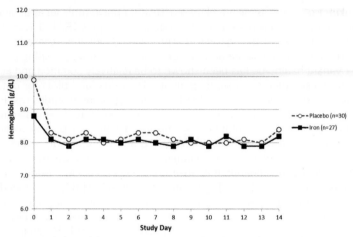

FIGURE 3.—Daily hemoglobin concentration among the subgroup of subjects who received six total doses ($n = 57$). Baseline hemoglobin was significantly higher for placebo group as compared with iron group ($p = 0.03$). (Reprinted from Pieracci FM, Stovall RT, Jaouen B, et al. A multicenter, randomized clinical trial of IV iron supplementation for anemia of traumatic critical illness. *Crit Care Med.* 2014;42:2048-2057, with permission from Society of Critical Care Medicine and Lippincott Williams & Wilkins)

551.5 ng/mL, respectively, $p < 0.01$). There was no significant difference between groups in transferrin saturation, erythrocyte zinc protoporphyrin concentration, hemoglobin concentration, or packed RBC transfusion requirement. There was no significant difference between groups in the risk of infection, length of stay, or mortality.

Conclusions.—Iron supplementation increased the serum ferritin concentration significantly, but it had no discernible effect on transferrin saturation, iron-deficient erythropoiesis, hemoglobin concentration, or packed RBC transfusion requirement. Based on these data, routine IV iron supplementation of anemic, critically ill trauma patients cannot be recommended (NCT 01180894) (Fig 3).

▶ Anemia is extremely common among critically ill patients. The etiology of intensive care unit (ICU) anemia is multifactorial, including acute and chronic blood loss, hemodilution, and inflammation. Inflammation induces cytokine-mediated alterations in erythrocyte longevity, erythropoietin synthesis, and iron metabolism. The authors of this selection previously reported that most critically ill surgical patients become both hypoferremic and hyperferritinemic within 48 hours of ICU admission.[1] Furthermore, more than half of these patients show evidence of iron-deficient erythropoiesis, as indicated by an increase in erythrocyte zinc protoporphyrin concentration, suggesting that iron supplementation may be beneficial. This was a multicenter, randomized, single-blind, placebo-controlled trial involving 4 state-verified, American College of Surgeons-certified, level I trauma centers.

Eligible patients included those admitted to the ICU with a primary diagnosis of trauma. The inclusion criteria were (1) anemia (latest hemoglobin concentration <12 g/dL); (2) age 18 years old or older; (3) ≤72 hours from ICU admission; and (4) expected ICU length of stay ≥5 days. In this multicenter, randomized, controlled trial of anemic, critically ill trauma patients, iron sucrose, 100 mg intravenously 3 times weekly for up to 2 weeks, did not impact functional iron deficiency, iron deficiency anemia, anemia, or packed red blood cell transfusion requirement. Iron supplementation at this level did not increase the risk of infection. Fig 3 is included depicting the serial hemoglobin measurements in the 2 study groups. Based on these data, routine intravenous iron supplementation of anemic, critically ill trauma patients cannot be recommended. This study is a wonderful example of the importance of multicenter collaborative research in answering basic clinical questions and extending the scope of evidenced-based patient care.

D. W. Mozingo, MD

Reference

1. Pieracci FM, Eachempati SR, Henderson P, et al. Prevalence of hypoferremia and iron-deficient erythropoiesis in anemic critically ill patients, and correlation with severity of illness. *Crit Care Med.* 2006;34:A132.

Early lung ultrasonography predicts the occurrence of acute respiratory distress syndrome in blunt trauma patients
Leblanc D, Bouvet C, Degiovanni F, et al (Université d'Angers, France)
Intensive Care Med 40:1468-1474, 2014

Purpose.—Extent of lung contusion on initial computed tomography (CT) scan predicts the occurrence of acute respiratory distress syndrome (ARDS) in blunt chest trauma patients. We hypothesized that lung ultrasonography (LUS) on admission could also predict subsequent ARDS.

Methods.—Forty-five blunt trauma patients were prospectively studied. Clinical examination, chest radiography, and LUS were performed on arrival at the emergency room. Lung contusion extent was quantified using a LUS score and compared to CT scan measurements. The ability of the LUS score to predict ARDS was tested using the area under the receiver operating characteristic curve (AUC-ROC). The diagnostic accuracy of LUS was compared to that of combined clinical examination and chest radiography for pneumothorax, lung contusion, and hemothorax, with thoracic CT scan as reference.

Results.—Lung contusion extent assessed by LUS on admission was predictive of the occurrence of ARDS within 72 h (AUC-ROC = 0.78 [95% CI 0.64—0.92]). The extent of lung contusion on LUS correlated well with CT scan measurements (Spearman's coefficient = 0.82). A LUS score of 6 out of 16 was the best threshold to predict ARDS, with a 58% [95% CI 36—77] sensitivity and a 96% [95% CI 76—100] specificity.

The diagnostic accuracy of LUS was higher than that of combined clinical examination and chest radiography: (AUC-ROC) 0.81 [95% CI 0.50−1.00] vs. 0.74 [0.48−1.00] ($p = 0.24$) for pneumothorax, 0.88 [0.76−1.00] vs. 0.69 [0.47−0.92] ($p < 0.05$) for lung contusion, and 0.84 [0.59−1.00] vs. 0.73 [0.51−0.94] ($p < 0.05$) for hemothorax.

Conclusions.—LUS on admission identifies patients at risk of developing ARDS after blunt trauma. In addition, LUS allows rapid and accurate diagnosis of common traumatic thoracic injuries.

▶ Lung contusion is a frequent thoracic injury in blunt chest trauma, and it is associated with increased morbidity and mortality. Direct damage of the lung causes both local and systemic inflammatory responses that can lead to acute respiratory distress syndrome (ARDS) and multiple organ failure. The initial size of the lung contusion seems to play a key role in these mechanisms. CT scans can predict the development of ARDS, but the measurement of lung contusion volume requires 3-dimensional modeling that is not always available. In addition, severely injured patients may have hemodynamic instability preventing transport to the CT suite. Thus, bedside ultrasonography could be an alternative diagnostic tool to assess the extent of lung contusion. The authors of this selection hypothesized that early assessment of lung contusion extent using lung ultrasound scan could predict the occurrence of ARDS in blunt trauma patients. The authors conducted a prospective observational study to evaluate the ability of lung ultrasound scan performed on admission of trauma patients to predict the development of ARDS. The authors confirmed that lung ultrasonography is accurate in assessing the extent of lung contusion. In addition, this study found that lung ultrasound scan performed on admission can predict the occurrence of subsequent ARDS. They found that a lung ultrasound score of 6 or more of 16 was predictive of ARDS. Whereas the specificity of this score was good, its sensitivity was relatively weak for predicting severe to moderate and severe to mild ARDS, respectively, 64% and 58%; however, overprediction in this setting would not have adverse consequences. The results of this study suggest that lung ultrasound scan could be added to the Extended Focused Assessment with Sonography for Trauma, not only for lung contusion diagnosis but also for the diagnosis of hemothorax and pneumothorax.

D. W. Mozingo, MD

5 Transplantation

Introduction

Organ transplantation has become an oversight experiment for performance and quality measures applied to clinical medicine. There is an extraordinary amount of information available from many databases about the people giving and receiving organ transplants. This information leads to many interesting publications, displaying extraordinary insights, glaring biases, or still inadequate clinical information. The fact also remains that organ availability has remained static for the past decade, with demand (especially for kidneys) continuing to increase. Barring some form of major breakthrough in regenerative, reparative medicine, or xenotransplantation, the demand for human organs will only continue to increase, putting more performance pressures on the existing transplant systems.

This year's literature selections illustrate some of these pressures. The first 3 selections bring different perspectives on the field. The first article by Adler et al is an analysis of kidney transplant center outcomes grouped by economic competition. The conclusion derived was that greater competition for deceased organs and patients leads to greater utilization of "lower quality" deceased donor kidneys, increased risk for recipient mortality, and graft failure. The analysis is limited in not doing an "intent-to-treat" analysis of the population. Not normalizing post-transplant outcomes to time spent on dialysis (quite protracted in some of the areas with higher local competition) will lead to quite spurious conclusions. The second article, by Schold, addressed the impact of "oversight" upon the benefit and availability of kidney transplantation and queried what should be "appropriate" endpoints to measure effectiveness in our transplant oversight system. The Scientific Registry of Transplant Recipients (SRTR) releases performance program specific reports that are used by OPTN/UNOS to monitor the quality of the transplantation system and by CMS to assure that individual programs continue to meet the performance expectations of the conditions of participation. Individual transplant programs are stratified as performing above expected, as expected, and lower than expected for post-transplant graft and patient survival. When assessed on an intent to treat (an individual being placed on the wait list), patient survival is significantly improved by being transplanted, irrespective of center performance. There is obviously a statistical difference in survival within transplanted individuals, as well, as that is how groups were stratified. The telling point was in growth of transplant availability for individuals. In those programs flagged for subpar performance, growth in number of procedures was lowest. This paper asked the question: What should be the appropriate comparator for transplant program performance—other programs doing similar procedures or care for the intended beneficiary? Using an intent-to-treat analytic tool would dramatically alter the presentation of information to the public. The final article on this topic is the benefit of "low quality" kidneys, as these are the organs least commonly used after being retrieved for the purpose of transplantation. As noted in the first article, the use of lower quality kidneys can be viewed pejoratively. All deceased donor kidneys are now stratified by a calculated index, and the bottom percentiles are often not used for transplantation. However, the authors analyzed the mortality risk of staying on dialysis vs receiving a "not so good" kidney. While the risk of mortality increases immediately after the transplant procedure, survival benefit rapidly overtakes the risk of remaining on dialysis within 8 months for the 70-80% of available kidneys, and within 18 months for the 80-90% and 20 months for recipients of the 90-100% kidneys. There is some selection bias at play in the database, in that women (smaller) are more likely to be recipients of the kidneys with less predicted functional reserve.

The analysis of intent to treat and use of essentially all retrieved kidneys makes a compelling case to expand kidney transplantation as a form of therapy. The current demographics of organ donors do not necessarily match the demographics of those individuals who die in the US. There is a need to gain acceptance of organ donation within the various ethnic communities. Using a before-and-after survey of community acceptance of organ donation, the authors of paper 4 demonstrated the benefit of using a focused campaign in schools, church, and media within the Hispanic community. A significant increase in understanding of the benefits accrued by organ donation and willingness to participate should serve as an impetus to develop culturally specific tools for improving organ availability from the increasingly diverse population in the US.

Despite the survival benefit associated with kidney transplantation, there are multiple system issues that either impair access to transplant care or do not maximize organ availability of existing donors. The paper by Patzer et al analyzed CMS data on dialysis units to discern likelihood of receiving a kidney transplant. An extraordinary diversity of accessibility to organ transplantation was found, including the common differentiators: geography, ethnicity, for profit status of dialysis facility, and financial and social status discriminators. What is distressing about this analysis is that these issues have been known for decades, and few inroads have been made. In fact, in this study, there were 99 dialysis units identified that had with no transplants performed over the four-year time period. One can quibble with standards and metrics, but the heterogeneity of access to life-saving and life-prolonging care is staggering. Paper 6 describes a cooperative effort between the agencies charged with retrieving organs from deceased individuals and centers that accept those organs for transplantation. Developing and meeting fairly basic donor management goals resulted in increased use of organs from extended criteria donors. This paper illustrates that improvements within the existing system can provide significant (albeit incremental) benefit.

Live donors represent a pool for kidney transplantation that has almost no limit. However, as there is no therapeutic benefit associated with donor nephrectomy, the consequences of the procedure have undergone renewed scrutiny. The RELIVE study (paper 7) analyzes the outcomes after live kidney donation performed between 1963 and 2005 at 3 US live donor centers. It provides an interesting insight into donors' perception of what they experienced. This study reports on pre- and post-donation depression. Of those kidney donors who reported pre-donation depression, the self-reported incidence of post-donation depression was twice that of those without the history. Other studies report a higher rate of post-donation psychological consequences, which may have faded in the memories of these individuals. It is encouraging that such events are remembered as relatively infrequent. Paper 8 assesses the risk that a live kidney donor will develop end-stage kidney failure. It created a significant buzz in the medical community because it purported to show that there is a significantly increased risk for renal failure if one has previously donated a kidney (compared to "matched" healthy non-donor controls). The incidence of ESRD in the kidney donor group is still less than the general population, even though higher than their matched controls. This is useful information to give healthy people as they contemplate kidney donation. Yes, having a solitary kidney puts you at higher risk for kidney failure should something stress your kidneys. However, the risk of developing renal failure still appears to be less than the general population (not having passed the donation evaluation process). Others have criticized the analysis for not finding appropriate controls for the donors, but irrespective of the "appropriate" control, it is intuitive that with reduced renal mass, an individual is at higher risk for renal failure should some damage occur to the remaining kidney. This "fact" needs to be incorporated into the informed consent process as one proceeds toward donation. The final paper in this trilogy of kidney donor consequences is about donor costs. A common statement told to live donors is that the cost of donation is not their responsibility. While the medical costs may be routed into an organ cost center, there are considerable "living" and travel costs in the donation process. Klarenbach et al did a prospective assessment of the economic consequences associated with the donation process. The authors found significant heterogeneity amongst people, but the mean cost was over $3000 per donor (including lost wages, travel expenses, and sundry medications). Fifteen percent of donors reported cost >$8000, and almost 10% had to pay for living assistance during their recovery period. Live donation has enough risks for donors without having them pay considerable sums to partake in the donation process.

Long-term outcomes after kidney transplantation continue to be less than one would hope. While early, post-procedure results have become quite impressive, but for a variety of reasons grafts continue to fail as time progresses. The report by Nabakow assessed the impact of isolated glomerular inflammation or glomerular inflammation in association with cellular or antibody upon graft function contrasted to the population with either no rejection or isolated cellular rejection. While this group represented slightly less than 10% of the transplanted patients, there was a significantly worsened outcome irrespective of whether an active immunologic reaction was recognized. Isolated glomerulitis resulted in significant loss of function over the observation period, irrespective of therapeutic efforts. Challenges associated with long-term maintenance of kidney function will require recognition of specific pathology and effective tools to counter progression.

There are challenges associated with all organs transplanted. A major issue for liver transplantation has been that the current allocation system mandates that the "sickest" potential recipient be first offered an individual liver. As sick people's health deteriorates and they eventually die, the question is more frequently being raised: When does one determine that a transplant is futile? This is a problem for every program, but one that was addressed by the experience of UCLA in paper 11. Futility for the very sick (MELD>40) was defined as either death within the transplant hospitalization or within 90 days. They contrasted the people who met the futility criteria to those who survived to discharge or past 90 days. Only 22% of patients with MELD>40 met the futility criteria. The magnitude of the MELD score, serious infection within 30 days of procedure, cardiac risk, and significant comorbidities were the 4 variables that on multivariate analysis were associated with futility. Of these variables, only infection and potentially the MELD score are modifiable. The need for better information to guide care is pivotal in avoidance of a futile transplant. However, appropriate definitions and adequate data are central to this discussion. Another tactic has been to use tools from other disciplines such as frailty. The "frail" are less likely to be able to withstand even the wait to obtain a liver transplant. In the paper by Lai et al, wait-list mortality was assessed for patients with a MELD >12 and stratified by standard functional frailty scores. Those deemed "frail" were twice as likely to die or be removed from the wait-list as the "nonfrail." Using the standard frailty scores, 17% of the wait list was deemed frail. How fixed is this condition? With nutrition and therapy, is it possible to reverse this designation? The final paper uses "objective" CT findings as a morphometric measure of muscle wasting. The conclusion that morphometric age predicted mortality better than chronologic age only reinforces that sick, debilitated people tolerate big operations and immunosuppression less well than those who are in better shape. The challenge is to improve outcomes and to improve the condition of those who have to go through the perioperative liver transplant period.

As with kidney transplantation, a major problem for recipients of liver transplantation is the relative paucity of organs. A variety of tactics have been generated to address this problem. The simplest one is to double the number of available livers by splitting a deceased donor liver into two lobes. As described by the Cleveland Clinic program in paper 14, recipients of split livers get comparable long-term results as whole grafts, albeit with a higher technical complication, compared with whole liver transplants. However, the true limiting factor for this technical tour de force is that relatively few organs can be split and matched with recipients. Only 25 adult individuals over an eight-year period benefited from the extra effort of splitting a deceased donor liver to benefit adults. The use of split livers for children is an ongoing process that benefits a few more individuals. While this practice benefits a few individuals and should be pursued, there are relatively few who benefit. Assuming that whole deceased livers cannot be significantly increased, the other major source of organs is from live liver donation. This source of organs has been cautiously reexamined after the highly publicized donor deaths of the past decade. The morbidity of hepatectomy appears to be proportional to the amount of liver removed. This was confirmed by the Kyoto experience in paper 15, as 140/208 adult liver transplant recipients received a left-lobe graft. The left-lobe donors had a quicker time to normalization of serum LFTs and lesser morbidity than right-lobe donors. However, it appeared that left-lobe recipients required significantly less liver mass, with a lower body weight and higher percentage of women. An analysis of the Nationwide Inpatient Sample (NIS) database attempted to get to similar information in paper 16. Standard billing codes were used by the authors to study 555 donors of the 2783 performed in the US. The complication rate during the donation hospitalization was 23%, with the majority being minor complications. This data report illustrates many limitations of "big data" and especially data predicated upon billing/coding information. Compared to A2ALL (NIH group charged with studying live liver donation), the complication rates in the liver donor population are lower and biliary leaks considerably less frequent in national pooled data vs procedures performed in the highly selected centers of the NIH study. Reasons for this discrepancy are legion and the most important are probably methodological, as the NIS data only tracks coding event during the liver donor admission. However, there are many other differences in terms of definition, mechanism for identification, and capture of the variables that account for differences.

Early outcomes after liver transplantation continue to be dominated by the severity of illness, as noted in the prior selections. However, long-term outcomes after liver transplantation continue to be influenced by recurrent disease and immunological events. The 2 common indications for liver transplantation include HCV and hepatocellular carcinoma (HCCa). Huge strides in HCV treatment over the past few years will be able to be evaluated in recipient outcomes within the next few years. However, the HCCa indication continues to be a major national indication for liver transplantation, especially as screening becomes more practiced in the community. The cancer survival benefit of transplantation compared with other forms of therapy has been demonstrated repetitively. However, as the wait-list population continues to age, many query whether an increasing age of the recipient will diminish the survival benefit of the recipient. Kim et al used OPTN to address this issue in paper 17. They found that HCCa-disease specific survival was identical between age groups, but that overall 5-year survival after liver transplantation was diminished in the >65 years group with HCCa by 7%. This analysis confirms the need for good medical evaluation of recipients, as management of medical comorbidities becomes the dominant factor for survival after stratification of the cancer is completed. Antibodies directed against alloantigens have been demonstrated to be a major predictor of graft lost in extrahepatic organs. The role of the humoral immune response in liver transplantation has been a bit of an uncertainty. In a report from France in paper 18, donor specific antibodies (DSA) were studied in the stable/maintenance liver transplant population. Two-hundred sixty-seven recipients were identified having undergone a liver transplant at least 6 months prior to routine clinic visit. They found that in this population, 35 (13%) had DSA on first check (it was unknown how many of these individuals had preexisting alloantibody that persisted after the liver transplant). Twenty-five people kept the DSA throughout the 4-year surveillance, and in 10 the antibody became undetectable. Of those initially without detectable DSA, 21 (9%) developed antibodies during the surveillance period and had 5 antibody mediated rejections. Additionally, the liver biopsy fibrosis score in patients DSA was higher than in patients without DSA after removing patients with HCV or autoimmune diseases. While the exact role that DSA plays in the long-term outcome of liver transplant recipients is unknown, it appears to be clinically meaningful, if not a strong predictor of patient or graft survival.

The final 2 papers are to illustrate 2 major topics: one is that system changes need to be monitored to discern if a change produces the intended outcome. Several years ago, the Lung Allocation Score (LAS) was introduced with the goal of getting lungs to those who would "benefit" most. While there was a substantive decrease of wait-list mortality and no significant alteration in one-year graft function, little has been done with long-term survival. In paper 19, the authors reviewed the long-term OPTN data from before and after the introduction of the LAS. Although reconfirming the early benefit, analysis of long-term data demonstrated a significant death rate after the first year. This is an interesting observation in that LAS allocation change occurred at a similar time the Center for Medicare and Medicaid Services (CMS) changed the Conditions of Participation. How much of this "observation" is due to biology of lung disease or how much is related to administrative monitoring and reporting will remain to be seen. There are multiple factors that influence outcome reporting: Sorting biology from administrative and social pressure variables is becoming remarkably complex, but crucial. The final paper discusses the role of cellular therapies to induce a "tolerance" or immune hyporesponsive condition in the organ recipient. The goal of drug-free maintenance of graft acceptance has been a quest for quite some time. It seems now that the horizon may finally be getting closer. There have been several cellular methods to achieve this state, and some are moving closer to clinical application. Paper 20 describes some of the cellular mechanisms involved with the induction of mixed chimerism and organ maintenance. The authors demonstrated the pivotal role of myeloid-derived suppressor cells (MDSC) and NKT cells in mice. Breaking the balance of cell populations through antibody depletion broke tolerance, and restoration of MDSC was necessary to restore the immunologic unresponsive condition. Unfortunately, these studies are in mice, and applicability to humans remains to be done. What is becoming clear is that multiple immunologic manipulations may alter the immune response to a transplanted organ. Finding the most direct and reproducible tactic is still a goal worth pursuing.

Transplantation has established itself as a treatment that is cost effective and life prolonging contrasted with other forms of treatments for organ failure. Limitations in availability are a severe limitation to optimization of treatment. The biology barriers are still formidable, but oversight and social barriers are almost as difficult.

Timothy L. Pruett, MD

Increasing Organ Donation in Hispanic Americans: The Role of Media and Other Community Outreach Efforts

Salim A, Ley EJ, Berry C, et al (Cedars-Sinai Med Ctr, Los Angeles, CA; et al)
JAMA Surg 149:71-76, 2014

Importance.—The growing demand for organs continues to outpace supply. This gap is most pronounced in minority populations, who constitute more than 40% of the organ waiting list. Hispanic Americans are particularly less likely to donate compared with other minorities for reasons that remain poorly understood and difficult to change.

Objective.—To determine whether outreach interventions that target Hispanic Americans improve organ donation outcomes.

Design, Setting, and Participants.—Prospective before-after study of 4 southern California neighborhoods with a high percentage of Hispanic American residents. We conducted cross-sectional telephone surveys before and 2 years after outreach interventions. Respondents 18 years or older were drawn randomly from lists of Hispanic surnames. Awareness, perceptions, and beliefs regarding organ donation and intent to donate were measured and compared before and after interventions.

Intervention.—Television and radio commercials about organ donation and educational programs at 5 high schools and 4 Catholic churches.

Main Outcomes and Measures.—Number of survey participants who specify intent to donate.

Results.—A total of 402 preintervention and 654 postintervention individuals participated in the surveys. We observed a significant increase in awareness of and knowledge about organ donation and a significant increase in the intent to donate (17.7% vs 12.1%; adjusted odds ratio, 1.55 [95% CI, 1.06-2.26; P =.02]).

Conclusions and Relevance.—Focused donor outreach programs sustain awareness and knowledge and can significantly improve intent to donate organs in the Hispanic American population. These programs should continue to be evaluated and implemented to influence donor registration.

▶ The ethnic distribution of organ donors and those that die in US hospitals do not parallel each other. Individuals of color traditionally have a lower rate of organ donation than their white counterparts. This is despite a disproportionate rate of organ failure and need for transplantation in many of the ethnic communities. Culturally relevant approaches to organ donation education are essential for optimal willingness to be an organ donor if availability is to occur. One may quibble with methods used in this report, but the need for information in a culturally relevant format is an essential first step. The authors found that when using a basic approach of media, schools, and churches directed toward the Los Angeles Hispanic community, a significant increase in willingness to be an organ donor was achieved. At this juncture, willingness to donate does not transfer to increased organ availability, but it is a necessary first step.

T. L. Pruett, MD

Requirement for Interactions of Natural Killer T Cells and Myeloid-Derived Suppressor Cells for Transplantation Tolerance

Hongo D, Tang X, Baker J, et al (Stanford Univ School of Medicine, CA)
Am J Transplant 14:2467-2477, 2014

The goal of the study was to elucidate the cellular and molecular mechanisms by which a clinically applicable immune tolerance regimen of combined bone marrow and heart transplants in mice results in mixed chimerism and graft acceptance. The conditioning regimen of lymphoid irradiation and anti-T cell antibodies changed the balance of cells in the lymphoid tissues to create a tolerogenic microenvironment favoring the increase of natural killer T (NKT) cells, $CD4^+CD25^+$ regulatory T cells and $Gr-1^+CD11^+$ myeloid-derived suppressor cells (MDSCs), over conventional T cells (Tcons). The depletion of MDSCs abrogated chimerism and tolerance, and add back of these purified cells was restorative. The conditioning regimen activated the MDSCs as judged by the increased expression of arginase-1, IL-4Rα and programmed death ligand 1, and the activated cells gained the capacity to suppress the proliferation of Tcons to alloantigens in the mixed leukocyte reaction. MDSC activation was dependent on the presence of host invariant NKT cells. The conditioning regimen polarized the host invariant NKT cells toward IL-4 secretion, and MDSC activation was dependent on IL-4. In conclusion, there was a requirement for MDSCs for chimerism and tolerance, and their suppressive function was dependent on their interactions with NKT cells and IL-4.

▶ Finding ways to maintain stable graft function without immunosuppressive medications has been a holy grail for the transplant community. There have been many approaches—chimerism, antigen lack of recognition, and T cell modification to diminish antigen recognition. Continued efforts in the laboratory and clinics will hopefully yield positive clinical results for transplant recipients. This report discusses phenotypic changes induced by a tolerogenic conditioning regimen. It was found that myeloid-derived suppressor cells, rather than conventional regulatory T cells, were pivotal in the development of tolerance in mice. Mechanisms that will eventually lead to clinical application of cell-based immunosuppression will likely be quite disparate. Central to clinical application will be reproducibility and ease to generate the tolerogenic environment.

T. L. Pruett, MD

The Impact of Meeting Donor Management Goals on the Number of Organs Transplanted per Expanded Criteria Donor: A Prospective Study From the UNOS Region 5 Donor Management Goals Workgroup

Patel MS, Zatarain J, De La Cruz S, et al (Massachusetts General Hosp, Boston; Portland Veterans Affairs Med Ctr, OR; et al)

JAMA Surg 149:969-975, 2014

Importance.—The shortage of organs available for transplant has led to the use of expanded criteria donors (ECDs) to extend the donor pool. These donors are older and have more comorbidities and efforts to optimize the quality of their organs are needed.

Objective.—To determine the impact of meeting a standardized set of critical care end points, or donor management goals (DMGs), on the number of organs transplanted per donor in ECDs.

Design, Setting, and Participants.—Prospective interventional study from February 2010 to July 2013 of all ECDs managed by the 8 organ procurement organizations in the southwestern United States (United Network for Organ Sharing Region 5).

Interventions.—Implementation of 9 DMGs as a checklist to guide the management of every ECD. The DMGs represented normal cardiovascular, pulmonary, renal, and endocrine end points. Meeting the DMG bundle was defined a priori as achieving any 7 of the 9 end points and was recorded at the time of referral to the organ procurement organization, at the time of authorization for donation, 12 to 18 hours later, and prior to organ recovery.

Main Outcomes and Measures.—The primary outcome measure was 3 or more organs transplanted per donor and binary logistic regression was used to identify independent predictors with $P < .05$.

Results.—There were 671 ECDs with a mean (SD) number of 2.1 (1.3) organs transplanted per donor. Ten percent of the ECDs had met the DMG bundle at referral, 15% at the time of authorization, 33% at 12 to 18 hours, and 45% prior to recovery. Forty-three percent had 3 or more organs transplanted per donor. Independent predictors of 3 or more organs transplanted per donor were older age (odds ratio [OR] = 0.95 per year [95% CI, 0.93-0.97]), increased creatinine level (OR = 0.73 per mg/dL [95% CI, 0.63-0.85]), DMGs met prior to organ recovery (OR = 1.90 [95% CI, 1.35-2.68]), and a change in the number of DMGs achieved from referral to organ recovery (OR = 1.11 per additional DMG [95% CI, 1.00-1.23]).

Conclusions and Relevance.—Meeting DMGs prior to organ recovery with ECDs is associated with achieving 3 or more organs transplanted per donor. An increase in the number of critical care end points achieved throughout the care of a potential donor by both donor hospital and organ procurement organization is also associated with an increase in organ yield.

▶ Older people are more prone to die than younger individuals. Organs retrieved from older individuals are not used at the same frequency as organs from younger people. If national organ availability is to increase, an increased utilization of organs from older deceased donors will need to be part of the process. A large part of the failure to utilize revolves around the perception that the organs from older individuals are less able to withstand hypoperfusion and hypoxia. The organ retrieval programs with the southwest sector of the United States undertook an effort to achieve specific donor management goals in anticipation that organs from older donors would be more frequently used for transplantation. The goals (circulatory, respiratory, and general metabolic) were very achievable with good clinical management. The fact that multiple organ procurement organizations in the region improved organ utilization from donors that achieved management goals prior to organ retrieval showed the importance of donor management in the acceptability of organs for transplantation. What was not shown was the function of the organs that met goals. Was there more or less dialysis required from the transplanted kidneys from donors that failed to meet management goals? There is much to be learned about use of organs from nonideal donors, but optimizing management in the predonation period does much to make the organs appear more transplantable.

T. L. Pruett, MD

Association between kidney transplant center performance and the survival benefit of transplantation versus dialysis

Schold JD, Buccini LD, Goldfarb DA, et al (Case Western Reserve Univ, Cleveland, OH; et al)

Clin J Am Soc Nephrol 9:1773-1780, 2014

Background and Objectives.—Despite the benefits of kidney transplantation, the total number of transplants performed in the United States has stagnated since 2006. Transplant center quality metrics have been associated with a decline in transplant volume among low-performing centers. There are concerns that regulatory oversight may lead to risk aversion and lack of transplantation growth.

Design, Setting, Participants, & Measurements.—A retrospective cohort study of adults (age ≥18 years) wait-listed for kidney transplantation in the United States from 2003 to 2010 using the Scientific Registry of Transplant Recipients was conducted. The primary aim was to investigate whether measured center performance modifies the survival benefit of transplantation versus dialysis. Center performance was on the basis of the most recent Scientific Registry of Transplant Recipients evaluation at the time that patients were placed on the waiting list. The primary outcome was the time-dependent adjusted hazard ratio of death compared with remaining on the transplant waiting list.

Results.—Among 223,808 waitlisted patients, 59,199 and 32,764 patients received a deceased or living donor transplant, respectively. Median follow-up from listing was 43 months (25th percentile = 25 months, 75th percentile = 67 months), and there were 43,951 total patient deaths. Deceased donor transplantation was independently associated with lower mortality at each center performance level compared with remaining on the waiting list; adjusted hazard ratio was 0.24 (95% confidence interval, 0.21 to 0.27) among 11,972 patients listed at high-performing centers, adjusted hazard ratio was 0.32 (95% confidence interval, 0.31 to 0.33) among 203,797 patients listed at centers performing as expected, and adjusted hazard ratio was 0.40 (95% confidence interval, 0.35 to 0.45) among 8039 patients listed at low-performing centers. The survival benefit was significantly different by center performance (*P* value for interaction <0.001).

Conclusions.—Findings indicate that measured center performance modifies the survival benefit of kidney transplantation, but the benefit of transplantation remains highly significant even at centers with low measured quality. Policies that concurrently emphasize improved center performance with access to transplantation should be prioritized to improve ESRD population outcomes.

▶ Organ transplantation has been a national experiment in the area of public release of information relating to center performance. The issue of appropriate comparators becomes essential for this domain. As noted in prior articles, competition, oversight agencies, use of lower-quality organs, dialysis units, and ethnicity have all been thought to influence outcomes and access to care. The current article uses an intent-to-treat analysis of people on the national kidney wait list and compared survival benefit from kidney transplantation in centers "higher than," "as expected," and "lower than" the predicted outcomes used by Health Resources and Services Administration/Centers for Medicare & Medicaid Services to assess transplant outcomes. Under this analysis, the survival benefit in all programs was higher than staying on dialysis. The centers with above-expected outcomes had a statistically higher percentage of patients with a college education and younger age patients and almost significantly more with private insurance. This analysis begs the question as to what is the true comparator that should be used to judge transplant centers. What has been found is that programs under review for outcomes are much more likely to limit number of transplants and not benefit those in need. A discussion relating to appropriateness of risk-adjusted outcomes and to what comparators is central to long-term treatment of patients with kidney failure.

T. L. Pruett, MD

Dialysis Facility and Network Factors Associated With Low Kidney Transplantation Rates Among United States Dialysis Facilities
Patzer RE, Plantinga L, Krisher J, et al (Emory Univ School of Medicine, Atlanta, GA; Rollins School of Public Health, Atlanta, GA; Southeastern Kidney Council of ESRD Network 6, Raleigh, NC; et al)
Am J Transplant 14:1562-1572, 2014

Variability in transplant rates between different dialysis units has been noted, yet little is known about facility-level factors associated with low standardized transplant ratios (STRs) across the United States End-stage Renal Disease (ESRD) Network regions. We analyzed Centers for Medicare & Medicaid Services Dialysis Facility Report data from 2007 to 2010 to examine facility-level factors associated with low STRs using multivariable mixed models. Among 4098 dialysis facilities treating 305 698 patients, there was wide variability in facility-level STRs across the 18 ESRD Networks. Four-year average STRs ranged from 0.69 (95% confidence interval [CI]: 0.64—0.73) in Network 6 (Southeastern Kidney Council) to 1.61 (95% CI: 1.47—1.76) in Network 1 (New England). Factors significantly associated with a lower STR ($p < 0.0001$) included for-profit status, facilities with higher percentage black patients, patients with no health insurance and patients with diabetes. A greater number of facility staff, more transplant centers per 10 000 ESRD patients and a higher percentage of patients who were employed or utilized peritoneal dialysis were associated with higher STRs. The lowest performing dialysis facilities were in the Southeastern United States. Understanding the modifiable facility-level factors associated with low transplant rates may inform interventions to improve access to transplantation.

► Access to organ transplantation is a multifaceted process. The authors assessed the Centers for Medicare & Medicaid Services dialysis facility report to characterize heterogeneity of transplant care across the country. The authors reconfirmed that heterogeneity does exist, with geography, ethnicity, insurance status, for-profit status of the dialysis unit, and other factors found to be statistically significant as factors influencing access to transplantation. Although the analysis is inclusive of the breadth of information collected by the Centers for Medicare & Medicaid Services, state, regional, and cultural variables can only be inferred. There are wide differences in perception by physicians and patients regarding the idea that kidney transplantation is the optimal treatment for someone with end-stage renal disease. Only 23% of patients younger than 70 are on a wait list for a kidney. It is likely that many others would benefit. An unmeasured but significant variable is the likelihood of receiving a kidney. There are individuals that would go through with evaluation and listing if there was a realistic likelihood that an organ would become available. The negative influence of insufficient organs for the needs of the population makes the analysis of the most influential factors impeding kidney transplantation difficult.

T. L. Pruett, MD

Survival Benefit of Primary Deceased Donor Transplantation With High-KDPI Kidneys

Massie AB, Luo X, Chow EKH, et al (Johns Hopkins Univ School of Medicine, Baltimore, MD)
Am J Transplant 14:2310-2316, 2014

The Kidney Donor Profile Index (KDPI) has been introduced as an aid to evaluating deceased donor kidney offers, but the relative benefit of high-KDPI kidney transplantation (KT) versus the clinical alternative (remaining on the waitlist until receipt of a lower KDPI kidney) remains unknown. Using time-dependent Cox regression, we evaluated the mortality risk associated with high-KDPI KT (KDPI 71–80, 81–90 or 91–100) versus a conservative, lower KDPI approach (remain on waitlist until receipt of KT with KDPI 0–70, 0–80 or 0–90) in first-time adult registrants, adjusting for candidate characteristics. High-KDPI KT was associated with increased short-term but decreased long-term mortality risk. Recipients of KDPI 71–80 KT, KDPI 81–90 KT and KDPI 91–100 KT reached a "break-even point" of cumulative survival at 7.7, 18.0 and 19.8 months post-KT, respectively, and had a survival benefit thereafter. Cumulative survival at 5 years was better in all three high-KDPI groups than the conservative approach ($p < 0.01$ for each comparison). Benefit of high-KDPI KT was greatest in patients age >50 years and patients at centers with median wait time $\geq$33 months. Recipients of high-KDPI

KT can enjoy better long-term survival; a high-KDPI score does not automatically constitute a reason to reject a deceased donor kidney.

▶ Through an analysis of the same data source used in the first report, the authors concluded that transplantation of kidneys up to the highest Kidney Donor Profile Index (KDPI) (those kidneys with lowest theoretical ability to function in the recipient) conferred survival benefit for recipients. The caveat to this finding was that the breakeven point was increasingly longer after transplantation with high KDPI kidneys, but eventually a benefit was demonstrated. The authors concluded that the people who would derive benefit from high KDPI kidneys were those wait listed at centers with a long waiting time. This, of course, is the scenario at centers in competitive organ allocation areas. These 2 reports show the complexity of providing kidneys for the US population. It is crucial that the benefit of transplantation be made in the context of disease management of kidney failure and not as an end in itself. When viewed in this context, the disservice done to the public through inability to provide sufficient numbers of kidneys becomes a tragedy.

T. L. Pruett, MD

Risk of End-Stage Renal Disease Following Live Kidney Donation
Muzaale AD, Massie AB, Wang M-C, et al (Johns Hopkins Univ School of Medicine, Baltimore, MD; Johns Hopkins Bloomberg School of Public Health, Baltimore, MD; et al)
JAMA 311:579-586, 2014

Importance.—Risk of end-stage renal disease (ESRD) in kidney donors has been compared with risk faced by the general population, but the general population represents an unscreened, high-risk comparator. A comparison to similarly screened healthy nondonors would more properly estimate the sequelae of kidney donation.

Objectives.—To compare the risk of ESRD in kidney donors with that of a healthy cohort of nondonors who are at equally low risk of renal disease and free of contraindications to live donation and to stratify these comparisons by patient demographics.

Design, Settings, and Participants.—A cohort of 96 217 kidney donors in the United States between April 1994 and November 2011 and a cohort of 20 024 participants of the Third National Health and Nutrition Examination Survey (NHANES III) were linked to Centers for Medicare & Medicaid Services data to ascertain development of ESRD, which was defined as the initiation of maintenance dialysis, placement on the waiting list, or receipt of a living or deceased donor kidney transplant, whichever was identified first. Maximum follow-up was 15.0 years; median follow-up was 7.6 years (interquartile range [IQR], 3.9-11.5 years) for kidney donors and 15.0 years (IQR, 13.7-15.0 years) for matched healthy nondonors.

Main Outcomes and Measures.—Cumulative incidence and lifetime risk of ESRD.

Results.—Among live donors, with median follow-up of 7.6 years (maximum, 15.0), ESRD developed in 99 individuals in a mean (SD) of 8.6 (3.6) years after donation. Among matched healthy nondonors, with median follow-up of 15.0 years (maximum, 15.0), ESRD developed in 36 nondonors in 10.7 (3.2) years, drawn from 17 ESRD events in the unmatched healthy nondonor pool of 9364. Estimated risk of ESRD at 15 years after donation was 30.8 per 10 000 (95% CI, 24.3-38.5) in kidney donors and 3.9 per 10 000 (95% CI, 0.8-8.9) in their matched healthy nondonor counterparts ($P < .001$). This difference was observed in both black and white individuals, with an estimated risk of 74.7 per 10 000 black donors (95% CI, 47.8-105.8) vs 23.9 per 10 000 black nondonors (95% CI, 1.6-62.4; $P < .001$) and an estimated risk of 22.7 per 10 000 white donors (95% CI, 15.6-30.1) vs 0.0 white nondonors ($P < .001$). Estimated lifetime risk of ESRD was 90 per 10 000 donors, 326 per 10 000 unscreened nondonors (general population), and 14 per 10 000 healthy nondonors.

Conclusions and Relevance.—Compared with matched healthy nondonors, kidney donors had an increased risk of ESRD over a median of 7.6 years; however, the magnitude of the absolute risk increase was small. These findings may help inform discussions with persons considering live kidney donation.

▶ This article addresses another major risk for the live donor: the risk of developing end-stage renal disease (ESRD). Using large databases, the authors determined that there was an increased risk of requiring therapy for ESRD in the group of individuals having previously donated a kidney. In matched individuals in separate databases, the 15-year ESRD risk for kidney donors was 0.3%, and for matched nonkidney donors was 0.04%. There were differences attributed to the ethnicity of the donor. Although there are differences in the datasets, they did not match the kidney donors to nondonors with family members having renal disease (or at least in proportion to numbers of related donors). Although flawed in many ways, this analysis provides useful information for discussion with potential donors. It is disingenuous for transplant teams to tell healthy people that removing one kidney is inconsequential to the risk of renal failure. The risk for the nondonating matched population is probably higher than that reported in this report because of "genes." However, it is helpful to have a number to give when telling those that pass the donor screening that they have a low risk for kidney failure and even losing a kidney; It is still about 10-fold lower than that of the general population.

T. L. Pruett, MD

Emotional Well-Being of Living Kidney Donors: Findings From the RELIVE Study

Jowsey SG, the RELIVE Study Group (Mayo Clinic, Rochester, MN; et al)
Am J Transplant 14:2535-2544, 2014

Following kidney donation, short-term quality of life outcomes compare favorably to US normative data but long-term effects on mood are not known. In the Renal and Lung Living Donors Evaluation Study (RELIVE), records from donations performed 1963–2005 were reviewed for depression and antidepressant use predonation. Postdonation, in a cross-sectional cohort design 2010–2012, donors completed the Patient Health Questionnaire (PHQ-9) depression screening instrument, the Life Orientation Test-Revised, 36-Item Short Form Health Survey and donation experience questions. Of 6909 eligible donors, 3470 were contacted and 2455 participated (71%). The percent with depressive symptoms (8%; PHQ-9>10) was similar to National Health and Nutrition Examination Survey participants (7%, $p = 0.30$). Predonation psychiatric disorders were more common in unrelated than related donors ($p = 0.05$). Postdonation predictors of depressive symptoms included nonwhite race (OR $= 2.00$, $p = 0.020$), younger age at donation (OR $= 1.33$ per 10 years, $p = 0.002$), longer recovery time from donation (OR $= 1.74$, $p = 0.0009$), greater financial burden (OR $= 1.32$, $p - 0.013$) and feeling morally obligated to donate (OR $= 1.23$, $p = 0.003$). While cross-sectional prevalence of depression is comparable to population normative data, some factors identifiable around time of donation, including longer recovery, financial stressors, younger age and moral obligation to donate may identify donorsmore likely to develop future depression, providing an opportunity for intervention.

▶ This article addresses one of the major psychological complications associated with live kidney donation—depression. From a large group of past live donors, a standardized series of demographic and psychological questions were asked. The self-reported incidence of significant postdonation depression was 8% in the group with a history of depressive symptoms before donation, twice the rate of the group without such history. Additionally, being younger at the time of donation, having a prolonged time to recovery, donating as a sense of duty, and ethnic minority added to risk for postdonation depression. Even though this was a large population, relatively few individuals self-reported the outcome. Also, the composition of current live kidney donors differs significantly from that of the study group, with more unrelated donors and virtually all donation procedures being performed laparoscopically. Still, this article highlights that undergoing an operation can have significant psychological consequences and identifies a group of individuals that are predisposed to have significant depressive symptoms. Inclusion of psychological surveillance tools in routine postdonation follow-up may be useful in managing known and predictable deleterious events.

T. L. Pruett, MD

Economic Consequences Incurred by Living Kidney Donors: A Canadian Multi-Center Prospective Study

Klarenbach S, Gill JS, Knoll G, et al (Inst of Health Economics, Edmonton, Alberta, Canada; Univ of British Columbia, Vancouver, Canada; Univ of Ottawa, Ontario, Canada; et al)
Am J Transplant 14:916-922, 2014

Some living kidney donors incur economic consequences as a result of donation; however, these costs are poorly quantified. We developed a framework to comprehensively assess economic consequences from the donor perspective including out-of-pocket cost, lost wages and home productivity loss. We prospectively enrolled 100 living kidney donors from seven Canadian centers between 2004 and 2008 and collected and valued economic consequences ($CAD 2008) at 3 months and 1 year after donation. Almost all (96%) donors experienced economic consequences, with 94% reporting travel costs and 47% reporting lost pay. The average and median costs of lost pay were $2144 (SD 4167) and $0 (25th–75th percentile 0, 2794), respectively. For other expenses (travel, accommodation, medication and medical), mean and median costs were $1780 (SD 2504) and $821 (25th–75th percentile 242, 2271), respectively. From the donor perspective, mean cost was $3268 (SD 4704); one-third of donors incurred cost >$3000, and 15% >$8000. The majority of donors (83%) reported inability to perform usual household activities for an average duration of 33 days; 8% reported out-of-pocket costs for assistance with these activities. The economic impact of living kidney donation for some individuals is large. We advocate for programs to reimburse living donors for their legitimate costs.

▶ It has been a general premise that a live kidney donor should not incur financial loss in addition to risk (actual or potential) and pain associated with the donor nephrectomy. The costs of evaluation, hospitalization, and follow-up are covered under most standard medical processes and not the responsibility of the donor. However, significant nonmedical costs are not routinely assessed or reimbursed under current live-donation systems. This prospective analysis of 100 live Canadian donors provides scope of financial losses in a series of kidney donors. The negative financial impact of being an organ donor is significant. Although the mean out-of-pocket and lost wages was $3268, 15% of live donors had losses of greater than $8000 in costs/lost revenue. This report used the donor's recollection regarding financial impact and not actual receipts. What was not measured in this study was the financial impact on total family income, accounting for time off work for those closely involved with the donor's operation and recovery. The financial impact of organ donation has considerable variability but is a significant barrier toward live donation. This study begins to put numbers to the obvious.

T. L. Pruett, MD

Long-Term Kidney Allograft Survival in Patients With Transplant Glomerulitis

Nabokow A, Dobronravov VA, Khrabrova M, et al (Nephrology Ctr of Lower Saxony, Hann. Muenden, Germany; 1st St. Petersburg Pavlov State Med Univ, Russian Federation; et al)
Transplantation 99:331-339, 2015

Background.—Renal transplant glomerulitis (G) is associated with acute antibody-mediated rejection (ABMR) in the presence of donor-specific antibodies. However, the long-term prognosis of isolated G (isG) in the absence of donor-specific antibodies or G in combination with T cell–mediated rejection (TCMR) remains unexplored.

Methods.—Seventy recipients with G were included in this retrospective study and subdivided into 3 groups: isG, G with TCMR (G + TCMR), and G with acute ABMR. The control groups were: patients with TCMR Banff type I or II without G (TCMR) and patients without rejection (NR). Kaplan-Meier death-censored survival plots and Cox regression were used to analyze graft survival. The combined graft survival endpoint was defined as a return to dialysis or estimated glomerular filtration rate less than 15 mL/min/1.73 m^2. The median follow-up was 37 (14; 77) months from biopsy.

Results.—Graft survival was significantly lower in patients with G than in the NR and TCMR groups. No significant differences were observed among the isG, G + TCMR, and ABMR groups. Graft survival was lower in the G + TCMR group than in the TCMR group. Glomerulitis was independently associated with the risk of adverse graft outcome in a multivariate Cox regression model adjusted for other confounders (hazard ratio, 4.52 [95% confidence interval, 2.37-8.68] vs controls; $P < 0.001$).

Conclusions.—Glomerulitis is strongly associated with increased risk of graft failure. Graft survival in patients with isG that do not meet the Banff criteria for acute/active ABMR and in patients with G accompanying TCMR is comparable to the ABMR group.

▶ Barriers to long-term kidney survival after kidney transplantation are many. In this single-center series, the impact of biopsy-demonstrated glomerulitis was assessed, irrespective of donor-specific antibody, association with T-cell rejection, or an isolated glomerulitis. The authors found that irrespective of associated pathology, glomerulitis was a poor prognostic finding. Fortunately, the percentage of kidney recipients with any form of glomerulitis was less than 10%. Although an early differential in outcome was seen (antibody-mediated rejection worse than glomerulitis with T-cell-mediated rejection worse than glomerulitis alone), after 7 years all patients had equally poor outcomes—significantly different than those of the nonglomerulitis groups.

Vascular inflammation within the glomerulus of a kidney transplant is a poor prognostic finding. The finding begs that effective strategies be generated.

Finding ways to maintain kidney function over the years demands understanding of a diverse biology.

T. L. Pruett, MD

Market Competition Influences Renal Transplantation Risk and Outcomes
Adler JT, Sethi RKV, Yeh H, et al (Brigham and Women's Hosp, Boston, MA; Massachusetts General Hosp, Boston; et al)
Ann Surg 260:550-557, 2014

Objective.—To evaluate the impact of market competition on patient mortality and graft failure after kidney transplantation.

Background.—Kidneys are initially allocated within 58 donation service areas (DSAs), which have varying numbers of transplant centers. Market competition is generally considered beneficial.

Methods.—The Scientific Registry of Transplant Recipients database was queried and the Herfindahl-Hirschman index (HHI), a measure of market competition, was calculated for each DSA from 2003 to 2012. Receipt of low-quality kidneys (Kidney Donor Profile Index ≥ 85) was modeled with multivariable logistic regression, and Cox proportional hazards models were created for graft failure and patient mortality.

Results.—A total of 127,355 adult renal transplants were performed. DSAs were categorized as 7 no (HHI = 1), 17 low (HHI − 0.52–0.97), 17 medium (HHI = 0.33–0.51), or 17 high (HHI = 0.09–0.32) competition. For deceased donor kidney transplantation, increasing market competition was significantly associated with mortality [hazard ratio (HR): 1.11, $P = 0.01$], graft failure (HR: 1.18, $P = 0.0001$), and greater use of low-quality kidneys (odds ratio = 1.39, $P < 0.0001$). This was not true for living donor kidney transplantation (mortality HR: 0.94, $P = 0.48$; graft failure HR: 0.99, $P = 0.89$). Competition was associated with longer waitlists ($P = 0.04$) but not with the number of transplants per capita in a DSA ($P = 0.21$).

Conclusions.—Increasing market competition is associated with increased patient mortality and graft failure and the use of riskier kidneys. These results may represent more aggressive transplantation and tolerance of greater risk for patients who otherwise have poor alternatives. Market competition should be better studied to ensure optimal outcomes.

▶ The authors make an interesting interpretation of data surrounding national experience with kidney transplantation. Through an analysis of the numbers of transplant centers in a specific organ distribution area, use of kidneys, recipient survival, and average quality of organs, the authors concluded that increased numbers of competing transplant centers for existing deceased donor kidneys led to use of lesser quality kidneys and inferior outcomes. Although this may be true in a simplistic evaluation, virtually every study comparing dialysis with transplantation with a spectrum of quality kidneys has shown a survival benefit. More than half of all the kidney transplants performed in the United States occur in the high-competition areas, and an argument could be made that more availability should exist for the person with end-stage renal disease. In this study, the authors should have done an intent-to-treat survival analysis of dialysis vs transplantation. The conclusion would probably have been different in that additional life-years would have been greater with transplantation over dialysis for virtually all potential kidney function. Survival certainly would be improved if all recipients had received a kidney with high potential function. However, this is not the state of organ availability in the United States. Virtually all kidneys must be used, as the benefit outweighs the risk of staying on dialysis without a transplant.

T. L. Pruett, MD

Split Liver Transplantation Using Hemiliver Graft in the MELD Era: A Single Center Experience in the United States
Hashimoto K, Quintini C, Aucejo FN, et al (Cleveland Clinic, OH)
Am J Transplant 14:2072-2080, 2014

Under the "sickest first" Model for End-Stage Liver Disease (MELD) allocation, livers amenable to splitting are most often allocated to patients unsuitable for split liver transplantation (SLT). Our experience with SLT using hemilivers was reviewed. From April 2004 to June 2012, we used 25 lobar grafts (10 left lobes and 15 right lobes) for adult-sized recipients. Twelve recipients were transplanted with primary offers, and 13 were transplanted with leftover grafts. Six grafts were shared with other centers. The data were compared with matched whole liver grafts (n = 121). In 92% of donors, the livers were split *in situ*. Hemiliver recipients with severe portal hypertension had a greater graft-torecipient weight ratio than those without severe portal hypertension (1.96% vs. 1.40%, $p < 0.05$). Hemiliver recipients experienced biliary complications more frequently (32.0% vs. 10.7%, $p = 0.01$); however, the 5-year graft survival for hemilivers was comparable to whole livers (80.0% vs. 81.5%, $p = 0.43$). The secondary recipients with leftover grafts did not have increased incidences of graft failure ($p = 0.99$) or surgical complications ($p = 0.43$) compared to the primary recipients. In conclusion, while routine application is still controversial due to various challenges, hemiliver SLT can achieve excellent outcomes under the MELD allocation.

▶ In an era of insufficient quantity of livers available for those waiting, methods to increase numbers of organs become increasingly important. The prospect of transplanting two individuals from a single deceased donor liver is an attractive option. The Cleveland Clinic is a busy program with experience in all facets of the procedure. It is surprising that only 25 adults benefited from hemiliver transplantation. In fact, only 48 of 1089 deceased donor liver transplants done over the 8-year period were split grafts. This is illustrative of the limitations of split livers to address the needs of adults. The reported results are comparable to those of full-sized grafts, with the expected increased biliary complications.

However long-term patient survival is identical to that seen with a complete liver. Although numbers of split livers transplanted should increase as the experience with live liver transplantation is reestablished in the United States, it is unlikely that a serious impact on wait list morbidity and mortality will occur because of limited numbers of organs suitable to split.

T. L. Pruett, MD

Perioperative Complications After Live-Donor Hepatectomy

Hall EC, Boyarsky BJ, Deshpande NA, et al (Johns Hopkins Univ School of Medicine, Baltimore, MD; et al)
JAMA Surg 149:288-291, 2014

Current studies of complications following donor hepatectomy may not be generalizable to all hospitals performing this procedure. To address this, live liver donors were identified in the Nationwide Inpatient Sample (2000-2008). Complications after donor hepatectomy were categorized using *International Classification of Diseases, Ninth Revision* codes and risk factors for complications were tested using logistic regression. Negative binomial regression models were used to estimate the increase in length of stay and hospital charge associated with complications. Among 555 donors (representing 2783 donors nationwide), 23% had 1 or more complications and 5% had a major complication. The most common complications were ileus (27%) and atelectasis (26%). No patient or hospital factors were associated with complications. Having any complication was associated with increased length of stay (incidence rate ratio, 1.36; 95% CI, 1.16-1.58; $P < .001$) and hospital charge (incidence rate ratio, 1.25; 95% CI, 1.09-1.44; $P = .002$). Approximately 25% of liver donors have complications immediately postoperatively but most are minor, lending support to current practices in live liver donation and donor selection.

▶ Information about a procedure is essential for adequate informed consent. This is particularly true when the proposed procedure is for organ donation. In the latter case, the potential donor will derive no therapeutic value from undergoing a major operative procedure, so he or she should understand the consequences of the procedure to make a good decision about whether to proceed with the donation. This report queried the Nationwide Inpatient Sample database for outcomes from donor hepatectomy. A total of 555 living liver donors were identified and International Classification of Diseases, Ninth Revision codes queried for the donation hospitalization. This is an interesting methodology to attempt validation of either single-center or study reports. The authors found that the incidence of complications was a bit less than that of self-reporting (23 vs 38% in Adult-to-Adult Living Donor Liver Transplantation Cohort Study). This represents the differences between how coders and researchers code events. Most adverse events were classified as Clavien grade 1 or 2. The significant finding in this report is the failure to find biliary complications or leaks in the donors. In large part, it is a methodologic issue: Often donor leaks are found after the initial hospitalization. The leaks occur because of ischemia or necrosis of the suture lines or sloughing of relatively ischemic areas of liver along the transection line. The importance of this report is in a random sampling of US live donations that coded complications, although occurring in greater than 1 in 5 donors, they are for the most part minor. The true complication rate is obviously higher, as a small percentage of donors are readmitted. This is an interesting report about what the outside observer (hospital coder) sees during the donation hospitalization.

T. L. Pruett, MD

Donor morbidity in right and left hemiliver living donor liver transplantation: the impact of graft selection and surgical innovation on donor safety

Iwasaki J, Iida T, Mizumoto M, et al (Kyoto Univ, Japan)
Transpl Int 27:1205-1213, 2014

This study investigated adequate liver graft selection for donor safety by comparing postoperative donor liver function and morbidity between the right and left hemilivers (RL and LL, respectively) of living donors. Between April 2006 and March 2012, RL (n = 168) and LL (n = 140) donor operations were performed for liver transplantation at Kyoto University Hospital. Postoperative hyperbilirubinemia and coagulopathy persisted in RL donors, whereas the liver function of LL donors normalized more rapidly. The overall complication rate of the RL donors was significantly higher than that of the LL donors (59.5% vs. 30.7%; $P < 0.001$). There were no significant differences in severe complications worse than Clavien grade IIIa or in biliary complication rates between the two donor groups. In April 2006, we introduced an innovative surgical procedure: hilar dissection preserving the blood supply to the bile duct during donor hepatectomy. Compared with our previous outcomes (1990-2006), the biliary complication rate of the RL donors decreased from 12.2% to 7.2%, and the severity of these complications was significantly lower. In conclusion, LL donors demonstrated good recovery in postoperative liver function and lower morbidity, and our surgical innovations reduced the severity of biliary complications in living donors.

▶ Live liver donation is becoming a necessity in areas of the country where average MELD at transplantation is high or death on the wait list is too high. A basic premise of the operation is to do the minimum to produce a reliable favorable outcome for the liver recipient. In the adult liver transplant experience described in this article, left lobe grafts resulted in fewer donor complications and a more prompt return of liver function than removal of the right lobe. The major discriminator regarding who was chosen to receive a right or left lobe graft was the sex of the recipient. Women recipients received more than 70% of the left lobe grafts and men approximately the same for right lobe grafts. The graft/recipient weight was significantly lower in left lobe grafts, despite the left lobe recipients in this report being on average 10 kg less than the right lobe recipients. Certainly a left hepatectomy is less morbid for the donor, however, if the intent of donation is to give sufficient liver mass to support the recipient. The optimal approach requires discernment of the minimal amount of liver needed to produce a reliably favorable outcome. After that is obtained, the donor surgeon should perform the least morbid operation to obtain a sufficiently sized graft—optimally a left lobe if feasible.

T. L. Pruett, MD

Morphometric Age and Mortality After Liver Transplant

Waits SA, Kim EK, Terjimanian MN, et al (Univ of Michigan Med School, Ann Arbor; et al)
JAMA Surg 149:335-340, 2014

Importance.—Morphometric assessment has emerged as a strong predictor of postoperative morbidity and mortality. However, a gap exists in translating this knowledge to bedside decision making. We introduced a novel measure of patient-centered surgical risk assessment: morphometric age.

Objective.—To investigate the relationship between morphometric age and posttransplant survival.

Data Sources.—Medical records of recipients of deceased-donor liver transplants (study population) and kidney donors/trauma patients (morphometric age control population).

Study Selection.—A retrospective cohort study of 348 liver transplant patients and 3313 control patients. We assessed medical records for validated morphometric characteristics of aging (psoas area, psoas density, and abdominal aortic calcification). We created a model (stratified by sex) for a morphometric age equation, which we then calculated for the control population using multivariate linear regression modeling (covariates). These models were then applied to the study population to determine each patient's morphometric age.

Data Extraction and Synthesis.—All analytic steps related to measuring morphometric characteristics were obtained via custom algorithms programmed into commercially available software. An independent observer confirmed all algorithm outputs. Trained assistants performed medical record review to obtain patient characteristics.

Results.—Cox proportional hazards regression model showed that morphometric age was a significant independent predictor of overall mortality (hazard ratio, 1.03 per morphometric year [95% CI, 1.02-1.04; $P < .001$]) after liver transplant. Chronologic age was not a significant covariate for survival (hazard ratio, 1.02 per year [95% CI, 0.99-1.04; $P = .21$]). Morphometric age stratified patients at high and low risk for mortality. For example, patients in the middle chronologic age tertile who jumped to the oldest morphometric tertile have worse outcomes than those who jumped to the youngest morphometric tertile (74.4% vs 93.2% survival at 1 year [$P = .03$]; 45.2% vs 75.0% at 5 years [$P = .03$]).

Conclusions and Relevance.—Morphometric age correlated with mortality after liver transplant with better discrimination than chronologic age. Assigning a morphometric age to potential liver transplant recipients could improve prediction of postoperative mortality risk.

▶ Similar to the frailty measure study, this study attempts to correlate recipient muscle mass with survival. In this instance, it was after the transplant has occurred. The authors found that individuals with muscle wasting, associated with a higher morphometric age, were more likely to die after liver transplantation than with a morphometric age approximating the actual chronologic age. As in the frailty report, the important analysis resides in how much of the morphometric age is reversible? If it possible to improve the outcomes of individuals on the wait list through exercise and nutrition, then strategies need to be developed to improve outcomes. If morphometric age is fixed, it is not suggested that one should let these individuals die, unless prognosis reaches the definition of futility, a conclusion that is not suggested. There is general recognition that prognosis after liver transplantation is not homogeneous, and strategies to better stratify patients would be beneficial. The role of functional measures as frailty or objective morphometrics is still being worked out.

T. L. Pruett, MD

Prevalence, Incidence and Risk Factors for Donor-Specific Anti-HLA Antibodies in Maintenance Liver Transplant Patients
Del Bello A, Congy-Jolivet N, Muscari F, et al (CHU Rangueil, Toulouse, France; Université Paul Sabatier, Toulouse, France; et al)
Am J Transplant 14:867-875, 2014

Although large retrospective studies have identified the presence of donor-specific antibodies (DSAs) to be a risk factor for rejection and impaired survival after liver transplantation, the long-term predicted pathogenic potential of individual DSAs after liver transplantation remains unclear. We investigated the incidence, prevalence and consequences of DSAs in maintenance liver transplant (LT) recipients. Two hundred sixty-seven LT recipients, who had undergone transplantation at least 6 months previously and had been screened for DSAs at least twice using single-antigen bead technology, were included and tested annually for the presence of DSAs. At a median of 51 months (min—max: 6—220) after an LT, 13% of patients had DSAs. At a median of 36.5 months (min—max: 2—45) after the first screening, 9% of patients have developed *de novo* DSAs. The sole predictive factor for the emergence of *de novo* DSAs was retransplantation (OR 3.75; 95% CI 1.28—11.05, $p = 0.025$). Five out of 21 patients with *de novo* DSAs (23.8%) developed an antibody-mediated rejection. Fibrosis score was higher among patients with DSAs. In conclusion, monitoring for the development of DSAs in maintenance LT patients is useful in case of graft dysfunction and to identify patients with a high risk of developing liver fibrosis.

▶ The role of the humoral response in liver transplantation is starting to take a turn. For years, the mantra has been that antibodies directed against alloantigens on the donor liver are of no significant clinical consequence. Over the last several years, there have been reports that challenge that supposition. This report supports the notion that long-term consequences of a humoral immune response generated against the donor liver may be detrimental. Although this may seem intuitive, it has not been accepted transplantation for the presence of antibodies directed against donor antigens. The authors did not have information about whether these antibodies had formed before the transplant event (in keeping with the supposition that such antibodies were irrelevant, so why measure them?). In assessing 267 liver recipients, it was found that 35 (13%) had donor-specific antibody(ies) (DSA) during the stable/maintenance phase of the transplant experience. Ten of these patients lost the alloantibody and became free of DSA. DSA developed in 21 of 232 individuals who on first screen did not have donor antibody. Antibody that was more likely to persist was directed against class II major histocompatibility complex and had high mean fluorescence intensity. Patients that had DSA had an increased fibrosis score on liver biopsy, suggesting that the immune response was somehow damaging the liver graft. The only predictive factor for those that had new acquisition of DSA was having a prior liver transplant. There is increasing interest of the immune response to liver allografts, and most likely there will be a measureable clinical outcome that is associated with the development of a humoral response to the allograft.

T. L. Pruett, MD

Increasing Age and Survival after Orthotopic Liver Transplantation for Patients with Hepatocellular Cancer

Kim J, Ko ME, Nelson RA, et al (City of Hope Comprehensive Cancer Ctr, Duarte, CA; et al)
J Am Coll Surg 218:431-438, 2014

Background.—Orthotopic liver transplantation (OLT) is the gold standard treatment for patients with early hepatocellular carcinoma (HCC). There are concerns about the efficacy of OLT for HCC in older patients, who we hypothesized might have poorer outcomes. Therefore, we sought to examine advanced age and its impact on OLT outcomes.

Study Design.—The United Network for Organ Sharing database was queried for patients who underwent OLT for HCC from 1987 to 2009. Patients were divided into 3 age groups: 35 to 49 years old, 50 to 64 years old, and 65 years or older, and patient characteristics were compared. Univariate and multivariate analyses were performed to assess the impact of age on OLT outcomes.

Results.—Of 10,238 patients with OLT for HCC, 16.5% (n = 1,688) of patients were 35 to 49 years old, 67.8% (n = 6,937) were 35 to 49 years old, and 15.8% (n = 1,613) were 65 years and older. By Kaplan-Meier method, the 50- to 64-year-old age group had the highest overall survival, despite having one of the highest rates of hepatitis C positivity (70%), but this group also had the lowest rate of diabetes mellitus (8.7%). The lowest overall survival was observed in the 65-year or older age group (*p* < 0.001). Finally, there was no difference in disease-specific survival among the age groups (*p* = 0.858), and patients aged 65 years and older had the highest rate of death from nonhepatic causes (17.5%).

Conclusions.—Although OS was prolonged in younger patients who underwent OLT for HCC, there was no observed difference in disease-specific survival among the age groups. Our results suggest that carefully selected patients 65 years of age and older can derive equal benefit from OLT for HCC when compared with their younger counterparts.

▶ Liver transplantation is the recognized best treatment for individuals with small hepatocellular carcinoma (HCCa). Currently, approximately 20% of donated livers are allocated to individuals with HCCa. There is ongoing debate regarding the right allocation weight to give individuals with HCCa. The current report attempts to address the issue by addressing outcomes in the elderly. It is projected that an ever-increasing number of individuals will get HCCa as they age. The question then becomes: What is the relative risk of tumor recurrence in the elderly population? The analysis of the United Network for Organ Sharing database did not show any difference in tumor recurrence with age. Although it is not surprising that the older population of liver recipients died with a greater frequency, the tumor-specific recurrence and attribution was not higher in the older age group. Those looking for easy ways to exclude the elderly are going to have to look past tumor recurrence.

T. L. Pruett, MD

Liver transplantation in highest acuity recipients: identifying factors to avoid futility
Petrowsky H, Rana A, Kaldas FM, et al (David Geffen School of Medicine at Univ of California, Los Angeles; Kaiser Permanente Los Angeles Med Ctr, CA)
Ann Surg 259:1186-1194, 2014

Objective.—To identify medical predictors of futility in recipients with laboratory Model of End-Stage Liver Disease (MELD) scores of 40 or more at the time of orthotopic liver transplantation (OLT).

Background.—Although the survival benefit for transplant patients with the highest MELD scores is indisputable, the medical and economic effort to bring these highest acuity recipients through OLT presents a major challenge for every transplant center.

Methods.—This study was undertaken to analyze outcomes in patients with MELD scores of 40 or more undergoing OLT during the period February 2002 to December 2010. The analysis was focused on futile outcome (3-month or in-hospital mortality) and long-term posttransplant outcome. Independent predictors of futility and failure-free survival were identified and a futility risk model was created.

Results.—During the study period, 1522 adult cadaveric OLTs were performed, and 169 patients (13%) had a MELD score of 40 or more. The overall 1, 3, 5, and 8-year patient survivals were 72%, 64%, 60%, and 56%. Futile outcome occurred in 37 patients (22%). MELD score, pretransplant septic shock, cardiac risk, and comorbidities were independent predictors of futile outcome. Using all 4 factors, the futility risk model had a good discriminatory ability (c-statistic 0.75). Recipient age per year, life-threatening postoperative complications, hepatitis C, and metabolic syndrome were independent predictors for long-term survival in nonfutile patients (Harrels c-statistic 0.72).

Conclusions.—Short- and long-term outcomes of recipients with MELD scores of 40 or more are primarily determined by disease-specific factors. Cardiac risk, pretransplant septic shock, and comorbidities are the most important predictors and can be used for risk stratification in these highest acuity recipients.

▶ The shortage of organs generates ethical dilemmas regarding who should or should not get a liver. Most individuals feel that transplanting an organ into an individual who is likely to die is not a good use of a transplantable organ. The authors sought to define which people met a reasonable definition of futility. The authors assessed wait-listed people with Model of End-Stage Liver Disease scores greater than 40 and assessed those who either died within 90 days or in the hospital. The authors derived variables that are consistent with experience. The real question is what constitutes futility. Not deriving the benefit of survival is the most fundamental element; however, it is likely that other definitions should be used. The authors bring up an extraordinarily important question that needs to be addressed by each program.

T. L. Pruett, MD

Frailty Predicts Waitlist Mortality in Liver Transplant Candidates

Lai JC, Feng S, Terrault NA, et al (Univ of California-San Francisco)
Am J Transplant 14:1870-1879, 2014

We aimed to determine whether frailty, a validated geriatric construct of increased vulnerability to physiologic stressors, predicts mortality in liver transplant candidates. Consecutive adult outpatients listed for liver transplant with laboratory Model for End-Stage Liver Disease (MELD) ≥12 at a single center (97% recruitment rate) underwent four frailty assessments: Fried Frailty, Short Physical Performance Battery (SPPB), Activities of Daily Living (ADL) and Instrumental ADL (IADL) scales. Competing risks models associated frailty with waitlist mortality (death/delisting for being too sick for liver transplant). Two hundred ninety-four listed liver transplant patients with MELD ≥12, median age 60 years and MELD 15 were followed for 12 months. By Fried Frailty score ≥3, 17% were frail; 11/51 (22%) of the frail versus 25/243 (10%) of the not frail died/were delisted ($p = 0.03$). Each 1-unit increase in the Fried Frailty score was associated with a 45% (95% confidence interval, 4−202) increased risk of waitlist mortality adjusted for MELD. Similarly, the adjusted risk of waitlist mortality associated with each 1-unit decrease (i.e. increasing frailty) in the Short Physical Performance Battery (hazard ratio 1.19, 95% confidence interval 1.07−1.32). Frailty is prevalent in liver transplant candidates. It strongly predicts waitlist mortality, even after adjustment for liver disease severity demonstrating the applicability and importance of the frailty construct in this population.

▶ People on a wait list for liver transplantation are, by definition, sick. However, there are varying degrees of disease. Frailty is an interesting measure that has been popularized in geriatrics literature. In this study, people who were being wait-listed for liver transplantation were ranked on a frailty score. Not surprisingly, those that were frailer fared less well than nonfrail. It was shown that the frailer the wait-listed patient, the risk of removal from the list or death was twice that of the nonfrail. This study is important not so much as to who should be excluded from waiting for transplantation but rather who should receive extra attention to minimize wait-list morbidity. Our system has much to learn regarding optimal management of people with chronic liver disease.

T. L. Pruett, MD

Impact of the Lung Allocation Score on Survival Beyond 1 Year
Maxwell BG, Levitt JE, Goldstein BA, et al (Stanford Univ School of Medicine, Stanford, CA; et al)
Am J Transplant 14:2288-2294, 2014

Implementation of the lung allocation score (LAS) in 2005 led to transplantation of older and sicker patients without altering 1-year survival. However, long-term survival has not been assessed and emphasizing the 1-year survival metric may actually sustain 1-year survival while not reflecting worsening longer-term survival. Therefore, we assessed overall and conditional 1-year survival; and the effect of crossing the 1-year threshold on hazard of death in three temporal cohorts: historical (1995−2000), pre-LAS (2001−2005) and post-LAS (2005−2010). One-year survival post-LAS remained similar to pre-LAS (83.1% vs. 82.1%) and better than historical controls (75%). Overall survival in the pre and post-LAS cohorts was also similar. However, long-term survival among patients surviving beyond 1 year was worse than pre-LAS and similar to historical controls. Also, the hazard of death increased significantly in months 13 (1.44, 95% CI 1.10–1.87) and 14 (1.43, 95% CI 1.09–1.87) post-LAS but not in the other cohorts. While implementation of the LAS has not reduced overall survival, decreased survival among patients surviving beyond 1 year in the post-LAS cohort and the increased mortality occurring immediately after 1 year suggest a potential negative long-term effect of the LAS and an unintended consequence of increased emphasis on the 1-year survival metric.

▶ The current transplant environment is one that is consumed with development of system approaches to outcomes after transplantation. We are routinely readjusting the allocation systems to make the ranking of individual candidates more transparent and fair. This article looks at the very real issue of what happens after 1 year from transplantation and finds that outcomes after lung transplantation have suffered. This discussion does not revolve around getting a candidate through a big procedure. Rather, it accounts for the fact that we want people to live for "quite a while" after the transplant experience. Although early survival was unchanged by changing the allocation schema, long-term results suffered. It is not the goal of the national allocation to only garner short-term benefit. Documentation is important for appropriate metrics.

T. L. Pruett, MD

6 Surgical Infections

Introduction

Infection after a surgical procedure is an unwanted event and has recently become a major focus for "quality" initiatives by government and other payers. One would hope that the major driver of this initiative is to improve the lives of those operated upon, but there is a significant economic element that pushes the anti-surgical infection agenda. The effect of infection upon operated individuals is significant, but very often the major element tracked by payers is the added resources that must be used in order to deal with an infectious event. Paper 1 is such a report, discussing outcomes after procedures performed at 129 VA hospitals in 2010. From the VA database, it was found that surgical site infection (SSI) increased costs by a factor of 1.43. A deep SSI was more expensive and had a cost increase of 1.93, whereas a superficial SSI was 1.25. Over 54 000 procedures were used to draw these conclusions; however, there are some things in the data that don't make much sense. The overall SSI rate was only 3%, despite reporting only 54.4% as clean cases. As will be seen later, this number is very low for surgical procedures with intraoperative contamination. Yes, infections are expensive, but the paper did not report the most fundamental cost, that of human life. Perioperative mortality in those with and without SSI should have been reported. One can surmise that mortality with an infectious complication was greater than those without SSI; however, from this report we only know costs for the VA are increased if a SSI is identified. It is suspected that the financial costs are much more stratified, as the cost of a superficial wound infection is the cost of labor and materials until skin closure has occurred. On the other extreme, infection resulting in mortality often includes ICU time, recurrent procedures, and an extensive pharmacy use. If one had analyzed the costs associated with those who died, the cost differential would have been much more substantial.

One of the attributes of modern healthcare change is the increasing public disclosure of performance metrics. This makes data accuracy and risk adjustment understanding mandatory, so that meaningful outcome comparisons are possible. Paper 2 explores some of the variables currently collected by the current American College of Surgeons, National Surgical Quality Improvement Program (ACS NSQIP). They demonstrated that quality/hospital rankings are not significantly altered if one excludes surgical wound classification. This seems more than counterintuitive, as the aggregate body of medical teaching and the data within the NSQIP database supports the fact that SSI rates increase as the amount of bacterial contamination increases. However, the huge numbers found in "big data" (over 440 000 procedures in this report) often obscure important variables, especially if a subset analysis demonstrates that wound classification is entered inconsistently. This was done with nephrectomy and demonstrated that, despite clear definitions, the data entered into the system appeared inconsistent with the reported outcomes. However, a major issue for hospital systems is the inconsistent use of entered data to produce outcome information. Methodology matters. Paper 3 demonstrates the impact of 2 different methodologies applied to the same patient population. Reported patient outcomes of the same patient population were compared from facilities reporting to both ACS NSQIP and the CDC National Healthcare Safety Network (NHSN). Despite using the same definition for SSI, the reported rates after colorectal procedures in the same population of patients were 5.7% for NHSN and 13.5% for ACS NSQIP. This difference would impact hospital rankings and quality reimbursement strategies (while delivering the same quality of care). The manuscript explains and discusses many of the methodological differences in data collection and manipulation. The importance for the reader is to recognize that 1) outcome data will be made public in the current era, 2) the methodology used to collect and present the "data" will greatly influence the incidence of seemingly equally defined outcomes, and 3) those who fail to recognize the impact of data management will be at a significant disadvantage in quality and payment systems.

Another theme in the surgical literature is about system efforts to address/reduce common problems. Accountability, system changes, and self-reporting are all thought to be fundamental to these process improvements (as touted for the airline industry). This approach has been applied to the prevention of surgical- and hospital-acquired infections, particularly ventilator-associated pneumonia and catheter-related blood stream infection. To study the various portions of the quality metrics, the VA system correlated outcomes with several of these process elements (paper 4). The VA system had introduced a "bundle" of specific preventive procedures to minimize the risk of these 2 hospital acquired infections, and from 2009 to 2011, the frequency of VAP and CR-BSI decreased across the VA system. Self-reported adherence to the "bundle" was not associated with diminished infection rates in the surgical intensive care facility. In fact, self-reported adherence to the "bundle" was negatively associated with these infections. In the airline industry, self-reporting is a central pillar of safety. It is unclear what role self-reporting has in quality maintenance. Did the reduction of these targeted infections result from implementation of "strategic bundles," or was the reduction a consequence of system recognition by an educated work force and implementation of other approaches? If the latter, establishment of quality process identifiers that facilitate system performance will not correlate with the outcome. This paper raises many interesting thoughts on process surveillance for prevention of undesired outcomes. Paper 5 is another report of the use of a "bundle" to address SSI. The authors were charged with reducing colorectal SSI after ACS NSQIP reported that the colorectal SSI at their institution was outside expected rates. In response, a "bundle" was developed and introduced for people undergoing colorectal procedures. The results were spectacular, with a SSI reduction of >300%. The authors attribute the reduction to the implemented bundle (chlorhexidine prep shower, mechanical and antibiotic bowel prep, IV antibiotic, wound protector...). The difficult part of this paper is not in the results, but in the rationale for the success of the methods. There is no compliance data or measures of adherence to the "bundle." Some of the implemented processes were designed to minimize skin/environmental contamination, others to eradicate contamination from the fecal flora. Presumably, the fecal flora modulation was the most predictive, but without assessment of adherence, adequacy of bowel prep, and other measures, it is impossible to attribute power to the processes. For efficiency measures, it is important to weed out inefficient "bundle" elements and focus only on those elements that result in major changes. Getting process measures right is a major challenge for any QAPI program. Another national agenda "quality" item is readmission after a surgical procedure. Again, the VA looked at their national database for insight (paper 6). From over 59 000 surgical procedures performed at 112 VA facilities, 11.9% of people were readmitted within 30 days of discharge. Over half of these admissions were for SSI. However, 28% of postoperative complications were recognized only after discharge had occurred. People with multiple comorbidities and complications recognized in the hospital were more likely to be readmitted, but there was wide variation. The existing data collection system was inefficient in identifying those individuals who would ultimately require hospitalization to manage perioperative events/complications. Discharge from the hospital was not a good endpoint for the absence of complications.

Surgeons have always touted that importance of technique is a major predictor of postoperative outcomes. The impact of technique can vary greatly by the predisposition of the viewer. A review of the ACS NSQIP database (paper 7) compared procedures performed using minimally invasive vs open surgical techniques. Not surprisingly, procedures that were performed through minimally invasive techniques had fewer surgical site infections. The authors used a propensity matching of comorbidities in order to balance the groups. However, as the authors chose institutions where minimally invasive surgery (MIS) was prevalent, the reader should query why an open technique was selected. Was there some anatomic or system reason why the procedure was performed open vs via MIS? The increased risk of SSI may well have superceded a greater risk associated with anatomic inability of an MIS approach, faulty equipment, or other such factors. One would think that in a center where both options are common and available that the average surgeon would choose the less-invasive modality to perform a procedure. To state that the open and MIS groups are equivalent patient populations is a bit incredulous. One can agree that doing a procedure with less manipulation is likely to result in lower rates of SSI, but it is not necessarily that one approach is superior to another, but what the variables are that make one approach superior to the other. The discussion should be more about when the choice of approach should favor a specific approach. Unfortunately, the database does not record those variables. Cigarette smoking is one of the major behavior variables that is often poorly collected and stratified in large databases. While the current trend is for less of the US population to smoke, still almost 20% of adults continue to smoke. Of those, about 80% smoke every day. What is the effect in large databases of not accurately stratifying for this variable? Paper 8 is a meta-analysis of the medical literature about cigarette smoking and surgical outcomes. The authors demonstrate a statistically significant increased propensity risk for wound complications and infections in those patients with a smoking history. But what should we tell our patients? For an elective surgical procedure, does the time of smoking cessation need to vary by duration and amount of cigarette smoking? How does one reliably risk stratify and validate the reliability of this important variable? Much of the current push toward "pay for performance" will be dramatically influenced by reliable and predictable outcome models. Existing databases that use billing and coding data have gaps in known important variables that must be understood by the practitioners.

The next 4 papers (9, 10, 11, and 12) are about surgical conduct of operative procedures and practical or theoretical impact upon SSI. Maintaining a barrier between bacteria on the surgeon and the patient wound has been a central tenet to prevent SSI since the time of Lister. Paper 9 measured bacteria on gown and gloves at various times in the conduct of joint replacement surgery. The study demonstrated that cloth gowns are more likely to become contaminated during the conduct of a clean operation and had almost universal penetrability to bacteria as compared to paper/disposable gowns. Interestingly, almost a quarter of operative gloves had bacteria identified on the palm after an hour of surgery. This was reduced almost in half by glove exchange. They recommended that only paper gowns be used in device surgery and that gloves be changed immediately prior to handling of the implant. Unfortunately, the authors did not comment upon the number of bacterial colonies identified, the infection rate, and whether there was a correlation between surgeon bacteria vs bacteria on the patient skin. Paper 10 purported to compare different skin preparation solutions and the specific role of isopropyl alcohol for effectiveness to prevent SSI. This was an interesting approach, as the procedures assessed were clean-contaminated procedures that should have had the major bacterial inoculum introduced into the wound through planned transgression into the patient's bacterial flora and not through skin contamination. The fact that no benefit was observed by the inclusion of alcohol with either chlorhexidine- or iodine-based skin antisepsis was not surprising. Skin preparation is important, but its contribution is proportional to the remaining numbers of bacteria in the surgical wound from all causes, skin often being a minor contributor. Paper 11 expands the barrier concept beyond the gloves and skin preparation to the notion of placing a sterile barrier between the skin, subcutaneous tissues, and fascia and the wound. The circular "wound protector," those sterile plastic barriers extending from below the fascia and extending well beyond the skin edges, has been hypothesized to be beneficial for decades. This paper reports the results of a randomized trial of circular wound edge protection (CWEP) vs standard towel blocking of a laparotomy wound. An overall benefit was seen with CWEP, but not in the case of clean laparotomy, where it would be expected to show no benefit. The benefit was fairly striking in the case of clean-contaminated and contaminated procedures giving credence to the concept that keeping bacteria to a minimum within the wound at the time of closure can reduce the risk of subsequent SSI. In keeping with the theme of minimizing bacteria within the wound, paper 12 addresses the role of the various elements of colon preparation and SSI prior to elective colorectal preparation. It is hard to believe that we continue to have to reinvent the premise that reduction of wound contamination is beneficial. Analyzing the elective colorectal procedures in the state of Michigan, the authors found that reduction of SSI was greatest when mechanical removal of fecal material and oral antibiotics were given prior to the colorectal procedure. What cannot be assessed is whether future innovations may result in reductions in wound contamination in the absence of the rigorous bowel preparation; however, in the absence of demonstrating such efficiency, mechanical preparation and oral antibiotics continues to be best practice.

The next series of papers is about individual patient predispositions and convention in the surgical management diseases. Unlike the results of homogenized "big data," paper 13 points out the heterogeneity of the individual patient to withstand stress. The authors looked for bacteria in mesenteric lymph nodes before and after esophagectomy. Those individuals with bacterial translocation after esophagectomy were more likely to experience postoperative infectious complications than individuals undergoing the procedure without translocation, without obvious differences in the patient populations with and without translocation. This paper raises many interesting observations, but the question is raised whether it is possible to predict and then alter this predisposition and if it would translate into less morbidity for the person undergoing the procedure. Host defenses are an important variable that must be characterized, and none of the "standard" variables collected accounted for the variance. The predisposition for infectious complications after splenectomy is thought to be relatively uniform. However, paper 14 assessed outcomes from the Swedish health registry and identified various predispositions for infectious complications after splenectomy. Those with traumatic splenectomy had less infectious morbidity than those where the spleen was removed for malignancy. Vaccination did not appear to alter the aggregate infectious morbidity, although the database did not capture the specific organisms within the vaccination profile. Not all diseases thought to be "surgical" infections are necessarily best treated by surgical intervention. Paper 15 readdresses management of acute appendicitis. While conservative management of acute appendicitis has been discussed for decades, the authors undertook a study of stratifying individuals seen for right lower quadrant pain to receive oral antibiotics and outpatient therapy. The conclusion was that 11.9% failed conservative management and required operative intervention within the first week. Another 10% required operation over the next 2 years, but 83% of individuals did not require an operation. It is easily to extrapolate that best therapy should start with the nonoperative approach with expectant management. Another bout of antibiotics was required for 13% of patients, but again the majority of patients were successfully treated with oral antibiotics alone. The outcomes in this study were excellent with no mortality and only one deep SSI. Predictive capacity for need of operative intervention could not be made by traditional signs and symptoms but was better with composite scores for appendicitis (Alvarado and Anderson scores). It is likely that many people were spared perioperative morbidities with this type of therapy algorithm. Paper 16 addresses a similar type of approach to acute diverticulitis, assessing need for operative intervention and recurrent readmissions. This study was not prospective, but rather a registry analysis of the Ontario health registry. Using coding discharge diagnosis, the authors assessed the group initially treated nonoperatively and with no planned surgery following resolution of acute diverticulitis. The 5-year need for readmission was 9%, and the need for operation was less than 2%. Complicated diverticular disease, abscess with percutaneous drainage, was more likely to result in need for operation than inflammation without significant abscess. However, the notion is given again that diseases once thought to mandate surgical intervention can have durable resolutions without surgical risks. Learning judgment on when a patient is best served by operative appendectomy, colectomy, or splenectomy is central to future medical understanding. Individual predisposition to complications and poor outcomes is central to optimal patient care.

The final series of papers looks at some of the translational research areas. While so much research has been about the patient, it is important to remember that the microbiome continues to adapt to the environment and is important for infection therapy. The current explosion of multidrug resistant organisms is a major manifestation of this problem. However, other specific "virulence" factors continue to play a role. Paper 17 looks at the organisms associated with *Clostridium difficile* colitis. The authors found that patients suffering from recurrent *C. difficile* colitis were more likely to be infected with an organism with binary toxin gene and *tcdC* gene mutations. This is particularly interesting in that the authors did not assess whether traits continued to be found in the bacteria associated with recurrences. It is unclear whether the toxin from the first infection lowers the infectious inoculum/changes the host environment for subsequent infection or is just more difficult to eradicate. Irrespective of the actual mechanism by which recurrent colitis is induced, the important message is that there is a significant bacterial influence upon the propensity for recurrence. One of the intriguing issues surrounding serious injury is the interplay between the microbiome and the injured host. Paper 18 addresses burn injury, antibiotics, and bacteria. In this model, burn injury was associated with increased bacteria within the gut. Treatment with antimicrobial agents decreased the numbers of bacteria, but increased translocation, gut permeability, and impaired phagocytic capacity of cells in the gut mucosa and pulmonary alveoli. The authors demonstrated physiologic and immunologic interactions between stress and rapid changes in gut bacterial population. It was not clear if the products of bacterial death or other factors were the causative agents in this phenomenon. The authors demonstrated that suspending dead bacteria in the animal drinking water markedly reduced the antibiotic-induced alterations. In many respects, this paper answers very few questions but exposes the breadth of mammalian changes induced by burn stress and the significant impact of a "simple" intervention-like antibiotic therapy. How dead bacteria affect the gut or immune system to modify the measured outcomes is uncertain. This article reemphasizes the complexity of the interactions between stress and infection and how much more work needs to be done to understand the changes. Paper 19 goes a bit deeper into changes induced by stress, looking at changes in amino acids in T cells. The authors assessed the effect of stress (laparotomy) upon T cell arginine in mice. They demonstrated that the decrease in intracellular arginine was coincident with an increase in myeloid-derived suppressor cells of arginase 1. The authors performed a variety of arginase 1 inhibition and passive transfer studies to demonstrate a correlation between these cells and an impaired ability to control infection. It is unclear how the immunologic effects addressed in the last 2 chapters are related, but one would surmise that the degree of immunologic impact would vary by the degree of stress/infection in both magnitude and duration of change. There are many adaptive and/or potentially injurious physiologic and immunologic responses induced in the infected/injured mammal that will eventually need reconciliation or at least unified understanding. The plethora of information relating to infection, stress, and immunity is staggering and often conflicting. In order to end with the diversity of human patients, paper 20 describes patients admitted to a trauma ICU, who were assessed for genetic variation in the *TLR1* gene. The authors found that 2 of the *TLR1* gene polymorphisms were associated with an increased risk of infection and mortality. This is not an unexpected finding, as the innate immune system is central to stress and injury responses. However, causality for this finding is lacking in this report. Gene studies are remarkably sensitive as they impact an individual's life, insurability, and family, and the findings of this study need to be confirmed before assuming the findings veracity. Even if the conclusion is true, rather than stating that the subset population with these genes are doomed to have worse outcomes, it is the role of physicians to discern whether alternative delivery of care could avoid the observed morbidity and mortality.

We are living in a peculiar age. The era of "big data" is transforming healthcare into an industrial business model. The problem with this approach is that necessary "data" for predictive outcomes is remarkably fluid and not currently available. Drawing conclusions from large data sets is fraught with risk for missing very important information. Technology produces change in outcomes, and the prediction of the impact of those changes from existing models is exceedingly low. Surgical infections are going to continue to be outcomes that are measured within the government, payment, and quality systems. Data should be accurate, and the management of the information generated is essential for all publicly released information. However, patients should be given "best care" irrespective of projection models and current observations.

Timothy L. Pruett, MD

Glove and Gown Effects on Intraoperative Bacterial Contamination
Ward WG Sr, Cooper JM, Lippert D, et al (Wake Forest Univ Health Sciences, Winston Salem, NC; Wexner Med Ctr at The Ohio State Univ, Columbus; Univ of Wisconsin School of Medicine and Public Health, Madison; et al)
Ann Surg 259:591-597, 2014

Objective.—Experiments were performed to determine the risk of bacterial contamination associated with changing outer gloves and using disposable spunlace paper versus reusable cloth gowns.

Background.—Despite decades of research, there remains a lack of consensus regarding certain aspects of optimal aseptic technique including outer glove exchange while double-gloving and surgical gown type selection.

Methods.—In an initial glove study, 102 surgical team members were randomized to exchange or retain outer gloves 1 hour into clean orthopedic procedures; cultures were obtained 15 minutes later from the palm of the surgeon's dominant gloved hand and from the surgical gown sleeve. Surgical gown type selection was recorded. A laboratory strike-through study investigating bacterial transmission through cloth and paper gowns was performed with coagulase-negative staphylococci. In a follow-up glove study, 251 surgical team members, all wearing paper gowns, were randomized as in the first glove study.

Results.—Glove study 1 revealed 4-fold higher levels of baseline bacterial contamination (31% vs 7%) on the sleeve of surgical team members wearing cloth gowns than those using paper gowns [odds ratio (95% confidence interval): 4.64 (1.72—12.53); $P = 0.0016$]. The bacterial strike-through study revealed that 26 of 27 cloth gowns allowed bacterial transmission through the material compared with 0 of 27 paper gowns ($P < 0.001$). In glove study 2, surgeons retaining outer gloves 1 hour into the case had a subsequent positive glove contamination rate of 23% compared with 13%

among surgeons exchanging their original outer glove [odds ratio (95% confidence interval): 1.97 (1.02–3.80); $P = 0.0419$].

Conclusions.—Paper gowns demonstrated less bacterial transmission in the laboratory and lower rates of contamination in the operating room. Disposable paper gowns are recommended for all surgical cases, especially those involving implants, because of the heightened risk of infection. Outer glove exchange just before handling implant materials is also recommended to minimize intraoperative contamination.

▶ A premise of aseptic technique is to place barriers between the bacterial flora of the operating team and the patient wound. The usual manner in which this is performed is gown and gloves for the operating team. With the implantation of mechanical devices, prevention of device infection takes on great significance. Often teams exchange gloves immediately before implantation of prosthetic devices. The purpose of this article was to discern bacterial retrieval from the surgeon's sleeve and palm during retention or exchange of gloves in the performance of a clean orthopedic case. The initial finding that was striking for the rate of sleeve contamination was associated with reusable, cloth gowns. Cloth gowns rapidly lost the ability to serve as a barrier for bacteria with bacterial penetrance of 96% on a strike-through test (compared with 0% for disposable gowns). Less convincing was the finding that glove exchange resulted in a lower frequency of positive cultures from the hand of the surgeon. Fortunately, these findings are intuitively consistent, such that the final recommendation that surgeons only wear disposable gowns and put on clean gloves immediately prior to handling/implanting a surgical device seems sound. It would have been more convincing had the authors reported whether any of the implanted devices became infected and if there was any correlation with bacterial inoculum on the operative team.

T. L. Pruett, MD

Comparative Effectiveness of Skin Antiseptic Agents in Reducing Surgical Site Infections: A Report from the Washington State Surgical Care and Outcomes Assessment Program
Hakkarainen TW, for the Surgical Care and Outcomes Assessment Program Collaborative (Univ of Washington Med Ctr, Seattle; et al)
J Am Coll Surg 218:336-344, 2014

Background.—Surgical site infections (SSI) are an important source of morbidity and mortality. Chlorhexidine in isopropyl alcohol is effective in preventing central venous-catheter associated infections, but its effectiveness in reducing SSI in clean-contaminated procedures is uncertain. Surgical studies to date have had contradictory results. We aimed to further evaluate the relationship of commonly used antiseptic agents and SSI, and to determine if isopropyl alcohol has a unique effect.

Study Design.—We performed a prospective cohort analysis to evaluate the relationship of commonly used skin antiseptic agents and SSI for patients undergoing mostly clean-contaminated surgery from January 2011 through June 2012. Multivariate regression modeling predicted expected rates of SSI. Risk adjusted event rates (RAERs) of SSI were compared across groups using proportionality testing.

Results.—Among 7,669 patients, the rate of SSI was 4.6%. The RAERs were 0.85 ($p = 0.28$) for chlorhexidine (CHG), 1.10 ($p = 0.06$) for chlorhexidine in isopropyl alcohol (CHG+IPA), 0.98 ($p = 0.96$) for povidone-iodine (PVI), and 0.93 ($p = 0.51$) for iodine-povacrylex in isopropyl alcohol (IPC+IPA). The RAERs were 0.91 ($p = 0.39$) for the non-IPA group and 1.10 ($p = 0.07$) for the IPA group. Among elective colorectal patients, the RAERs were 0.90 ($p = 0.48$) for CHG, 1.04 ($p = 0.67$) for CHG+IPA, 1.04 ($p = 0.85$) for PVI, and 1.00 ($p = 0.99$) for IPC+IPA.

Conclusions.—For clean-contaminated surgical cases, this large-scale state cohort study did not demonstrate superiority of any commonly used skin antiseptic agent in reducing the risk of SSI, nor did it find any unique effect of isopropyl alcohol. These results do not support the use of more expensive skin preparation agents.

▶ Since the time of Lister, a cardinal rule of surgery is to place barriers between the patient's wound and operating team and to disinfect the patient's skin of microbes that can be introduced into the surgical wound. The use of a variety of antiseptics in preparation of the surgical site is central to the concept of keeping bacteria from the wound. This study assessed surgical site infection in more than 7600 patients for comparison with skin preparation techniques in surgical procedures classified as clean-contaminated. Not surprisingly, there were no significant differences among the types of skin preparation. The predominance of bacteria introduced into the wound was probably not from the skin but the controlled bacterial inoculum after entry into a contaminated space. Any real difference in antiseptic capacity or durability of skin flora reduction would have been overwhelmed by the intraoperative introduction of bacteria caused by violation of natural host defense mechanisms. A better population to study this question would have been in clean implant cases, such as knee or hip replacements. The many variables that enter into the clinical consequence of surgical site infection need to be stratified if meaningful reductions in rates are to occur.

T. L. Pruett, MD

Effect of Minimally Invasive Surgery on the Risk for Surgical Site Infections: Results From the National Surgical Quality Improvement Program (NSQIP) Database
Gandaglia G, Ghani KR, Sood A, et al (Univ of Montreal Health Ctr, Quebec, Canada; Univ of Michigan, Ann Arbor; Henry Ford Health System, Detroit, MI; et al)
JAMA Surg 149:1039-1044, 2014

Importance.—Surgical site infection (SSI) represents the second most common cause of hospital-acquired infection and the most common type of infection in patients undergoing surgery. However, evidence is scarce regarding the effect of the surgical approach (open surgery vs minimally invasive surgery [MIS]) on the risk for SSIs.

Objective.—To evaluate the role of the surgical approach on the risk for SSIs in a large contemporary cohort of patients undergoing surgery across different specialties.

Design, Setting, and Participants.—The American College of Surgeons National Surgical Quality Improvement Program database is a national, prospective perioperative database specifically developed to assess quality of surgical care. We queried the database from January 1, 2005, through December 31, 2011, for patients undergoing appendectomy (n = 97 780), colectomy (n = 118 407), hysterectomy (n = 26 639), or radical prostatectomy (n = 11 183).

Exposures.—Thirty-day SSIs.

Main Outcomes and Measures.—We abstracted the data on 30-day SSIs and compared patients undergoing open procedures and MIS using propensity score matching. Logistic regression analyses of the matched cohorts tested the association between the surgical approach and risk for SSIs.

Results.—The overall 30-day rates of SSIs were 5.4% for appendectomy, 12.1% for colectomy, 2.8% for hysterectomy, and 1.7% for prostatectomy. After propensity score matching, MIS was associated with lower rates of postoperative SSIs in patients undergoing MIS vs open procedures for appendectomy (3.8% vs 7.0%; $P < .001$), colectomy (9.3% vs 15.0%; $P < .001$), hysterectomy (1.8% vs 3.9%; $P < .001$), and radical prostatectomy (1.0% vs 2.4%; $P < .001$). In logistic regression analyses, MIS was associated with lower odds of SSIs in patients treated with appendectomy (odds ratio [OR], 0.52 [95% CI, 0.48-0.58]; $P < .001$), colectomy (OR, 0.58 [95% CI, 0.55-0.61]; $P < .001$), hysterectomy (OR, 0.44 [95% CI, 0.37-0.53]; $P < .001$), and radical prostatectomy (OR, 0.39 [95% CI, 0.25-0.61]; $P < .001$).

Conclusions and Relevance.—The proportion of patients developing SSIs within 30 days after surgery can be substantial and depends on the type of surgery. Minimally invasive surgery is significantly associated with reduced odds of SSIs. This advantage should be considered when assessing the overall benefits of minimally invasive techniques.

▶ There has always been a degree of competition between surgeons that their way of performing an operation is best, especially so with the advent of minimally invasive surgery (MIS) and robotic surgery. In the current analysis using American College of Surgeons National Surgical Quality Improvement Program (ACS-NSQIP) data, the authors showed significantly fewer superficial, deep, and (most) organ space infections for 4 common procedures. This data analysis fails on an intent-to-treat analysis, stratification by socioeconomic variables, and payer groups. On the whole, it makes sense that smaller wounds are less likely to develop infections, until one confounds the analysis with complexity variables. It is likely that in the group with straightforward laparoscopic appendectomy or colectomy, for example, the complexity of surgery was less than in those individuals in whom the procedure had to be performed through an open approach. This is especially likely, as one of the inclusion criteria was that MIS was well penetrated into the practice system. Although lower risk of surgical site infection exists with MIS, the heterogeneity of infectious outcomes may be more reflective of heterogeneity of anatomy and disease complexity than the specific technique. Appropriate risk adjustment for surgical findings is not in this analysis nor captured in the ACS NSQIP database.

T. L. Pruett, MD

Preoperative Smoking Status and Postoperative Complications: A Systematic Review and Meta-analysis

Grønkjær M, Eliasen M, Skov-Ettrup LS, et al (Univ of Southern Denmark, Copenhagen, Denmark; et al)

Ann Surg 259:52-71, 2014

Objective.—To systematically review and summarize the evidence of an association between preoperative smoking status and postoperative complications elaborated on complication type.

Background.—The conclusions of studies examining the association between preoperative smoking and postoperative complications are inconsistent, thus there is a need for a review and meta-analysis to summarize the existing evidence.

Methods.—A systematic review and meta-analysis based on a search in MEDLINE, EMBASE, CINAHL, and PsycINFO. Included were original studies of the association between smoking status and postoperative complications occurring within 30 days of operation. In total, 9354 studies were identified and reviewed for eligibility and data were extracted. Forest plots and summarized relative risks (RR) including 95% confidence intervals (CIs) were estimated for various complication types.

Results.—Of the 9354 identified studies, 107 studies were included in the meta-analyses and based on these, 157 data sets were extracted. Preoperative smoking was associated with an increased risk of various postoperative complications including general morbidity (RR = 1.52, 95% CI: 1.33–1.74), wound complications (RR = 2.15, 95% CI: 1.87–2.49), general infections (RR = 1.54, 95% CI: 1.32–1.79), pulmonary complications (RR = 1.73, 95% CI: 1.35–2.23), neurological complications (RR = 1.38, 95% CI: 1.01–1.88), and admission to intensive care unit (RR = 1.60, 95% CI: 1.14–2.25). Preoperative smoking status was not observed to be associated with postoperative mortality, cardiovascular complications, bleedings, anastomotic leakage, or allograft rejection.

Conclusions.—Preoperative smoking was found to be associated with an increased risk of the following postoperative complications: general morbidity, wound complications, general infections, pulmonary complications, neurological complications, and admission to the intensive care unit.

▶ Smoking is a variable that is inconsistently captured in most data systems. Its importance is only partially captured in this meta-analysis with wound complications being a highly significant negative outcome in people with preoperative smoking. Although most complications are surgical site infections, there is small but real increase in wound dehiscence that is not captured in this analysis. The down side of this report is the real paucity of information that would lead to meaningful risk stratification: How many cigarettes and for how long is deleterious? How long does one need to stop to alter the increased wound complication rate? How long to modify the lung complications? Clear risk stratification is rarely a binary question, but for ease of data systems that is how comorbidities are usually classified.

T. L. Pruett, MD

Mandated Self-reporting of Ventilator-Associated Pneumonia Bundle and Catheter-Related Bloodstream Infection Bundle Compliance and Infection Rates

Helmick RA, Knofsky ML, Braxton CC, et al (Baylor College of Medicine, Houston, TX; et al)
JAMA Surg 149:1003-1007, 2014

Importance.—As quality measures increasingly become tied to payment, evaluating the most effective ways to provide high-quality care becomes more important.

Objectives.—To determine whether mandated reporting for ventilator and catheter bundle compliance is correlated with decreased infection rates, and to determine whether labor-intensive audits are correlated with compliance.

Design, Setting, and Participants.—Multiyear retrospective review of aggregated data from all patients admitted to 15 intensive care units in a Veterans Affairs hospital setting (the Veterans Integrated Service Network 16) from 2009 to 2011.

Exposures.—Ventilator-associated pneumonia and catheter-related bloodstream infections.

Main Outcomes and Measures.—Mean rates of ventilator-associated pneumonia and catheter-related bloodstream infection were analyzed by year. Relationships between infection rates, self-reported compliance, and audits were analyzed by Pearson correlation.

Results.—During the study period, ventilator-associated pneumonia decreased from 2.50 to 1.60 infections per 1000 ventilator days ($P = .07$). The rate of pneumonia was not correlated with self-reported compliance overall ($R = 0.19$) or by individual year (2009, $R = 0.30$; 2010, $R = 0.24$; 2011, $R = 0.46$); there was a correlation in cardiac intensive care units ($R = -0.70$) but not other types of intensive care units (mixed, $R = -0.18$; medical, $R = 0.42$; surgical, $R = 0.34$). Catheter-related bloodstream infections decreased from 2.38 to 0.73 infections per 1000 catheter days ($P = .04$). The rate of catheter infection was not correlated with self-reported compliance overall ($R = -0.18$), by individual year (2009, $R = -0.39$; 2010, $R = -0.42$; 2011, $R = 0.37$), or by intensive care unit type (mixed, $R = -0.19$; cardiac, $R = 0.55$; medical, $R = 0.17$; surgical, $R = -0.44$).

Conclusions and Relevance.—Current mandated self-reported compliance and audit measures are poorly correlated with decreased ventilator-associated pneumonia or catheter-related bloodstream infection.

▶ The current emphasis on quality and performance has led to adoption of many process elements to reduce untoward infectious events. Ventilator-associated pneumonia (VAP) and catheter-related blood stream infections (CRBSI) are 2 commonly tracked and reported events. The Veterans Affairs system has been attempting to find the right bundles to minimize risk of these outcomes and to find process monitoring compliance. In 2005 to 2006 the Veterans Affairs system mandated self-reported compliance with the bundles that are thought to influence development of VAP and CRBSI. This report assessed self-reported compliance and observed rate of VAP and CRBSI. After introduction of the bundles, the rates of VAP and CRBSI decreased. However, neither self-reported nor audited compliance rates correlated with this decrease. It was observed that the numbers of ventilator days and catheter days decreased during this time without sufficient explanation. It is important to address other associated issues, such as duration of intubation, rate of reintubation, nutritional status, length of time with catheter, overall survival, and length of stay associated with this population. Certainly, there can be an overuse of resources that are trimmed when attention or bundles are brought to the issue.

T. L. Pruett, MD

Dead Bacteria Reverse Antibiotic-Induced Host Defense Impairment in Burns

Chen L-W, Chen P-H, Fung C-P, et al (Veterans General Hosp, Taipei, Taiwan; Natl Yang-Ming Univ, Taipei, Taiwan; et al)
J Am Coll Surg 219:606-619, 2014

Background.—Burn patients can incur high rates of hospital-acquired infections. The mechanism of antibiotic exposure on inducing infection vulnerability has not been determined. This study aimed to examine the effects of antibiotic treatment on host defense mechanisms.

Study Design.—First we treated C57/BL6 mice with combined antibiotic treatment after 30% to 35% total body surface area burn. Animals were sacrificed at 48 hours after sham or thermal injury treatment. Bacterial counts in intestinal lumen and mucosa were measured. Next, we treated animals with or without oral dead *Escherichia coli* or *Staphylococcus aureus* supplementation to stimulate Toll-like receptor in the intestinal mucosa. Toll-like receptor 4, antibacterial protein expression, nuclear factor (NF)-κB DNA-binding activity, and bacteria-killing activity in the intestinal mucosa; intestinal permeability; bacterial translocation to mesenteric lymph nodes; *Klebsiella pneumoniae* translocation; interleukin-6 in the blood; and phagocytic activity of alveolar macrophages, were assessed.

Results.—Thermal injury increased microflora and NF-κB DNA-binding activity of the intestine. Systemic antibiotic treatment decreased gut microflora and increased bacterial translocation to mesenteric lymph nodes, intestinal permeability, and interleukin-6 levels in the blood. Antibiotic treatment also decreased bacteria-killing activity in intestinal mucosa and phagocytic activity of alveolar macrophages. Oral dead *E coli* and *S aureus* supplementation induced NF-κB DNA-binding activity, Toll-like receptor 4, and antibacterial protein expression of the intestinal mucosa.

Conclusions.—Taken together with the fact that dead bacteria reversed antibiotic-induced *K pneumoniae* translocation and intestinal and pulmonary defense impairment, we conclude that combined antibiotic treatment results in systemic host defense impairment in burns through the decrease in intestinal flora. We suggest that dead bacteria supplementation could induce nondefensin protein expression and reverse antibiotic-induced gut and lung defense impairment in burn patients.

▶ The prevention of infection in surgical patients is an important part of surgical care. Infection proclivity can be altered by seemingly unrelated therapeutic interventions. The use of antibiotics in burn patients is such an example. This report shows the significant relationship between scald burn, gut bacterial populations, antimicrobial therapy, and gut permeability. The authors also found that 2×10^6 dead bacteria in animals' drinking water would alter changes in luminal bacteria, gut permeability, immune function, pulmonary alveolar phagocytic activity, and other physiologic events. This series of experiments was methodic and convincing. From a practical standpoint, the report left the reader a bit uncertain about how the practitioner should modify immunomodulation to benefit the patient. The authors found that a burn was associated with increased gut bacteria and that antibiotics were associated with reduced numbers. However, the salutatory effect of dead bacteria in the drinking water was left remarkably vague. The authors did not address how the bacteria were killed—heat, formalin, or mechanical—nor did they describe the variation, time, and quantity of water that the mice consumed. One must assume that antibiotics resulted in dead bacteria within the gut, probably in numbers far exceeding the dead bacteria in the water. What is different between antibiotic-killed bacteria and the mechanism used by the authors? This report is motivation to determine immunologic adjunct methods to address the proclivity for infection after thermal burns but one that still leaves many questions unanswered.

T. L. Pruett, MD

The Relationship Between Timing of Surgical Complications and Hospital Readmission

Morris MS, Deierhoi RJ, Richman JS, et al (Birmingham Veterans Administration Hosp, AL; et al)
JAMA Surg 149:348-354, 2014

Importance.—Readmissions after surgery are costly and may reflect quality of care in the index hospitalization.

Objectives.—To determine the timing of postoperative complications with respect to hospital discharge and the frequency of readmission stratified by predischarge and postdischarge occurrence of complications.

Design, Setting, and Participants.—This is a retrospective cohort study of national Veterans Affairs Surgical Quality Improvement Program preoperative risk and outcome data on the Surgical Care Improvement Project cohort for operations performed from January 2005 to August 2009, including colorectal, arthroplasty, vascular, and gynecologic procedures. The association between timing of complication with respect to index hospitalization and 30-day readmission was modeled using generalized estimating equations.

Main Outcome and Measure.—All-cause readmission within 30 days of the index surgical hospitalization discharge.

Results.—Our study of 59 273 surgical procedures performed at 112 Department of Veterans Affairs (VA) hospitals found an overall complication rate of 22.6% (predischarge complications, 71.9%; postdischarge complications, 28.1%). The proportion of postdischarge complications varied significantly, from 8.7% for respiratory complications to 55.7% for surgical site infection ($P < .001$). The overall 30-day readmission rate was 11.9%, of which only 56.0% of readmissions were associated with a currently assessed complication. Readmission was predicted by patient comorbid conditions, procedure factors, and the occurrence of postoperative complications. Multivariable generalized estimating equation models of readmission adjusting for patient and procedure characteristics, hospital, and index length of stay found that the occurrence of postdischarge complications had the highest odds of readmission (odds ratio, 7.4-20.8) compared with predischarge complications (odds ratio, 0.9-1.48).

Conclusions and Relevance.—More than one-quarter of assessed complications are diagnosed after hospital discharge and strongly predict readmission. Hospital discharge is an insufficient end point for quality assessment. Although readmission is associated with complications, almost half of readmissions are not associated with a complication currently assessed by the Veterans Affairs Surgical Quality Improvement Program.

▶ One of the major negative outcomes that is receiving significant attention is readmission to the hospital. Again, Veterans Affairs is trying to "best" manage the population that they serve, and an analysis of 4.5 years of surgical discharges was performed for all-cause readmission within 30 days of discharge from surgery. It was found that 11.9% of surgical patients were readmitted within 30 days of initial discharge with more than half being for surgical site infection (SSI). The authors noted that people with multiple pre-existing comorbidities had an increased hazard ration for readmission. Also, those with emergency surgery, increased American Society of Anesthesiologists class, and longer and more complex procedures had more complications. This finding is not really surprising, as sick people are less able to withstand significant stress; however, that statement has little to do with whether the people received the best procedure and preventive measures for SSI. Although readmission is certainly something to be avoided, one runs the balance between prolonged hospitalizations to address issues and higher rates of readmission for events that take time to evolve. This sort of analysis is interesting but only with appropriate risk adjustment of accurately collected information. It is interesting that the SSI rate in this cohort is at least 6% (50 + % of 11.9%), whereas the assessment of the cost of SSI was only 3.2%.

T. L. Pruett, MD

A Comparison of 2 Surgical Site Infection Monitoring Systems
Ju MH, Ko CY, Hall BL, et al (American College of Surgeons, Chicago, IL; et al)
JAMA Surg 150:51-57, 2015

Importance.—Surgical site infection (SSI) has emerged as the leading publicly reported surgical outcome and is tied to payment determinations. Many hospitals monitor SSIs using the American College of Surgeons National Surgical Quality Improvement Program (ACS NSQIP), in addition to mandatory participation (for most states) in the Centers for Disease Control and Prevention's National Healthcare Safety Network (NHSN), which has resulted in duplication of effort and incongruent data.

Objective.—To identify discrepancies in the implementation of the NHSN and the ACS NSQIP at hospitals that may be affecting the respective SSI rates.

Design, Setting, and Participants.—A pilot sample of hospitals that participate in both the NHSN and the ACS NSQIP.

Interventions.—For each hospital, observed rates and risk-adjusted observed to expected ratios for year 2012 colon SSIs were collected from both programs. The implementation methods of both programs were identified, including telephone interviews with infection preventionists who collect data for the NHSN at each hospital.

Main Outcomes and Measures.—Collection methods and colon SSI rates for the NHSN at each hospital were compared with those of the ACS NSQIP.

Results.—Of 16 hospitals, 11 were teaching hospitals with at least 500 beds. The mean observed colon SSI rates were dissimilar between the 2 programs, 5.7% (range, 2.0%-14.5%) for the NHSN vs 13.5% (range, 4.6%-26.7%) for the ACS NSQIP. The mean difference between the NHSN and the ACS NSQIP was 8.3% (range, 1.6%-18.8%), with the

ACS NSQIP rate always higher. The correlation between the observed to expected ratios for the 2 programs was nonsignificant (Pearson product moment correlation, $\rho = 0.4465$; $P = .08$). The NHSN collection methods were dissimilar among interviewed hospitals. An SSI managed as an outpatient case would usually be missed under the current NHSN practices.

Conclusions and Relevance.—Colon SSI rates from the NHSN and the ACS NSQIP cannot be used interchangeably to evaluate hospital performance and determine reimbursement. Hospitals should not use the ACS NSQIP colon SSI rates for the NHSN reports because that would likely result in the hospital being an outlier for performance. It is imperative to reconcile SSI monitoring, develop consistent definitions, and establish one reliable method. The current state hinders hospital improvement efforts by adding unnecessary confusion to the already complex arena of perioperative improvement.

▶ Methodology is still the crux of risk adjustment, and when payments are predicated on risk-adjusted quality, alignment of outcomes and methodology becomes central. At 16 hospitals using 2 separate performance tracking systems (National Healthcare Safety Network [NHSN] and American College of Surgeons National Surgical Quality Improvement Program [ACS NSQIP]), rates of SSI after colon operations were compared. The authors found that the reported rates of SSI (in the same patient population) were always significantly higher using NSQIP compared with NHSN. The conclusion was that hospitals need to know the relative predictive value of each methodology and align reporting with the desired end. For the sake of public disclosure and hospital ranking using ACS NSQIP SSI results comparing with other hospitals reporting with NHSN, the NSQIP reporter will have system-based higher rates of SSI and rank significantly lower. The importance of this report is to re-emphasize the importance of methodology. Using the same definition of SSI in the same patient population, different rates of SSI were obtained using different methods. Understanding methodology, definitions, and process is central in this day of pay for performance.

T. L. Pruett, MD

Effect of Wound Classification on Risk Adjustment in American College of Surgeons NSQIP
Ju MH, Cohen ME, Bilimoria KY, et al (American College of Surgeons, Chicago, IL; et al)
J Am Coll Surg 219:371-381, 2014

Background.—Surgical wound classification has been used in risk-adjustment models. However, it can be subjective and could potentially improperly bias hospital quality comparisons. The objective is to examine the effect of wound classification on hospital performance risk-adjustment models.

Study Design.—Retrospective review of the 2011 American College of Surgeons NSQIP database was conducted for the following wound classification categories: clean, clean-contaminated, contaminated, and dirty-infected. To assess the influence of wound classification on risk adjustment, 2 models were developed for all outcomes: 1 including and 1 excluding wound classification. For each model, hospital postoperative complications were estimated using hierarchical multivariable regression methods. Absolute changes in hospital rank, correlations of odds ratios, and outlier status agreement between models were examined.

Results.—Of the 442,149 cases performed in 315 hospitals: 53.6% were classified as clean; 34.2% as clean-contaminated; 6.7% as contaminated; and 5.5% as dirty-infected. The surgical site infection rate was highest in dirty-infected (8.5%) and lowest in clean (1.8%) cases. For overall surgical site infection, the absolute change in risk-adjusted hospital performance rank between models, including vs excluding wound classification, was minimal (mean 4.5 of 315 positions). The correlations between odds ratios of the 2 performance models were nearly perfect ($R = 0.9976$, $p < 0.0001$), and outlier status agreement was excellent ($\kappa = 0.95ss08$, $p < 0.0001$). Similar findings were observed in models of subgroups of surgical site infections and other postoperative outcomes.

Conclusions.—In circumstances where alternate information is available for risk adjustment, there appear to be minimal differences in performance models that include vs exclude wound classification. Therefore, the American College of Surgeons NSQIP is critically evaluating the continued use of wound classification in hospital performance risk-adjustment models.

▶ Risk adjustment is an important event when comparing outcomes between groups. This is the basis of the Centers of Excellence and Pay for Performance. The challenge for all risk adjustment efforts is to find appropriate information that stratifies performers. The current analysis evaluates the effect of using (or not) wound classification as a predictor of hospital rank. To the end that *surgical site infection (SSI)* is an outcome incorporated into hospital rankings, it makes sense to risk stratify. The authors show that eliminating the wound classification in the risk adjustment models did not really change hospital ranking.

Several factors should be noted in this conclusion. First, the recognized SSI rate is very low (2% to 8% from clean to dirty cases) and the relative numbers of higher risk procedures (SSI rate > 5%) is relatively small (< 15% of cases). It is difficult to show differences in cases where little differences exist. The authors did not state whether risk adjustment was different if wound classification was preserved in facilities that had a higher proportion of significantly contaminated wounds. It may be that a volume threshold needs to be achieved prior to showing a correlation. SSI occurs because bacteria are in a wound. The trick is developing a scoring system that reliably predicts which wound has significant contamination. This brings the second question: How reliable of a metric is the current practice of wound classification? A risk adjustment tool that is inconsistently applied will not appropriately stratify performance. The data supplied for the nephrectomy classification suggest that there may be such heterogeneity of application that the tool may be meaningless. However, if one still uses SSI as a quality metric, those facilities that will have a higher SSI will need NOT be adversely penalized because of inappropriate application of the metric. The impact of technique (open vs minimally invasive) and complexity of the procedure will likewise impact the risk for SSI.

T. L. Pruett, MD

Costs Associated With Surgical Site Infections in Veterans Affairs Hospitals

Schweizer ML, Cullen JJ, Perencevich EN, et al (Iowa City Veterans Affairs Health Care System; et al)
JAMA Surg 149:575-581, 2014

Importance.—Surgical site infections (SSIs) are potentially preventable complications that are associated with excess morbidity and mortality.

Objective.—To determine the excess costs associated with total, deep, and superficial SSIs among all operations and for high-volume surgical specialties.

Design, Setting, and Participants.—Surgical patients from 129 Veterans Affairs (VA) hospitals were included. The Veterans Health Administration Decision Support System and VA Surgical Quality Improvement Program databases were used to assess costs associated with SSIs among VA patients who underwent surgery in fiscal year 2010.

Main Outcomes and Measures.—Linear mixed-effects models were used to evaluate incremental costs associated with SSIs, controlling for patient risk factors, surgical risk factors, and hospital-level variation in costs. Costs of the index hospitalization and subsequent 30-day readmissions were included. Additional analysis determined potential cost savings of quality improvement programs to reduce SSI rates at hospitals with the highest risk-adjusted SSI rates.

Results.—Among 54 233 VA patients who underwent surgery, 1756 (3.2%) experienced an SSI. Overall, 0.8% of the cohort had a deep SSI, and 2.4% had a superficial SSI. The mean unadjusted costs were $31 580 and $52 620 for patients without and with an SSI, respectively. In the risk-adjusted analyses, the relative costs were 1.43 times greater for patients with an SSI than for patients without an SSI (95% CI, 1.34-1.52; difference, $11 876). Deep SSIs were associated with 1.93 times greater costs (95% CI, 1.71-2.18; difference, $25 721), and superficial SSIs were associated with 1.25 times greater costs (95% CI, 1.17-1.35; difference, $7003). Among the highest-volume specialties, the greatest mean cost attributable to SSIs was $23 755 among patients undergoing neurosurgery, followed by patients undergoing orthopedic surgery, general surgery, peripheral vascular surgery, and urologic surgery. If hospitals in the highest 10th percentile (ie, the worst hospitals) reduced their SSI rates to the rates of the hospitals in the 50th percentile, the Veterans Health Administration would save approximately $6.7 million per year.

Conclusions and Relevance.—Surgical site infections are associated with significant excess costs. Among analyzed surgery types, deep SSIs and SSIs among neurosurgery patients are associated with the highest risk-adjusted costs. Large potential savings per year may be achieved by decreasing SSI rates.

▶ The era of big data provides many insights into the practice of surgery. A focus of many overseers is preventing the preventable. Surgical site infections (SSI) fall squarely within this domain. In this analysis of SSI within the Veterans Affairs (VA) hospitals, the cost of SSI was assessed. Of the more than 50 000 procedures analyzed, the relative cost associated with an identified SSI was increased 1.43 times. Deep SSI had 1.93 times greater cost. The authors concluded that the VA could save significant money by decreasing SSI.

However, one must query whether the data collection is accurate. The methodology for identification is through record reviews by trained nurses. The aggregate SSI rate was 3.2%, superficial SSI was 2.4%, and deep infections 0.8%. A total of 45% of the procedures without SSI were contaminated in some form, whereas in those with SSI, 64% of wounds had recognized contamination. Compared with historical data, these outcomes are already remarkably low: 2.1% SSI for clean, 4.4% for clean-contaminated, 5.9% for contaminated, and 3.9% SSI in dirty wounds. What was the cost associated with a patient that died with an SSI? The VA should be asking itself whether these rates are in fact true, although the resource utilization data suggest that it may not be relevant if the primary outcome is cost.

T. L. Pruett, MD

Multicenter Double-Blinded Randomized Controlled Trial of Standard Abdominal Wound Edge Protection With Surgical Dressings Versus Coverage With a Sterile Circular Polyethylene Drape for Prevention of Surgical Site Infections: A CHIR-Net Trial (BaFO; NCT01181206)

Mihaljevic AL, Schirren R, Özer M, et al (Technische Universität München, Munich, Germany; et al)

Ann Surg 260:730-737, 2014

Objective.—To determine whether circular plastic wound edge protectors (CWEPs) significantly reduce the rate of surgical site infections (SSIs) in comparison to standard surgical towels in patients undergoing laparotomy.

Background.—SSIs cause substantial morbidity, prolonged hospitalization, and costs and remain one of the most frequent surgical complications. CWEPs have been proposed as a measure to reduce the incidence of SSIs.

Methods.—In this randomized controlled, multicenter, 2-arm, parallel-group design, patient- and observer-blinded trial patients undergoing open elective abdominal surgery were assigned to either intraoperative wound coverage with a CWEP or standard coverage with surgical towels. Primary endpoint was superiority of intervention over control in terms of the incidence of SSIs within a 30-day postoperative period.

Results.—Between September 2010 and November 2012, 608 patients undergoing laparotomy were randomized at 16 centers across Germany. Three patients in the device group and 11 patients in the control group did not undergo laparotomy. Patients' and procedural characteristics were well balanced between the 2 groups. Forty-eight patients discontinued the study prematurely, mainly because of relaparotomy (control, n = 9; intervention, n = 9) and death (control, n = 4; intervention, n = 7). A total of 79 patients experienced SSIs within 30 days of surgery, 27 of 274 (9.9%) in the device group and 52 of 272 (19.1%) in the control group (odds ratio = 0.462, 95% confidence interval: 0.281−0.762; $P = 0.002$). Subgroup analyses indicate that the effect could be more pronounced in colorectal surgery, and in clean contaminated/contaminated surgeries.

▶ Another technique for barrier formation is the use of circular wound edge protectors (CWEP). These devices have been postulated as beneficial for years. The current report is on a multicenter randomized study on the role of CWEP in elective open abdominal surgery. The concept is to place a sterile barrier between skin, subcutaneous fat, and fascia and the abdominal viscera as the source of microbes into the wound. A total of 80% of the procedures were classified as clean-contaminated and 18% clean. The rate of surgical site infection (SSI) was significant (19% in control and 9.9% with CWEP) overall—certainly results that are higher than typical chart review findings. However, irrespective of type of analysis, the risk of SSI was lower with the use of CWEP vs the control use of towels around the wound. The conclusion supported the routine use of the CWEP in clean contaminated and contaminated procedures. Benefit was not seen in clean abdominal cases.

T. L. Pruett, MD

A Statewide Colectomy Experience: The Role of Full Bowel Preparation in Preventing Surgical Site Infection
Kim EK, Sheetz KH, Bonn J, et al (Univ of Michigan, Ann Arbor)
Ann Surg 259:310-314, 2014

Objective.—To assess the utility of full bowel preparation with oral nonabsorbable antibiotics in preventing infectious complications after elective colectomy.

Background.—Bowel preparation before elective colectomy remains controversial. We hypothesize that mechanical bowel preparation with nonabsorbable oral antibiotics is associated with a decreased rate of postoperative infectious complications when compared with no bowel preparation.

Methods.—Patient and clinical data were obtained from the Michigan Surgical Quality Collaborative−Colectomy Best Practices Project.

Propensity score analysis was used to match elective colectomy cases based on primary exposure variable—full bowel preparation (mechanical bowel preparation with nonabsorbable oral antibiotics) or no bowel preparation (neither mechanical bowel preparation given nor nonabsorbable oral antibiotic given). The primary outcomes for this study were occurrence of surgical site infection and *Clostridium difficile* colitis.

Results.—In total, 2475 cases met the study criteria. Propensity analysis created 957 paired cases (n = 1914) differing only by the type of bowel preparation. Patients receiving full preparation were less likely to have any surgical site infection (5.0% vs 9.7%; $P = 0.0001$), organ space infection (1.6% vs 3.1%; $P = 0.024$), and superficial surgical site infection (3.0% vs 6.0%; $P = 0.001$). Patients receiving full preparation were also less likely to develop postoperative *C difficile* colitis (0.5% vs 1.8%, $P = 0.01$).

Conclusions.—In the state of Michigan, full bowel preparation is associated with decreased infectious complications after elective colectomy. Within this context, the Michigan Surgical Quality Collaborative recommends full bowel preparation before elective colectomy.

▶ Reducing the size of the bacterial inoculum during the surgical procedure has been the cornerstone of surgical site infection (SSI) prevention. The current study looked at retrospective data comparing colorectal outcomes with or without a full (mechanical plus topical antibiotics) bowel preparation. Many have tried to get away from this old preparation, as the mechanical removal of fecal material is uncomfortable for patients, and the use of oral antibiotics to reduce bacterial numbers can be replaced by parenteral therapy. Using statewide data, the authors found that full mechanical and oral antibiotic preparation (plus intravenous antibiotics) still significantly reduced the risk of all forms of SSI roughly in half. This report just reiterates what has already been known, that by reducing the numbers of bacteria within the wound, the aggregate risk of SSI is diminished. Until studies show a significantly improved SSI from alternative preparations for colorectal surgery, then the old time preparation still results in fewest SSI.

T. L. Pruett, MD

The NOTA Study (Non Operative Treatment for Acute Appendicitis): Prospective Study on the Efficacy and Safety of Antibiotics (Amoxicillin and Clavulanic Acid) for Treating Patients With Right Lower Quadrant Abdominal Pain and Long-Term Follow-up of Conservatively Treated Suspected Appendicitis

Di Saverio S, Sibilio A, Giorgini E, et al (Maggiore Hosp Regional Trauma Ctr, Bologna, Italy; et al)
Ann Surg 260:109-117, 2014

Objectives.—To assess the safety and efficacy of antibiotics treatment for suspected acute uncomplicated appendicitis and to monitor the long term follow-up of non-operated patients.

Background.—Right lower quadrant abdominal pain is a common cause of emergency department admission. The natural history of acute appendicitis nonoperatively treated with antibiotics remains unclear.

Methods.—In 2010, a total of 159 patients [mean AIR (Appendicitis Inflammatory Response) score = 4.9 and mean Alvarado score = 5.2] with suspected appendicitis were enrolled and underwent nonoperative management (NOM) with amoxicillin/clavulanate. The follow-up period was 2 years.

Results.—Short-term (7 days) NOM failure rate was 11.9%. All patients with initial failures were operated within 7 days. At 15 days, no recurrences were recorded. After 2 years, the overall recurrence rate was 13.8% (22/159); 14 of 22 patients were successfully treated with further cycle of amoxicillin/clavulanate. No major side effects occurred. Abdominal pain assessed by the Numeric Rating Scale and the visual analog scale; median Numeric Rating Scale score was 3 at 5 days and 2 after 7 days. Mean length of stay of nonoperatively managed patients was 0.4 days, and mean sick leave period was 5.8 days. Long-term efficacy of NOM treatment was 83% (118 patients recurrence free and 14 patients with recurrence nonoperatively managed). None of the single factors forming the Alvarado or AIR score were independent predictors of failure of NOM or long-term recurrence. Alvarado and AIR scores were the only independent predictive factors of NOM failure after multivariate analysis, but both did not correlate with recurrences. Overall costs of NOM and antibiotics were €316.20 per patient.

Conclusions.—Antibiotics for suspected acute appendicitis are safe and effective and may avoid unnecessary appendectomy, reducing operation rate, surgical risks, and overall costs. After 2 years of follow-up, recurrences of nonoperatively treated right lower quadrant abdominal pain are less than 14% and may be safely and effectively treated with further antibiotics.

▶ The judgment algorithm for surgical intervention for various diseases is being re-examined. Acute appendicitis has always been the domain of the surgeon, but history and thoughtful reflection may teach us to think differently. The experience reported notes that most individuals with clinical appendicitis can effectively be treated with oral antibiotics and observation with a fairly low recidivism rate. In this interesting report, 100% of the initial patient population was treated nonoperatively, and only 11.9% required surgical intervention within or after the first week. Another 10% had a relapse within the first 6 months (most effectively retreated with antibiotics) with another 3% recurrences throughout the 2 years from incident presentation. Operative removal of the appendix is not essential in the management of acute appendicitis. The clinical acumen used in this study led to very little morbidity and no mortality. Nineteen of 159 people had an appendectomy within the first week. Of the 22 recurrent episodes of appendicitis, only 8 required subsequent appendectomy and all within the 6 to 12 months from the sentinel event. Timely intervention and diligent follow-up are central in management. However, the benefit for most patients, along with the absence of operative morbidities, makes this algorithm an important management strategy for those with symptoms and signs of acute appendicitis.

T. L. Pruett, MD

The Preventive Surgical Site Infection Bundle in Colorectal Surgery: An Effective Approach to Surgical Site Infection Reduction and Health Care Cost Savings

Keenan JE, Speicher PJ, Thacker JKM, et al (Duke Univ Med Ctr, Durham, NC; et al)
JAMA Surg 149:1045-1052, 2014

Importance.—Surgical site infections (SSIs) in colorectal surgery are associated with increased morbidity and health care costs.

Objective.—To determine the effect of a preventive SSI bundle (hereafter bundle) on SSI rates and costs in colorectal surgery.

Design.—Retrospective study of institutional clinical and cost data. The study period was January 1, 2008, to December 31, 2012, and outcomes were assessed and compared before and after implementation of the bundle on July 1, 2011.

Setting and Participants.—Academic tertiary referral center among 559 patients who underwent major elective colorectal surgery.

Main Outcomes and Measures.—The primary outcome was the rate of superficial SSIs before and after implementation of the bundle. Secondary outcomes included deep SSIs, organ-space SSIs, wound disruption, postoperative sepsis, length of stay, 30-day readmission, and variable direct costs of the index admission.

Results.—Of 559 patients in the study, 346 (61.9%) and 213 (38.1%) underwent their operation before and after implementation of the bundle, respectively. Groups were matched on their propensity to be treated with the bundle to account for significant differences in the preimplementation and postimplementation characteristics. Comparison of the matched groups revealed that implementation of the bundle was associated with reduced superficial SSIs (19.3% vs 5.7%, $P < .001$) and postoperative sepsis (8.5% vs 2.4%, $P = .009$). No significant difference was observed in deep SSIs, organ-space SSIs, wound disruption, length of stay, 30-day readmission, or variable direct costs between the matched groups. However, in a subgroup analysis of the postbundle period, superficial SSI occurrence was associated with a 35.5% increase in variable direct costs ($13 253 vs $9779, $P = .001$) and a 71.7% increase in length of stay (7.9 vs 4.6 days, $P < .001$).

Conclusions and Relevance.—The preventive SSI bundle was associated with a substantial reduction in SSIs after colorectal surgery. The increased costs associated with SSIs support that the bundle represents an effective approach to reduce health care costs.

▶ The purpose of quality assessment is to intervene in a timely fashion with process improvements. This report is the consequence of being flagged within the American College of Surgeons National Surgical Quality Improvement Program as being an outlier. Duke University was identified as being outside the "norm" for colorectal surgical site infections (SSI) and engaged in implementation of a bundle program to decrease that rate. The implemented bundle consisted of numerous barrier and wound/operative site protections and several modulation/prophylaxis elements. These elements address different parts of operative risks, probably with significant alterations upon outcomes. With start of the process, there was a striking reduction in SSI (superficial SSI reduced from 19% to 5.7% with no significant change in deep or organ space SSI). However, the behavior modifications that were induced by introducing the bundle and recognition that SSI in colorectal cases were not measured. It is also unknown the degree of compliance by the colorectal team with these bundle elements. While on the face, the introduction of the colorectal bundle produced the desired effect; however, experience from other bundle implementation must make one cautious about cause-and-effect relationship. More importantly, it is important to recognize a hierarchy of significance of the elements. In fact, one easy measure regarding attention to background elements would be bacterial characteristics of the SSI. Many elements of the bundle were designed to keep skin bacteria from the wound. Many were designed to minimize fecal contamination. Wound cultures would have helped establish a hierarchy of the elements regarding what part of the behavior alteration was being addressed. Finding the right components of processes with appropriate measures of effectiveness is central to process improvement in the clinical arena.

T. L. Pruett, MD

Risk of Readmission and Emergency Surgery Following Nonoperative Management of Colonic Diverticulitis: A Population-Based Analysis
Li D, de Mestral C, Baxter NN, et al (Univ of Toronto, Ontario, Canada; et al)
Ann Surg 260:423-431, 2014

Objective.—To characterize the clinical course of patients with diverticulitis after nonoperative management and determine factors associated with readmission and subsequent emergency surgery.

Background.—Clinical course of this disease remains poorly understood; indications for elective colectomy are unclear.

Methods.—This was a retrospective cohort study of patients managed nonoperatively after a first episode of diverticulitis in Ontario, Canada (2002–2012). Time-to-event analysis and Fine and Gray multivariable regression were used to characterize the risks of readmission and emergency surgery for diverticulitis, accounting for death and elective colectomy as competing events.

Results.—A total of 14,124 patients were followed for a median of 3.9 years (maximum 10, interquartile range: 1.7−6.4). Five-year cumulative incidence was 9.0% for readmission, 1.9% for emergency surgery, and 14.1% for all-cause mortality. Patients younger than 50 years had higher incidence of readmission than patients aged 50 years and older (10.5% vs 8.4%; $P < 0.001$) but not emergency surgery (1.8% vs 2.0%; $P = 0.52$). Patients with complicated disease (abscess, perforation) were at increased risk of readmission than those with uncomplicated disease (12.0% vs 8.2%; $P < 0.001$), as well as increased risk of emergency surgery (4.3% vs 1.4%, $P < 0.001$). In multivariable regression, complicated disease and number of prior admissions were associated with increased risk of emergency surgery, yet age less than 50 years was not. Risks associated with complicated disease were nonproportional over time, being highest immediately after discharge and decreasing thereafter.

Conclusions.—Absolute risks of readmission and emergency surgery are low after nonoperative management of diverticulitis, providing evidence for the practice of deferring colectomy for patients without persistent symptoms or multiple recurrences.

▶ More efforts to mine large registries are used in this report. Using provincial hospital data, the admission and operative history of individuals with diverticulitis were assessed over a 10-year period. Roughly a quarter of patients had operative interventions within the first few months; however, for the individuals who were treated conservatively (antibiotics with or without tube drainage of an abscess) and subsequently discharged, only 8% of patients had another admission for diverticulitis. The indications for elective surgery were not clearly captured, but complexity of disease was associated with need for further intervention. However, most patients appeared to resolve the acute inflammation without the need for operative intervention. Like appendicitis, conservative management is likely to be definitive in most cases. Whether outpatient therapy with oral antibiotics would have benefit in this population is not clear. However, elements involved in good judgment for best recovery and fewest complications are not available in large databases.

T. L. Pruett, MD

The Detection of Intraoperative Bacterial Translocation in the Mesenteric Lymph Nodes Is Useful in Predicting Patients at High Risk for Postoperative Infectious Complications After Esophagectomy

Nishigaki E, Abe T, Yokoyama Y, et al (Nagoya Univ Graduate School of Medicine, Japan; et al)
Ann Surg 259:477-484, 2014

Objective.—To investigate the incidence of BT in the mesenteric lymph node and bacteremia after an esophagectomy using a bacterium-specific ribosomal RNA-targeted reverse-transcriptase quantitative polymerase chain reaction (RT-qPCR).

Background.—There is little evidence regarding the occurrence of bacterial translocation (BT) and its correlation to postoperative infectious complications after an esophagectomy.

Methods.—Eighteen patients with esophageal cancer were studied. Mesenteric lymph nodes were harvested from the jejunal mesentery before surgical mobilization (MLN-1) and after the restoration of bowel continuity (MLN-2). Blood and sputum were also sampled before surgery (Blood-1 and Sputum-1) and on postoperative day 1 (Blood-2 and Sputum-2).

Results.—The detection rates of bacteria in the MLN-2 (56%) and Blood-2 (56%) were significantly higher than those in the MLN-1 (17%) and Blood-1 (22%), indicating that surgical stress induces BT. The detection rate was not different between Sputum-1 (80%) and Sputum-2 (78%). There was an 80% sequence homology between the RT-qPCR products in the MLN-2 and Blood-2, whereas the homology was only 20% between Blood-2 and Sputum-2. In the patients with positive bacteria in the MLN-2 sample, there was a greater incidence of postoperative infectious complications than in patients without bacteria in the MLN-2 sample ($P = 0.04$). The postoperative hospital stay was also longer ($P = 0.037$) for patients with positive bacteria in the MLN-2 sample.

Conclusions.—BT frequently occurs during esophagectomies, and postoperative bacteremia is likely to be gut-derived. Patients with positive bacteria in the MLN-2 sample should be carefully managed because these patients are more susceptible to postoperative infectious complications.

▶ It is known that bacteria can be detected in mesenteric lymph nodes (MLN) after a variety of stresses. This study adds new insights into the significance, but not the causality, of bacterial translocation. In this study of patients undergoing esophagectomy, bacterial ribosomal DNA in MLN, blood, and sputum was assessed by polymerase chain reaction. More than half the patients had MLN bacteria detected at the end of the operation and of those with detectable bacteremia, 100% homology was found with the bacteria in the MLN (and a much lower homology with bacteria in the sputum). Patients with translocation and detectable bacteria in the blood (but without conventional positive cultures) had more complications than those without translocation. Whether translocation is an associated event or causal event is not clear. It would have been helpful if other data had been provided such as association with the Charlson Comorbidity Index, *Acute Physiology and Chronic Health Evaluation* score, frailty index, or nutritional parameters. Many clinical predictive and associative tools may also be correlated with complications and translocation. The interface between biologic observations and clinical outcomes is interesting but of uncertain consequence.

T. L. Pruett, MD

Splenectomy and the risk of sepsis: a population-based cohort study

Edgren G, Almqvist R, Hartman M, et al (Karolinska Institutet, Stockholm, Sweden; Harvard School of Public Health, Boston, MA Karolinska Univ Hosp, Stockholm, Sweden; et al)
Ann Surg 260:1081-1087, 2014

Objective.—We sought to estimate the long-term risk of sepsis in patients who underwent splenectomy before, during, and after implementation of vaccination.

Background.—Because patients who have undergone splenectomy are considered at increased risk of bacterial sepsis, they typically receive vaccination, education, and occasionally antibiotic prophylaxis. However, the extent to which these interventions have actually reduced the risk of sepsis remains unclear.

Methods.—Retrospective cohort study encompassing all patients in the Swedish national inpatient register, who underwent splenectomy in 1970-2009. Patients were followed for hospitalization for or death from sepsis, as identified using national inpatient and cause of death registers. Relative risks, comparing patients to the background population were expressed as standardized incidence ratios (SIRs) and standardized mortality ratios (SMRs).

Results.—Altogether, 20,132 splenectomized patients were included. The overall SIR for hospitalization for sepsis was 5.7 [95% confidence interval (CI), 5.6-6.0]. However, risks depended on the indication for splenectomy, with SIRs varying from 3.4 (95% CI, 3.0-3.8) for trauma patients to 18 (95% CI, 16-19) for patients with hematologic malignancies. SMRs ranged from 3.1 (95% CI, 2.1-4.3) for trauma to 8.7 (95% CI, 6.8-11) for hematologic disease. In regression analyses adjusting for age at splenectomy, follow-up time, sex, and calendar year of splenectomy, there were no significant risk decreases after implementation of routine vaccination, except for in patients with malignant and non-malignant hematologic disease.

Conclusions.—The risk of hospitalization or death from sepsis is high in patients who previously underwent splenectomy and depends on the indication for splenectomy. The effectiveness of current vaccination practices warrants further evaluation.

▶ A portion of surgical judgment is to know the consequences of what surgical procedure is performed. Removal of the spleen is recognized as being associated with an overwhelming sepsis syndrome, and it is routine to vaccinate people with polysaccharide capsular antigens of *Streptococcus pneumoniae*, Haemophilus influenzae, and Neisseria meningitidis with the expectation that risk will be ameliorated. The current "big data" attempt to address this question was made using the Swedish national health database. Analyzing results of splenectomy over 3 decades, the incidence of hospitalization and infectious death was assessed in those individuals undergoing splenectomy for a variety of causes. Stratification by indication found various results. Not surprisingly, infectious deaths from sepsis were highest in malignancies (hematologic and nonhematologic). This is not surprising, as this population would have had a disproportionate number of individuals undergoing chemotherapy with associated leucopenia and infection. The trauma population had a significantly lower rate of both hospitalization and mortality. Unfortunately, the incidence of the overwhelming infections is lost in other infections in this population. Etiologies and comorbidities were lost. The rate of infections of pathogens included within the vaccines was not reported. The vaccines may well have reduced infections by the specific pathogens; however, the information is not available in a large database. This article represents one of the overstretch conclusions that can be generated by large databases.

T. L. Pruett, MD

Toll-Like Receptor 1 Polymorphisms and Associated Outcomes in Sepsis After Traumatic Injury: A Candidate Gene Association Study
Thompson CM, Holden TD, Rona G, et al (Univ of Washington, Seattle)
Ann Surg 259:179-185, 2014

Objective.—To determine whether single nucleotide polymorphisms (SNPs) in *TLR1* are associated with mortality, specifically sepsis-associated mortality, in a traumatically injured population.

Background.—Innate immune responses mediated by toll-like receptors (TLRs) induce early inflammatory responses to pathogen and damage-associated molecular patterns. Genetic variation in TLRs has been associated with susceptibility and outcomes in a number of infectious and noninfectious disease states.

Methods.—Patients admitted to the trauma intensive care unit at a level 1 trauma center serving 4 states were enrolled and followed for development of infection, sepsis, and death. Genomic DNA was genotyped and logistic regression analysis was performed to determine associations between *TLR1* SNPs and mortality. We further examined for associations between *TLR1* SNPs and mortality in subgroups on the basis of the presence of sepsis and the type of sepsis-associated organism.

Results.—We enrolled 1961 patients. $TLR1_{-7202G}$ ($rs5743551$) was associated with increased mortality after traumatic injury and this association was primarily observed in the subset of patients who developed sepsis [adjusted odds ratio (OR): 3.16; 95% confidence interval (CI): 1.43–6.97, $P = 0.004$]. This association persisted after further restriction to gram-positive sepsis. $TLR1_{742A/G(Asn248Ser)}$ ($rs4833095$), a coding SNP in LD with $TLR1_{-7202G}$, was also associated with mortality in gram-positive sepsis (adjusted OR: 4.16; 95% CI: 1.22–14.19, $P = 0.023$).

Conclusions.—Genetic variation in *TLR1* is associated with increased mortality in patients with sepsis after traumatic injury and may represent a novel marker of risk for death in critically injured patients.

▶ This article shows that variations in the fundamental elements of innate immunity are associated with differences in clinical outcomes. The authors show that a variation in toll-like receptor 1 (TLR 1) is retrospectively found in people who have died after admission to a trauma intensive care unit. In this analysis, it was found that people with $TLR1_{-7202G}$ had a propensity to die from infection that exceeded the other polymorphisms studied. This study reconfirms the complexity of the mammalian response to trauma/stress/risk for infection. This is a genome-type study that does not state the functional status of *TLR1*. It is uncertain whether this polymorphism has a similar binding capacity and signaling as the others and whether it is transported and expressed at the same frequency as the other polymorphisms. In a day of individualized medicine, the variables associated with clinical conditions will typically overwhelm the small amount of knowledge that is available about any one biologic variable.

T. L. Pruett, MD

Single Nucleotide Polymorphisms of the *tcdC* Gene and Presence of the Binary Toxin Gene Predict Recurrent Episodes of *Clostridium difficile* Infection
Stewart DB, Berg AS, Hegarty JP (The Pennsylvania State Univ College of Medicine, Hershey)
Ann Surg 260:299-304, 2014

Objective.—To identify *Clostridium difficile* genotypes, which are associated with recurrent *C difficile* infection (RCDI).

Background.—Reliable bacterial genetic factors predicting RCDI are currently lacking.

Methods.—Inpatients and outpatients 18 years or older treated at our institution for *C difficile* infection (CDI) of any severity were consecutively enrolled. CDI was defined as symptoms of colitis with a positive PCR stool test. Each bacterial isolate was studied for virulence factors: *tcdC* mutations, including single nucleotide polymorphisms (SNPs) via PCR, the presence of genes for toxins A, B and binary toxin using restriction fragment length polymorphism, and identification of ribotype by PCR. χ^2 tests, *t* tests, and logistic and linear regression were used to determine which virulence factors predicted RCDI and the need for hospital admission, with corrections made for multiple statistical comparisons.

Results.—Seventy-three patients (male: 52%; mean age: 66 ± 15 years) were studied. Binary toxin gene ($P = 0.03$) was associated with at least 1 episode of RCDI, as was the presence of SNPs C184T ($P = 0.006$) and A117T ($P = 0.003$). The presence of the binary toxin gene with either of these *tcdC* SNPs increased RCDI by 80% ($P = 0.0002$) but did not predict the need for hospital admission. None of the other virulence factors, including ribotype 027, were predictive of RCDI.

Conclusions.—The presence of the binary toxin gene and *tcdC* SNPs C184T and A117T strongly predict RCDI. The presence of both *tcdC*

SNPs and the binary toxin gene significantly increased the risk of RCDI, which might warrant longer antibiotic courses to eradicate the infection.

▶ Hospital-acquired infection is a significant morbidity for surgical patients. *Clostridium difficile* infection (CDI) has become particularly problematic in a variety of geographic locales. Initially, studies of CDI found successful treatment in more than 90% of patients. However, relapse is becoming increasingly frequent, and in this report recurrent CDI was an extraordinary 42%. The article assesses *C difficile* toxin and promoter region to correlate with CDI recurrence. The authors found that the presence of the binary toxin gene in combination with specific nucleotide changes in the *tcdC* promoter gene was highly predictive of recurrent CDI after treatment. The rationale for why recurrence should be more common in this group is not fully explained in the report. Although this is an important observation, that bacterial and not host factors are associated with adverse outcomes, there are several more fundamental issues associated with the population that need clarification. The treatment dose and duration were not mentioned, nor was there even an acknowledgment that courses followed routine treatment guidelines. Recurrent CDI is thought to be caused by reinfection (with bacterial spores) or failure to eradicate the initial population of bacteria. The authors did not provide bacterial information about the recurrent bacteria associated with infection. It is unclear what role the toxin or promoter plays in the inability eradicate or possibly change in reinfection propensity. This is an interesting paper, but it again stresses the need to correlate laboratory biology with what are currently thought to be relevant factors in clinical disease.

T. L. Pruett, MD

The Central Role of Arginine Catabolism in T-Cell Dysfunction and Increased Susceptibility to Infection After Physical Injury

Zhu X, Pribis JP, Rodriguez PC, et al (Univ of Pittsburgh, PA; Louisiana State Univ Health Sciences Ctr, New Orleans)
Ann Surg 259:171-178, 2014

Objective.—To explore the hypothesis that decreased arginine availability by myeloid-derived suppressor cells (MDSCs) is a cause of T-cell dysfunction after physical injury (PI).

Background.—Arginine is an essential amino acid for normal T-cell function whose availability becomes limited after PI. MDSCs expressing arginase 1 are induced by PI. T-cell dysfunction after PI seems to increase the risk of infection but the mechanisms that cause it are unclear.

Methods.—PI was created using a standard laparotomy model. Phenotypical and functional alterations in T cellswere evaluated in vivo. MDSCs expressing arginase 1 were measured by flow cytometry. Infection after PI was created by intraperitoneal injection of *Listeria monocytogenes*. N^{ω}-Hydroxy-*Nor*-L-arginine (*Nor*-NOHA) was used as an arginase inhibitor. The effect of arginine depletion on T-cell function and susceptibility to infection was assessed through adoptive transfer of MDSC or injection of arginase into noninjured mice.

Results.—PI caused a decrease in intracellular arginine in T cells, loss of the T-cell receptor (TCR) CD3-ζ chain, inhibition of in vivo T-cell proliferation, memory, and cytotoxicity. PI exponentially increased bacterial growth and mortality to *L. monocytogenes*. T-cell dysfunction and increased infection were reversed by arginase inhibitor *Nor*-NOHA but were reproduced by adoptively transferring MDSC or injecting arginase 1 to noninjured mice.

Conclusions.—Arginine availability is decreased after PI coinciding with an induction of MDSC expressing arginase 1. Decreased arginine may inhibit T-cell function and increase susceptibility to infection after injury.

▶ The immune system is altered by stress. Using conventional assays of T-cell response, it has long been known that physical injury is associated with a diminished response to conventional stimuli. Because infection is such a significant variable after operations, there have been many efforts to understand and devise mechanisms for effective intervention. This report is along this theme. Animals were injured by performing a laparotomy. T cells diminished, immune response to an antigen for which the animal had received a vaccination was diminished, and it was associated with a diminution of intracellular arginine. This finding could be replicated by passive transfer of cells or artificial reduction of arginine and somewhat inhibited by arginase-1 blockade. Although a very interesting progression and logic, the authors acknowledge the remarkable multiplicity of pathways that are likely to be operative. The immunologic balances between proinflammatory and counterregulatory immune responses are legion. While understanding how cell populations and activities shift with various stimuli, the reasons and sequelae of changes in amino acid substrate in lymphocytes is still far from being understood.

T. L. Pruett, MD

7 Endocrine

Voice Outcomes after Total Thyroidectomy, Partial Thyroidectomy, or Non-Neck Surgery Using a Prospective Multifactorial Assessment
Vicente DA, Solomon NP, Avital I, et al (Walter Reed Natl Military Med Ctr, Bethesda, MD; Univ of the Health Sciences, Bethesda, MD; et al)
J Am Coll Surg 219:152-163, 2014

Background.—Voice alteration remains a significant complication of thyroid surgery. We present a comparison of voice outcomes between total thyroidectomy (TT), partial thyroidectomy (PT), and non-neck (NN) surgery using a multifactorial voice-outcomes classification tool.

Study Design.—Patients with normal voice (n = 112) were enrolled between July 2004 and March 2009. The patients underwent TT (n = 54), PT (n = 35), or NN (n = 23) surgery under general endotracheal anesthesia as part of a prospective observational study involving serial multimodality voice evaluation preoperatively, and at 2 weeks, 3 months, and 6 months postoperatively. Patients with adverse voice outcomes were grouped into the negative voice outcomes (NegVO) category, including patients with objective (abnormality on videolaryngostroboscopy and substantial voice dysfunction) and subjective (normal videolaryngostroboscopy but with notable voice impairment) NegVO. Voice outcomes were compared among study groups.

Results.—Negative voice outcomes occurred in 46% (95% CI, 34−59%) and 14% (95% CI, 6−30%) of TT and PT groups, respectively. No NegVOs were observed after NN surgery. Early NegVOs were more common in the TT group than in the NN or PT groups ($p < 0.001$). Most voice disturbances resolved by 6 months (TT 84%; PT 92%) with no difference in NegVO among all groups ($p = 0.23$). Black race and significant changes in certain voice outcomes measures at the 2-week follow-up visit were identified as predictors of late (3 to 6 months) NegVO.

Conclusions.—This comprehensive voice outcomes study revealed that the extent of thyroidectomy impacts voice outcomes in the early postoperative period, and identified risk factors for late NegVO in post-thyroidectomy patients who should be considered for early voice rehabilitation referral (Fig 3).

▶ The authors present the results of a prospective observational study examining voice changes after thyroid surgery. The study is carefully done and has utility; however, it seems that although the authors claim that all operations were

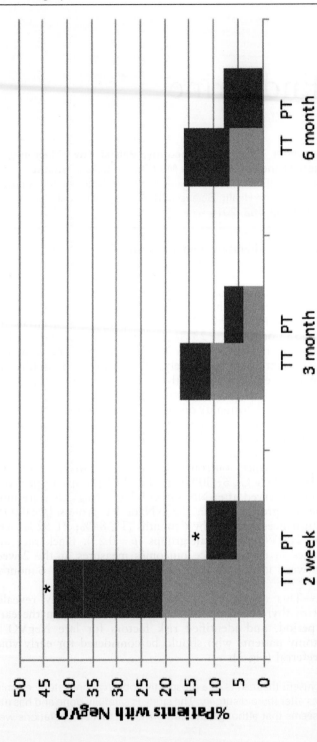

FIGURE 3.—Incidence of voice outcomes for total thyroidectomy (TT) and partial thyroidectomy (PT) groups at each time point. Total thyroidectomy group with significantly more negative voice outcomes (NegVO) (p = 0.030), objective NegVO* (p = 0.002), subjective NegVO* (p = 0.017) than PT at 2-week follow-up visit. Black bar, subjective negative voice outcomes; gray bar, objective negative voice outcomes. (Reprinted from the Journal of the American College of Surgeons. Vicente DA, Solomon NP, Avital I, et al. Voice outcomes after total thyroidectomy, partial thyroidectomy, or non-neck surgery using a prospective multifactorial assessment. J Am Coll Surg. 2014;219:152-163, Copyright 2014, with permission from American College of Surgeons.)

performed by experienced endocrine surgeons, only 112 operations were done over a period of nearly 5 years, which would not qualify this center as a high-volume center. Nevertheless, the study is well done, as each patient underwent voice recording and computerized voice analysis preoperatively and then at 3 points postoperatively (2 weeks and 3 and 6 months) as well as video laryng-ostroboscopy. There are several messages here. First, if questioned closely, nearly half of patients undergoing total thyroidectomy will report voice changes at a 2-week postoperative visit (vs just a more than 10% of patients undergoing hemithyroidectomy), as shown in Fig 3 included here. Fortunately, most of these negative voice outcomes resolve by the 3- and 6-month follow-up. How-ever, at 6 months, approximately 15% of patients undergoing total thyroidec-tomy will still have either a perception of or objective findings of a negative voice outcome. And these data are not associated with recurrent laryngeal nerve injury.

Does this knowledge help treat postoperative patients undergoing thyroid surgery? The authors recommend early referral to speech pathology to help mit-igate the long-term effects of subtle voice changes. Although no outcome data are given to support this finding, which would imply that nearly half of patients undergoing total thyroidectomy may require referral (which seems like a lot), those patients who have significant early voice complaints (and certainly those with suspected recurrent laryngeal nerve injury) should have an early referral to a voice specialist.

T. J. Fahey, MD

BRAF V600E and *TERT* Promoter Mutations Cooperatively Identify the Most Aggressive Papillary Thyroid Cancer With Highest Recurrence

Xing M, Liu R, Liu X, et al (Johns Hopkins Univ School of Medicine, Baltimore, MD)
J Clin Oncol 32:2718-2726, 2014

Purpose.—To investigate the prognostic value of the *BRAF* V600E mutation and the recently identified *TERT* promoter mutation chr5:1,295,228C>T (C228T), individually and in their coexistence, in papillary thyroid cancer (PTC).

Patients and Methods.—We performed a retrospective study of the rela-tionship of *BRAF* and *TERT* C228T mutations with clinicopathologic outcomes of PTC in 507 patients (365 women and 142 men) age 45.9 ± 14.0 years (mean ± SD) with a median follow-up of 24 months (interquartile range, 8 to 78 months).

Results.—Coexisting *BRAF* V600E and *TERT* C228T mutations were more commonly associated with high-risk clinicopathologic characteris-tics of PTC than they were individually. Tumor recurrence rates were 25.8% (50 of 194;77.60 recurrences per 1,000 person-years; 95% CI, 58.81 to 102.38) versus 9.6% (30 of 313; 22.88 recurrences per 1,000 person-years; 95% CI, 16.00 to 32.72) in *BRAF* mutation—positive versus —negative patients (hazard ratio [HR], 3.22; 95% CI, 2.05 to 5.07) and

47.5% (29 of 61; 108.55 recurrences per 1,000 person-years; 95% CI, 75.43 to 156.20) versus 11.4% (51 of 446; 30.21 recurrences per 1,000 person-years; 95% CI, 22.96 to 39.74) in *TERT* mutation–positive versus –negative patients (HR, 3.46; 95% CI, 2.19 to 5.45). Recurrence rates were 68.6% (24 of 35; 211.76 recurrences per 1,000 person-years; 95% CI, 141.94 to 315.94) versus 8.7% (25 of 287; 21.60 recurrences per 1,000 person-years; 95% CI, 14.59 to 31.97) in patients harboring both mutations versus patients harboring neither mutation (HR, 8.51; 95% CI, 4.84 to 14.97), which remained significant after clinicopathologic cofactor adjustments. Disease free patient survival curves displayed a moderate decline with *BRAF* V600E or *TERT* C228T alone but a sharp decline with two coexisting mutations.

Conclusion.—Coexisting *BRAF* V600E and *TERT* C228T mutations form a novel genetic background that defines PTC with the worst clinicopathologic outcomes, providing unique prognostic and therapeutic implications.

▶ This study from the Hopkins group is an excellent study that will have far-reaching implications. The study documents a clear increase in recurrence in papillary thyroid carcinomas that harbor both *BRAF* and *TERT* mutations. This is summarized nicely in Fig 2 from the original article. The effect of *BRAF* mutations alone on recurrence has been debated because *BRAF* mutations are seen almost exclusively in classical variant papillary thyroid cancer (PTC). The data shown in Fig 2 of the original article indicate that the negative effect of the presence of both *BRAF* and *TERT* mutations on recurrence-free survival hold for both classical and follicular variant PTC. Fortunately (and logically given the overall excellent outcomes of PTC), the number of tumors that contain both mutations is low (only 35 of 507 or 6.9%). The mechanism by which the combination of these 2 mutations leads to increased recurrence rates is not established—and not necessarily even causative at this point. Interestingly, the combination of the 2 mutations was not associated with an increase in vascular invasion in classical PTC, despite an association with a substantial increase in distant metastasis.

Because diagnostic mutation panels are likely to include both *BRAF* and *TERT* in examining FNA specimens going forward, the management of patients who have nodules that harbor both mutations should probably be more aggressive, although this definitely requires further study.

T. J. Fahey, MD

The Effect of Extent of Surgery and Number of Lymph Node Metastases on Overall Survival in Patients with Medullary Thyroid Cancer
Esfandiari NH, Hughes DT, Yin H, et al (Univ of Michigan, Ann Arbor)
J Clin Endocrinol Metab 99:448-454, 2014

Context.—Total thyroidectomy with central lymph node dissection is recommended in patients with medullary thyroid cancer (MTC). However, the relationship between disease severity and extent of resection on overall survival remains unknown.

Objective.—The aim of the study was to identify the effect of surgery on overall survival in MTC patients.

Methods.—Using data from 2968 patients with MTC diagnosed between 1998 and 2005 from the National Cancer Database, we determined the relationship between the number of cervical lymph node metastases, tumor size, distant metastases, and extent of surgery on overall survival in patients with MTC.

Results.—Older patient age (5.69 [95% CI, 3.34—9.72]), larger tumor size (2.89 [95% CI, 2.14—3.90]), presence of distant metastases (5.68 [95% CI, 4.61—6.99]), and number of positive regional lymph nodes (for ≥16 lymph nodes, 3.40 [95% CI, 2.41—4.79]) were independently associated with decreased survival. Overall survival rate for patients with cervical lymph nodes resected and negative, cervical lymph nodes not resected, and 1—5, 6—10, 11—16, and ≥16 cervical lymph node metastases was 90, 76, 74, 61, 69, and 55%, respectively. There was no difference in survival based on surgical intervention in patients with tumor size ≤2 cm without distant metastases. In patients with tumor size >2.0 cm and no distant metastases, all surgical treatments resulted in a significant improvement in survival compared to no surgery (*P* < .001). In patients with distant metastases, only total thyroidectomy with regional lymph node resection resulted in a significant improvement in survival (*P* < .001).

Conclusions.—The number of lymph node metastases should be incorporated into MTC staging. The extent of surgery in patients with MTC should be tailored to tumor size and distant metastases.

▶ The authors here turn to the National Cancer Database to try to answer the question as to whether extent of local/regional surgery matters in patients with medullary thyroid cancer (MTC) who have either suspected low level of disease or, at the other end of the spectrum, known metastatic disease. Specifically they are trying to address the following questions: (1) Are thorough lymph node dissections useful in patients with metastatic MTC? and (2) Is a prophylactic central neck dissection necessary in low-risk patients? Finally they aimed to assess the relationship between the number of lymph node metastases and outcome.

The fact that the study depends on a large administrative database to answer these questions is limiting. Although the authors acknowledge this issue in the discussion, I do not think it is given enough attention. The only outcome that can be ascertained from the database is survival. Thus, the incidence and influence of recurrence on long-term survival cannot be determined. This is important, as the curves following mortality shown in Fig 1 of the original article (included here) have not leveled off for the earlier stage disease, suggesting that long-term follow-up will identify increased mortality. On the other hand, it does appear that in the most advanced stage tumors, locoregional control may be helpful in prolonging life. Finally, the data shown in Fig 1 of the original article do demonstrate that there appears to be a correlation between number of lymph nodes involved and survival.

So in sum, it would appear that the authors have answered question 1 in the affirmative—a thorough neck operation does appear to enhance survival in patients with MTC and metastatic disease. Although the authors claim to have answered question 2 (indicating that local/regional LN dissection is not necessary), the data presented do not support this conclusion, and I would recommend continued prophylactic central neck dissection for virtually all MTC until this is studied in a more prospective fashion, or at least in a large series that includes data on recurrence.

T. J. Fahey, MD

Nodules in Autoimmune Thyroiditis Are Associated With Increased Risk of Thyroid Cancer in Surgical Series But Not in Cytological Series: Evidence for Selection Bias

Castagna MG, Belardini V, Memmo S, et al (Univ of Siena, Italy)
J Clin Endocrinol Metab 99:3193-3198, 2014

Background.—The association of thyroid cancer and autoimmune thyroiditis (AIT) has been widely addressed, with conflicting results in surgical and cytological series, likely affected by selection bias.

Objective.—The objective of the study was to evaluate the association between the cytological features suggestive or indicative of malignancy and AIT in 2504 consecutive patients (2029 females and 475 males, mean age 58.3 ± 14.1 y) undergoing fine-needle aspiration cytology for thyroid nodules.

Patients.—Based on the clinical diagnosis, patients were divided into four groups: AIT with nodules (N-AIT, 14.9%); nodular Graves disease (N-GD, 2.8%); nodular goiter and negative thyroid antibodies (NGAb−, 68.4%); and nodular goiter with positive thyroid antibodies (NGAb+, 13.9%).

Results.—The prevalence of patients with cytological features suggestive (Thy4) or indicative of malignancy (Thy5) was 4.5% in the N-AIT group, not different compared with the other groups (N-GD, 5.6%; NGAb−, 5.0%; NGAb+, 4.3%). No difference was also found in the other categories (Thy2 and Thy3). When the same analysis was performed in the subgroup of patients (14.3%) with a histological confirmation, we found that the prevalence of differentiated thyroid cancer was significantly higher ($P=.01$) in the N-AIT group (67.8%) compared with the other groups (N-GD, 40.0%; NGAb−, 37.2%; NGAb+, 36.9%).

Conclusions.—The results of our cytological series do not support a link between N-AIT and thyroid cancer. The association between cancer and N-AIT found in the histology-based series is likely due to a selection bias represented by the fact that the prevalent indication for surgery in the N-AIT group was suspicious cytology (60.7% of patients) more frequently than in the other groups.

▶ This article attempts to take a new look at the age-old problem of whether there is an increased risk of cancer with chronic lymphocytic thyroiditis. The authors have a clear bias toward the supposition that the association between thyroiditis in malignant nodules is a product of selection bias from surgical series. The data presented indicate that patients referred for surgery with nodular autoimmune thyroid disease are referred more commonly because of a suspicious thyroid cytology (Bethesda IV or V), as opposed to being symptomatic due to a goiter, for example. Thus the authors conclude that there is no link between autoimmune thyroiditis and thyroid cancer. The logic behind this reasoning escapes me. How does the fact that there is a higher likelihood of finding cancer in nodules referred because of suspicious cytology translate to a conclusion that there is no link between the 2 entities? The more pertinent comparison would be the total number of cancers in Bethesda IV, V, and VI nodules in patients with or without autoimmune cytology, yet these data are not presented in the article.

Although the article delineates that patients referred for thyroidectomy with autoimmune thyroiditis are more likely to be referred because of a suspicious nodule, it does not answer the question regarding whether a link exists between autoimmune thyroiditis and the development of thyroid cancer.

T. J. Fahey, MD

Highly Accurate Diagnosis of Cancer in Thyroid Nodules With Follicular Neoplasm/Suspicious for a Follicular Neoplasm Cytology by ThyroSeq v2 Next-Generation Sequencing Assay
Nikiforov YE, Carty SE, Chiosea SI, et al (Univ of Pittsburgh, PA; et al)
Cancer 120:3627-3634, 2014

Background.—Fine-needle aspiration (FNA) cytology is a common approach to evaluating thyroid nodules, although 20% to 30% of FNAs have indeterminate cytology, which hampers the appropriate management of these patients. Follicular (or oncocytic) neoplasm/suspicious for a follicular (or oncocytic) neoplasm (FN/SFN) is a common indeterminate diagnosis with a cancer risk of approximately 15% to 30%. In this study, the authors tested whether the most complete next-generation sequencing (NGS) panel of genetic markers could significantly improve cancer diagnosis in these nodules.

Methods.—The evaluation of 143 consecutive FNA samples with a cytologic diagnosis of FN/SFN from patients with known surgical outcomes included 91 retrospective samples and 52 prospective samples. Analyses were performed on a proprietary sequencer using the targeted ThyroSeq v2 NGS panel, which simultaneously tests for point mutations in 13 genes and for 42 types of gene fusions that occur in thyroid cancer.

The expression of 8 genes was used to assess the cellular composition of FNA samples.

Results.—In the entire cohort, histologic analysis revealed 104 benign nodules and 39 malignant nodules. The most common point mutations involved the neuroblastoma RAS viral oncogene homolog (*NRAS*), followed by the Kirsten rat sarcoma viral oncogene homolog (*KRAS*), the telomerase reverse transcriptase (*TERT*) gene, and the thyroid-stimulating hormone receptor (*TSHR*) gene. The identified fusions involved the thyroid adenoma associated (*THADA*) gene; the peroxisome proliferator-activated receptor γ (*PPARG*) gene; and the neurotrophic tyrosine kinase, receptor, type 3 (*NTRK3*) gene. Performance characteristics were similar in the retrospective and prospective groups. Among all FN/SFN nodules, preoperative ThyroSeq v2 performed with 90% sensitivity (95% confidence interval [CI], 80%-99%), 93% specificity (95% CI, 88%-98%), a positive predictive value of 83% (95% CI, 72%-95%), a negative predictive value of 96% (95% CI, 92%-100%), and 92% accuracy (95% CI, 88%-97%).

Conclusions.—The current results indicate that comprehensive genotyping of thyroid nodules using a broad NGS panel provides a highly accurate diagnosis for nodules with FN/SFN cytology and should facilitate the optimal management of these patients.

▶ The application of next-generation sequencing to the diagnostic dilemma of indeterminate thyroid nodules has resulted in the development of the ThyroSeq panel for detecting mutations in thyroid nodules undergoing FNA. Thyroseq v2 essentially covers all known mutations associated with thyroid cancer and thus seems like the perfect complement to cytology for differentiating benign and malignant thyroid nodules. However, this study reports on a highly selected group of patients—they have already had a molecular test before going to surgery—and thus raises the question as to whether the test will perform as well in other hands in previously untested patients. An independent study is definitely needed before widespread application. Although I am enthusiastic about the application of Thyroseq to thyroid nodule diagnosis, ultimately this test will likely bring up new dilemmas. Perhaps the most important of these will be in regard to the extent of surgery in patients who present with a thyroid nodule that has had 1 of the 3 ras mutations identified. It is likely that these patients will now be routinely subjected to total thyroidectomy, which may in fact be overtreatment for many of them because many of these nodules will prove to be nonthreatening follicular variant of papillary thyroid carcinoma, and at least 20% will not have cancer at all. Nevertheless, mutation panel testing has now entered a new phase that will likely remain an integral component of thyroid nodule diagnosis for many years to come.

T. J. Fahey, MD

Examining National Outcomes after Thyroidectomy with Nerve Monitoring

Chung TK, Rosenthal EL, Porterfield JR, et al (Univ of Alabama at Birmingham)
J Am Coll Surg 219:765-770, 2014

Background.—Previous intraoperative nerve monitoring (IONM) studies have demonstrated modest-to-no benefit and did not include a nationwide sample of hospitals representative of broad thyroidectomy practices. This national study was designed to compare vocal cord paralysis (VCP) rates between thyroidectomy with IONM and without monitoring (conventional).

Study Design.—We performed a retrospective analysis of 243,527 thyroidectomies during 2008 to 2011 using the Nationwide Inpatient Sample.

Results.—Use of IONM increased yearly throughout the study period (2.6% [2008], 5.6% [2009], 6.1% [2010], 6.9% [2011]) and during this time, VCP rates in the IONM group initially increased year-over-year (0.9% [2008], 2.4% [2009], 2.5% [2010], 1.4% [2011]). In unadjusted analyses, IONM was associated with significantly higher VCP rates (conventional 1.4% vs IONM 1.9%, $p < 0.001$). After propensity score matching, IONM remained associated with higher VCP rates in partial thyroidectomy and lower VCP rates for total thyroidectomy with neck dissection. Hospital-level analysis revealed that VCP rates were not explained by differential laryngoscopy rates, decreasing the likelihood of ascertainment bias. Additionally, for hospitals in which IONM was applied to more than 50% of thyroidectomies, lower VCP rates were observed (1.1%) compared with hospitals that applied IONM to less than 50% (1.6%, $p = 0.016$). Higher hospital volume correlated with lower VCP rates in both groups (<75, 75 to 299, >300 thyroidectomies/year: IONM, 2.1%, 1.7%, 1.7%; conventional, 1.5%, 1.3%, 1.0%, respectively).

Conclusions.—According to this study, IONM has not been broadly adopted into practice. Overall, IONM was associated with a higher rate of VCP even after correction for numerous confounders. In particular, low institutional use of IONM and use in partial thyroidectomies are associated with higher rates of VCP. Further studies are warranted to support the broader application of IONM in patients where benefit can be reliably achieved.

▶ This provocative paper analyzes recurrent laryngeal nerve (RLN) injury using the Nationwide Inpatient Sample database in patients undergoing thyroidectomy with and without associated intraoperative nerve monitoring (IONM). The data presented document that IONM utilization is slowly increasing over the time period analyzed. However, this increase in use was not associated with an overall decrease in RLN injury rates compared with operations performed without IONM. This was particularly true for patients undergoing hemithyroidectomy, although the use of IONM did prove to be associated with lower RLN injury rates in patients undergoing total thyroidectomy and central neck dissection. The most obvious explanation for this, which the authors include in the discussion, is that patients who had an RLN injury that was recognized at the time of surgery would likely not go on to a total thyroidectomy and thus would be placed in the hemithyroidectomy group.

Overall, this study is useful in that it highlights the fact that IONM has not been widely adopted into practice. Furthermore, it would appear that if it is going to be incorporated into surgical practice, it would be better to make it a routine part of the surgery—especially if it is to be adopted for use in total thyroidectomy with a central neck dissection. As is the case with much new technology, occasional or casual use may be associated with worse outcomes rather than realizing the benefits of IONM. Finally, although the cost of IONM does not appear to substantially increase the overall cost of thyroidectomy ($11 409 vs $11 200), at this point, it does not appear that it will be cost-effective for most everyday thyroid operations.

T. J. Fahey, MD

Centralized Molecular Testing for Oncogenic Gene Mutations Complements the Local Cytopathologic Diagnosis of Thyroid Nodules

Beaudenon-Huibregtse S, Alexander EK, Guttler RB, et al (Asuragen Inc, Austin, TX; Brigham and Women's Hosp and Harvard Med School, Boston, MA; Santa Monica Thyroid Ctr, CA)
Thyroid 24:1479-1487, 2014

Background.—Molecular testing for oncogenic gene mutations and chromosomal rearrangements plays a growing role in the optimal management of thyroid nodules, yet lacks standardized testing modalities and systematic validation data. Our objective was to assess the performance of molecular cytology on preoperative thyroid nodule fine-needle aspirates (FNAs) across a broad range of variables, including independent collection sites, clinical practices, and anatomic pathology interpretations.

Methods.—Single-pass FNAs were prospectively collected from 806 nodules 1 cm or larger by ultrasonography at five independent sites across the United States. Specimens were shipped in a nucleic acid stabilization solution and tested at a centralized clinical laboratory. Seventeen genetic alterations (*BRAF, KRAS, HRAS,* and *NRAS* mutations, *PAX8-PPARG* and *RET-PTC* rearrangements) were evaluated by multiplex polymerase chain reaction and liquid bead array cytometry in 769 FNAs that met inclusion criteria. Cytology, histology, and clinical care followed local procedures and practices. All results were double-blinded.

Results.—Thirty-two specimens (4.2%) failed to yield sufficient nucleic acid to generate molecular data. A single genetic alteration was detected in 80% of cytology malignant cases, 21% of indeterminate, 7.8% of nondiagnostic, and 3.5% of benign cases. Among 109 nodules with surgical histology reference standard, oncogenic mutations were present in 50% of malignant nodules missed by cytology. There were 14 cancers not identified by cytology or molecular tests, including 5 carcinomas with histologic sizes less than 1 cm (3 multifocal) and 8 noninvasive follicular variants of papillary carcinoma (4 encapsulated). No mutations were detected in 89% of the nodules benign by histopathology with 6 false-positive molecular results in 5 adenomas (2—5.5 cm) and 1 cystic nodule with an incidental papillary microcarcinoma (0.15 cm). The posttest probability of thyroid cancer was 100% for nodules positive for *BRAF* or *RET-PTC*, 70% for *RAS* or *PAX8-PPARG*, and 88% for molecular cytology overall.

Conclusions.—Centralized and standardized molecular testing for genetic alterations associated with a high risk of malignancy efficiently complements the local cytopathologic diagnosis of thyroid nodule aspirates in the clinical setting. Actionable molecular cytology can improve the personalized surgical and medical management of patients with thyroid cancers, facilitating one-stage total thyroidectomy and reducing the number of unnecessary diagnostic surgeries.

▶ Molecular testing for indeterminate thyroid nodules can be done by gene expression analysis (most commonly Afirma) or identification of mutations known to be present in thyroid cancers. Here the authors present the data from Asuragen's mutation profile. The differences between the Asuragen test and Thyroseq[1] are in the way that mutations are identified; the Asuragen test assayed here uses a multiplex polymerase chain reaction, which is considerably less sophisticated than the RNA-seq platform used in Thyroseq. The advantages are that it is simpler and easier to run (and probably less expensive). The disadvantage is that it does not cover as many of the mutations known to exist in thyroid cancers. Nevertheless, it does cover most known mutations, and two-thirds of histopathologically proven cancers had mutations detected by the Asuragen test. The overall sensitivity for cancer was 66% with a specificity of 89%. There were 6 "false-positive" molecular results, 2 *PAX8-PPARG*, 2 *HRAS*, and 2 *NRAS* mutations, that were identified in ultimately benign nodules. Three of these were in adenomas, and the remaining 3 in theoretically nonneoplastic nodules. This is not surprising because both *RAS* mutations and *PAX8-PPARG* mutations have been described and identified in histologically benign nodules previously.

Overall, the authors conclude that there is value in mutation analysis, and this study adds to the growing body of literature that indicates that this is now becoming a reality. The new dilemma for endocrinologists, surgeons, and their patients will be whether to proceed with a hemithyroidectomy or total thyroidectomy when a *RAS* or *PAX8-PPARG* mutation is identified.

T. J. Fahey, MD

Reference

1. Nikiforov YE, Carty SE, Chiosea SI, et al. Highly accurate diagnosis of cancer in thyroid nodules with follicular neoplasm/suspicious for a follicular neoplasm cytology by ThyroSeq v2 next-generation sequencing assay. *Cancer.* 2014;120: 3627-3634.

Identification of the transforming *STRN-ALK* fusion as a potential therapeutic target in the aggressive forms of thyroid cancer

Kelly LM, Barila G, Liu P, et al (Univ of Pittsburgh School of Medicine, PA; Med College of Wisconsin, Milwaukee)
Proc Natl Acad Sci U S A 111:4233-4238, 2014

Thyroid cancer is a common endocrine malignancy that encompasses well-differentiated as well as dedifferentiated cancer types. The latter tumors have high mortality and lack effective therapies. Using a paired-end RNA-sequencing approach, we report the discovery of rearrangements involving the anaplastic lymphoma kinase (*ALK*) gene in thyroid cancer. The most common of these involves a fusion between *ALK* and the striatin (*STRN*) gene, which is the result of a complex rearrangement involving the short arm of chromosome 2. *STRN-ALK* leads to constitutive activation of ALK kinase via dimerization mediated by the coiled-coil domain of STRN and to a kinase-dependent, thyroid-stimulating hormone-independent proliferation of thyroid cells. Moreover, expression of STRN-ALK transforms cells in vitro and induces tumor formation in nude mice. The kinase activity of STRN-ALK and the ALK-induced cell growth can be blocked by the ALK inhibitors crizotinib and TAE684. In addition to well-differentiated papillary cancer, *STRN-ALK* was found with a higher prevalence in poorly differentiated and anaplastic thyroid cancers, and it did not overlap with other known driver mutations in these tumors. Our data demonstrate that *STRN-ALK* fusion occurs in a subset of patients with highly aggressive types of thyroid cancer and provide initial evidence suggesting that it may represent a therapeutic target for these patients.

▶ Identifying mutations in thyroid cancers without known driver mutations has been a goal of many groups for some time. Dr Nikiforova, due to his excellent comprehensive approach to cataloging molecular events in thyroid cancer, and his group report here the presence of a previously characterized fusion gene, *STRN-ALK*, in thyroid cancer. The overall prevalence of this mutation in PTC is low—3 of 256 tumors, or 1.2%. However, the fusion gene was present in a higher percentage of poorly differentiated thyroid cancers (9% of 35) and in 1 of 24 anaplastic thyroid cancers, suggesting that it may lead to more aggressive thyroid cancer. The authors report finding a different ALK fusion gene, *EML4-ALK*, in 1 of the well-differentiated tumors as well. The implications of identifying the *STRN-ALK* fusion in thyroid cancers, even if only in a very low percentage, are important because small-molecule inhibitors of the ALK tyrosine kinase have already been developed for the treatment of patients with other cancers. Thus, identification of ALK fusion genes, especially in those tumors that are recurrent or poorly differentiated, will instantly lead to new treatment options.

T. J. Fahey, MD

Determination of the Optimal Time Interval for Repeat Evaluation After a Benign Thyroid Nodule Aspiration

Nou E, Kwong N, Alexander LK, et al (Harvard Med School, Boston, MA)
J Clin Endocrinol Metab 99:510-516, 2014

Introduction.—The optimal timing for repeat evaluation of a cytologically benign thyroid nodule greater than 1 cm is uncertain. Arguably, the most important determinant is the disease-specific mortality resulting from an undetected thyroid cancer. Presently there exist no data that evaluate this important end point.

Methods.—We studied the long-term status of all patients evaluated in our thyroid nodule clinic between 1995 and 2003 with initially benign fine-needle aspiration (FNA) cytology. The follow-up interval was defined from the time of the initial benign FNA to any one of the following factors: thyroidectomy, death, or the most recent clinic visit documented anywhere in our health care system. We sought to determine the optimal timing for repeat assessment based on the identification of falsely benign malignancy and, most important, disease-related mortality due to a missed diagnosis.

Results.—One thousand three hundred sixty-nine patients with 2010 cytologically benign nodules were followed up for an average of 8.5 years (range 0.25−18 y). Thirty deaths were documented, although zero were attributed to thyroid cancer. Eighteen false-negative thyroid malignancies were identified and removed at a mean 4.5 years (range 0.3−10 y) after the initial benign aspiration. None had distant metastasis, and all are alive presently at an average of 11 years after the initial falsely benign FNA. Separate analysis demonstrates that patients with initially benign nodules who subsequently sought thyroidectomy for compressive symptoms did so an average of 4.5 years later.

Conclusions.—An initially benign FNA confers negligable mortality risk during long-term follow-up despite a low risk of identifying several such nodules as thyroid cancer. Because such malignancies appear adequately treated despite detection at a mean 4.5 years after falsely benign cytology, these data support a recommendation for repeat thyroid nodule evaluation 2−4 years after the initial benign FNA.

▶ This article attempts to address a question that is encountered in practice every day in the care of patients with thyroid nodules. It is one of those topics for which most surgeons have a standard practice that has developed but one that is probably not based in objective data. Here the authors demonstrate that it is unlikely that patients will develop a thyroid malignancy after an initial benign cytology and that even if one is eventually found, it is even more unlikely that the patient will die of thyroid cancer. Although the authors state that disease-specific mortality is arguably the most important outcome, their follow-up is not really long enough to truly assess that parameter. Because no deaths were attributable to thyroid cancer despite a mean of 4.5 years time elapsed since initial biopsy to time of excision, the authors conclude that a repeat aspirate can be performed in 2 to 4 years' time. Although the authors provide some good clinical data, this number does not appear to be based on any real data from the study. The problem with 2 to 4 years is that if a nodule is misdiagnosed on initial fine-needle aspiration (FNA) and subsequently turns out to be malignant, then the physician or surgeon making such a recommendation can easily be criticized for delay in diagnosis. Because the false-negative rate in the current study was in the accepted range for most benign thyroid cytology reports (1%–2%), it would seem to make more sense to repeat the FNA some time early (6–18 months) and then be content to observe unless there were ultrasonographic changes in the nodule that prompted repeat biopsy. Although the data provided are useful, using it as a basis for deciding when to repeat a biopsy is perhaps a little bit of a stretch.

T. J. Fahey, MD

Negative Parafibromin Staining Predicts Malignant Behavior in Atypical Parathyroid Adenomas

Kruijff S, Sidhu SB, Sywak MS, et al (Univ of Sydney, New South Wales, Australia; et al)
Ann Surg Oncol 21:426-433, 2014

Background.—The histopathological criteria for carcinoma proposed by the World Health Organization (WHO) are imperfect predictors of the malignant potential of parathyroid tumors. Negative parafibromin (PF) and positive protein gene product 9.5 (PGP9.5) staining are markers of *CDC73* mutation and occur commonly in carcinoma but rarely in adenomas. We investigated whether PF and PGP9.5 staining could be used to predict the behavior of atypical parathyroid adenomas—tumors with atypical features that do not fulfill WHO criteria for malignancy.

Methods.—Long-term outcomes were compared across four groups: group A, WHO-positive criteria/PF-negative staining; group B, WHO$^+$/PF$^+$, group C; WHO$^-$/PF$^-$; and group D, WHO$^-$/PF$^+$.

Results.—Eighty-one patients were included in the period 1999–2012: group A ($n = 13$), group B ($n = 14$), group C ($n = 21$), and group D ($n = 33$). Mortality and recurrence rates, respectively, for group A were 15 and 38 %, for group B 7 and 36 %, for group C 0 and 10 %, and for group D 0 and 0 %. The PGP9.5$^+$ ratios for groups A to D were 85, 78, 71, and 12 %, further informing prognosis. Five-year disease-free survival for groups A to D were 55, 80, 78, and 100 %, respectively. Tumor recurrence was significantly associated with PF ($p = 0.048$) and PGP9.5 ($p = 0.003$) staining.

Conclusions.—Although WHO criteria are essential to differentiate parathyroid carcinoma from benign tumors, the presence of negative PF staining in an atypical adenoma predicts outcome better, whereas PF-positive atypical adenomas do not recur and can be considered benign.

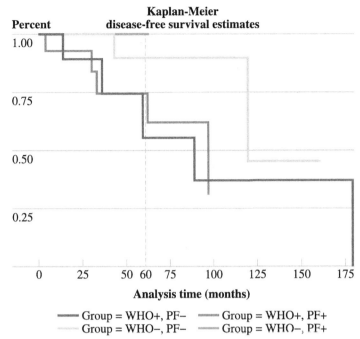

FIGURE 5.—Kaplan—Meier curves for groups a (WHO⁺PF⁻), b (WHO⁺PF⁺), c (WHO⁻PF⁻), and d (WHO⁻PF⁺). (With kind permission from Springer Science+Business Media. Kruijff S, Sidhu SB, Sywak MS, et al. Negative parafibromin staining predicts malignant behavior in atypical parathyroid adenomas. *Ann Surg Oncol.* 2014;21:426-433, with permission from Society of Surgical Oncology.)

PF-negative atypical adenomas have a low but real recurrence risk and should be considered tumors of low malignant potential (Fig 5).

▶ Parathyroid carcinoma is a rare tumor, and even atypical parathyroid adenomas are rare. The Sydney group details their considerable experience with parathyroid carcinoma and atypical parathyroid adenomas in this report and shows the importance of parafibromin staining in helping direct treatment for patients who present with atypical adenomas. Fig 5 shows the disease-free survival of patients with World Health Organization (WHO) criteria carcinoma and the effect of including parafibromin staining. It is apparent from the figure that a pathologic diagnosis of parathyroid carcinoma remains the most important driver of outcome. However, in those tumors that do not meet WHO criteria for carcinoma—and these are the atypical adenomas that ultimately are treatment dilemmas—the presence of parafibromin staining can reassure the physician and patient that it is safe to watch and that recurrence is unlikely. The major problem with using parafibromin staining is that it is a difficult immunostain to master, and the authors point this out. This will likely limit its widespread adoption, as very few centers see enough atypical adenomas or parathyroid carcinomas in a year to maintain a level of expertise in the immunostaining. Given the recent explosion in capability for DNA testing of clinical specimens, it would seem that immunostaining for parafibromin will soon be replaced by a DNA test looking at CDC73.

T. J. Fahey, MD

Primary Hyperparathyroidism With Negative Imaging: A Significant Clinical Problem
Wachtel H, Bartlett EK, Kelz RR, et al (Hosp of the Univ of Pennsylvania, Philadelphia)
Ann Surg 260:474-482, 2014

Objective.—To compare the outcomes for patients undergoing parathyroidectomy for primary hyperparathyroidism by imaging results.

Background.—Preoperative imaging plays an increasingly important role in the evaluation of primary hyperparathyroidism, and surgical referral may be predicated upon successful imaging.

Methods.—We performed a retrospective study of patients undergoing initial parathyroidectomy for primary hyperparathyroidism (2002–2014). Patients were classified as nonlocalized when preoperative imaging failed to identify affected gland(s) and localized if successful. Primary outcome was cure, defined as eucalcemia postoperatively. Intraoperative success, defined by intraoperative parathyroid hormone criteria, and complication rates were also analyzed. Localized and nonlocalized patients were matched (1:1) utilizing a propensity score. Logistic regression determined factors associated with localization in the matched cohort.

Results.—Of 2185 patients, 38.3% (n = 836) were nonlocalized. Nonlocalized patients had smaller parathyroids by size (1.2 vs 1.6 cm, $P < 0.001$) and mass (250 vs 537 mg, $P < 0.001$), higher incidence of hyperplasia (12.8% vs 5.4%, $P < 0.001$) and lower incidence of single adenoma (73.6 vs 86.0%, $P < 0.001$) compared with localized patients. There was no difference in intraoperative success (93.9 vs 95.6%, $P = 0.073$) or cure rates (96.2% vs 97.7%, $P = 0.291$) between nonlocalized and localized groups. In a propensity-matched cohort of 452 patients, there was no significant difference in cure rates (97.8 vs 97.4%, $P = 0.760$) between nonlocalized patients and matched localized controls.

Conclusions.—Nonlocalization of abnormal glands preoperatively is not associated with a decreased surgical cure rate for primary hyperparathyroidism. Referral for surgical evaluation should be based on biochemical diagnosis rather than localization by imaging.

▶ Debate about the role of localization studies in primary hyperparathyroidism has once again become a hot topic. The point of this paper is not to argue for or against localization studies but simply to point out that lack of localization does not mean patients with primary hyperparathyroidism should not be referred for surgery. Nonlocalized disease in primary hyperparathyroidism has probably increased—despite better imaging techniques—because of earlier diagnosis and increased prevalence of small gland disease. Despite this, however, the authors demonstrate nicely that surgery for primary hyperparathyroidism is equally effective in experienced hands whether the disease is localized or not. Experience is probably the most important and underemphasized aspect of the success noted in the article.

The discussion at the end of the article regarding whether localization is necessary at all is enlightening and should be read with the article for those interested. I strongly agree with Dr Fraker: If you are going to perform parathyroidectomy under local anesthesia, it is much easier to do with a high likelihood of a single gland that has already been identified by preoperative imaging. Finally, even if you are a minimalist when it comes to imaging, a preoperative ultrasound should be considered a mandatory part of the workup to be sure that there is no thyroid disease that requires workup as well.

T. J. Fahey, MD

Patients With Apparently Nonfunctioning Adrenal Incidentalomas May Be at Increased Cardiovascular Risk Due to Excessive Cortisol Secretion

Androulakis II, Kaltsas GA, Kollias GE, et al (Natl Univ of Athens, Greece; et al)

J Clin Endocrinol Metab 99:2754-2762, 2014

Context.—Although adrenal incidentalomas (AIs) are associated with a high prevalence of cardiovascular risk (CVR) factors, it is not clear whether patients with nonfunctioning AI (NFAI) have increased CVR.

Objective.—Our objective was to investigate CVR in patients with NFAI.

Design and Setting.—This case-control study was performed in a tertiary general hospital.

Subjects.—Subjects included 60 normotensive euglycemic patients with AI and 32 healthy controls (C) with normal adrenal imaging.

Main Outcome Measures.—All participants underwent adrenal imaging, biochemical and hormonal evaluation, and the following investigations: 1) measurement of carotid intima-media thickness (IMT) and flow-mediated dilatation, 2) 2-hour 75-gram oral glucose tolerance test and calculation of insulin resistance indices (homeostasis model assessment, quantitative insulin sensitivity check, and Matsuda indices), 3) iv ACTH stimulation test, 4) low-dose dexamethasone suppression test, and 5) NaCl (0.9%) post-dexamethasone saline infusion test.

Results.—Based on cutoffs obtained from controls, autonomous cortisol secretion was documented in 26 patients (cortisol-secreting AI [CSAI] group), whereas 34 exhibited adequate cortisol and aldosterone suppression (NFAI group). IMT measurements were higher and flow-mediated vasodilatation was lower in the CSAI group compared with both NFAI and C and in the NFAI group compared with C. The homeostasis model assessment index was higher and quantitative insulin sensitivity check index and Matsuda indices were lower in the CSAI and NFAI groups compared with C as well as in CSAI compared with the NFAI group. The area under the curve for cortisol after ACTH stimulation was higher in the CSAI group compared with the NFAI group and C and in the NFAI group compared with C. In the CSAI group, IMT correlated with cortisol, urinary free cortisol, and cortisol after a low-dose dexamethasone suppression test, whereas in the NFAI group, IMT correlated with area under the curve for cortisol after ACTH stimulation and urinary free cortisol.

Conclusions.—Patients with CSAI without hypertension, diabetes, and/ or dyslipidemia exhibit adverse metabolic and CVR factors. In addition, NFAIs are apparently associated with increased insulin resistance and endothelial dysfunction that correlate with subtle but not autonomous cortisol excess.

▶ This is the third report examining adrenal incidentalomas and their relationship to cardiovascular disease included this year, all from the *Journal of Clinical Endocrinology and Metabolism*. Although the numbers of patients included in this study are not very high, the study is perhaps the most comprehensive in its evaluation, as the authors took care to measure objective measures of cardiovascular risk at the start and completion of the study. This is best seen in Fig 2 from the original article, which shows that both adrenal incidentalomas associated with mild cortisol excess (subclinical Cushing's, cortisol-secreting adrenal incidentalomas [CSAI] in figure) and those that do not show evidence for excess cortisol secretion (nonfunctioning adrenal incidentalomas [NFAI] in the figure) are associated with increased cardiovascular risk as measured by carotid intima-media thickness (IMT) and flow-mediated vasodilatation (FMD). Both of these parameters have been associated with risk of cardiovascular disease—IMT, as a marker for structural vascular changes, is associated with atherosclerosis, and FMD, as a marker for functional properties, has been correlated with endothelial dysfunction and also predicts the presence of atherosclerosis. Furthermore, incidentalomas, regardless of whether associated with cortisol excess (CSAI or NFAI), were also associated with insulin resistance. The importance of this study is that it examined patients with adrenal incidentalomas that did not have previously documented cardiovascular disease or evidence for abnormal glucose homeostasis. The authors hypothesize—and their data support their hypothesis—that even nonfunctioning incidentalomas may have abnormal responses to adrenocorticotropic hormone stimulation. There are prior studies that have indicated that adrenalectomy is not protective for atherosclerotic risk factors in patients with incidentalomas.[1] However, this study did not carefully document excess cortisol production or document existing changes such as IMT or FMD. Clearly, a prospective trial is needed in determining the best treatment course for such patients. If the adrenal adenoma is not causative, then other courses of action should be pursued to prevent cardiovascular morbidity in these patients.

T. J. Fahey, MD

Reference

1. Sereg M, Szappanos A, Toke J, et al. Atherosclerotic risk factors and complications in patients with non-functioning adrenal adenomas treated with or without adrenalectomy: a long-term follow-up study. *Eur J Endocrinol.* 2009;160:647-655.

Aldosteronoma resolution score predicts long-term resolution of hypertension

Aronova A, Gordon BL, Finnerty BM, et al (Weill Cornell Med College, NY)
Surgery 156:1387-1393, 2014

Background.—The Aldosteronoma Resolution Score (ARS) takes into consideration four, readily available, preoperative clinical parameters in predicting the likelihood of resolution of hypertension in patients 6 months after undergoing unilateral adrenalectomy for aldosterone-producing adenoma (APA). We sought to determine the durability of this predictive model after 1 year.

Methods.—Sixty patients who underwent unilateral adrenalectomy for APA at a single institution between 2004 and 2013 were reviewed retrospectively. Patients who were normotensive without any antihypertensive medication requirement at greater than 1-year follow-up were considered to have complete resolution of hypertension.

Results.—Forty-seven patients had data available for analysis. Median follow-up was 1,135 days (371—3,202). Forty-five percent of patients had complete resolution, 45% had improvement, and 10% had no improvement in hypertension. Applying the ARS, we found there was

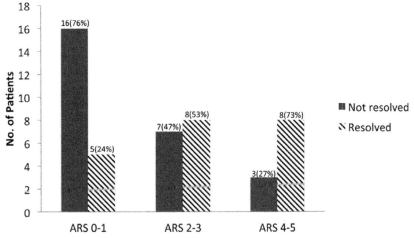

FIGURE 1.—Patient outcomes by composite ARS. (Reprinted from Surgery. Aronova A, Gordon BL, Finnerty BM, et al. Aldosteronoma resolution score predicts long-term resolution of hypertension. *Surgery.* 2014;156:1387-1393, Copyright 2014, with permission from Elsevier.)

complete resolution of hypertension in 73% of patients with ARS 4–5, 53% of patients with ARS 2–3, and 24% of patients with ARS 0–1 compared with 75% ($P=.9$), 46% ($P=.66$), and 28% ($P=.76$), respectively, in the original cohort used to create the ARS.

Conclusion.—Most patients (90%) have long-term improvement or complete resolution of hypertension after unilateral adrenalectomy for APA. The ARS predicts accurately a patient's likelihood of complete resolution of hypertension beyond 1 year (Fig 1).

▶ Patients with primary hyperaldosteronism who are facing surgery frequently want to know if they are going to be cured after the operation. The Aldosteronoma Resolution Score (ARS) distilled the experience of 2 large endocrine centers into a reproducible score to estimate for patients' likelihoods of resolution of hypertension after adrenalectomy. The ARS assigns 1 point each for a body mass index less than 25, female sex, and duration of hypertension less than 6 years and 2 points if the number of preoperative antihypertensive medications is less than 2. A composite score greater than 4 predicts a high likelihood of resolution of hypertension at 6 months. Here the authors examined outcomes at 1 year or more after surgery to determine if the ARS was able to predict long-term resolution of hypertension. The data presented in Fig 1 (included here) summarize the findings. It can be seen that large, male patients with longstanding hypertension and who are on 3 or more antihypertensive medications have the least likelihood of being off blood pressure medications after surgery (approximately 25%). It is notable that even patients with the best predictive scores still have an approximately 25% chance of having complete resolution of their hypertension. It is also reassuring to know that these percentages are virtually identical to those seen in the original study,[1] both validating the original data and indicating that the ARS has long-term prognostic value.

T. J. Fahey, MD

Reference

1. Zarnegar R, Young WF Jr, Lee J, et al. The aldosteronoma resolution score: predicting complete resolution of hypertension after adrenalectomy for aldosteronoma. *Ann Surg.* 2008;247:511-518.

Cortisol as a Marker for Increased Mortality in Patients with Incidental Adrenocortical Adenomas
Debono M, Bradburn M, Bull M, et al (Univ of Sheffield, South Yorkshire, UK; Royal Hallamshire Hosp, South Yorkshire, UK)
J Clin Endocrinol Metab 99:4462-4470, 2014

Context.—Incidental benign adrenocortical adenomas, adrenal incidentalomas are found in 4.5% of abdominal computed tomography scans, with the incidence increasing to 10% in patients older than 70 years of age. These incidentalomas frequently show evidence of excess cortisol secretion but without overt Cushing's syndrome. The mortality rate is increased in Cushing's syndrome.

Objective.—This study sought to investigate whether patients with adrenal incidentalomas have an increased mortality.

Design.—This was a retrospective, longitudinal cohort study.

Setting.—The study was carried out in an Endocrine Investigation Unit in a University Teaching Hospital.

Patients.—Two hundred seventy-two consecutive patients with an incidental adrenal mass underwent a dedicated diagnostic protocol, which included dexamethasone testing for hypercortisolism between 2005 and 2013. Overall survival was assessed in 206 patients with a benign, adrenocortical adenoma.

Main Outcome Measures.—Survival analysis was carried out by using Kaplan-Meier curves and the effect of dexamethasone cortisol estimated by Cox-regression analysis. Cause-specific mortality was ascertained from death certificates and compared with local and national data.

Results.—Eighteen of 206 patients died and the mean time (SD) from diagnosis to death was 3.2 (1.7) years. Seventeen of 18 patients who died had a post dexamethasone cortisol >1.8 μg/dL and there was a significant decrease in survival rate with increasing dexamethasone cortisol levels ($P = .001$). Compared with the <1.8 μg/dL group, the hazard ratio (95% confidence interval) for the 1.8–5μg/dL group was 12.0 (1.6–92.6) whereas that of the >5 μg/dL group was 22.0 (2.6–188.3). Fifty percent and 33% of deaths were secondary to circulatory or respiratory/infective causes, respectively.

Conclusions.—Patients with adrenal incidentalomas and a post-dexamethasone serum cortisol >1.8 μg/dL have increased mortality, mainly related to cardiovascular disease and infection.

▶ This report strongly suggests that adrenal incidentalomas associated with significant alteration of the pituitary-adrenal axis are associated with increased risk of mortality. The increase in mortality is a result of increased events in cardiovascular disease and infectious disease as shown in Fig 3 of the original article. Interestingly, the authors here also note that the rate of hypercortisolism is higher in adrenal nodules that have reached 2.5 cm in size (compared with 2.4 cm noted in the Italian study by Morelli et al[1]). The implications of the results noted in this study strongly advocate for surgical excision of adrenal nodules—regardless of whether incidentally discovered—that are associated with evidence for excess cortisol secretion, even if it is just on an altered dexamethasone suppression test. This study and the Morelli et al[1] study offer compelling data to obtain a dexamethasone suppression test on all patients with adrenal incidentalomas, especially those over 2 cm. Of course, both studies are from Europe, and whether the level of alteration in the pituitary-adrenal axis will hold up here in the United States (with a more obese population) is something that is worthy of study. Nevertheless, the data are compelling enough to spur the ordering of a dexamethasone suppression test in patients who present with an adrenal incidentaloma.

T. J. Fahey, MD

Reference

1. Morelli V, Reimondo G, Giordano R, et al. Long-term follow-up in adrenal incidentalomas: an Italian multicenter study. *J Clin Endocrinol Metab.* 2014;99: 827-834.

Long-Term Follow-Up in Adrenal Incidentalomas: An Italian Multicenter Study

Morelli V, Reimondo G, Giordano R, et al (Univ of Milan, Italy; Ospedale San Luigi, Orbassano, Italy; Univ of Turin, Italy; et al)
J Clin Endocrinol Metab 99:827-834, 2014

Context.—The long-term consequences of subclinical hypercortisolism (SH) in patients with adrenal incidentalomas (AIs) are unknown.

Setting and Patients.—In this retrospective multicentric study, 206 AI patients with a ≥5-year follow-up (median, 72.3 mo; range, 60–186 mo) were enrolled.

Intervention and Main Outcome Measures.—Adrenocortical function, adenoma size, metabolic changes, and incident cardiovascular events (CVEs) were assessed. We diagnosed SH in 11.6% of patients in the presence of cortisol after a 1 mg-dexamethasone suppression test >5 μg/dL (138 nmol/L) or at least two of the following: low ACTH, increased urinary free cortisol, and 1 mg-dexamethasone suppression test >3 μg/dL (83 nmol/L).

Results.—At baseline, age and the prevalence of CVEs and type 2 diabetes mellitus were higher in patients with SH than in patients without SH (62.2 ± 11 y vs 58.5 ± 10 y; 20.5 vs 6%; and 33.3 vs 16.8%, respectively; $P < .05$). SH and type 2 diabetes mellitus were associated with prevalent CVEs (odds ratio [OR], 3.1; 95% confidence interval [CI], 1.1−9.0; and OR, 2.0; 95% CI, 1.2−3.3, respectively), regardless of age. At the end of the follow-up, SH was diagnosed in 15 patients who were without SH at baseline. An adenoma size >2.4 cm was associated with the risk of developing SH (sensitivity, 73.3%; specificity, 60.5%; $P = .014$). Weight, glycemic, lipidic, and blood pressure control worsened in 26, 25, 13, and 34% of patients, respectively. A new CVE occurred in 22 patients. SH was associated with the worsening of at least two metabolic parameters (OR, 3.32; 95% CI, 1.6−6.9) and with incident CVEs (OR, 2.7; 95% CI, 1.0−7.1), regardless of age and follow-up.

Conclusion.—SH is associated with the risk of incident CVEs. Besides the clinical follow-up, in patients with an AI >2.4 cm, a long-term biochemical follow-up is also required because of the risk of SH development.

▶ Patients who present with incidentally discovered adrenal nodules undergo biochemical workup, and, if results are negative, are told that observation is the best course. This article examines the long-term outcomes of patients with adrenal nodules with and without evidence for subclinical hypercortisolism and suggests that if there is evidence for subclinical hypercortisolism, these patients would probably be better served by excision of the offending adenoma. This relationship is more clearly established for adenomas that are initially measured at 2.4 cm or larger. The main adverse effect of observation is the development of cardiovascular events, which is defined in the study as either coronary heart disease or ischemic or hemorrhagic stroke. Although the percent of patients who actually go on to develop a cardiovascular event is actually still reasonably low (around 15%), this is substantially higher than expected and than that seen in those patients without subclinical hypercortisolism. It should be noted—and the authors do acknowledge this in the discussion—that the observed effects may be more pronounced than reported because the study group included only those patients who were deemed arbitrarily to be suitable for observation, meaning some patients were advised to have surgery on the basis of perceived risk by their physician. Although the study is not perfect, it does highlight the fact that patients with adrenal incidentalomas should be followed for possible development of subclinical hypercortisolism, especially if the size is greater than 2.4 cm. Finally, although the authors do not state this in the conclusions, it would appear that patients with subclinical hypercortisolism should be strongly considered for surgery, even if they have an adenoma that is less than 4 cm. This article provides important data for those of us who face the dilemma about whether to advise surgery for patients with adrenal incidentalomas.

T. J. Fahey, MD

Accuracy of Adrenal Imaging and Adrenal Venous Sampling in Predicting Surgical Cure of Primary Aldosteronism
Lim V, Guo Q, Grant CS, et al (Mayo Clinic, Rochester, MN; Chinese PLA General Hosp, Beijing, People's Republic of China)
J Clin Endocrinol Metab 99:2712-2719, 2014

Context.—The accurate distinction between unilateral and bilateral adrenal disease in patients with primary aldosteronism (PA) guides surgical management. Adrenal venous sampling (AVS), the criterion standard localization procedure, is not readily available at many centers throughout the world.

Objective.—The objective of the study was to determine factors most consistent with surgically curable PA.

Design.—This was a retrospective observational study.

Setting.—The study was conducted at the Mayo Clinic (Rochester, Minnesota), a tertiary referral center.

Patients.—All patients who underwent unilateral adrenalectomy for treatment of PA between January 1993 and December 2011 participated in the study.

Intervention.—The intervention in the study was unilateral adrenalectomy.

Main Outcome Measures.—Variables associated with the prediction of unilateral disease were measured.

Results.—Over 19 years, 263 patients underwent unilateral adrenalectomy for the treatment of PA. Long-term postoperative follow-up was obtained in 143 patients (54.4%). The overall effective cure rate of PA was 95.5% in those patients sent for adrenalectomy for presumptive unilateral disease. In patients with cured PA, defined as the resolution of autonomous aldosterone secretion, hypertension was cured in 53 (41.7%) and improved in 59 (46.5%) patients. PA was not cured with unilateral adrenalectomy in six patients (4.2%). Adrenal imaging and AVS were concordant to the surgically documented side in 58.6% and 97.1% of the patients, respectively. Although there was no statistically significant difference in mean age between the inaccurate vs the accurate adrenal imaging group, we found that the minimum age in the former was 35.1 years.

Conclusions.—Using adrenal imaging and AVS, the effective surgical cure rate for PA was 95.5%. Although the overall accuracy of computed tomography and magnetic resonance imaging in detecting unilateral adrenal disease was poor at 58.6%, adrenal imaging performed well in those patients younger than 35 years of age.

▶ This study from the Mayo clinic addresses the question of whether cross-sectional imaging with CT or MRI is adequate for localization prior to adrenalectomy for primary aldosteronism or whether adrenal vein sampling (AVS) should be pursued. Although the authors do not outright make a recommendation, the suggestion is very strong that AVS should be used, as it correlated with the correct side at surgery in 97% of patients vs just 58.6% of patients who had only cross-sectional imaging. Most of the time that cross-sectional imaging was inaccurate, the inaccuracy was caused by designating a patient as having bilateral disease (Table 4 in the original article). As can be seen in the table in the original article, only in 7 of 133 patients (5%) did the cross-sectional imaging predict the wrong side. The implications of these data are considerable for endocrinologists and hypertension specialists as well as surgeons. Essentially, all patients who present with documented primary aldosteronism should undergo adrenal vein sampling, as cross-sectional imaging will miss unilateral disease one-third of the time. Patients whose disease was localized to unilateral disease by CT or MRI in this series had properly localized disease 92% of the time! The authors suggest that because no patient younger than 35 who had unilateral disease identified by CT or MRI was localized wrongly, younger patients (< 35) can skip the adrenal vein sampling.

The authors are surprisingly noncommittal in their recommendations here. In general, I recommend AVS in all patients with primary aldosteronism unless there is an extenuating circumstance (severe contrast allergy), with the possible exception of very young patients (in their 20s) who have an obvious adrenal adenoma with a normal contralateral gland on cross-sectional imaging. Any abnormalities in the contralateral gland—and it is important to review these images yourself—will mandate AVS.

T. J. Fahey, MD

Both preoperative alpha and calcium channel blockade impact intraoperative hemodynamic stability similarly in the management of pheochromocytoma
Brunaud L, Boutami M, Nguyen-Thi P-L, et al (Univ de Lorraine, Nancy, France; Université de Nantes, Nantes, France; et al)
Surgery 156:1410-1418, 2014

Background.—Alpha-blockade is the standard management preoperatively to prevent intraoperative hemodynamic instability (IHD) during resection of a pheochromocytoma. Calcium channel blockers also have been shown to lessen the risk of IHD. We aim to determine differences between these classes of antihypertensive agents in minimizing IHD.

Methods.—This was a retrospective analysis from a tri-institutional database. Inclusion criteria were unilateral transabdominal adrenalectomy for pheochromocytomas between 2002 and 2012. IHD was defined as at least one systolic blood pressure (SBP) measurement >160 mm Hg and at least one episode of mean arterial pressure 60 mm Hg.

Results.—A total of 155 patients were included: 110 receiving calcium channel blockers, 41 alpha-blockade, and 4 no medication. Intraoperatively, mean maximal SBP was less after alpha-blockade ($P < .0001$) as well as the incidence and duration of episodes of SBP >200 mm Hg ($P < .01$); however, severe hypotensive episodes (MAP < 60 mm Hg) were more frequent ($P < .001$) and longer ($P < .0001$) with alpha-blockade. Consequently, intraoperative vasoactive drugs were used more frequently ($P = .03$), and mean fluid volume infused was larger ($P < .001$). Fifty-four patients had IHD, but these were independent of type of preoperative medication used. Familial disease was the only independent predictor of IHD.

Conclusion.—IHD was independent of type of preoperative medical management but was dependent on familial disease. These findings broaden options for clinicians in the preoperative management of pheochromocytoma.

▶ Preparation of patients with pheochromocytomas for surgery has long depended on alpha blockade with phenoxybenzamine for hemodynamic stabilization. Increasingly, it has become difficult to obtain phenoxybenzamine in the United States, and some patients tolerate the side effects poorly, especially at the higher doses. The use of calcium channel blockers to prepare patients for surgery for pheochromocytoma resection was first reported by the legendary French surgeon, Charles Proye at the American Association of Endocrine Surgeons meeting in 1989. Since then, there has been widespread adoption of the use of nicardipine to prepare patients with pheochromocytomas in France, whereas US surgeons have continued to utilize phenoxybenzamine almost exclusively. This study compares intraoperative hemodynamics in patients prepared with nicardipine vs those prepared with phenoxybenzamine. The data indicate that for smaller tumors, there is little difference: Nicardipine has equal benefits as phenoxybenzamine. For larger tumors (> 3 cm), alpha blockade was associated with significantly lower and shorter peak intraoperative blood pressures but also with significantly lower and longer hypotensive episodes following tumor removal. I have gone almost exclusively to the use of nicardipine in preparing patients for resection of pheochromocytomas because it is equally safe and easier to use than phenoxybenzamine with the possible exception of large, very active tumors. A prospective study to compare nicardipine and phenoxybenzamine for larger tumors would be welcome to sort out the best preoperative management for these patients.

T. J. Fahey, MD

Long-Term Survival After Adrenalectomy for Stage I/II Adrenocortical Carcinoma (ACC): A Retrospective Comparative Cohort Study of Laparoscopic Versus Open Approach

Donatini G, Caiazzo R, Do Cao C, et al (Lille Regional Univ Hosp, France)
Ann Surg Oncol 21:284-291, 2014

Background.—Laparoscopic adrenalectomy (LA) is the standard treatment for benign adrenal lesions. The laparoscopic approach has also been increasingly accepted for adrenal metastases but remains controversial for adrenocortical carcinoma (ACC). In a retrospective cohort study we compared the outcome of LA versus open adrenalectomy (OA) in the treatment of stage I and II ACC.

Methods.—This was a double cohort study comparing the outcome of patients with stage I/II ACC and a tumor size <10 cm submitted to LA or OA at Lille University Hospital referral center from 1985 to 2011. Main outcomes analyzed were: postoperative morbidity, overall survival, and disease-free survival.

Results.—Among 111 consecutive patients operated on for ACC, 34 met the inclusion criteria. LA and OA were performed in 13 and 21 patients, respectively. Baseline patient characteristics (gender, age, tumor size, hormonal secretion) were similar between groups. There was no difference in postoperative morbidity, but patients in LA group were discharged earlier ($p < 0.02$). After a similar follow-up (66 ± 52 for LA and 51 ± 43 months for OA), Kaplan—Meier estimates of disease-specific survival and disease-free survival were identical in both groups ($p = 0.65$, $p = 0.96$, respectively).

Conclusions.—LA was associated with a shorter length of stay and did not compromise the long-term oncological outcome of patients operated on for stage I/II ACC ≤ 10 cm ACC. Our results suggest that LA can be safely proposed to patients with potentially malignant adrenal lesions smaller than 10 cm and without evidence of extra-adrenal extension (Fig 4).

▶ This study compares a relatively small number of patients (although one of the larger series for this disease) who underwent laparoscopic vs open adrenalectomy for adrenal cortical carcinoma. The authors show that the laparoscopic approach is both feasible and safe and leads to equivalent outcomes, as seen in

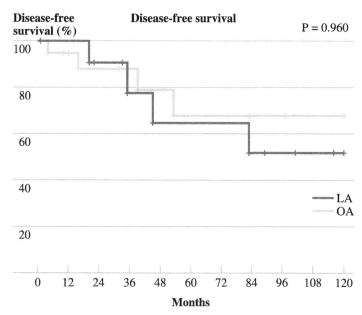

FIGURE 4.—Disease-free survival. (With kind permission from Springer Science+Business Media. Donatini G, Caiazzo R, Do Cao C, et al. Long-term survival after adrenalectomy for stage I/II adrenocortical carcinoma (ACC): A retrospective comparative cohort study of laparoscopic versus open approach. *Ann Surg Oncol.* 2014;21:284-291,with permission from Society of Surgical Oncology.)

Fig 4. This is in contradistinction to the data presented from the Michigan and MD Anderson groups who are both vocal opponents of the laparoscopic approach for adrenal cortical cancer resection. Why the different conclusions? The answer lies in 2 important aspects. First, the group from Lille selected their patients—only patients with stage I or II tumors were considered, and only tumors that were less than 10 cm were approached laparoscopically. Second, and in my opinion most importantly, only experienced laparoscopic adrenal surgeons were operating in the study from Lille. This is the most important difference between the report here and the reports from Michigan and MD Anderson. The latter groups analyzed data from patients who had been operated on from all over (without any assessment of the experience of the surgeons) who were then referred in for additional treatment. Surgical resection of larger adrenal masses should be performed by experienced surgeons only—whether laparoscopic or open—as this will undoubtedly lead to the best outcomes for the patient. Nevertheless, the main flaw of this study is that it is a small retrospective study. Ultimately, only a prospective randomized trial will definitively answer this question.

T. J. Fahey, MD

Adjuvant Therapies and Patient and Tumor Characteristics Associated With Survival of Adult Patients With Adrenocortical Carcinoma

Else T, Williams AR, Sabolch A, et al (Univ of Michigan Hosp and Health Systems, Ann Arbor; Univ of Michigan Med School, Ann Arbor)
J Clin Endocrinol Metab 99:455-461, 2014

Context.—Adrenocortical carcinoma is a rare malignant endocrine neoplasia. Studies regarding outcome and prognostic factors rely on fairly small studies. Here we summarize the experience with patients with a diagnosis of adrenocortical carcinoma from a large tertiary referral center.

Objective.—The objective of the study was to identify prognostic factors in patients with adrenocortical carcinoma and evaluate adjuvant treatment strategies.

Design.—Patient data were collected in a retrospective single-center study. Epidemiological, patient, and tumor characteristics were analyzed for prognostic factors regarding overall and recurrence-free survival in Cox regression models (multivariable and univariable).

Results.—Three hundred ninety-one adult patients with the diagnosis of adrenocortical carcinoma were identified. Median overall survival was 35.2 months. Cortisol production [hazard ratio (HR) 1.4, HR 1.5], tumor stage (HR stage 3 of 2.1 and 2.1, HR stage 4 of 4.8), and tumor grade (HR 2.4 and 2.0) were identified as negative prognostic factors (HR for death, HR for recurrence). Mitotane therapy increases recurrence-free survival, an effect that was significantly further improved by adjuvant radiation therapy but did not impact overall survival. Patients with open adrenalectomy had improved overall survival.

Conclusions.—This study increases the evidence for adverse risk factors (cortisol production, high tumor stage, and high tumor grade) and suggests the following therapy approach: adrenocortical carcinoma patients should be treated with open adrenalectomy. Adjuvant therapy, particularly mitotane therapy in conjunction with radiation, should be considered to delay tumor recurrence.

▶ This study of adrenocortical carcinoma (ACC) is a retrospective review of a single center's large experience with ACC. As expected, tumor stage and grade are important predictors of survival. In contradistinction to some previous studies, cortisol production was identified as an adverse prognostic risk factor. Overall survival remains poor, even for stage 1 and 2 tumors, and interestingly stage 2 tumors had somewhat better overall 5-year survival (40%) than stage 1 (27%). Mitotane was given to 40% of the patients and increased recurrence-free survival but not overall survival. Adjuvant radiation therapy helped to reduce local recurrence but also had no effect on overall survival.

Overall, although the article reports on a large number of patients, the message is that not much is new in our fight against ACC. The authors once again recommend open adrenalectomy and suggest that this improves survival, although the data supporting this stance are not presented in the article. It is surprising, really, that this statement is in the abstract and repeated in the article because, once again, the unwritten bias in the article is that the patients seen in this study have been operated on by a variety of surgeons, many with uncertain experience with laparoscopic adrenalectomy. The standard recommendation to pursue open surgery followed by mitotane therapy could easily be refuted based on the data presented in this article. There remains much to be done in identifying new treatments for these patients.

T. J. Fahey, MD

Adrenalectomy Outcomes Are Superior with the Participation of Residents and Fellows
Seib CD, Greenblatt DY, Campbell MJ, et al (Univ of California, San Francisco; Sharp Rees-Stealy Med Group, San Diego, CA; Univy of California, Davis)
J Am Coll Surg 219:53-61, 2014

Background.—Adrenalectomy is a complex procedure performed in many settings, with and without residents and fellows. Patients often ask, "Will trainees be participating in my operation?" and seek reassurance that their care will not be adversely affected. The purpose of this study was to determine the association between trainee participation and adrenalectomy perioperative outcomes.

Study Design.—We performed a cohort study of patients who underwent adrenalectomy from the 2005 to 2011 American College of Surgeons NSQIP database. Trainee participation was classified as none, resident, or fellow, based on postgraduate year of the assisting surgeon. Associations between trainee participation and outcomes were determined via multivariate linear and logistic regression.

Results.—Of 3,694 adrenalectomies, 732 (19.8%) were performed by an attending surgeon with no trainee, 2,315 (62.7%) involved a resident, and 647 (17.5%) involved a fellow. The participation of fellows was associated with fewer serious complications (7.9% with no trainee, 6.0% with residents, and 2.8% with fellows; $p < 0.001$). In a multivariate model, the odds of serious 30-day morbidity were lower when attending surgeons operated with residents (odds ratio = 0.63; 95% CI, 0.45−0.89). Fellow participation was associated with significantly lower odds of overall (odds ratio = 0.51; 95% CI, 0.32−0.82) and serious (odds ratio = 0.31; 95% CI, 0.17−0.57) morbidity. There was no significant association between trainee participation and 30-day mortality.

Conclusions.—In this analysis of multi-institutional data, the participation of residents and fellows was associated with decreased odds of perioperative adrenalectomy complications. Attending surgeons performing adrenalectomies with trainee assistance should reassure patients of the equivalent or superior care they are receiving.

▶ This is an interesting paper that will serve its stated purpose well. Specifically, the authors set out to examine whether there was increased morbidity by involving trainees in operations and showed exactly the opposite—that the morbidity of the procedure is actually decreased by the involvement of train-ees, and particularly advanced-level trainees (senior residents or fellow). The major criticism of this article is that surgeons with trainees—and particularly fel-lows—are likely to be located in major academic centers and be the busiest endocrine surgeons. Certainly to be eligible to host an endocrine surgery fel-lowship requires an adequate case number to permit training both fellows and residents. So it seems entirely possible, if not likely, that the analysis may simply be examining outcomes of higher volume surgeons vs lower volume sur-geons. Without some accounting for numbers of cases between the groups, it is hard to entirely believe the results. Nevertheless, the article demonstrates that the presence of trainees in the operating room and involved in the care of patients undergoing laparoscopic adrenalectomy is overall better, not worse. This will undoubtedly be useful when faced with questions, and sometimes ultimatums, from patients that their care be rendered without involvement of residents or fellows.

T. J. Fahey, MD

Regional lymphadenectomy is indicated in the surgical treatment of pancreatic neuroendocrine tumors (PNETs)
Hashim YM, Trinkaus KM, Linehan DC, et al (Barnes-Jewish Hosp and Washington Univ School of Medicine, St Louis, MO; Washington Univ School of Medicine, St Louis, MO)
Ann Surg 259:197-203, 2014

Objective.—To explore the prognostic importance and preoperative predictors of lymph node metastasis in an effort to guide surgical decision making in patients with pancreatic neuroendocrine tumors (PNETs).

Background.—PNETs are uncommon, and the natural history of the disease is not well described. As a result, there remains controversy regard-ing the optimal management of regional lymph nodes during resection of the primary tumor.

Methods.—A retrospective review of a prospectively maintained data-base of patients who underwent surgery for locoregional PNET between 1994 and 2012 was performed. Logistic regression was used to identify predictors of nodal metastasis. Overall survival (OS) and disease free sur-vival (DFS) were calculated using Kaplan Meier method. Results were expressed as p-values and odds ratio estimates with 95% confidence intervals.

Results.—One-hundred thirty six patients were identified, of whom 50 (38%) patients had nodal metastasis. The frequency of lymph node meta-stasis was higher for: larger tumors (> 1.5 cm (OR = 4.7), tumors of the head as compared to body-tail of the pancreas (OR = 2.8), tumors with Ki-67 > 20% (OR = 6.7), and tumors with lymph vascular invasion (OR = 3.6), (p value <0.05). Median DFS was lower for patients with nodal metastases (4.5 v 14.6 years, $p < 0.0001$).

Conclusions.—Lymph node metastasis is predictive of poor outcomes in patients with PNETs. Preoperative variables are not able to reliably predict patients where the probability of lymph node involvement was less than 12%. These data support inclusion of regional lymphadenectomy in patients undergoing pancreatic resections for PNET.

▶ Management of incidentally discovered pancreatic neuroendocrine tumors (PNETs) remains a challenge for clinicians, the options being observation vs localized excision vs major pancreatic resection. Here the group from Washington University report their experience with PNETs focusing on predictors for lymph node metastasis. The presumption is that lymph node metastases are associated with worse outcome, and thus if patients with tumors that are more likely to have lymph node metastases can be identified, then the recommendation for extent of surgery can be made more knowledgeably. Of course, it should be noted that some studies have not been able to identify the presence of lymph node metastases as a risk factor for worse outcome, thus complicating the question considerably.[1] The study is a retrospective review of 136 PNETs resected over an 18-year period of which 98% did have lymph node resections included with the initial surgery. What is not noted in the article is whether any (or how many) patients were observed with PNETs during this time period. This is important because it may introduce a significant bias into the results if the number is significant. The authors note that size and location of tumor, as well as Ki-67 index and the pathologic presence of lymphovascular invasion are associated with lymph node metastases. None of these is particularly surprising, except for tumor location. The number of lymph nodes excised in tumors of the body/tail was approximately half that for head, and although the authors do some complex mathematical modeling to indicate that this is not significant, it does raise the question as to whether location is really important. Of the significant factors, a Ki-67 index > 20% was the most powerful predictor of LN metastases, which is also not surprising because this will identify the more aggressive tumors.

Finally, the authors did find an association between the presence of lymph node metastases and disease-free survival, and this was a substantial difference (4.5 vs 14.6 years) for patients with and without lymph node metastases, respectively. Although the data in this series do support the authors' conclusions, the study highlights the need for better methods to stratify patients with PNETs at the time of diagnosis. Finally, the morbidity of major pancreatic resection for each patient must be taken into account when considering the surgical options. Larger prospective studies are needed to properly answer the question of extent of resection in PNETs.

T. J. Fahey, MD

Reference

1. Bilimoria KY, Talamonti MS, Tomlinson JS, et al. Prognostic score predicting survival after resection of pancreatic neuroendocrine tumors: analysis of 3851 patients. *Ann Surg.* 2008;247:490-500.

Lanreotide in Metastatic Enteropancreatic Neuroendocrine Tumors

Caplin ME, for the CLARINET Investigators (Royal Free Hosp, London, UK)
N Engl J Med 371:224-233, 2014

Background.—Somatostatin analogues are commonly used to treat symptoms associated with hormone hypersecretion in neuroendocrine tumors; however, data on their antitumor effects are limited.

Methods.—We conducted a randomized, double-blind, placebo-controlled, multinational study of the somatostatin analogue lanreotide in patients with advanced, well-differentiated or moderately differentiated, nonfunctioning, somatostatin receptor—positive neuroendocrine tumors of grade 1 or 2 (a tumor proliferation index [on staining for the Ki-67 antigen] of <10%) and documented disease-progression status. The tumors originated in the pancreas, midgut, or hindgut or were of unknown origin. Patients were randomly assigned to receive an extended-release aqueous-gel formulation of lanreotide (Autogel [known in the United States as Depot], Ipsen) at a dose of 120 mg (101 patients) or placebo (103 patients) once every 28 days for 96 weeks. The primary end point was progression-free survival, defined as the time to disease progression (according to the Response Evaluation Criteria in Solid Tumors, version 1.0) or death. Secondary end points included overall survival, quality of life (assessed with the European Organization for Research and Treatment of Cancer questionnaires QLQ-C30 and QLQ-GI.NET21), and safety.

Results.—Most patients (96%) had no tumor progression in the 3 to 6 months before randomization, and 33% had hepatic tumor volumes greater than 25%. Lanreotide, as compared with placebo, was associated with significantly prolonged progression-free survival (median not reached vs. median of 18.0 months, $P < 0.001$ by the stratified log-rank test; hazard ratio for progression or death, 0.47; 95% confidence interval [CI], 0.30 to 0.73). The estimated rates of progression-free survival at 24 months were 65.1% (95% CI, 54.0 to 74.1) in the lanreotide group and 33.0% (95% CI, 23.0 to 43.3) in the placebo group. The therapeutic effect in predefined subgroups was generally consistent with that in the overall population, with the exception of small subgroups in which confidence intervals were wide. There were no significant between-group differences in quality of life or overall survival. The most common treatment-related adverse event was diarrhea (in 26% of the patients in the lanreotide group and 9% of those in the placebo group).

Conclusions.—Lanreotide was associated with significantly prolonged progression-free survival among patients with metastatic enteropancreatic neuroendocrine tumors of grade 1 or 2 (Ki-67 <10%). (Funded by Ipsen; CLARINET ClinicalTrials.gov number, NCT00353496; EudraCT 2005-004904-35.)

▶ This fairly large, randomized prospective study examines the role of routine lanreotide in patients with well- or moderately differentiated neuroendocrine tumors of gastrointestinal sites (pancreas, small and large intestine) that had metastatic disease or unresectable primary disease. The study documents that treatment with lanreotide does lead to prolongation of progression-free survival in these patients. A couple of things are worth noting: 204 patients were randomized from 48 sites in 14 countries over the course of 7 years—that is approximately 4 patients per site over 4 years. Only 40% of the patients in either arm had their primary tumor resected. This seems abysmally low. Additionally, these tumors were all relatively stable; only 5% in each group had demonstrated any evidence for progression before enrollment. So although the outcomes reported here are very positive, it is important to realize that this is a highly selected group of patients and tumors who had indolent disease to begin with. One has to wonder whether treatment with a somatostatin analogue in these patients at this time point in their disease is necessary. Should treatment with lanreotide or other somatostatin analogs wait until there are signs of progression? This must be the focus of trials for these interventions in the future.

T. J. Fahey, MD

A Single Institution's Experience with Surgical Cytoreduction of Stage IV, Well-Differentiated, Small Bowel Neuroendocrine Tumors

Boudreaux JP, Wang Y-Z, Diebold AE, et al (Univ Med Ctr, New Orleans, LA; et al)
J Am Coll Surg 218:837-845, 2014

Background.—Well-differentiated neuroendocrine tumors (NETs) of the gastrointestinal tract are rare, slowgrowing neoplasms. Clinical outcomes in a group of stage IV, well-differentiated patients with NETs with small bowel primaries undergoing cytoreductive surgery and multidisciplinary management at a single center were evaluated.

Study Design.—The charts of 189 consecutive patients who underwent surgical cytoreduction for their small bowel NETs were reviewed. Information on the extent of disease, complications, and Kaplan-Meier survival were collected from the patient records.

Results.—A total of 189 patients underwent 229 cytoreductive operations. Ten percent of patients required an intraoperative blood transfusion and 3% (6 of 229) had other intraoperative complications. For all 229 procedures performed, mean (±SD) stay in the ICU was 4 ± 3 days and in the hospital was 9 ± 10 days. Before discharge, 51% of patients had no postoperative complications and 39% of patients had only minor complications. In a 30-day follow-up period from discharge, 85% of patients had no additional complications and 13% had only minor complications. The 30-day postoperative death rate was 3% (5 of 189). Mean survival from histologic diagnosis of NET was 236 months. The 5-, 10-, and 20-year Kaplan-Meier survival rates from diagnosis were 87%, 77%, and 41%, respectively.

Conclusions.—Cytoreductive surgery in patients with well-differentiated midgut NETs has low mortality and complication rates and is associated with prolonged survival. We believe that cytoreductive surgery is a key component in the care of patients with NETs.

▶ This article from Dr Woltering's group was presented at the Southern Surgical and reports on the role of surgery in patients with Stage IV small intestinal NETs. The results reported here are impressive, as this group of patients with known metastatic disease had a mean survival from the time of diagnosis of 236 months. However, the study suffers from all of the problems associated with retrospective studies of this nature. Clearly there is a selection bias in the patients who are selected—or select themselves—to undergo long, difficult operations (the mean operative time was 6.3 hours). In one-third of the patients, an R0 resection was achieved, and it might be expected that this group had the best outcomes for survival. Unfortunately, the survival data are not stratified by the degree of resection (of the remaining patients, one-third had an R1 resection and one-third had an R2 resection), missing a chance to perhaps demonstrate why an aggressive surgical approach is warranted in these patients. Although better data are needed from the surgical community to support aggressive surgery (especially as more medical therapies for NETs emerge), the authors demonstrate that in their series, cytoreductive surgery, when performed with low morbidity and mortality, is associated with prolonged survival in patients who are candidates for an aggressive surgical approach.

T. J. Fahey, MD

Multicenter Clinical Experience With the Afirma Gene Expression Classifier
Alexander EK, Schorr M, Klopper J, et al (Brigham and Women's Hosp and Harvard Med School, Boston, MA; Univ of Colorado School of Medicine, Aurora; et al)
J Clin Endocrinol Metab 99:119-125, 2014

Background.—Increasingly, patients with thyroid nodule cytology labeled atypical (or follicular lesion) of undetermined significance (AUS/FLUS) or follicular neoplasm (FN) undergo diagnostic analysis with the Afirma gene expression classifier (GEC). No long-term, multisite analysis of Afirma GEC performance has yet been performed.

Methods.—We analyzed all patients who had received Afirma GEC testing at five academic medical centers between 2010 and 2013. Nodule and patient characteristics, fine needle aspiration cytology, Afirma GEC results, and subsequent clinical or surgical follow-up were obtained for 339 patients. Results were analyzed for pooled test performance, impact on clinical care, and site-to-site variation.

Results.—Three hundred thirty-nine patients underwent Afirma GEC testing of cytologically indeterminate nodules (165 AUS/FLUS; 161 FN; 13 suspicious for malignancy) and 174 of 339 (51%) indeterminate nodules were GEC benign, whereas 148 GEC were suspicious (44%). GEC results significantly altered care recommendations, as 4 of 175 GEC benign were recommended for surgery in comparison to 141 of 149 GEC suspicious (*P* < .01). Of 121 Cyto Indeterminate/GEC Suspicious nodules surgically removed, 53 (44%) were malignant. Variability in site-to-site GEC performance was confirmed, as the proportion of GEC benign varied up to 29% (*P* = .58), whereas the malignancy rate in nodules cytologically indeterminate/GEC suspicious varied up to 47% (*P* = .11). Seventy-one of 174 GEC benign nodules had documented clinical follow-up for an average of 8.5 months, in which 1 of 71 nodules proved cancerous.

Conclusions.—These multicenter, clinical experience data confirm originally published Afirma GEC test performance and demonstrate its substantial impact on clinical care recommendations. Although nonsignificant site-to-site variation exists, such differences should be anticipated by the practicing clinician. Follow-up of GEC benign nodules thus far confirm the clinical utility of this diagnostic test.

▶ Use of the Afirma test in clinical practice has been widely adopted in many centers around the country. This follow-up study addresses 2 questions: (1) How do the results provided by an Afirma report affect recommendations for surgery, and (2) what is the malignancy rate seen in a suspicious report. Fig 1 in the original article documents that doctors appear to be recommending—and patients are following these recommendations—that surgery is not necessary for a benign Afirma designation, and conversely that surgery is very likely to be recommended for a suspicious report. The malignancy rate in patients who underwent operation with an Afirma suspicious nodule was 44% overall—48% for Bethesda III nodules and 37% for a Bethesda IV nodule. This number is very close to the company's published rate for malignancy of around 40%. The report provides confirmation of what to expect for a suspicious report, but the follow-up is far too short to provide meaningful data for patients with an Afirma benign report. Furthermore, despite the fact that the samples were all collected from 5 prominent academic medical centers, there was very substantial variation in the rate of a benign designation between the centers—from as low as 38% to as high as 71%—for Bethesda III and IV nodules. This finding highlights once again the need for physicians to know their own cytopathologists' malignancy rates for Bethesda III and IV nodules to truly understand and calculate what their negative and positive predictive value of the Afirma test is for their patient population. In some cases, this has led to the realization that the test adds little to the standard cytology report (if, for instance, a Bethesda III nodule has a risk of malignancy of 30%-40% in your institution).

T. J. Fahey, MD

8 Nutrition

Limited long-term survival after in-hospital intestinal failure requiring total parenteral nutrition
Oterdoom LH, ten Dam SM, de Groot SDW, et al (VU Univ Med Ctr, Amsterdam, Netherlands)
Am J Clin Nutr 100:1102-1107, 2014

Background.—Total parenteral nutrition (TPN) is an invasive and advanced rescue feeding technique that has acceptable short-term survival although at costs of substantial risks. Survival after the clinical use of TPN >6 mo is unknown.

Objective.—We determined long-term survival after clinical TPN use in a consecutive cohort who were attending an academic hospital.

Design.—The study included a prospective cohort with a retrospective analysis of all 537 consecutive episodes of TPN in 437 patients between January 2010 and April 2012. Follow-up was until October 2013 with a total follow-up of 608 patient-years. Survival was analyzed by using Kaplan-Meier and Cox regression.

Results.—Survival was 58% in 437 patients with a first-time use of TPN at an average of 1.5 y after the initiation of TPN. The mortality rate was 30 deaths/100 patient-years. Older age, admission at an intensive care unit or a nonsurgical department, lower body mass index, and an underlying malignancy were positively associated with mortality.

Conclusion.—TPN use, if correctly indicated, is a clinical sign of intestinal failure and a surrogate marker for markedly increased risk of mortality even >1.5 y after TPN use. This trial was registered at clinicaltrials.gov as NCT02189993 with protocol identification name TPN-01.

▶ The use of total parenteral nutrition (TPN) in a hospital setting is done for patients who cannot eat and cannot take adequate amounts of enteral nutrition by tube feeding. These patients are, by definition, quite ill. On a surgical service, such patients may have a cause that is operable and potentially resolvable when the patient recovers. In the nonsurgical patient, the underlying cause is often unsolvable and the use of TPN is palliative for nutrition purposes. The nonsurgical patient stays in the hospital longer receiving TPN for a longer period as demonstrated by this study. This retrospective review from a prospective database demonstrated that older age, intensive care admission, lower body mass index, nonsurgical department admission, and an underlying malignancy were significantly associated with greater risk of mortality. This article provides some useful baseline information as to the long-term monitoring of patients that receive TPN for an average of around 7 days in hospital and what happens to them on long-term follow-up. It would have been useful to have the causes of mortality in these patients and to look at a survival curve for those who were discharged from the hospital.

J. M. Daly, MD

Peripherally Inserted Central Catheter for Use in Home Parenteral Nutrition: A 4-Year Follow-Up Study
Christensen LD, Rasmussen HH, Vinter-Jensen L (Aalborg Univ Hosp, Denmark)
JPEN J Parenter Enteral Nutr 38:1003-1006, 2014

Background.—Peripherally inserted central catheters (PICCs) are a relatively new device for home parenteral nutrition (HPN). Usually, tunneled central catheters such as the Hickman catheter are used for this purpose. However, severe complications (eg, pneumothorax) have been reported in association with the insertion of the central catheter. In contrast, PICCs may offer some advantages due to the peripheral insertion. There are only few studies on the use of PICCs for HPN.

Method.—A retrospective study (2008—2012) was performed in our Center for Nutrition and Bowel Disease. Patients receiving parenteral nutrition through PICCs were identified, their files examined, and indication, dwell time, cause of removal, and complications recorded.

Results.—Fifty-six patients (aged 28—81 years) had a total of 94 lines. Total catheter days were 9859. Mean catheter days per patient were 179.1, and mean dwell time of each line was 104.9 days (longest, 572 days). There were no major complications in relation to the insertion of the catheters. The catheters were removed due to catheter-related sepsis, mechanical reasons, and thrombotic complications in 1.7, 2.1, and 0.2 per 1000 catheter days, respectively.

Conclusion.—This study demonstrates that PICCs are appropriate for use in HPN for at least 3—4 months (a period that sometimes unexpectedly becomes long term). The complications equal those reported for tunneled central catheters. We conclude that PICCs are a relevant alternative to patients receiving HPN, especially if they cannot handle a central line. At present, the choice of catheter must be determined on an individual basis.

▶ From their local register, the authors retrospectively identified 56 patients receiving a peripherally inserted central venous catheter (PICC) for home parenteral nutrition from 2008 through January 2012. A total of 94 PICCs were used for 56 patients. The mean dwell time was 105 days, with a maximal dwell time of 572 days. The mean dwell time per patient was 176 days. Seventeen catheters were removed due to suspected catheter sepsis, giving an incidence of 1.7 per 1000 catheter years; they had a mean dwell time of 93 days. Eight of these 17 catheters were from 2 patients. The bacteria were isolated in 15 of the 17 cases and included *Staphylococcus aureus*, coagulase-negative staphylococci, *Pseudomonas aeruginosa*, different Gram-negative bacteria, and *Candida albicans*.

Obviously, PICC lines have been used for some time for home antibiotics and other medications, but less often for home parenteral nutrition. Clearly, a prospective, randomized trial would be indicated to determine if one method (central vs peripheral) is better.

J. M. Daly, MD

Preventing Bloodstream Infection in Patients Receiving Home Parenteral Nutrition
Muir A, Holden C, Sexton E, et al (Birmingham Children's Hosp NHS Foundation Trust, UK)
J Pediatr Gastroenterol Nutr 59:177-181, 2014

Patients receiving home parenteral nutrition (HPN) are at particularly high risk of methicillin-sensitive *Staphylococcus aureus* (MSSA) catheter-related bloodstream infections (CRBSI). We developed a multidisciplinary enhanced care pathway encompassing a number of minimal cost interventions involving line/exit site care, training for staff and parents, multidisciplinary discharge planning, and monitoring compliance. Implementation reduced the mean rates of MSSA CRBSI (from 0.93, 95% CI 0.25—1.61, to 0.23, 95% CI —0.06 to 0.52, per 1000 parenteral nutrition [PN] days) and all-cause CRBSI (from 1.98, 95% CI 0.77—3.19, to 0.45, 95% CI 0.10—0.80, per 1000 PN days). A similar approach could be applied to preventing health care-associated infections in other complex, vulnerable patient groups.

▶ Home parenteral nutrition is lifesaving but is wrought with problems related to catheter-based blood stream infections. The occurrence of these infections is related to the prolonged duration of an indwelling catheter, the presence of other portal sites of infection in these children with ineffective intestinal absorptive capacity, and the very nature of being at home with multiple caregivers.

Thus, it is important that multidisciplinary home nutrition teams have reduction of catheter-based infection as their primary goal. This home parenteral nutrition pathway demonstrated that the mean rates of catheter-related blood stream infection before and during implementation were 1.98 and 1.82 per 1000 catheter days, respectively, compared with 8.6 per 1000 days in another study. *Staphylococcus aureus* was the pathogen most commonly isolated at all stages. Following implementation of this pathway, the rate of methicillin-resistant *S aureus* decreased from 0.93 per 1000 parenteral nutrition days to 0.23 per 1000 days. Closer multidisciplinary working is central to this pathway. Methicillin-sensitive *S aureus* catheter-related bloodstream infections were often preceded by local signs of infection at the catheter exit site for a short period beforehand. Because of their pathway, an exit site swab was taken and empiric topical mupirocin commenced immediately.

This study is important because it shows the benefit of multidisciplinary teams working in concert to develop critical pathways that improve patient care.

J. M. Daly, MD

Trial of the Route of Early Nutritional Support in Critically Ill Adults

Harvey SE, for the CALORIES Trial Investigators (Guy's and St. Thomas' NHS Foundation Trust, London, UK; et al)
N Engl J Med 371:1673-1684, 2014

Background.—Uncertainty exists about the most effective route for delivery of early nutritional support in critically ill adults. We hypothesized that delivery through the parenteral route is superior to that through the enteral route.

Methods.—We conducted a pragmatic, randomized trial involving adults with an unplanned admission to one of 33 English intensive care units. We randomly assigned patients who could be fed through either the parenteral or the enteral route to a delivery route, with nutritional support initiated within 36 hours after admission and continued for up to 5 days. The primary outcome was all-cause mortality at 30 days.

Results.—We enrolled 2400 patients; 2388 (99.5%) were included in the analysis (1191 in the parenteral group and 1197 in the enteral group). By 30 days, 393 of 1188 patients (33.1%) in the parenteral group and 409 of 1195 patients (34.2%) in the enteral group had died (relative risk in parenteral group, 0.97; 95% confidence interval, 0.86 to 1.08; $P = 0.57$). There were significant reductions in the parenteral group, as compared with the enteral group, in rates of hypoglycemia (44 patients [3.7%] vs. 74 patients [6.2%]; $P = 0.006$) and vomiting (100 patients [8.4%] vs. 194 patients [16.2%]; $P < 0.001$). There were no significant differences between the parenteral group and the enteral group in the mean number of treated infectious complications (0.22 vs. 0.21; $P = 0.72$), 90-day mortality (442 of 1184 patients [37.3%] vs. 464 of 1188 patients [39.1%], $P = 0.40$), in rates of 14 other secondary outcomes, or in rates of adverse events. Caloric intake was similar in the two groups, with the target intake not achieved in most patients.

Conclusions.—We found no significant difference in 30-day mortality associated with the route of delivery of early nutritional support in critically ill adults. (Funded by the United Kingdom National Institute for Health Research; CALORIES Current Controlled Trials number, ISRCTN17386141.)

▶ The authors provided the rationale for this well-designed, large (2388 patients), multi-institutional clinical trial comparing parenteral vs enteral nutrition in critically ill patients. As the authors stated in their preamble, "Currently, the enteral route is the mainstay, largely on the grounds of physiological rationale and modest evidence suggesting an association with fewer infections, yet it can also be associated with gastrointestinal intolerance and underfeeding. The parenteral route, though more invasive, more often secures delivery of the intended nutrition, but has been associated with greater risks and rates of complications." In this study, the route of delivery was used exclusively for at least 5 days and thereafter additional feedings could be given via oral or other routes. Thus, the question was: "Does the intake of calories make the difference, or is it the route of delivery?"

As the authors pointed out, there were no significant differences between the groups in the total calories administered, the duration of feeding, the 30- and 90-day mortality and many other parameters. There was less vomiting and less hypoglycemia in the parenteral group vs the enteral group.

This is an excellent, well-conducted clinical trail that gives important information for future use of nutritional support for critically ill patients in the intensive care unit.

J. M. Daly, MD

Early versus On-Demand Nasoenteric Tube Feeding in Acute Pancreatitis
Bakker OJ, for the Dutch Pancreatitis Study Group (Univ Med Ctr Utrecht, the Netherlands; et al)
N Engl J Med 371:1983-1993, 2014

Background.—Early enteral feeding through a nasoenteric feeding tube is often used in patients with severe acute pancreatitis to prevent gut-derived infections, but evidence to support this strategy is limited. We conducted a multicenter, randomized trial comparing early nasoenteric tube feeding with an oral diet at 72 hours after presentation to the emergency department in patients with acute pancreatitis.

Methods.—We enrolled patients with acute pancreatitis who were at high risk for complications on the basis of an Acute Physiology and Chronic Health Evaluation II score of 8 or higher (on a scale of 0 to 71, with higher scores indicating more severe disease), an Imrie or modified Glasgow score of 3 or higher (on a scale of 0 to 8, with higher scores indicating more severe disease), or a serum C-reactive protein level of more than 150 mg per liter. Patients were randomly assigned to nasoenteric tube feeding within 24 hours after randomization (early group) or to an oral diet initiated 72 hours after presentation (on-demand group), with tube feeding provided if the oral diet was not tolerated. The primary end point was a composite of major infection (infected pancreatic necrosis, bacteremia, or pneumonia) or death during 6 months of follow-up.

Results.—A total of 208 patients were enrolled at 19 Dutch hospitals. The primary end point occurred in 30 of 101 patients (30%) in the early group and in 28 of 104 (27%) in the on demand group (risk ratio, 1.07; 95% confidence interval, 0.79 to 1.44; $P = 0.76$). There were no significant differences between the early group and the on-demand group in the rate of major infection (25% and 26%, respectively; $P = 0.87$) or death (11% and 7%, respectively; $P = 0.33$). In the on-demand group, 72 patients (69%) tolerated an oral diet and did not require tube feeding.

Conclusions.—This trial did not show the superiority of early nasoenteric tube feeding, as compared with an oral diet after 72 hours, in reducing the rate of infection or death in patients with acute pancreatitis at high risk for complications. (Funded by the Netherlands Organization for Health Research and Development and others; PYTHON Current Controlled Trials number, ISRCTN18170985.)

▶ Previous reports have suggested that early enteral feeding may reduce infectious complications by improving the integrity of the intestinal mucosa and submucosa diminishing bacterial translocation. However, there remains some controversy regarding this issue.

Therefore, the Dutch Pancreatitis Group initiated a prospective, randomized trial in which more than 700 patients with severe pancreatitis were assessed and slightly more than 200 patients were randomized to early enteral tube feeding or to later feeding on demand. Necrotizing pancreatitis developed in 63% of the patients in the early group and in 62% of those in the on-demand group. A total of 18% of the patients in the early group and 19% of those in the on-demand group required intensive care unit admission. The primary composite end point of major infection or death occurred in 30 patients (30%) in the early group compared with 28 (27%) in the on-demand group. Major infections occurred in 25% of the patients in the early group and in 26% of those in the on-demand group. Mortality was 11% in the early group compared with 7% in the on-demand group. In the on-demand group, 32 patients (31%) required naso-enteral tube feeding; 72 patients (69%) tolerated an oral diet and did not require tube feeding. The on-demand tube-feeding strategy reduced the number of days to full tolerance of an oral diet (9 days with the early strategy vs 6 days with the on-demand strategy).

Thus, in this large, multi-institutional, prospective trial no statistical differences were noted between patients deliberately given early naso-enteral tube feeding compared with patients who were fed on demand. From this trial, one may assume that on-demand feeding should be the standard method of treating patients with severe pancreatitis reserving tube feeding for those patients who become unable to eat for several days and using total parenteral nutrition when tube feeding cannot be accomplished.

J. M. Daly, MD

Use of a concentrated enteral nutrition solution to increase calorie delivery to critically ill patients: a randomized, double-blind, clinical trial
Peake SL, for the TARGET investigators and the Australian and New Zealand Intensive Care Society Clinical Trials Group (Univ of Adelaide, Australia; et al)
Am J Clin Nutr 100:616-625, 2014

Background.—Critically ill patients typically receive ~60% of estimated calorie requirements.

Objectives.—We aimed to determine whether the substitution of a 1.5-kcal/mL enteral nutrition solution for a 1.0-kcal/mL solution resulted in greater calorie delivery to critically ill patients and establish the feasibility of conducting a multicenter, double-blind, randomized trial to evaluate the effect of an increased calorie delivery on clinical outcomes.

Design.—A prospective, randomized, double-blind, parallel-group, multicenter study was conducted in 5 Australian intensive care units. One hundred twelve mechanically ventilated patients expected to receive enteral nutrition for >2 d were randomly assigned to receive 1.5 ($n = 57$) or 1.0 ($n = 55$) kcal/mL enteral nutrition solution at a rate of 1 mL/kg ideal body weight per hour for 10 d. Protein and fiber contents in the 2 solutions were equivalent.

Results.—The 2 groups had similar baseline characteristics (1.5 compared with 1.0 kcal/mL). The mean ($\pm$ SD) age was 56.4 $\pm$ 16.8 compared with 56.5 $\pm$ 16.1 y, 74% compared with 75% were men, and the Acute Physiology and Chronic Health Evaluation II score was 23 $\pm$ 9.1 compared with 22 $\pm$ 8.9. The groups received similar volumes of enteral nutrition solution [1221 mL/d (95% CI: 1120, 1322 mL/d) compared with 1259 mL/d (95% CI: 1143, 1374 mL/d); $P = 0.628$], which led to a 46% increase in daily calories in the group given the 1.5-kcal/mL solution [1832 kcal/d (95% CI: 1681, 1984 kcal/d) compared with 1259 kcal/d (95% CI: 1143, 1374 kcal/d); $P < 0.001$]. The 1.5-kcal/mL solution was not associated with larger gastric residual volumes or diarrhea. In this feasibility study, there was a trend to a reduced 90-d mortality in patients given 1.5 kcal/mL [11 patients (20%) compared with 20 patients (37%); $P = 0.057$].

Conclusions.—The substitution of a 1.0- with a 1.5-kcal/mL enteral nutrition solution administered at the same rate resulted in a 46% greater calorie delivery without adverse effects. The results support the conduct of a large-scale trial to evaluate the effect of increased calorie delivery on clinically important outcomes in the critically ill. This trial was registered at Australian New Zealand Clinical Trials (http://www.anzctr.org.au/) as ACTRN 12611000793910.

▶ Enteral feeding in the intensive care unit is frequently done by protocol while assessing bowel function, gastric residual volumes, and blood glucose levels. Whatever the calorie/protein goal chosen, it is common not to be able to achieve that goal because of feeding interruptions secondary to tolerance and other reasons. The calorie requirement is usually estimated by using a variety of predictive equations, which are believed to approximate energy expenditure, with approximately 25 to 30 kcal per kg per day generally recommended. Results of this study in more than 100 patients at multiple institutions showed that calorie goals could more closely be achieved and that 50% more calories could be administered using the higher calorie solution. This enteral nutrition study successfully blinded the study intervention in this patient population, improving its believability. The concealment of the intervention was important to prevent inadvertent bias by the investigators. As the authors noted, in previous studies, blinding of the intervention has not been undertaken, which raises concerns about reported differences in outcomes, particularly when outcomes were subject to an ascertainment bias (eg, nosocomial infections and functional outcomes). They designed a double-blind enteral nutrition study using 2 commercially available enteral nutrition solutions that were similar in color, indistinguishable at the bedside, and delivered at the same flow rate and volume to both study groups.

This is an important clinical trial in that its methodology was rigorous using blinding in the protocol to avoid bias. Interestingly, they found a decrease in 90-day mortality in the experimental group. Further studies need to be carried out to evaluate this finding and determine whether reduction in late mortality is a consistent finding.

J. M. Daly, MD

Proactive Enteral Nutrition in Moderately Preterm Small for Gestational Age Infants: A Randomized Clinical Trial

Zecca E, Costa S, Barone G, et al (Catholic Univ of the Sacred Heart, Rome, Italy)
J Pediatr 165:1135-1139, 2014

Objective.—To investigate the efficacy of a proactive feeding regimen (PFR) in reducing hospital length of stay in a population of moderately preterm small for gestational age (SGA) infants.

Study Design.—SGA infants (z-score <-1.28) of gestational age (GA) 32-36 weeks and birth weight (BW) >1499 g were allocated at random to receive either a PFR, starting with 100 mL/kg/day and gradually increasing to 200 mL/kg/day by day 4, or a standard feeding regimen, starting with 60 mL/kg/day and gradually increasing to 170 mL/kg/ day by day 9. All infants received human milk.

Results.—A total of 72 infants were randomized to the 2 groups, 36 to the PFR group (mean GA, 35.1 ± 0.7 weeks; mean BW, 1761 ± 177 g) and 36 to the standard feeding regimen group (mean GA, 35.5 ± 1.2 weeks; mean BW, 1754 ± 212 g). Infants in the PFR group were discharged significantly earlier (mean, 9.8 ± 3.1 days vs 11.9 ± 4.7 days; $P = .029$). The need for intravenous fluids (2.8% vs 33.3%; $P = .0013$) and the incidence of hypoglycemia (0 vs 33.3%; $P = .00016$) were significantly lower in the PFR group. Feeding intolerance and fecal calprotectin levels did not differ between the 2 groups.

Conclusion.—A PFR in moderately preterm SGA infants is well tolerated and significantly reduces both the length of stay and the risk of neonatal hypoglycemia.

▶ The authors noted that small for gestational age (SGA) infants have increased neonatal morbidity and mortality and are at increased risk for short stature, cardiovascular disease, insulin resistance, diabetes, dyslipidemia, and poor cognitive performance. They designed a prospective, randomized study whereby SGA infants of gestational age 32 to 36 weeks and birth weight > 1499 g were allocated at random to receive either a preferred feeding regimen (PFR) starting with 100 mL/kg/day and gradually increasing to 200 mL/kg/day by day 4, or a standard feeding regimen, starting with 60 mL/kg/day and gradually increasing to 170 mL/kg/day by day 9. All infants received human milk. Length of stay was significantly shorter in the PFR group. Infants in the PFR group had less weight loss, significantly faster regain of body weight, and a significantly lower incidence of hypoglycemia.

Thus, the proactive feeding regimen appeared better than standard, but additional work is needed before the PFR becomes standard of care.

J. M. Daly, MD

Randomized Controlled Trial of Early Enteral Fat Supplement and Fish Oil to Promote Intestinal Adaptation in Premature Infants with an Enterostomy
Yang Q, Ayers K, Welch CD, et al (Wake Forest Univ Health Science, Winston-Salem, NC)
J Pediatr 165:274-279.e1, 2014

Objective.—To test the hypothesis that early enteral supplementing fat and fish oil decreases the duration of parenteral nutrition (PN) and increases enteral nutrition (EN) before bowel reanastomosis in premature infants with an enterostomy.

Study Design.—Premature infants (<2 months old) who had an enterostomy and tolerated enteral feeding at 20 mL/kg/day were randomized to usual care (control = 18) or early supplementing enteral fat supplement and fish oil (treatment = 18). Intravenous lipid was decreased as enteral fat intake was increased. Daily weight, clinical and nutrition data, and weekly length and head circumference were recorded. The primary outcomes were the duration of PN and volume of EN intake, and the secondary outcomes were weight gain (g/day), ostomy output (mL/kg/d), and serum conjugated bilirubin level (mg/dL) from initiating feeding to reanastomosis. Data were analyzed by Student t test or Wilcoxon rank sum test.

Results.—There were no differences in the duration of PN, ostomy output, and weight gain between the 2 groups before reanastomosis. However, supplemented infants received less intravenous lipid, had greater EN intake, and lower conjugated bilirubin before reanastomosis, and they also received greater total calorie, had fewer sepsis evaluations and less exposure to antibiotics and central venous catheters before reanastomosis, and had greater weight and length gain after reanastomosis (all $P < .05$).

Conclusion.—Early enteral feeding of a fat supplement and fish oil was associated with decreased exposure to intravenous lipid, increased EN intake, and reduced conjugated bilirubin before reanastomosis and improved weight and length gain after reanastomosis in premature infants with an enterostomy.

▶ Neonates, particularly low-birth-weight, premature infants, have a higher rate of necrotizing enterocolitis requiring surgery and the creation of an ostomy.

This can lead to a short gut syndrome and the need for long-term parenteral nutrition with its attendant consequences. It has been suggested that a high fat enteral diet might speed intestinal adaptation and reduce the need for parenteral nutrition. In this prospective, randomized trial, the eligibility criteria were the presence of a jejunostomy or ileostomy, preterm birth (birth prior to 37 completed weeks of gestation), and age less than 2 months. Infants in the control group received usual nutritional care. Infants in the treatment group received usual nutritional care plus enteral fat supplement and fish oil once they tolerated enteral feedings at 20 mL/kg/day. Compared with control patients, the treated infants had fewer sepsis evaluations, fewer days of antibiotics treatment, and shorter duration of central venous catheter use. These results suggest that early enteral fat supplementation for infants awaiting bowel reanastomosis is well tolerated and could have important clinical benefits. Clearly, additional studies should be done to confirm these results, but the conclusions are intriguing and deserve further investigation.

J. M. Daly, MD

Effects of Early Enteral Nutrition on Patients After Emergency Gastrointestinal Surgery: A Propensity Score Matching Analysis
Lee SH, Jang JY, Kim HW, et al (Yonsei Univ College of Medicine, Seoul, Korea; Yonsei Univ Wonju College of Medicine, Korea)
Medicine 93:e323, 2014

Early postoperative enteral feeding has been demonstrated to improve the outcome of patients who underwent surgery for gastrointestinal (GI) malignancies, trauma, perforation, and/or obstruction. Thus, this study was conducted to assess the efficacy of early postoperative enteral nutrition (EN) after emergency surgery in patients with GI perforation or strangulation.

The medical records of 484 patients, admitted between January 2007 and December 2012, were reviewed retrospectively. Patients were divided into 2 groups: the early EN (EEN, N = 77) group and the late EN (LEN, N = 407) group. The morbidity, mortality, length of hospital, and intensive care unit (ICU) stays were compared between the 2 groups. Propensity score matching was performed in order to adjust for any baseline differences.

Patients receiving EEN had reduced in-hospital mortality rates (EEN 4.5% vs LEN 19.4%; $P = 0.008$), pulmonary complications (EEN 4.5% vs LEN 19.4%; $P = 0.008$), lengths of hospital stay (median: 14.0, interquartile range: 8.0–24.0 vs median: 17.0, interquartile range: 11.0–26.0, $P = 0.048$), and more 28-day ICU-free days (median: 27.0, interquartile range: 25.0–27.0 vs median: 25.0, interquartile range: 22.0–27.0, $P = 0.042$) than those receiving LEN in an analysis using propensity score matching. The significant difference in survival between the 2 groups was also shown in the Kaplan–Meier survival curve ($P = 0.042$). In a further analysis using the Cox proportional hazard ratio after matching on the propensity score, EEN was associated with reduced in-hospital mortality (hazard ratio, 0.03; 95% confidence interval, 0.01–0.49; $P = 0.015$).

EEN is associated with beneficial effects, such as reduced in hospital mortality rates, pulmonary complications, lengths of hospital stay, and more 28-day ICU-free days, after emergency GI surgery.

▶ Many studies have evaluated the use of enteral nutrition initiated "early" after gastrointestinal surgery, after admission to an intensive care or burn unit, demonstrating that early enteral nutritional intervention results in significantly improved outcomes compared with late enteral nutrition support or no support. This study, although retrospective, is unique because enteral nutrition was examined as to whether it started "early" or late after emergency surgery. Patients receiving early enteral nutrition had reduced in-hospital mortality rates, lengths of hospital stay, pulmonary complications, and more 28-day intensive care unit (ICU)-free days than those receiving late enteral nutrition in an unmatched analysis. In the propensity-matched cohort, the early enteral nutrition group had significantly lower in-hospital mortality rates (4% vs 19%), pulmonary complications (4% vs 19%), reduced lengths of hospital stay (median: 14 vs median: 17), and more 28-day ICU-free days (median: 27 vs 25) than the late enteral nutrition group.

One must remember that this is a retrospective study subject to the bias that perhaps healthier patients received early nutrition and sicker patients received later nutrition intervention. Propensity-score analysis, although a good statistical technique, may not properly account for all variables such as these. Thus, we are left with an "association" not causation, and further studies (prospective and randomized) must be done to answer this intriguing question.

J. M. Daly, MD

Minimal enteral nutrition during neonatal hypothermia treatment for perinatal hypoxic-ischaemic encephalopathy is safe and feasible
Thyagarajan B, Tillqvist E, Baral V, et al (Princess Anne Hosp, Southampton, UK; Karolinska Hosp, Stockholm, Sweden; et al)
Acta Paediatr 104:146-151, 2015

Aim.—The safety and efficacy of enteral feeding during hypothermia treatment following hypoxic-ischaemic encephalopathy has not been studied before, resulting in variations in practice. Our study compared the benefits and safety of both early minimal and delayed enteral feeding during hypothermia treatment.

Methods.—Our retrospective cohort study, from January 2009 to December 2011, compared a Swedish cohort, who received early enteral feeding during hypothermia, and a UK cohort, who received delayed enteral feeding.

Results.—In Sweden (n = 51), enteral feeds were initiated at a median of 23.6 h and full oral feeding was achieved at 9 days (range 3–23). In the

UK (n = 34), the equivalent figures were 100 h and 8 days (range 3–13) (p = 0.01). Both groups achieved enteral feeding at a median 6 days. The median length of hospital stay was 13 days in Sweden and 10 days in the UK (p = 0.04). More babies were fully breastfeeding or breastfed and bottle-fed at discharge in Sweden (85%) than the UK (67%) (p = 0.08). There were no significant differences between the two groups regarding adverse events.

Conclusion.—Early minimal enteral feeding during hypothermia proved feasible, with no significant complications. Delayed enteral feeding did not affect time to full enteral feeding.

▶ Infants who suffer ischemic encephalopathy at birth are placed into a hypothermic condition to preserve organ function and reduce consequences of brain ischemia. The investigators designed a retrospective study involving cohorts of these infants from the United Kingdom and Sweden that followed similar hypothermia protocols but had different feeding practices during hypothermia treatment. Infants were cooled to a rectal temperature of 33.5°C. Rewarming was commenced after 72 hours of cooling by increasing the temperature by 0.5°C per hour to a temperature of 36.5°C. The authors note that enteral feeds can be tolerated by newborns with hypothermic ischemic encephalopathy receiving hypothermia without a significant increase in complications. This may be due to a gradual increase in intestinal blood flow in the first few days of postnatal life, which improves feeding tolerance. Interestingly, there were few differences between the UK and Swedish cohorts, but a prospective, randomized trial would be necessary to determine whether early or late minimal feeding makes a difference in outcomes for these children.

J. M. Daly, MD

Effects of Enteral Nutrition on the Barrier Function of the Intestinal Mucosa and Dopamine Receptor Expression in Rats With Traumatic Brain Injury
Zhang X, Jiang X (Fujian Med Univ, Fuzhou, China)
JPEN J Parenter Enteral Nutr 39:114-123, 2015

Background.—Impaired intestinal mucosal barrier (IMB) function is common in traumatic brain injury (TBI), but dopamine receptors (DRs) change in intestinal mucosa after TBI, and effects of enteral nutrition (EN) and supplements on IMB function remain unclear. Our purpose was to study the effects of EN and supplements on intestinal mucosal permeability (IMPB) and the expression of DRs DRD1 and DRD2 in the intestinal mucosa of rats with TBI.

Methods.—Forty-eight rats were divided into 8 groups; control, animals with TBI, dopamine group, animals with TBI treated with dopamine antagonist, EN alone, or EN combined with glutamine, probiotics, or a combination of probiotics and glutamine daily after TBI.

Results.—The IMPB was improved in the glutamine, probiotics, and combination groups. Including probiotics improved IMPB more than adding glutamine, and bacterial translocation in the intestines after TBI was reduced in the probiotics and combination groups (all *Ps* < .01). TBI led to elevated DRD1 and DRD2 mRNA and protein levels, which were reduced in the DA antagonist, glutamine, probiotics, and combination groups. DRD2 mRNA and protein levels in the probiotics and combination groups were decreased more than in the DA antagonist group (all *Ps* < .01). The increased IMPB after TBI correlated with increased DRD1 and DRD2 levels in the rat intestinal mucosa.

Conclusion.—EN supplemented with probiotics or combining glutamine and probiotics lowers the increased IMPB, bacterial translocation, and DRD1 and DRD2 mRNA and protein expression in rat intestinal mucosa caused by TBI.

▶ It has long been known that trauma, starvation, and sepsis seem to increase intestinal permeability to bacteria, leading to bacterial translocation and a subsequent gram-negative cascade and thus increasing mortality. In this study, the authors noted that the intestinal epithelia were damaged and their intestinal mucosal barrier function was impaired in rats that suffered total brain injury, leading to increased bacterial translocation. The application of the dopamine receptor antagonist, as well as enteral nutrition combined with either probiotics or probiotics and glutamine after total brain injury, reduced bacterial colony-forming units per gram of tissue in the intestines after injury. Enteral nutrition supplemented with probiotics or combined probiotics and glutamine significantly reduced bacterial translocation and lowered DRD2 mRNA and protein expression levels in rat intestinal mucosa compared with the effects of a dopamine receptor antagonist and enteral nutrition alone.

This study in animals is a bit confounded because intestinal translocation is not often documented in humans but easily seen in rats. Thus, it is unclear how relevant the study is to clinical situations. Nevertheless, these studies document mechanisms of action that provide much needed information for future drug development.

J. M. Daly, MD

Frequency of Aspirating Gastric Tubes for Patients Receiving Enteral Nutrition in the ICU: A Randomized Controlled Trial
Williams TA, Leslie G, Mills L, et al (ICU Royal Perth Hosp, Bentley, Western Australia; Curtin Univ, Perth, Western Australia; Royal Perth Hosp, Western Australia; et al)
JPEN J Parenter Enteral Nutr 38:809-816, 2014

Background.—Enteral nutrition (EN) tolerance is often monitored by aspirating stomach contents by syringe at prescribed intervals. No studies have been conducted to assess the most appropriate time interval for aspirating gastric tubes. We compared gastric tube aspirations every 4 hours (usual care) with a variable regimen (up to every 8 hours aspirations).

Methods.—This randomized controlled trial (RCT) enrolled patients who stayed in the intensive care unit (ICU) for >48 hours, had a gastric tube, and were likely to receive EN for 3 or more days. Patients were randomized (computer-generated randomization) to either the control (every 4 hours) or intervention group (variable regimen). The primary outcome was number of gastric tube aspirations per day from randomization until EN was ceased or up to 2 weeks postrandomization.

Results.—Following Institutional Ethics Committee approval, 357 patients were recruited (control group, n = 179; intervention group, n = 178). No differences were found in age, sex, worst APACHE II score, or time to start of EN. In the intention-to-treat analysis, the intervention group had fewer tube aspirations per day (3.4 versus 5.4 in the control group, $P < .001$). Vomiting/regurgitation was increased in the intervention group (2.1% versus 3.6%, $P = .02$). There were no other differences in complications.

Conclusion.—This is the first RCT to examine the frequency of gastric tube aspirations. The frequency of gastric tube aspirations was reduced in the variable-regimen group with no increase in risk to the patient. Reducing the frequency of aspirations saves nursing time, decreases risk of contamination of feeding circuit, and minimizes risk of body fluid exposure.

▶ It has been well established that enteral feeding is the best method of nutritional support in hospitalized patients who require such intervention. However, the risks of patient aspiration have made the measurement of gastric residual volumes mandatory in an effort to reduce vomiting and pulmonary aspiration. Yet it is unclear as to how often these measurements should be done, what is the maximum gastric volume that should be allowed before holding further feeding, and how gastric residual volume relates to pulmonary aspiration and subsequent pneumonia. In this study, patients were randomized to receive either tube aspiration every 4 hours (standard practice) or a variable regimen of up to 8 hourly gastric tube aspirations. Results of this prospective, randomized trial showed that the frequency of gastric tube aspirations was reduced in the variable regimen group with no increase in risk to patients using ventilator-associated pneumonia as the measure of risk. The proportion of patients who regurgitated or vomited tube feedings almost doubled, which might be considered a risk factor for further complications. The reduced frequency of aspirations saves nursing time, decreases risk of contamination of the Enteral nutrition circuit, and minimizes the risk of body fluid exposure. However, the increased frequency of vomiting that occurred with the variable regimen is worrisome, suggesting that this approach must be adapted slowly in hospitals to reduce pulmonary aspiration complications.

J. M. Daly, MD

Home enteral nutrition reduces complications, length of stay, and health care costs: results from a multicenter study
Klek S, Hermanowicz A, Dziwiszek G, et al (Stanley Dudrick's Memorial Hosp, Skawina, Poland; Med Univ of Bialystok, Poland; Home Enteral Nutrition Unit, Stomed, Ostroleka, Poland; et al)
Am J Clin Nutr 100:609-615, 2014

Background.—Home enteral nutrition (HEN) has always been recognized as a life-saving procedure, but with the ongoing economic crisis influencing health care, its cost-effectiveness has been questioned recently.

Objective.—The unique reimbursement situation in Poland enabled the otherwise ethically unacceptable, hence unavailable, comparison of the period of no-feeding and long-term feeding and the subsequent analyses of the clinical value of the latter and its cost-effectiveness.

Design.—The observational multicenter study in the group of 456 HEN patients [142 children: 55 girls and 87 boys, mean ($\pm$ SD) age 8.7 $\pm$ 5.9 y; 314 adults: 151 women and 163 men, mean age 59.3 $\pm$ 19.8 y] was performed between January 2007 and July 2013. Two 12-mo periods were compared. During the first period, patients were tube fed a homemade diet and were not monitored; during the other period, patients received HEN. HEN included tube feeding and complex monitoring by a nutrition support team. The number of complications, hospital admissions, length of hospital stay, biochemical and anthropometric variables, and costs of hospitalization were compared.

Results.—Implementation of HEN enabled weight gain and stabilized liver function in both age groups, but it hardly influenced the other tests. HEN implementation reduced the incidence of infectious complications (37.4% compared with 14.9%; $P < 0.001$, McNemar test), the number of hospital admissions [1.98 $\pm$ 2.42 (mean $\pm$ SD) before and 1.26 $\pm$ 2.18 after EN; $P < 0.001$, Wilcoxon's signed-rank test], and length of hospital stay (39.7 $\pm$ 71.9 compared with 11.9 $\pm$ 28.5 d; $P < 0.001$, Wilcoxon's signed-rank test). The mean annual costs ($) of hospitalization were reduced from 6500.20 $\pm$ 10,402.69 to 2072.58 $\pm$ 5497.00.

Conclusions.—The study showed that HEN improves clinical outcomes and decreases health care costs. It was impossible, however, to determine precisely which factor mattered more: the artificial diet itself or the introduction of complex care. This trial was registered at clinicaltrials.gov as NCT02122120.

► For many conditions, public health entities question the vigor and reimbursement of home interventions. Yet the cost of care over time is often reduced by such professional medical intervention. This study included both children and adults in a 12-month retrospective review and a 12-month prospective review comparing home enteral nutrition with an artificial formula and medical support versus a home-created diet given by a caregiver to patients at home.

Implementation of the artificial enteral diet in children enabled weight gain, increased the hemoglobin concentration, and stabilized liver function; in adults, it also increased body weight and helped the liver and kidneys to recover. The introduction of enteral nutrition reduced the incidence of infectious complications, especially pneumonia and urinary tract infection. Differences between the homemade and enteral nutrition diet periods were significant if all study participants were considered (37% compared with 15%), and when children were considered separately from adults. Enteral nutrition significantly reduced the number of hospital admissions and the length of hospital stay, both in children and in adults. Use of home enteral nutrition reduced the annual cost of care from approximately $6500 to slightly more than $2000. Studies such as these are important because they give longitudinal credence to the concept of adequate medical interventions at home, reducing the overall cost of care and hospital readmission.

J. M. Daly, MD

Enteral Energy and Macronutrients in End-Stage Liver Disease
Mouzaki M, Ng V, Kamath BM, et al (Hosp for Sick Children, Toronto, Ontario, Canada; et al)
JPEN J Parenter Enter Nutr 38:673-681, 2014

Protein-energy malnutrition is the most common comorbidity affecting adults and children with end-stage liver disease. Despite clear evidence linking malnutrition to poor outcomes before and after liver transplantation, nutrition rehabilitation is often inadequately emphasized in the clinical management of these patients. The primary aim of this review is to synthesize the available evidence supporting the current clinical guidelines on enteral nutrition support and, more important, to highlight the lack of evidence behind much of what is considered "standard of care" for the nutrition management of patients with cirrhosis. In addition, the mechanisms of malnutrition are reviewed, the limitations of tools used to assess body composition in this setting are discussed, and the differences in macronutrient metabolism between healthy subjects and patients with end-stage liver disease are explained. A summary of recommendations is provided.

▶ As the authors have stated, protein-energy malnutrition is common in patients with substantial liver dysfunction and cirrhosis. Difficulties arise when trying to feed too much, too fast to replenish the host because the liver cannot handle higher levels of carbohydrates, fat, and protein. In general, current guidelines put forth by the American Society of Parenteral and Enteral Nutrition suggest that carbohydrates should provide 45—60% of total daily calories, whereas fat requirements should provide 25%—30% of total daily calories. However, fat requirements vary among patients, depending on the degree of maldigestion and the metabolic efficiency of the type of fat consumed. Energy requirements are approximately 25—40 kcal/kg/d. However, there is significant variation in energy requirements among patients because of differences in muscle mass, disease severity, and other comorbidities. ASPEN guidelines recommend the use of standard enteral and parenteral formulations for critically ill adults with acute or chronic liver disease. It is suggested that formulas enriched in branched chain amino acids only be used in patients with refractory hepatic encephalopathy.

J. M. Daly, MD

Cardiorespiratory Events with Bolus versus Continuous Enteral Feeding in Healthy Preterm Infants

Corvaglia L, Martini S, Aceti A, et al (Univ of Bologna, Italy)
J Pediatr 165:1255-1257, 2014

We evaluated the effects of bolus vs continuous tube feeding on cardiorespiratory events, detected by polysomnographic monitoring, in healthy preterm infants. Continuous tube feeding resulted in a significant increase of apneas and apneas-related hypoxic episodes compared with bolus feeding.

▶ The proper method of enteral feeding in preterm infants is unclear. There are many proponents of continuous nasal-enteral feeding to allow better absorption of the formula and perhaps less reflux of formula and aspiration. In this study, preterm infants were randomized to orogastric bolus (10 minutes) or 3-hour continuous feeding. Thirty-three healthy preterm infants were enrolled. During continuous feeding, a greater number of apneas was observed, particularly of those lasting more than 20 seconds and not associated with bradycardic and/or hypoxic events. Furthermore, continuous feeding resulted in more mild (oxygen saturation measured by pulse oximetry 81%—85%) and short (#10 seconds) hypoxic episodes concomitant with cardiorespiratory events.

Thus, in healthy, preterm infants, bolus feeding is the preferred approach. It remains to be determined which method is superior in unhealthy preterm infants. I applaud the authors for an important study with proper physiologic measures to determine better outcomes.

J. M. Daly, MD

Causes and Consequences of Interrupted Enteral Nutrition: A Prospective Observational Study in Critically Ill Surgical Patients

Peev MP, Yeh DD, Quraishi SA, et al (Massachusetts General Hosp, Boston)
JPEN J Parenter Enteral Nutr 39:21-27, 2015

Background.—Malnutrition and underfeeding are major challenges in caring for critically ill patients. Our goal was to characterize interruptions in enteral nutrition (EN) delivery and their impact on caloric debt in the surgical intensive care unit (ICU).

Materials and Methods.—We performed a prospective, observational study of adults admitted to surgical ICUs at a Boston teaching hospital (March—December 2012). We categorized EN interruptions as "unavoidable" vs "avoidable" and compared caloric deficit between patients with

≥1 EN interruption (group 1) vs those without interruptions (group 2). Multivariable logistic regression was used to investigate the association of EN interruption with the risk of underfeeding. Poisson regression was used to investigate the association of EN interruption with length of stay (LOS) and mortality.

Results.—Ninety-four patients comprised the analytic cohort. Twenty-six percent of interruptions were deemed "avoidable." Group 1 (n = 64) had a significantly higher mean daily and cumulative caloric deficit vs group 2 (n = 30). Patients in group 1 were at a 3-fold increased risk of being underfed (adjusted odds ratio, 2.89; 95% confidence interval [CI], 1.03−8.11), had a 30% higher risk of prolonged ICU LOS (adjusted incident risk ratio [IRR], 1.27; 95% CI, 1.14−1.42), and had a 50% higher risk of prolonged hospital LOS (adjusted IRR, 1.53; 95% CI, 1.41−1.67) vs group 2.

Conclusions.—In our cohort of critically ill surgical patients, EN interruption was frequent, largely "unavoidable," and associated with undesirable outcomes. Future efforts to optimize nutrition in the surgical ICU may benefit from considering strategies that maximize nutrient delivery before and after clinically appropriate EN interruptions.

▶ Over the past 20 years, the pendulum has swung from attempting to use only total parenteral nutrition (TPN) for nutritional support to using predominantly enteral nutritional support in critically ill patients. The reasons are many, including higher infection rates in TPN patients, cost, and the commonsense approach that "when the gut works, use it."

It is common, however, that patients in an intensive care unit (ICU) setting have interruptions in their enteral support leading to protein and calorie deficits that are hard to make up for when only enteral nutrition is used. In this prospective observational study, the authors investigated the causes and consequences of enteral nutrition (EN) interruptions in surgical ICU patients. They demonstrated that the most common reasons for interruptions in EN were (1) (re)intubation/extubation, (2) major bedside interventions (tracheostomy/percutaneous endoscopic gastrostomy tube placement), and (3) for imaging studies. Only 26% of these interruptions were considered avoidable. Patients who had interruptions in their EN infusions experienced a significantly higher caloric deficit during their ICU stay and had longer ICU as well as hospital length of stay compared with patients who did not have any feeding interruptions. Of interest, the Acute Physiology and Chronic Health Evaluation scores in the group with interruptions was higher (although not significantly) than the group with fewer interruptions. Could it be that sicker patients are just simply harder to feed enterally?

Could TPN have been started in the group who was falling further behind in terms of their caloric and protein intake?

These and other questions remain to be answered.

J. M. Daly, MD

Refeeding Hypophosphatemia in Hospitalized Adolescents With Anorexia Nervosa: A Position Statement of the Society for Adolescent Health and Medicine

Society for Adolescent Health and Medicine (Hosp for Sick Children, Toronto, ON; Univ of California San Francisco; The Children's Hosp at Westmead, New South Wales, Australia; et al)
J Adolesc Health 55:455-457, 2014

Refeeding hypophosphatemia in hospitalized adolescents with anorexia nervosa is correlated with degree of malnutrition. Therefore, when initiating nutritional rehabilitation, clinicians should have a heightened awareness of the possibility of refeeding hypophosphatemia in severely malnourished patients (<70% median body mass index).

▶ Refeeding syndrome describes the clinical and metabolic derangements that can occur during the refeeding of a malnourished patient. It occurs in conditions associated with malnutrition, including anorexia nervosa. Refeeding syndrome is complex and consists of a variety of metabolic and clinical features. The clinical features include cardiac arrhythmias, cardiac failure or arrest, muscle weakness, hemolytic anemia, delirium, seizures, coma, and sudden death that can occur days to weeks after the initiation of nutritional rehabilitation. The hallmark biochemical feature of refeeding syndrome is hypophosphatemia, also referred to as refeeding hypophosphatemia. This significant problem was described in the 1970s when total parenteral nutrition (TPN) was first used to treat malnutrition. Although exact amounts of phosphate depend on the individual patient, at least 15—20 mEq of potassium phosphate or sodium acid phosphate should be added per liter of TPN to avoid this complication.

J. M. Daly, MD

Supplementation with olive oil, but not fish oil, improves cutaneous wound healing in stressed mice

Rosa A dos S, Bandeira LG, Monte-Alto-Costa A, et al (Rural Federal Univ of Rio de Janeiro, Seropédica, Brazil; State Univ of Rio de Janeiro, Brazil)
Wound Repair Regen 22:537-547, 2014

Supplementation with olive and fish oils reverses the effects of stress on behavioral activities and adrenal activation. However, previous studies have not shown whether supplementation with olive and fish oil could inhibit the effects of stress on cutaneous wound healing. Thus, this study investigated the effects of supplementation with fish or olive oil on cutaneous healing in stressed mice. Mice were subjected to rotational stress and treated with olive or fish oil daily until euthanasia. An excisional lesion was created on each mouse, and 14 days later, the lesions were analyzed.

In addition, murine skin fibroblasts were exposed to elevated epinephrine levels plus olive oil, and fibroblast activity was evaluated. In the in vivo studies, administration of olive oil, but not fish oil, inhibited stress-induced reduction in wound contraction, reepithelialization, hydroxyproline levels, and blood vessel density. Stress-induced increases in vascular endothelial growth factor expression and the numbers of macrophages and neutrophils were reversed only by olive oil. Both oils reversed stress induced increase in catecholamine levels and oxidative damage. In in vitro studies, olive oil treatment reversed the reduction in fibroblast migration and collagen deposition and the increase in lipid peroxidation induced by epinephrine. In conclusion, supplementation with olive oil, but not fish oil, improves cutaneous wound healing in chronically stressed mice.

▶ It has been suggested that diets supplemented with fish oils can reduce the inflammatory response to injury, thereby improving outcomes. In this experimental study, mice underwent a full-thickness excision of the skin and then were subjected to rotational cage stress. Controls were not stressed. In contrast to what the authors predicted, olive oil supplementation improved the rate of skin closure in stressed mice.

The authors noted that in spite of reducing norepinephrine levels, fish oil increased neutrophil and macrophage infiltration in both nonstressed and stressed mice. In addition, the norepinephrine levels in nonstressed or stressed mice treated with fish oil were greater than in nonstressed or stressed mice treated with olive oil. Thus, fish oil may directly enhance skin inflammation (ie, inflammatory cell migration) resulting in slower wound closure independent of catecholamine production. Thus, the results suggest that a diminution of the inflammatory response is important to reduce complications such as acute respiratory distress syndrome after injury with fish oil supplementation, but the healing wound may suffer.

Many more trials will be required with different models of injury to be certain of this hypothesis.

J. M. Daly, MD

Enteral Granulocyte-Colony Stimulating Factor and Erythropoietin Early in Life Improves Feeding Tolerance in Preterm Infants: A Randomized Controlled Trial
El-Ganzoury MM, Awad HA, El-Farrash RA, et al (Ain Shams Univ, Cairo, Egypt)
J Pediatr 165:1140-1145, 2014

Objective.—To evaluate the efficacy and safety of enteral recombinant human granulocyte colony-stimulating factor (rhG-CSF) and recombinant human erythropoietin (rhEPO) in preventing feeding intolerance.

Study Design.—An interventional randomized control trial was conducted in 90 preterm infants born at ≤33 weeks gestational age. The neonates were assigned to 4 groups; 20 received rhG-CSF, 20 received rhEPO, 20 received both, and 30 received distilled water (placebo control). The test solution was given at the beginning of enteral feeding and was discontinued when enteral intake reached 100 mL/kg/day or after a maximum of 7 days, whichever came first. Feeding tolerance and adverse effects of treatment were assessed. Serum granulocyte colony-stimulating factor and erythropoietin levels were measured on days 0 and 7 of treatment.

Results.—All neonates tolerated the treatment without side effects. Neonates who received rhG-CSF and/or rhEPO had better feeding tolerance, as reflected by earlier achievement of 75 mL/kg/day, 100 mL/kg/day, and full enteral feeding of 150 mL/kg/day with earlier weight gain and a shorter hospital stay ($P < .05$). The risk of necrotizing enterocolitis was reduced from 10% to 0% in all treatment groups ($P < .05$). There was a shorter duration of withholding of feeding secondary to feeding intolerance among neonates receiving both rhG-CSF and rhEPO compared with those receiving placebo ($P < .05$). Serum levels of granulocyte colony-stimulating factor and erythropoietin at 0 and 7 days did not differ across the treatment groups.

Conclusions.—Enteral administration of rhG-CSF and/or rhEPO improves feeding outcome and decreases the risk of necrotizing enterocolitis in preterm neonates. The mechanism may involve the prevention of villous atrophy.

▶ Necrotizing enterocolitis (NEC) is a devastating illness in preterm, low birthweight infants. The authors point out that in utero, infants swallow amniotic fluid containing important growth factors that may prevent intestinal atrophy. This study was a double-blind, randomized trial in 90 preterm infants of 33 weeks' gestational age. Infants were assigned to receive enteral granulocyte colony-stimulating factor (G-CSF) and/or erythropoietin (EPO) or water placebo. A single daily dose of enteral recombinant human (rh)G-CSF, and/or enteral rhEPO was given with the start of enteral feeding. This dose was calculated to provide the same amount of growth factors ingested by a fetus swallowing 200 mL/kg/day of amniotic fluid. Results of the trial showed that the risk of NEC was reduced from 10% in the placebo group to 0% in all treatment groups. Notably, neonates who received both enteral rhG-CSF and rhEPO showed a trend toward better feeding tolerance, both clinically and radiologically, compared with the other 2 groups.

This is an important study carried out in a solid clinical trial. The results have implications for the use of these growth factors combined with enteral nutrition in other situations in infants who actually develop necrotizing enterocolitis or those who require major intestinal resectional surgery.

J. M. Daly, MD

Parenteral Nutrition–Associated Liver Injury and Increased GRP94 Expression Prevented by ω-3 Fish Oil–Based Lipid Emulsion Supplementation

Zhu X, Xiao Z, Chen X, et al (Soochow Univ, Suzhou, Jiangsu, China)
J Pediatr Gastroenterol Nutr 59:708-713, 2014

Objective.—Parenteral nutrition in infants with gastrointestinal disorders can be lifesaving, but it is also associated with parenteral nutrition–associated liver disease. We investigated the effects of incorporating ω-3 fish oil in a parenteral nutrition mixture on signs of parenteral nutrition–associated liver disease and explored the mechanism involved in this process.

Methods.—Seven-day-old New Zealand rabbits were divided into 3 groups of 8, and for 1 week they were infused via the right jugular vein with standard total parenteral nutrition with soybean oil (TPN-soy) or TPN with ω-3 fish oil–based lipid emulsion (TPN-FO), or naturally nursed with rabbit milk (control). Serum and liver tissues were analyzed for serological indicators and pathology, respectively. Reverse-transcriptase polymerase chain reaction was used to evaluate the messenger RNA levels of the endoplasmic reticulum stress chaperone protein glucose-regulated protein 94 (GRP94) in liver tissues and GRP94 protein levels were compared through immunohistochemistry and Western blot assays.

Results.—TPN-soy animals had significantly higher serum total bilirubin, direct bilirubin, and γ-glutamyl transpeptidase and lower serum albumin than the controls ($P < 0.01$, each) or the TPN-FO group, which were similar to the controls ($P < 0.01$ cf. TPN). Damage to liver tissues of the TPN-FO group was much less than that of the TPN-soy group. GRP94 messenger RNA and protein levels in liver tissues of TPN-soy animals were significantly higher than that of the controls or TPN-FO rabbits, which were similar to the controls.

Conclusions.—Incorporating ω-3 fish oil in parenteral nutrition emulsion greatly prevented liver dysfunction and liver tissue damage in week-old rabbit kits, possibly by preventing endoplasmic reticulum stress.

▶ Parenteral nutrition is often life-saving for infants and children who require nutritional support because of a variety of pathophysiologic conditions. Its use, however, is not without inherent risks, among which is parenteral nutrition-associated liver disease (PNALD). As the authors stated, approximately 30% to 60% of the infants who require long-term parenteral nutrition develop PNALD, with abnormalities of liver function and hepatic damage. Thus, much research has taken place attempting to ameliorate PNALD in neonates and infants receiving parenteral nutrition. Among the methods tried is the use of different fatty acids (omega-3 fatty acids) in fish oil instead of soybean oil. Compared with control 7-day-old rabbits, soy total parenteral nutrition (TPN) animals had significantly higher serum total bilirubin, direct bilirubin, and gamma-glutamyl transpeptidase levels, but lower albumin ($P < .01$). In the fish oil TPN group, only mild hepatic steatosis and inflammatory cell infiltration were found; the morphology of hepatocytes was normal, and there was no cholangiectasis, bile duct epithelial hyperplasia, or cholestasis.

Thus, as others have stated, it may be very beneficial to alter the fatty acid composition of lipid and oil administered to neonates. Clearly, more study is necessary.

J. M. Daly, MD

Randomized Clinical Trial of New Intravenous Lipid (SMOFlipid 20%) Versus Medium-Chain Triglycerides/Long-Chain Triglycerides in Adult Patients Undergoing Gastrointestinal Surgery

Wu M-H, Wang M-Y, Yang C-Y, et al (Natl Taiwan Univ Hosp, Taipei)
JPEN J Parenter Enteral Nutr 38:800-808, 2014

Background.—SMOFlipid 20% is intravenous lipid emulsion (ILE) containing long-chain triglycerides (LCT), medium-chain triglycerides (MCT), olive oil, and fish oil as a mixed emulsion containing α-tocopherol. The aim was to assess the efficacy of this new ILE in gastrointestinal surgery compared with MCT/LCT.

Methods.—In this prospective study, 40 patients were randomized to SMOFlipid 20% or MCT/LCT (Lipovenoes 20%) group. Clinical and biochemistry data were collected. Inflammatory markers (CRP, IL-6, IL-10, TNF-α, TGF-β1) and oxidative stress (ROS and superoxide) were measured.

Results.—Thirty-five patients (17 males and 18 females) with a mean age of 57 years completed the study. The patients' demographic characteristics (age, gender, height, body weight, and BMI) were similar without significant differences between groups. The increment of triglyceride on day 6 from baseline was significantly lower in SMOFlipid group than in Lipovenoes MCT/LCT group. Inflammatory markers, as well as superoxide radical and total oxygen radical were not different between groups.

Conclusions.—Despite the comparable effect on inflammatory response, because of its well-balanced fatty acid pattern, relatively low n-6:n-3 ratio, and high vitamin E content, SMOFlipid had a better triglyceride-lowering effect as compared with MCT/LCT in adult patients undergoing gastrointestinal surgery.

▶ Search for the more perfect parenteral nutrition continues unabated. The solution should be designed to normalize the average serum profile, maximize accretion of protein for visceral synthesis (circulating proteins) and lean body mass, while improving lipid profiles in patients requiring such solutions for prolonged periods. This study tested a new formula containing long-chain triglycerides, medium-chain triglycerides, olive oil, and fish oil as a mixed emulsion containing alpha tocopherol. The investigators hypothesized that using this new, experimental formula, there would be a reduction in circulating inflammatory markers, which was not the case. There did seem to be a better normalization of serum triglycerides and other circulating lipid components using the new experimental solution.

Studies such as these are valuable providing good baseline information to develop a better parenteral nutrient solution.

J. M. Daly, MD

Effect of Repeated Fasting/Refeeding on Obesity Development and Health Complications in Rats Arising from Reduced Nest

Mozeš Š, Šefčíková Z, Raček Ľ (Slovak Academy of Sciences, Šoltésovej, Kosice)
Dig Dis Sci 60:354-361, 2014

Background.—Overnutrition during postnatal life represents a risk factor for later obesity and associated metabolic disorders.

Aim.—We investigated the interaction between postnatal and later-life nutrition on body composition, blood pressure and the jejunal enzyme activities in male Sprague—Dawley rats.

Methods.—From birth, we adjusted the number of pups in the nest to 4 (small litters—SL; overfeeding) or to 10 pups (normal litters—NL; controls), and from day 50 until 70, the SL (SL-R) and NL (NL-R) rats were subjected to 1 day fasting and 1 day refeeding cycles (RFR). Their body composition was determined by magnetic resonance imaging, and enzyme activity was assayed histochemically.

Results.—At 50 and 70 days, SL rats were found to be overweight ($p < 0.001$), with higher adiposity ($p < 0.001$) and blood pressure ($p < 0.01$). Moreover, despite significantly decreased daily food intake during RFR (SL-R 39%, NL-R 23%), higher fat deposition ($p < 0.001$) and blood pressure ($p < 0.05$) was detected in SL-R rats. Activity of alkaline phosphatase (AP) functionally involved in lipid absorption was significantly higher in SL than NL rats ($p < 0.001$) but substantially decreased in RFR groups (SL-R $p < 0.001$, NL-R $p < 0.01$). However, despite these enzymatic adaptations to reduced food intake, the SL-R rats displayed significantly higher AP activity in comparison with NL-R rats ($p < 0.01$) on day 70.

Conclusions.—Our results demonstrate that postnatal overfeeding predisposes the ontogeny of intestinal function, which may promote the probability of obesity risk. Accordingly, in these animals, efficient fat deposition and elevated blood pressure were not diminished in response to dietary restrictions in later life.

▶ Obesity has been described as a genetic, epigenetic, and environmental problem with early-life eating habits and development of fat stores predictive of obesity in later life. It is important to understand these various influences on the development of obesity to create methods to reduce this public health scourge. This animal study sought to understand the effects of early eating volume on early obesity and later body fat composition.

From day 10 until day 50 of age, the smaller liter pups became heavier than those raised in normal liter nests and displayed significantly higher weight gain as well as increased both absolute and relative weight of the fat tissues during these phases. In addition, these changes persisted despite episodes of fasting and refeeding into later life. Thus, the authors concluded that neonatal overfeeding sets the stage for later obesity development.

It would be interesting to know whether sustained low-calorie diets later in life or any nutritional alterations or exercise could significantly alter this pattern of fat deposition that seemed to persist.

J. M. Daly, MD

Fish-Oil Fat Emulsion Supplementation Reduces the Risk of Retinopathy in Very Low Birth Weight Infants: A Prospective, Randomized Study
Pawlik D, Lauterbach R, Walczak M, et al (Jagiellonian Univ Med College, Kraków, Poland; Univ of Missouri School of Medicine, Columbia)
JPEN J Parenter Enter Nutr 38:711-716, 2014

Background.—Preliminary studies suggest that fish-oil lipid emulsion given parenterally to very preterm infants reduces the severity of retinopathy (ROP) and cholestasis.

Methods.—Infants weighing <1250 g at birth were randomly allocated to 2 groups: an experimental group of 60 infants that received an intravenous (IV) soybean, olive oil, and fish oil emulsion, and a control group of 70 infants that was given a parenteral soybean and olive oil emulsion. Plasma and erythrocyte concentrations of docosahexaenoic acid (DHA) were determined using a high-performance liquid chromatography—mass spectrometry analysis.

Results.—Nine infants in the fish oil group required laser therapy for ROP compared with 22 infants in the standard intralipid group (risk ratio [RR], 0.48; 95% confidence interval [CI], 0.24—0.96). Three infants in the fish oil group developed cholestasis compared with 20 infants in the standard intralipid group (RR, 0.18; 95% CI, 0.055—0.56). The mean plasma DHA concentrations in treated infants were 2.9-fold higher in the fish oil group than in control infants on the 7th and 14th days of life. The mean DHA content in erythrocytes of treated infants was 4.5-fold and 2.7-fold higher compared with controls at 7 and 14 days of age.

Conclusions.—Premature infants receiving an IV fat emulsion containing fish oil had less ROP requiring laser treatment and less cholestasis than those receiving a standard lipid emulsion. These infants also had higher plasma and erythrocyte DHA levels at 7 and 14 days, suggesting potential long-term neurodevelopmental benefits.

▶ Preterm, low-birth-weight infants have a high risk of developing retinopathy requiring frequent laser therapy. The ability to feed them enterally with adequate calories is often difficult. Thus, the ability to provide total parenteral nutrition with appropriate nutrients is critical to their survival and development. All infants with birth weights of < 1250 g, who were delivered at < 32 weeks of gestation and who were admitted to the neonatal intensive care unit, were eligible for this study. Infants whose parents gave informed consent were randomly assigned to an experimental group that received an intravenous emulsion proportioned to contain a 50% volume of soybean and olive oil and a 50% volume of fish oil and a control group that was given a 20% soybean and olive oil emulsion. Of the 19 infants who developed retinopathy in the experimental group, in 10 patients, a spontaneous regression was observed, whereas in the control group of 26 infants with diagnosed retinopathy of prematurity (ROP), in 22 patients, the progression of disease required treatment. Laser therapy for ROP was used twice as often in the control group (n = 22 vs 9, respectively). Also, cholestasis was diagnosed 6 times more frequently in the control group (n = 20 vs 3, respectively). Finally, docosahexaenoic acid (DHA) plasma and red cell levels were significantly increased in the experimental group compared with controls.

This is an excellent prospective, randomized trial in a group of infants that is difficult to manage. None of the infants developed coagulopathy due to the increased DHA levels. Although further work needs to be done, I recommend this article to all who treat neonates.

J. M. Daly, MD

High-Protein Enteral Nutrition Enriched With Immune-Modulating Nutrients vs Standard High-Protein Enteral Nutrition and Nosocomial Infections in the ICU: A Randomized Clinical Trial

van Zanten ARH, Sztark F, Kaisers UX, et al (Gelderse Vallei Hosp, Ede, the Netherlands; Groupe Hôpital Pellegrin — CHU Bordeaux, France; Universitätsklinikum Leipzig, Germany; et al)
JAMA 312:514-524, 2014

Importance.—Enteral administration of immune-modulating nutrients (eg, glutamine, omega-3 fatty acids, selenium, and antioxidants) has been suggested to reduce infections and improve recovery from critical illness. However, controversy exists on the use of immune-modulating enteral nutrition, reflected by lack of consensus in guidelines.

Objective.—To determine whether high-protein enteral nutrition enriched with immune-modulating nutrients (IMHP) reduces the incidence of infections compared with standard high-protein enteral nutrition (HP) in mechanically ventilated critically ill patients.

Design, Setting, and Participants.—The MetaPlus study, a randomized, double-blind, multicenter trial, was conducted from February 2010 through April 2012 including a 6-month follow-up period in 14 intensive care units (ICUs) in the Netherlands, Germany, France, and Belgium. A total of 301 adult patients who were expected to be ventilated for more than 72 hours and to require enteral nutrition for more than 72 hours were randomized to the IMHP (n = 152) or HP (n = 149) group and included in an intention-to-treat analysis, performed for the total population as well as predefined medical, surgical, and trauma subpopulations.

Interventions.—High-protein enteral nutrition enriched with immune-modulating nutrients vs standard high-protein enteral nutrition, initiated within 48 hours of ICU admission and continued during the ICU stay for a maximum of 28 days.

Main Outcomes and Measures.—The primary outcome measure was incidence of new infections according to the Centers for Disease Control and Prevention (CDC) definitions. Secondary end points included mortality, Sequential Organ Failure Assessment (SOFA) scores, mechanical ventilation duration, ICU and hospital lengths of stay, and subtypes of infections according CDC definitions.

Results.—There were no statistically significant differences in incidence of new infections between the groups: 53% (95% CI, 44%-61%) in the IMHP group vs 52% (95% CI, 44%-61%) in the HP group ($P = .96$). No statistically significant differences were observed in other end points, except for a higher 6-month mortality rate in the medical subgroup: 54% (95% CI, 40%-67%) in the IMHP group vs 35% (95% CI, 22%-49%) in the HP group ($P = .04$), with a hazard ratio of 1.57 (95% CI, 1.03-2.39; $P = .04$) for 6-month mortality adjusted for age and Acute Physiology and Chronic Health Evaluation II score comparing the groups.

Conclusions and Relevance.—Among adult patients breathing with the aid of mechanical ventilation in the ICU, IMHP compared with HP did not improve infectious complications or other clinical end points and may be harmful as suggested by increased adjusted mortality at 6 months. These findings do not support the use of IMHP nutrients in these patients.

Trial Registration.—trialregister.nl Identifier: NTR2181.

▶ Studies of enteral nutrition with or without immune-supplementing formulas have had conflicting results. In malnourished, elective surgical patients with upper gastrointestinal cancer, single-institution and meta-analysis studies have shown positive results in reducing infectious complications. In critically ill patients in the intensive care unit (ICU), however, some studies and meta-analyses have shown harm or no benefit. Often variables such as patient selection, amount of calorie and protein feeding, and quantitative amounts of immune agents in the diet have confounded results. In this randomized, double-blind multicenter trial comparing immune modulating high-protein diets (IMHP) with high-protein (HP) diets in a heterogeneous ICU group of patients, there was no effect of the nutritional formulae on infectious complications. Within a mean of 3 days, 70% of target energy intake was reached in IMHP patients and 80% in HP patients demonstrating adequacy of feeding.

Why are there differences across these multiple studies over the past 30 years? The answer is unclear. It appears that overall, the mortality across studies for both control and experimental groups has declined, making it harder to demonstrate differences with a single intervention such as an immune-modulating enteral formula. In the current high-protein enteral feeding protocol, a fair amount of glutamine was given in the control group, and it may be that once a certain level is reached, further augmentation is not necessary. Nevertheless, the results of this well-conducted study call into questions the current guidelines for feeding ICU patients.

J. M. Daly, MD

Definition, prevalence, and outcome of feeding intolerance in intensive care: a systematic review and meta-analysis
Blaser AR, Starkopf J, Kirsimägi Ü, et al (Univ of Tartu, Estonia; Tartu Univ Hosp, Estonia; et al)
Acta Anaesthesiol Scand 58:914-922, 2014

Clinicians and researchers frequently use the phrase 'feeding intolerance' (FI) as a descriptive term in enterally fed critically ill patients. We aimed to: (1) determine what is the most accepted definition of FI; (2) estimate the prevalence of FI; and (3) evaluate whether FI is associated with important outcomes. Systematic searches of peer-reviewed publications using PubMed, MEDLINE, and Web of Science were performed with studies reporting FI extracted. We identified 72 studies defining FI. In 33 studies, the definition was based on large gastric residual volumes (GRVs) together with other gastrointestinal symptoms, while 30 studies relied solely on large GRVs, six studies used inadequate delivery of enteral nutrition (EN) as a threshold, and three studies gastrointestinal symptoms without reference to GRV. The median volume used to define a 'large' GRV was 250 ml (ranges from 75 to 500 ml). The pooled proportion ($n = 31$ studies) of FI was 38.3% (95% CI 30.7—46.2). Five studies reported outcomes, all of them observed adverse outcome in FI patients. In three studies, respectively, FI was associated with increased mortality and ICU length-of-stay. In summary, FI is inconsistently defined but appears to occur frequently. There are preliminary data indicating that FI is associated with adverse outcomes. A standard definition of FI is required to determine the accuracy of these preliminary data.

▶ As the authors have stated, the term "feeding intolerance" (FI) is poorly understood, not only in conversation among physicians but also in the published literature. Because of this, the authors performed a systemic review of the literature. The prevalence of FI in 31 studies ranged from 2% to 75%, with the pooled proportion of 38%. The differences among the FI definition categories were not significant, whereas the largest variance was observed in 2 categories, including large gastric residual volumes. However, these data are based on various definitions and study inclusion criteria; therefore, substantial heterogeneity was observed among all of the studies. Pooling the studies according to the category of definition did not reduce the heterogeneity as described in the article. Interestingly, with postpyloric feeding, there was a 17% incidence of feeding intolerance compared with 37% feeding intolerance in those fed intragastrically.

It is recognized that many patients do not receive the full dosage of enteral feedings as prescribed based on their needs, but instead "intolerance" and feeding interruptions result in major calorie and protein deficits relative to needs. Better definitions are needed, but more important is to understand the causes and solutions for feeding intolerance.

J. M. Daly, MD

A.S.P.E.N. Clinical Guidelines: Support of Pediatric Patients With Intestinal Failure at Risk of Parenteral Nutrition—Associated Liver Disease
Wales PW, Allen N, Worthington P, et al (Univ of Toronto, Ontario, Canada; Children's Mercy Hosp, Kansas City, MO; Thomas Jefferson Univ Hosp, Philadelphia, PA; et al)
JPEN J Parenter Enter Nutr 38:538-557, 2014

Background.—Children with severe intestinal failure and prolonged dependence on parenteral nutrition are susceptible to the development of parenteral nutrition—associated liver disease (PNALD). The purpose of this clinical guideline is to develop recommendations for the care of children with PN-dependent intestinal failure that have the potential to prevent PNALD or improve its treatment.

Method.—A systematic review of the best available evidence to answer a series of questions regarding clinical management of children with intestinal failure receiving parenteral or enteral nutrition was undertaken and evaluated using concepts adopted from the Grading of Recommendations, Assessment, Development, and Evaluation (GRADE) Working Group. A consensus process was used to develop the clinical guideline recommendations prior to external and internal review and approval by the American Society for Parenteral and Enteral Nutrition Board of Directors.

Questions.—(1) Is ethanol lock effective in preventing bloodstream infection and catheter removal in children at risk of PNALD? (2) What fat emulsion strategies can be used in pediatric patients with intestinal failure to reduce the risk of or treat PNALD? (3) Can enteral ursodeoxycholic acid improve the treatment of PNALD in pediatric patients with intestinal failure? (4) Are PNALD outcomes improved when patients are managed by a multidisciplinary intestinal rehabilitation team?

▶ Clinical Guidelines are often created by groups of individuals with expertise in certain areas under the aegis of a professional organization. As such, they provide the most comprehensive critique of existing published knowledge on a given subject. The development of parenteral nutrition associated liver disease (PNALD) in children with intestinal failure is a major unresolved problem.

The Committee asked and then answered the following 4 questions:

Question 1: Is ethanol lock effective in preventing bloodstream infection and catheter removal in children at risk of PNALD? (Tables 2 and 3 in the original article.)

Recommendation: A suggestion is made to use ethanol lock to prevent central line-associated bloodstream infection and to reduce catheter replacements in children at risk of PNALD.

Evidence: Low and very low

Recommendation Grade: Weak

Question 2: What fat emulsion strategies can be used in pediatric patients with intestinal failure to reduce the risk of or treat PNALD? (Tables 4 and 5 in the original article.)

Recommendation: Because the only IV fat emulsion available for use in the United States is soy-based fat emulsion (SOE), a suggestion is made to reduce the dose of SOE to ≤1 g/kg/d to treat cholestasis in children with PNALD. The quality of evidence supporting this recommendation is very low.

Question 3: Can enteral ursodeoxycholic acid (UDCA) improve the treatment of PNALD in pediatric patients with intestinal failure? (Tables 6 and 7 in the original article.)

Recommendation: A suggestion is made to use UDCA for the treatment of elevated liver enzymes in children with PNALD. The evidence is of very low quality and confounded with the presence of enteral feeding in conjunction with treatment with UDCA.

Evidence: Very low

Recommendation: Weak

Question 4: Are PNALD outcomes improved when patients are managed by a multidisciplinary intestinal rehabilitation team? (Tables 8 and 9 in the original article.)

Recommendation: A suggestion is made to refer patients with parenteral nutrition-dependent intestinal failure to multidisciplinary intestinal rehabilitation programs. The evidence on this topic is of very low quality, but the improvement in survival is compelling, and the risk to the child of treatment with multidisciplinary practice is not increased.

Evidence: Very low

Recommendation: Weak

I recommend this article for all readers interested in parenteral nutrition therapy for children and adults.

J. M. Daly, MD

Neonates With Short Bowel Syndrome: An Optimistic Future for Parenteral Nutrition Independence

Fallon EM, Mitchell PD, Nehra D, et al (Boston Children's Hosp and Harvard Med School, MA)

JAMA Surg 149:663-670, 2014

Importance.—The introduction of hepatoprotective strategies and multidisciplinary management has significantly improved the outcome of neonates with short bowel syndrome (SBS) who require parenteral nutrition (PN).

Objective.—To determine the probability of weaning from PN based on intestinal length in neonates with SBS amidst the new era of hepatoprotective strategies and multidisciplinary management.

Design, Setting, and Participants.—Retrospective medical record review at a single-center academic institution. Neonates with no more than 100 cm of small intestine at a corrected gestational age of no more than 30 days who were diagnosed with a surgical gastrointestinal disease and PN dependent for at least 2 weeks were included. Data were collected from January 1, 2004, through June 1, 2012.

Exposure.—Neonates with SBS requiring PN.

Main Outcomes and Measures.—The probability of wean from PN without reinitiation for at least 1 year, as determined by logistic regression. Predictors of wean were evaluated using exact conditional logistic regression. Predictors of time to wean were determined by Cox proportional hazards regression.

Results.—Sixty-three patients with a median (25th percentile, 75th percentile [interquartile range (IQR)]) gestational age of 31 (27, 35) weeks, birth weight of 1423 (895, 2445) g, small intestinal length of 41.0 (24.0, 65.0) cm, and predicted length of 29.0% (17.1%, 45.5%) underwent analysis. Fifty-one patients (81%) received a fish oil-based lipid emulsion (1 g/kg/d), 40 (63%) were weaned, 11 (17%) remained PN dependent, 4 (6%) underwent transplant, and 8 (13%) died while on PN. Excluding patients who underwent transplant or died, the median (IQR) small intestinal length was 55.0 (28.0, 75.0) cm in weaned and 26.0 (14.0, 41.0) cm in PN-dependent patients ($P=.006$), with 40 of 51 (78%) weaned by study end. The cumulative probability of wean for patients with at least 50 cm of small intestine was 88% after 12 and 96% after 24 months. Patients with less than 50 cm of small intestine had a cumulative probability of wean of 23% after 12, 38% after 24, and 71% after 57 months. Small intestinal length was found to be the primary predictor of wean. Notable predictors of time to wean included the amount of small intestine remaining (hazard ratio, 1.94 [95% CI, 1.45-2.58] per 20 cm of intestine; $P < .001$), entirety of care within our institution (3.27 [1.59-6.72]; $P=.001$), and intestinal lengthening procedure (0.19 [0.04-0.84]; $P=.03$).

Conclusions and Relevance.—The majority of patients will wean from PN despite short intestinal length, likely as a result of new management strategies combined with a multidisciplinary team approach.

▶ There has long been pessimism for neonates and adults with severe short bowel syndrome as to whether they can ever be weaned from the total parenteral nutrition (PN) that is necessary for their survival. Specific nutrients such as glutamine, growth hormone, and other nutrient substrates have been used to help with a weaning process. This retrospective review studied 63 neonates of whom 40 (63%) were weaned from PN, 11 (17%) remained PN-dependent at the end of the study, 4 (6%) underwent multivisceral transplant, and 8 (13%) died while on PN. These 4 cohorts did not differ according to patient demographics, diagnosis, and/or PN initiation. Excluding those infants who underwent transplant ($n = 4$) or who died ($n = 8$), the median small intestinal length in patients weaned from PN ($n = 40$) was 55 cm compared with 26 cm in PN-dependent patients.

Overall, 40 of 51 patients (78%) were weaned by study end, after excluding patients who underwent transplant and who died. Intestinal length was found to be the primary predictor of weaning from PN. Collectively, these patients were similar with the exception of the frequency of gastroschisis, which was 3% in weaned vs 27% in PN-dependent patients. Thus, some optimism is justified in treating infants with short-bowel syndrome. Surgical procedures, such as intestinal lengthening and strictureplasty, also clearly play a role in weaning these patients from PN.

J. M. Daly, MD

Preliminary Findings of Long-Term Neurodevelopmental Outcomes of Infants Treated With Intravenous Fat Emulsion Reduction for the Management of Parenteral Nutrition—Associated Cholestasis

Blackmer AB, Warschausky S, Siddiqui S, et al (Univ of Michigan College of Pharmacy, Ann Arbor; Univ of Michigan Health System, Ann Arbor; Univ of Michigan, Ann Arbor; et al)
JPEN J Parenter Enteral Nutr 39:34-46, 2015

Introduction.—Parenteral nutrition—associated cholestasis (PNAC) is linked with the administration of soybean-based intravenous fat emulsion (IVFE). IVFE reduction (IFER) may be an effective management strategy for PNAC; however, long-term associated neurodevelopmental outcomes (NDOs) for infants undergoing IFER have not been measured previously. This single-institution, prospective study examined the risk for negative NDOs and key predictors of NDOs associated with IFER.

Methods.—Patients (2—5 years) treated with soybean-based IFER as neonates underwent NDO measurements, including Ages and Stages Questionnaires—3 (ASQ-3), Parents' Evaluations of Developmental Status (PEDS), and Behavior Assessment System for Children, Second Edition Preschool, Parent (BASC-2 PRS-P). The relationship between NDOs and predictive variables was evaluated.

Results.—A total of 25 children had a complete PEDS survey, and 17 were found to be "not at risk." The BASC-2 PRS-P evaluation (n = 18 patients) showed that all 4 composite domains fell within the normative developmental range, and 67%—89% of patients were observed to be "typically developing." For the primary outcome measure, ASQ-3, 82.4%—94.4% of patients were "not at risk." Logistical regression analyses were performed to examine risk factors contributing to negative NDOs. Of children completing all NDO studies, IFER-related variables (eg, development of essential fatty acid deficiency, duration of IFER, and mean IVFE dose) were not found to be predictors of adverse NDOs.

Conclusions.—This study represents the first report of NDOs in pediatric patients treated with IFER. IFER-treated patients score within the normative range most of the time. IFER-related variables were *not* found to be associated with negative NDOs. The results set the stage for a larger, multicenter, prospective study.

▶ The risk of parenteral nutrition-associated liver disease (cholestasis) is significant with the use of long-term parenteral nutrition. One strategy that has been suggested to reduce this risk is the reduction in dose of soybean-based fat emulsion. However, the long-term neurodevelopmental outcomes associated with this strategy are unknown to date. This single-institution study represents the first published report of neurodevelopmental outcomes in pediatric patients treated with reduced doses of soy bean-based fat emulsion with intravenous fat emulsion reduction (IFER). Importantly, most patients were found to be not at risk, and in those with negative neurodevelopment outcomes, regression analysis showed that IFER-related variables were not predictive of neurodevelopmental or behavioral outcomes. Further work is required to determine if lower doses of soy bean oil fat emulsion is safe for children receiving long-term parenteral nutrition.

J. M. Daly, MD

Enteral Arginine Partially Ameliorates Parenteral Nutrition—Induced Small Intestinal Atrophy and Stimulates Hepatic Protein Synthesis in Neonatal Piglets

Dinesh OC, Dodge ME, Baldwin MP, et al (Memorial Univ of Newfoundland, St John's, Newfoundland & Labrador, Canada)
JPEN J Parenter Enter Nutr 38:973-981, 2014

Background.—Arginine is an indispensable amino acid in neonates; de novo synthesis of arginine occurs in the small intestine (SI) but is reduced during parenteral nutrition (PN), limiting the arginine available to the mucosa. We assessed the effects of route of intake and dietary concentration of arginine on protein synthesis, superior mesenteric artery (SMA) blood flow, and SI morphology.

Methods.—Piglets (n = 18, 14−17 days old) were given complete PN for 3 days to induce SI atrophy, then switched to 1 of 3 treatments: arginine-free PN plus an intragastric (IG) infusion of high arginine $(1.6 \text{ g·kg}^{-1}\text{·d}^{-1}$, IG-H Arg) or low arginine $(0.6 \text{ g·kg}^{-1}\text{·d}^{-1}$, IG-L Arg) or complete high-arginine PN $(1.6 \text{ g·kg}^{-1}\text{·d}^{-1}$, IV-H Arg).

Results.—Enteral arginine, irrespective of amount provided, stimulated hepatic protein synthesis compared with intravenous delivery of arginine $(P = .01)$. SMA blood flow declined for all groups following the initiation of PN. After 48 hours on the test diets, all groups reached low constant levels, but the IV-H group was significantly higher than both IG groups $(P < .05)$. Despite greater blood flow, the SI morphological characteristics in IV-H Arg pigs were not significantly improved over the other groups. IV-H Arg pigs had higher plasma concentrations of indispensable amino acids (tyrosine, isoleucine, and valine) compared with IG-H Arg, despite identical amino acid intakes.

Conclusions.—Intravenous delivery of arginine sustained the best SMA blood flow, whereas even a moderate amount of enteral arginine stimulated liver protein synthesis and maintained SI growth, independent of blood flow.

▶ Necrotizing enterocolitis is a devastating complication in neonates that occurs more often in low-birth-weight babies. The exact etiology is unclear, but intestinal ischemia may play a significant role. Arginine is known to be conditionally essential in neonates. In addition, through its metabolism to nitrous oxide, arginine can stimulate blood flow to organs. Thus, the authors studied intestinal blood flow and other factors when piglets were given enteral or parenteral arginine.

Enteral arginine, irrespective of the amount provided, stimulated hepatic protein synthesis compared with intravenous delivery of arginine. However, despite greater superior mesenteric arterial blood flow, small intestinal morphological characteristics in pigs receiving intravenous arginine were not significantly improved over the other groups. Arginine is important in both protein synthesis, and blood flow and may help in the prevention of necrotizing enterocolitis.

J. M. Daly, MD

9 Gastrointestinal

Preoperative Enoxaparin Versus Postoperative Semuloparin Thromboprophylaxis in Major Abdominal Surgery: A Randomized Controlled Trial
Kakkar AK, Agnelli G, Fisher W, et al (Thrombosis Res Inst and Univ College London, UK; Univ of Perugia, Italy; McGill Univ Health Centre, Montreal, Quebec, Canada; et al)
Ann Surg 259:1073-1079, 2014

Objective.—To compare efficacy and safety of thromboprophylaxis with semuloparin started postoperatively versus enoxaparin started preoperatively in major abdominal surgery.

Background.—Venous thromboembolism is an important complication following major abdominal surgery. Semuloparin is a novel ultra-low-molecular-weight heparin with high antifactor Xa and minimal antifactor IIa activity.

Methods.—In this double-blind noninferiority trial, adult patients undergoing major abdominal or pelvic operation under general anesthesia lasting more than 45 minutes were assigned to either daily enoxaparin 40 mg commenced preoperatively or daily semuloparin 20 mg commenced postoperatively, for 7 to 10 days. Patients underwent bilateral leg venography between 7 and 11 days postsurgery. The primary efficacy end point was the composite of any deep vein thrombosis, nonfatal pulmonary embolism, or all-cause death. The primary safety outcome was bleeding. Both were independently adjudicated.

Results.—In total, 4413 patients were randomized; 3030 (1499 in the enoxaparin and 1531 in the semuloparin groups) were evaluable for the primary efficacy end point, which occurred in 97 patients (6.3%) in the semuloparin group and 82 patients (5.5%) in the enoxaparin group [odds ratio (OR) = 1.16, 95% confidence interval (CI): 0.84−1.59]. On the basis of a noninferiority margin of 1.25, postoperative semuloparin did not demonstrate noninferiority to preoperative enoxaparin. Major bleeding occurred in 63 of 2175 patients (2.9%) in the semuloparin group and 98 of 2177 patients (4.5%) in the enoxaparin group (OR = 0.63, 95% CI: 0.46−0.87).

Conclusions.—Semuloparin commenced postoperatively did not demonstrate noninferiority to enoxaparin initiated preoperatively for thromboprophylaxis after major abdominal surgery (Fig 2).

▶ Most patients undergoing major abdominal operations should receive some type of deep vein thrombosis (DVT) prophylaxis. This trial is a large randomized

247

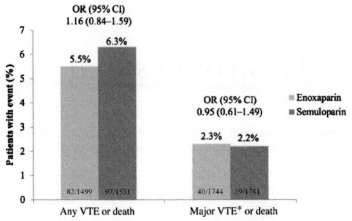

FIGURE 2.—Primary and secondary efficacy parameters by treatment group. *Including any proximal DVT, symptomatic distal DVT, and nonfatal PE. (Reprinted from Kakkar AK, Agnelli G, Fisher W, et al. Preoperative enoxaparin versus postoperative semuloparin thromboprophylaxis in major abdominal surgery: a randomized controlled trial. *Ann Surg.* 2014;259:1073-1079, © 2014, Southeastern Surgical Congress.)

trial comparing 2 low-molecular-weight heparins, enoxaparin (Lovenox) and semuloparin. The enoxaparin treatment was initiated preoperatively and the semuloparin postoperatively and continued for 7 to 10 days. This trial enrolled more than 4400 patients and found that these drugs were equivalent with regard to postoperative DVT as seen by lower-extremity venography or pulmonary embolus (Fig 2). Bleeding events were lower in the semuloparin group but ranged between 2.9% and 4.5%. The ability to make a decision regarding chemical DVT prophylaxis postoperatively has some advantages, allowing the surgeon to make a decision about prophylaxis depending on the findings and difficulty of the operation. Many continue to discuss the efficacy of prophylaxis, but the data consistently suggest that prophylaxis is important, decreases complications and deaths, and is safe with regard to postoperative bleeding. The hospitals in which you operate should be able to provide rates of DVT and pulmonary embolism in the facility and even give you data on your own patients.

J. Hines, MD

Impact of postoperative non-steroidal anti-inflammatory drugs on adverse events after gastrointestinal surgery
STARSurg Collaborative (Univ of Leeds, UK; Univ of Cardiff, UK; Univ of Liverpool, UK; et al)
Br J Surg 101:1413-1423, 2014

Background.—Recent evidence has suggested an association between postoperative non-steroidal anti-inflammatory drugs (NSAIDs) and increased operation-specific complications. This study aimed to determine

NSAID dose	Complication type	Odds ratio	P
Any dose	All	0·72 (0·52, 0·99)	0·041
	Major	0·94 (0·54, 1·73)	0·817
	Minor	0·73 (0·53, 1·04)	0·057
Low dose	All	0·81 (0·53, 1·26)	0·334
	Major	0·61 (0·30, 1·66)	0·230
	Minor	0·95 (0·60, 1·49)	0·817
High dose	All	0·64 (0·42, 0·95)	0·032
	Major	1·27 (0·68, 2·72)	0·447
	Minor	0·57 (0·39, 0·89)	0·009
Any dose	Anastomotic leak	1·30 (0·61, 2·68)	0·481
	Cardiovascular event	0·71 (0·25, 4·13)	0·517
	Surgical-site infection	0·94 (0·58, 1·66)	0·792
	Intra-abdominal abscess	0·49 (0·19, 2·58)	0·200

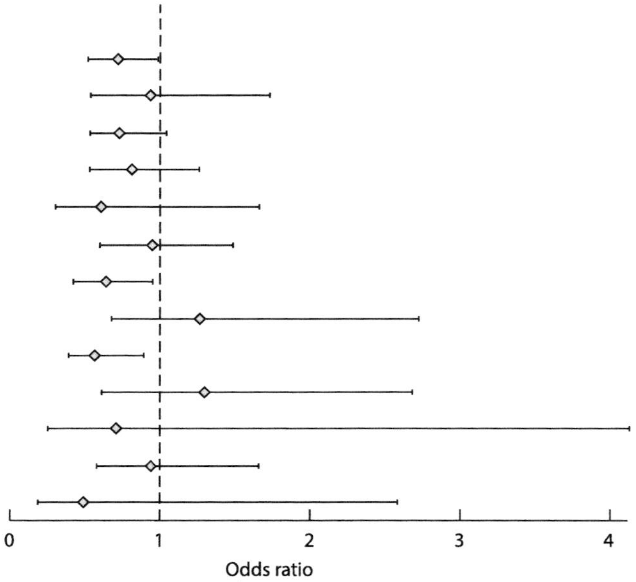

FIGURE 2.—Adjusted outcome measures from risk-adjusted propensity score-matched models for complication type according to non-steroidal anti-inflammatory drug (NSAID) dose. Odds ratios are shown with 95 per cent confidence intervals. (Reprinted from STARSurg Collaborative. Impact of postoperative non-steroidal anti-inflammatory drugs on adverse events after gastrointestinal surgery. *Br J Surg.* 2014;101:1413-1423, © British Journal of Surgery Society Ltd. Reproduced with permission. Permission is granted by John Wiley & Sons Ltd on behalf of the BJSS Ltd.)

the safety profile following gastrointestinal surgery across a multicentre setting in the UK.

Methods.—This multicentre study was carried out during a 2-week interval in September—October 2013. Consecutive adults undergoing elective or emergency gastrointestinal resection were included. The study was powered to detect a 10 per cent increase in major complications (grade III—V according to the Dindo—Clavien classification). The effect of administration of NSAIDs on the day of surgery or the following 2 days was risk-adjusted using propensity score matching and multivariable logistic regression to produce adjusted odds ratios (ORs). The type of NSAID and the dose were registered.

Results.—Across 109 centres, early postoperative NSAIDs were administered to 242 (16·1 per cent) of 1503 patients. Complications occurred in 981 patients (65·3 per cent), which were major in 257 (17·1 per cent) and minor (Dindo—Clavien grade I—II) in 724 (48·2 per cent). Propensity score matching created well balanced groups. Treatment with NSAIDs was associated with a reduction in overall complications (OR 0·72, 95 per cent confidence interval 0·52 to 0·99; $P = 0·041$). This effect predominately comprised a reduction in minor complications with high-dose NSAIDs (OR 0·57, 0·39 to 0·89; $P = 0·009$).

Conclusion.—Early use of NSAIDs is associated with a reduction in postoperative adverse events following major gastrointestinal surgery (Fig 2).

▶ Postoperative pain management after gastrointestinal surgery most commonly includes narcotics, but this can impact intestinal function and in this way slow recovery. The use of nonsteroidal anti-inflammatory drugs (NSAIDs) for postoperative pain control is common by our gynecology colleagues. This study suggests that NSAIDs—namely ibuprofen—is quite helpful and, in fact, decreases morbidity after gastrointestinal surgery (Fig 2). Specifically, the group found in this multicenter site study of more than 1500 patients that anastomotic leaks were no higher in the NSAID-treated group and the improvements in complication rates mostly came when the patients were treated with high-dose ibuprofen. Overall, there was a 28% decrease in overall complications in the patients given NSAIDs. The addition of NSAIDs to your postoperative treatment regimen can be beneficial for your patients and may actually provide benefit over narcotics alone.

J. Hines, MD

Variation in triggers and use of perioperative blood transfusion in major gastrointestinal surgery
Ejaz A, Spolverato G, Kim Y, et al (The Johns Hopkins Univ School of Medicine, Baltimore, MD; et al)
Br J Surg 101:1424-1433, 2014

Background.—The decision to perform intraoperative blood transfusion is subject to a variety of clinical and laboratory factors. This study examined variation in haemoglobin (Hb) triggers and overall utilization of intraoperative blood transfusion, as well as the impact of transfusion on perioperative outcomes.

Methods.—The study included all patients who underwent pancreatic, hepatic or colorectal resection between 2010 and 2013 at Johns Hopkins Hospital, Baltimore, Maryland. Data on Hb levels that triggered an intraoperative or postoperative transfusion and overall perioperative blood utilization were obtained and analysed.

Results.—Intraoperative transfusion was employed in 437 (15.6 per cent) of the 2806 patients identified. Older patients (odds ratio (OR) 1.68), patients with multiple co-morbidities (Charlson co-morbidity score 4 or above; OR 1.66) and those with a lower preoperative Hb level (OR 4.95) were at increased risk of intraoperative blood transfusion (all $P < 0.001$). The Hb level employed to trigger transfusion varied by sex, race and service (all $P < 0.001$). A total of 105 patients (24.0 per cent of patients transfused) had an intraoperative transfusion with a liberal Hb trigger (10 g/dl or more); the majority of these patients (78; 74.3 per cent) did not require any additional postoperative transfusion. Patients who received an intraoperative transfusion were at greater risk of perioperative complications (OR 1.55; $P = 0.002$), although patients transfused with a restrictive Hb trigger (less than 10 g/dl) showed no increased risk of perioperative morbidity compared with those transfused with a liberal Hb trigger (OR 1.22; $P = 0.514$).

Conclusion.—Use of perioperative blood transfusion varies among surgeons and type of operation. Nearly one in four patients received a blood transfusion with a liberal intraoperative transfusion Hb trigger of 10 g/dl or more. Intraoperative blood transfusion was associated with higher risk of perioperative morbidity.

► The use of packed red blood cells in the perioperative period has been the focus of reassessment during the past few years. There is a general consensus that a hemoglobin (Hgb) of 10 g/dL is not necessary, and there may be some advantage in allowing a lower blood count. A blood transfusion triggers a subclinical inflammatory response that can contribute to an increased perioperative complication rate. This article examined blood transfusion trends at the Johns Hopkins Hospital. The study found that gender, race, and surgical service influenced the trigger to transfuse. Patients who received a blood transfusion had a 55% higher risk of complication. It is difficult to attribute the transfusion to the complication, but instead transfusion is likely a surrogate for a more difficult operation and patient with more comorbidities. The authors conclude that a trigger Hgb of 10 g/dL is probably not required and a more liberal approach allowing Hgb of 7 or 8 g/dL is safe.

J. Hines, MD

A Comparative Study on Comprehensive, Objective Outcomes of Laparoscopic Heller Myotomy With Per-Oral Endoscopic Myotomy (POEM) for Achalasia

Bhayani NH, Kurian AA, Dunst CM, et al (Division of Gastrointestinal and Minimally Invasive Surgery, Portland, OR; Oregon Health and Sciences Univ, Portland)

Ann Surg 259:1098-1103, 2014

Objective.—To compare symptomatic and objective outcomes between HM and POEM.

Background.—The surgical gold standard for achalasia is laparoscopic Heller myotomy (HM) and partial fundoplication. Per-oral endoscopic myotomy (POEM) is a less invasive flexible endoscopic alternative. We compare their safety and efficacy.

Methods.—Data on consecutive HMs and POEMs for achalasia from 2007 to 2012 were collected. Primary outcomes: swallowing function—1 and 6 months after surgery. Secondary outcomes: operative time, complications, postoperative gastro-esophageal reflux disease (GERD).

Results.—There were 101 patients: 64 HMs (42% Toupet and 58% Dor fundoplications) and 37 POEMs. Presenting symptoms were comparable. Median operative time (149 vs 120 min, $P < 0.001$) and mean hospitalization (2.2 vs 1.1 days, $P < 0.0001$) were significantly higher for HMs. Postoperative morbidity was comparable. One-month Eckardt scores were significantly better for POEMs (1.8 vs 0.8, $P < 0.0001$). At 6 months, both groups had sustained similar improvements in their Eckardt scores (1.7 vs 1.2, $P = 0.1$).

Both groups had significant improvements in postmyotomy lower esophageal sphincter profiles. Postmyotomy resting pressures were higher for POEMs than for HMs (16 vs 7.1 mm Hg, $P = 0.006$). Postmyotomy relaxation pressures and distal esophageal contraction amplitudes were not significantly different between groups. Routine postoperative 24-hour pH testing was obtained in 48% Hellers and 76% POEMs. Postoperatively, 39% of POEMs and 32% of HM had abnormal acid exposure ($P = 0.7$).

Conclusions.—POEM is an endoscopic therapy for achalasia with a shorter hospitalization than HM. Patient symptoms and esophageal physiology are improved equally with both procedures. Postoperative esophageal acid exposure is the same for both. The POEM is comparable with laparoscopic HM for safe and effective treatment of achalasia (Fig 2).

▶ Per oral endoscopic myotomy (POEM) is evolving into an acceptable approach for achalasia.[1] To date, smaller case and safety series have been reported, but this article from Oregon provides better comparison data to Heller myotomy. The POEM procedure involves cutting the inner circular fibers using a submucosal tunnel and leaving the longitudinal fibers intact. Overall, the POEM approach offers relief from dysphagia similar to that of a Heller myotomy and may result in less gastroesophageal reflux after the procedure. Because

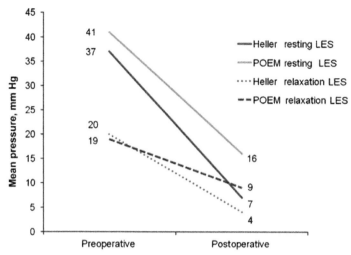

FIGURE 2.—Manometry, before and after myotomy. (Reprinted from Bhayani NH, Kurian AA, Dunst CM, et al. A comparative study on comprehensive, objective outcomes of laparoscopic heller myotomy with Per-Oral Endoscopic Myotomy (POEM) for achalasia. *Ann Surg.* 2014;259:1098-1103, © 2014, Southeastern Surgical Congress.)

the longitudinal fibers are left intact and the hiatus is not disrupted, patients are left with a higher resting lower esophageal sphincter pressure (Fig 2). Despite this, patients report excellent relief of symptoms. The POEM may allow patients to escape the intermittent need for antacid therapy. The surgical community should embrace this new technology soon to keep this advancement as a part of our armamentarium before gastroenterologist in our communities offer this alternative.

J. Hines, MD

Reference

1. Wang L, Li Y-M, Li L. Meta-analysis of randomized and controlled treatment trials for achalasia. *Dig Dis Sci.* 2009;54:2303-2311.

Outcomes of operations for benign foregut disease in elderly patients: A National Surgical Quality Improvement Program database analysis

Molena D, Mungo B, Stem M, et al (Johns Hopkins Univ School of Medicine, Baltimore, MD)
Surgery 156:352-360, 2014

Background.—The development of minimally invasive operative techniques and improvement in postoperative care has made surgery a viable option to a greater number of elderly patients. Our objective was to evaluate the outcomes of laparoscopic and open foregut operation in relation to the patient age.

TABLE 3.—Multivariable Logistic Regression Analysis for 30-day mortality for all Patients

Variable	30-Day Mortality (n = 93), OR, 95% CI	P Value
Age, years		
<65	Reference	
65−69	1.45 (0.62−3.41)	.394
70−74	2.70 (1.34−5.44)	.005*
75−79	2.80 (1.35−5.81)	.006*
≥80	6.12 (3.41−10.99)	<.001*
Admission-procedure		
Elective-lap	Reference	
Elective-open	2.94 (1.80−4.78)	<.001*
Emergent-lap	4.19 (1.38−12.74)	.012*
Emergent-open	6.34 (3.21−12.51)	<.001*
C-statistic	0.85	

The 30-day mortality model was adjusted for age, interaction term of admission and procedure type, and ASA.
ASA, American Society of Anesthesiology; CI, confidence interval; OR, odds ratio; open, laparotomy and thoracotomy.
*Statistically significant.
Reprinted from Surgery. Molena D, Mungo B, Stem M, et al. Outcomes of operations for benign foregut disease in elderly patients: A National Surgical Quality Improvement Program database analysis. *Surgery.* 2014;156:352-360, Copyright 2014, with permission from Elsevier.

Methods.—Patients who underwent gastric fundoplication, paraesophageal hernia repair, and Heller myotomy were identified via the National Surgical Quality Improvement Program (NSQIP) database (2005−2011). Patient characteristics and outcomes were compared between five age groups (group I: ≤65 years, II: 65−69 years; III: 70−74 years; IV: 75−79 years; and V: ≥80 years). Multivariable logistic regression analysis was used to predict the impact of age and operative approach on the studied outcomes.

Results.—A total of 19,388 patients were identified. Advanced age was associated with increased rate of 30-day mortality, overall morbidity, serious morbidity, and extended length of stay, regardless of the operative approach. After we adjusted for other variables, advanced age was associated with increased odds of 30-day mortality compared with patients <65 years (III: odds ratio 2.70, 95% confidence interval 1.34−5.44, P = .01; IV: 2.80, 1.35−5.81, P = .01; V: 6.12, 3.41−10.99, P < .001).

Conclusion.—Surgery for benign foregut disease in elderly patients carries a burden of mortality and morbidity that needs to be acknowledged (Table 3).

▶ How are we doing with foregut operations in the elderly? This is a comprehensive analysis from National Surgical Quality Improvement Program hospitals examining the outcome of nearly 20 000 elderly patients undergoing fundoplication, paraesophageal hernia repair, or Heller myotomy. These are common procedures in the elderly groups, and this study identified increasing mortality with increasing age with a 6-fold higher mortality rate in patients 80 years and older (Table 3). Overall, the mortality rate was 0.5%, and patients undergoing a laparoscopic procedure had lower morbidity. Despite this, an open operation was more likely to be performed in the elderly with nearly one-third of the patients older than 80 receiving an open operation. Regardless of the approach, the availability of minimally invasive surgery should not influence the indications or recommendation of operation. The surgery should be performed by necessity as indicated by the preoperative evaluation, and for paraesophageal hernias the indications appear to be evolving with few patients requiring intervention.

J. Hines, MD

Does Hospital Accreditation Impact Bariatric Surgery Safety?
Morton JM, Garg T, Nguyen N (Stanford School of Medicine, CA; Univ of California, Irvine)
Ann Surg 260:504-509, 2014

Objective.—To evaluate the impact of hospital accreditation upon bariatric surgery outcomes.

Background.—Since 2004, the American College of Surgeons and the American Society of Metabolic and Bariatric Surgery have accredited bariatric hospitals. Few studies have evaluated the impact of hospital accreditation on all bariatric surgery outcomes.

Methods.—Bariatric surgery hospitalizations were identified using *International Classification of Diseases, Ninth Revision (ICD9)* codes in the 2010 Nationwide Inpatient Sample (NIS). Hospital names and American Hospital Association (AHA) codes were used to identify accredited bariatric centers. Relevant *ICD9* codes were used for identifying demographics, length of stay (LOS), total charges, mortality, complications, and failure to rescue (FTR) events.

Results.—There were 117,478 weighted bariatric patient discharges corresponding to 235 unique hospitals in the 2010 NIS data set. A total of 72,615 (61.8%) weighted discharges, corresponding to 145 (61.7%) named or AHA-identifiable hospitals were included. Among the 145 hospitals, 66 (45.5%) were unaccredited and 79 (54.5%) accredited. Compared with accredited centers, unaccredited centers had a higher mean LOS (2.25 vs 1.99 days, $P < 0.0001$), as well as total charges ($51,189 vs $42,212, $P < 0.0001$). Incidence of any complication was higher at unaccredited centers than at accredited centers (12.3% vs 11.3%, $P = 0.001$), as was mortality (0.13% vs 0.07%, $P = 0.019$) and FTR (0.97% vs 0.55%, $P = 0.046$). Multivariable logistic regression analysis identified unaccredited status as a positive predictor of incidence of complication [odds ratio (OR) = 1.08, $P < 0.0001$], as well as mortality (OR = 2.13, $P = 0.013$).

Conclusions and Relevance.—Hospital accreditation status is associated with safer outcomes, shorter LOS, and lower total charges after bariatric surgery (Table 5).

▶ Is your hospital an accredited center of excellence for bariatric surgery? The American College of Surgeons and the American Society of Metabolic and Bariatric Surgery initiated an accreditation process in 2004 whereby hospitals are

TABLE 5.—Summary of Postoperative Complications by Accreditation Status, 2010

	Unaccredited	Accredited	P
Blood transfusion	2.04	1.07	<0.0001
Abscess	0.51	0.21	<0.0001
Pulmonary embolism	0.08	0.04	0.087
Pneumonia	0.16	0.29	0.010
Other pulmonary	1.41	1.15	0.015
Wound	0.55	0.25	<0.0001
Spleen	0.29	0.06	<0.0001
Deep venous thrombosis	1.43	2.12	<0.0001
Genitourinary	1.11	1.08	0.755
Cardiac arrhythmia	2.91	3.79	<0.0001
Myocardial infarction	0.04	0.07	0.307
Stroke	0.00	0.02	0.146
GI leak	1.85	1.47	0.002
Reoperation	0.40	0.29	0.043
Other	6.47	4.73	<0.0001

"Other" includes complications of surgical and medical care, not elsewhere classified.
Reprinted from Morton JM, Garg T, Nguyen N. Does Hospital Accreditation Impact Bariatric Surgery Safety? *Ann Surg.* 2014;260:504-509. © 2014, Southeastern Surgical Congress.

designated as centers of excellence if they perform a high volume of bariatric surgery, defined as more than 125 cases per year, and are equipped with appropriate equipment, experienced surgeons, and a multidisciplinary team to care for patients.[1] Does it matter? It certainly seems so from this report that was presented at the annual American Surgical Association this year. Length of stay, complication rate (Table 5), cost, and mortality were higher at unaccredited hospitals. The death rate was actually almost twice that of accredited centers. Unaccredited status was the single-most important factor in patient outcomes. And surgical volume was not what made the difference—the surgical volume at both was equal. The process of accreditation and commitment to the requirements creates a culture of safety and can be a surrogate for local resources that can result in the rescue of patients who fail in the immediate postoperative period.

J. Hines, MD

Reference

1. American College of Surgeons. ACS BSCN accreditation program manual. 2013. http://www.mbsaqip.org. Accessed March 3, 2015.

Evaluation of progression prior to surgery after neoadjuvant chemoradiotherapy with computed tomography in esophageal cancer patients

Hulshoff JB, Smit JK, van der Jagt EJ, et al (Univ Med Ctr Groningen, The Netherlands)
Am J Surg 208:73-79, 2014

Background.—The risk of tumor progression during neoadjuvant chemoradiotherapy (CRT) in esophageal cancer (EC) is around 8% to

17%. We assessed the efficacy of computed tomography (CT) to identify these patients before esophagectomy.

Methods.—Ninety-seven patients with locally advanced EC treated with Carboplatin/Paclitaxel and 41.4 Gy neoadjuvantly were restaged with CT. Two radiologists reviewed pre- and post-CRT CT images. The primary outcome was detection of clinically relevant progressive disease. Missed metastases were defined as metastatic disease found during surgery or within 3 months after post-CRT CT.

Results.—Progressive disease was detected in 9 patients (9%). Both radiologists detected 5 patients with distant metastases (liver, $n = 4$; lung metastasis, $n = 1$), but missed progressive disease in 4 cases. One radiologist falsely assessed 2 metastatic lesions, but after agreement progressive disease was detected with sensitivity and specificity of 56% and 100%, respectively.

Conclusion.—CT is effective in detecting clinically relevant progressive disease in EC patients, after neoadjuvant treatment.

▶ Neoadjuvant therapy for esophageal cancer has become standard treatment for patients with locally advanced disease.[1] The evaluation of these patients should include an upper endoscopy, endoscopic ultrasound, and positron emission tomography/CT to establish the absence of distant disease. After a period of chemotherapy, patients will need to be restaged to judge the response to treatment and be certain that the cancer has not progressed before operation. The appropriate means for restaging has not been certain and can include repeating the entire preoperative staging protocol. This group evaluated the efficacy of 2-mm-slice CT to make this assessment and found that this is a reliable method to avoid futile surgery. Repeating endoscopic ultrasound is probably not necessary as long as the CT imaging is performed using up-to-date equipment. These particular nuances regarding the management of patients with esophageal cancer require multidisciplinary expertise working together to stratify the patient into the appropriate treatment plan.

J. Hines, MD

Reference

1. van Hagen P, Hulshof MC, van Lanschot JJ, et al. Preoperative chemoradiotherapy for esophageal or junctional cancer. *N Engl J Med.* 2012;366:2074-2084.

A Decade Analysis of Trends and Outcomes of Bariatric Surgery in Medicare Beneficiaries

Young MT, Jafari MD, Gebhart A, et al (Univ of California, Irvine)
J Am Coll Surg 219:480-488, 2014

Background.—In 2006, the Centers for Medicare and Medicaid Services issued a National Coverage Determination (NCD), which mandates that bariatric procedures be performed only at accredited centers. The aim of this study was to analyze outcomes of Medicare beneficiaries who underwent bariatric surgery before (2001 through 2005) vs after (2006 through 2010) implementation of the NCD.

Study Design.—The Nationwide Inpatient Sample database was used to analyze data on patients who underwent bariatric surgery between 2001 and 2010. Main outcomes measures were demographics, length of stay, risk-adjusted inpatient morbidity and mortality, and cost.

Results.—There were 775,040 patients who underwent bariatric surgery, with 16% of the patients Medicare beneficiaries. There was an overall trend for improved in-hospital mortality during the decade (0.35% in 2001 to 0.10% in 2010). Medicare patients who underwent bariatric surgery had higher rates of comorbidities and a higher rate of in-hospital mortality than non-Medicare patients. After the NCD, there was a significant reduction of the in-hospital mortality (0.56% vs 0.23%; $p < 0.01$) and serious morbidity (9.92% vs 6.98%; $p < 0.01$) for Medicare patients and a similar reduction of the in-hospital mortality (0.18% vs 0.08%; $p < 0.01$) and serious morbidity (6.84% vs 5.08%; $p < 0.01$) for non-Medicare patients. Compared with patients who underwent stapling bariatric procedures at accredited centers, patients at nonaccredited centers had higher risk-adjusted in-hospital mortality (odds ratio = 3.53; 95% CI, 1.01−6.52) and serious morbidity (odds ratio = 1.18; 95% CI, 1.07−1.30). After the NCD, use of bariatric surgery within Medicare beneficiaries increased by 71%.

Conclusions.—Outcomes of bariatric surgery in Medicare beneficiaries have improved substantially since the 2006 NCD. Facility accreditation appears to be a contributing factor to the observed improvement in outcomes.

▶ In 2006, the Centers for Medicare and Medicaid Services began limiting coverage to bariatric programs that were certified by the American College of Surgeons or the American Society for Metabolic and Bariatric Surgery. This change was controversial, and some believe it arbitrarily limited access without particular improvements in outcome for patients seeking these procedures. Early studies looking at the impact of this change suggested that these concerns may be valid. This study, however, refutes these concerns. Using the Nationwide Inpatient Sample database, some three-quarter million patients were analyzed. The authors found that patients receiving care at the certified center had significantly reduced morbidity and mortality. The risk-adjusted mortality was 3.5 times higher at nonaccredited centers. In addition, there appeared to be no impact on access to care between ethnic groups. Although significant resources, coordination, and effort are required for focused certified centers, the process leads to a culture of safety and improved outcomes. This updated analysis clearly demonstrates the value of the ACS Metabolic and Bariatric Surgery Accreditation and Quality Improvement Program.

J. Hines, MD

Randomized Pilot Trial of Bariatric Surgery Versus Intensive Medical Weight Management on Diabetes Remission in Type 2 Diabetic Patients Who Do NOT Meet NIH Criteria for Surgery and the Role of Soluble RAGE as a Novel Biomarker of Success
Parikh M, Chung M, Sheth S, et al (NYU School of Medicine/Bellevue Hosp; et al)
Ann Surg 260:617-624, 2014

Objective.—To compare bariatric surgery versus intensive medical weight management (MWM) in patients with type 2 diabetes mellitus (T2DM) who do not meet current National Institutes of Health criteria for bariatric surgery and to assess whether the soluble form of receptor for advanced glycation end products (sRAGE) is a biomarker to identify patients most likely to benefit from surgery.

Background.—There are few studies comparing surgery to MWM for patients with T2DM and BMI less than 35.

Methods.—Fifty-seven patients with T2DM and BMI 30 to 35, who otherwise met the criteria for bariatric surgery were randomized to MWM versus surgery (bypass, sleeve or band, based on patient preference). The primary outcomes assessed at 6 months were change in homeostatic model of insulin resistance (HOMA-IR) and diabetes remission. Secondary outcomes included changes in HbA1c, weight, and sRAGE.

Results.—The surgery group had improved HOMA-IR (-4.6 vs $+1.6$; $P = 0.0004$) and higher diabetes remission (65% vs 0%, $P < 0.0001$) than the MWM group at 6 months. Compared to MWM, the surgery group had lower HbA1c (6.2 vs 7.8, $P = 0.002$), lower fasting glucose (99.5 vs 157; $P = 0.0068$), and fewer T2DM medication requirements (20% vs 88%; $P < 0.0001$) at 6 months. The surgery group lost more weight (7.0 vs 1.0 BMI decrease, $P < 0.0001$). Higher baseline sRAGE was associated with better weight loss outcomes ($r = -0.641$; $P = 0.046$). There were no mortalities.

Conclusions.—Surgery was very effective short-term in patients with T2DM and BMI 30 to 35. Baseline sRAGE may predict patients most likely to benefit from surgery. These findings need to be confirmed with larger studies. ClinicalTrials.gov ID: NCT01423877 (Table 2).

▶ Can bariatric surgery help patients with body mass index (BMI) less than 35? Currently, patients with a BMI of 35 or greater are candidates for weight loss surgery, but many patients with lower BMIs harbor manifestations of metabolic syndrome including diabetes mellitus. This study randomly assigned patients to a medical weight management program or surgery. There was a mixture of surgical procedures that included bypass, sleeve, and band. The surgery group had a higher diabetes remission rate (65% vs 0%), lower hemoglobin A1c, and fewer diabetes medication requirements (Table 2). The patients who underwent a sleeve gastrectomy had the highest rate of diabetes remission, and overall there was a very low complication rate in the surgery group. This type of data is very important to expand the indications for bariatric surgery, which would likely

TABLE 2.—Primary Outcome Measures for MWM Versus Bariatric Surgery at 6 Months

	MWM (N = 24)	Surgery (N = 20)	P
HOMA-IR			
Pre	3.1 (2.6)	6.5 (3.9)	0.0032
Post	4.7 (4.9)	1.8 (1.2)	0.013
Change	+1.6 (4.9)	−4.6 (4.1)	0.0004
Diabetes remission			
Yes	0% (n = 0)	65% (n = 13)	<0.0001
No	100% (n = 24)	35% (n = 7)	
HbA1c			
Pre	7.7 (1.0)	7.4 (1.2)	0.274
Post	7.8 (1.7)	6.2 (0.9)	0.0002
Change	+0.1 (1.5)	−1.2 (1.1)	0.0027
Fasting glucose			
Pre	143.6 (46.9)	149.6 (45.5)	0.675
Post	156.9 (91.3)	99.5 (28.0)	0.0068
Change	+13.3 (77.8)	−50.1 (44.4)	0.0017
Glucose after OGTT			
Post	306.3 (108.1)	130.2 (78.0)	<0.0001
Requiring T2DM meds			
Yes	88% (n = 21)	20% (n = 4)	<0.0001
No	12% (n = 3)	80% (n = 16)	

Continuous data are presented as mean (SD) and were compared using a 2-sample *t* test. Diabetes medication and diabetes remission were compared using the Fisher's exact test.

Reprinted from Parikh M, Chung M, Sheth S, et al. Randomized Pilot Trial of Bariatric Surgery Versus Intensive Medical Weight Management on Diabetes Remission in Type 2 Diabetic Patients Who Do NOT Meet NIH Criteria for Surgery and the Role of Soluble RAGE as a Novel Biomarker of Success. *Ann Surg.* 2014;260:617-624, © 2014, Southeastern Surgical Congress.

come out of the National Institutes of Health. These procedures have again demonstrated durable benefit that impacts life expectancy, health care cost, and patients' lives.

J. Hines, MD

Comparative Effectiveness of Laparoscopic Adjustable Gastric Banding vs Laparoscopic Gastric Bypass

Arterburn D, Powers JD, Toh S, et al (Group Health Res Inst, Seattle, WA; Kaiser Permanente Colorado Inst for Health Res, Denver; Harvard Med School and Harvard Pilgrim Health Care Inst, Boston, MA; et al)
JAMA Surg 149:1279-1287, 2014

Importance.—Laparoscopic Roux-en-Y gastric bypass (RYGB) and laparoscopic adjustable gastric banding (AGB) are 2 of the most commonly performed bariatric procedures worldwide. However, few large, multisite studies have directly compared the benefits and harms of these procedures.

Objective.—To compare the effect of laparoscopic RYGB vs AGB on short- and long-term health outcomes.

Design, Setting, and Participants.—A retrospective cohort study of 7457 individuals 21 years or older who underwent laparoscopic bariatric surgery from January 1, 2005, through December 31, 2009, with follow-up through December 31, 2010. All individuals were participants in the Scalable Partnering Network, a network of 10 demographically and geographically distributed health care systems in the United States.

Main Outcomes and Measures.—The primary outcomes were (1) change in body mass index (BMI), (2) a composite end point of 30-day rate of major adverse outcomes (death, venous thromboembolism, subsequent intervention, and failure to discharge from the hospital), (3) subsequent hospitalization, and (4) subsequent intervention.

Results.—We identified 7457 patients who underwent laparoscopic AGB or RYGB procedures with a median follow-up time of 2.3 years (maximum, 6 years). The mean maximum BMI (calculated as weight in kilograms divided by height in meters squared) loss was 8.0 (95% CI, 7.8-8.3) for AGB patients and 14.8 (95% CI, 14.6-14.9) for RYGB patients ($P < .001$). In propensity score—adjusted models, the hazard ratio for AGB vs RYGB patients experiencing any 30-day major adverse event was 0.46 (95% CI, 0.27-0.80; $P = .006$). The hazard ratios comparing AGB vs RYGB patients experiencing subsequent intervention and hospitalization were 3.31 (95% CI, 2.65-4.14; $P < .001$) and 0.73 (95% CI, 0.61-0.88; $P < .001$), respectively.

Conclusions and Relevance.—In this large bariatric cohort from 10 health care systems, we found that RYGB resulted in much greater weight loss than AGB but had a higher risk of short-term complications and long-term subsequent hospitalizations. On the other hand, RYGB patients had a lower risk of long-term subsequent intervention procedures than AGB patients. Bariatric surgery candidates should be well informed of these benefits and risks when they make their decisions about treatment.

▶ Formulating a weight loss procedure plan for each patient requires consideration of the goals, risks, and desired endpoints. Each of the bariatric options provides advantages and disadvantages for the patient. This large multisite evaluation of gastric band and Roux-en-Y gastric bypass compares more than 7400 patients between 2005 and 2010. In the entire cohort, only 1 patient died as a result of a Roux-en-Y procedure. As expected, the Roux-en-Y group had a greater weight loss with an average maximum body mass index decrease of 14.8. The band patients had fewer early complications, however, but greater need for long-term interventions like adjustments for band malfunction, slippage, or erosion. As expected, many patients regained weight over time in both groups (Fig 4 in the original article). The report does not provide any information regarding the impact of surgery on metabolic syndrome conditions. Most would agree, however, that the Roux-en-Y gastric bypass offers greater remission rates of diabetes, hypertension, and dyslipidemias.

J. Hinoc, MD

Risk Factors for 30-Day Readmissions and Modifying Postoperative Care After Gastric Bypass Surgery

Tayne S, Merrill CA, Shah SN, et al (Tufts Univ School of Medicine, Boston, MA)

J Am Coll Surg 219:489-495, 2014

Background.—Although hospital 30-day readmissions policies currently focus on medical conditions, readmission penalties will be expanding to encompass surgical procedures, logically beginning with common and standardized procedures, such as gastric bypass. Therefore, understanding predictors of readmission is essential in lowering readmission rate for these procedures.

Study Design.—This is a retrospective case-control study of patients undergoing laparoscopic gastric bypass at Tufts Medical Center from 2007 to 2012. Variables analyzed included demographics, comorbidities, intraoperative events, postoperative complications, discharge disposition, and readmission diagnoses. Univariate analysis was used to identify factors associated with readmission, which were then subjected to multivariable logistic regression analysis.

Results.—We reviewed 358 patients undergoing laparoscopic gastric bypass, 119 readmits, and 239 controls. By univariate analysis, public insurance, body mass index >60 kg/m^2, duration of procedure, high American Society of Anesthesiologists (ASA) class, and discharge with visiting nurse services (VNA) were significantly associated with 30-day readmissions. In the regression model, duration of procedure, high ASA class, and discharge with visiting nurse services (VNA) remained significantly associated with readmission when controlling for other factors (odds ratio [OR] 1.523, 95% CI 1.314 to 1.766; OR 2.447, 95% CI 1.305 to 4.487; and OR 0.053 with 95% CI 0.011 to 0.266, respectively). The majority of readmissions occurred within the first week after discharge. Gastrointestinal-related issues were the most common diagnoses on readmission, and included anastomotic leaks, postoperative ileus, and bowel obstruction. The next 2 most common reasons for readmission were wound infection and fluid depletion.

Conclusions.—Using readmission risk, we can stratify patients into tiered clinical pathways. Because most readmissions occur within the first postdischarge week and are most commonly associated with dehydration, pain, or wound issues, focusing our postoperative protocols and patient education should further lower the incidence of readmission.

▶ Hospital readmission rates are now publically posted by the Centers for Medicare and Medicaid Services, and it is now penalizing for readmissions with heart failure, myocardial infarction, and pneumonia. This approach is not only fashioned to decrease health care expense but more importantly to improve patient care. Readmissions after gastric bypass are less common than other surgical procedures but nonetheless represent an opportunity for improvement. The group from Tufts has examined their rates of readmissions and report ways to improve on this issue. They found that high American Society of Anesthesiologists class and the need for home nursing care predicted which patients would be readmitted. They also found that for every 20-minute increase in duration of the operation the odds readmission increased by 50%. By categorizing patients, the authors suggest that specific accommodation, including quicker return to the clinic for postoperative evaluation and intervention, which includes intravenous hydration, be made for high-risk readmission patients.

J. Hines, MD

Laparoscopic versus open gastrectomy for gastric cancer: Long-term oncologic results
Lee J-H, Lee CM, Son S-Y, et al (Seoul Natl Univ Bundang Hosp, Gyeonggi-do, South Korea; et al)
Surgery 155:154-164, 2014

Background.—Data are lacking regarding the oncologic safety of laparoscopic gastrectomy (LG) for the treatment of gastric cancer. The aim of this study was to compare the long-term outcomes of LG with open gastrectomy (OG) for the treatment of gastric cancer.

Methods.—A total of 1,874 patients underwent curative distal or total gastrectomy for gastric adenocarcinoma between May 2003 and December 2009 and were included in this retrospective study. Recurrence-free survival and recurrence pattern were compared according to each tumor stage, and a subgroup analysis was performed in advanced gastric cancer patients who underwent D2 lymphadenectomy.

Results.—Of 1,874 patients, 816 were treated with OG and 1,058 with LG. No differences were observed in recurrence-free survival rates between the LG and the OG groups for any tumor stage. The number of harvested lymph nodes was similar between the two groups when analyzed according to tumor progression, operative procedure, and extent of lymphadenectomy. There were no differences between the 2 groups when we compared recurrence patterns after stratifying for tumor stage. The subgroup analysis in advanced gastric cancer patients who underwent D2 lymphadenectomy showed that there was no difference in the recurrence-free survival rates for any tumor stage between the 2 groups. Multivariate analysis indicated that the type of operative approach did not influence recurrence in either early or advanced gastric cancer patients.

Conclusion.—LG for gastric cancer is an oncologically safe procedure with comparable long-term outcomes with OG (Fig 1).

▶ For some time now, several reports have highlighted the safety of performing gastric resections for cancer laparoscopically. To date, however, the long-term oncologic outcomes have been unknown. Given the lack of data and the technical challenge, most gastrectomies are still performed with a open approach. This report from South Korea is a long-term retrospective analysis of more than 1800 patients who underwent an open or laparoscopic resection that included,

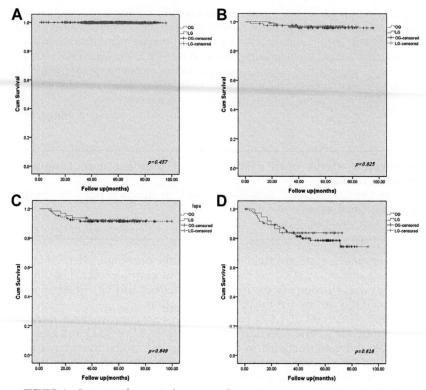

FIGURE 1.—Recurrence-free survival rates according to tumor stages. (*A*) Stage IA: the 5-year recurrence-free survival rate was 99.7% for the laparoscopy group, and 100% for the OG group. (*B*) Stage IB: 96.7% vs 95.9%. (*C*) Stage IIA: 92.2% vs 91.4%. (*D*) Stage IIB: 83.8% vs 78.6%. (*E*) Stage IIIA: 80.2% vs 73.7%. (*F*) Stage IIIB: 35.5% vs 49.0%. (*G*) Stage IIIC: 42.9% vs 37.6%. (Reprinted from Lee J-H, Lee C-M, Son S-Y, et al. Laparoscopic versus open gastrectomy for gastric cancer: long-term oncologic results. *Surgery*. 2014;155:154-164, Copyright 2014, with permission from Elsevier.)

in many cases, a more extensive D2 lymphadenectomy (Fig 1). The nodal harvests in the series were impressive and were always more than 30 nodes. There were no differences in the 5-year recurrence-free survival rates, according to tumor stage between the laparoscopic and open group (stage IB, 100% vs 95.6%, *P* = .276; stage IIA, 93.3% vs 91.9%, *P* = .832; stage IIB, 95.0% vs 80.3%, *P* = .145; stage IIIA, 78.4% vs 73.7%, *P* = .582; stage IIIB, 34.7% vs 49.0%, *P* = .629; stage IIIC, 42.1% vs 37.9%, *P* = .989). This is solid evidence that from an oncologic perspective, a laparoscopic resection for gastric cancer is at least as good as that of an open operation. Of course, with all advanced laparoscopic surgery, the surgeon needs to be adept with advanced techniques to duplicate results like these.

J. Hines, MD

Pure Single-Port Laparoscopic Distal Gastrectomy for Early Gastric Cancer: Comparative Study with Multi-Port Laparoscopic Distal Gastrectomy

Ahn S-H, Son S-Y, Jung do H, et al (Seoul Natl Univ College of Medicine, Seongnam, Korea; Seoul National Univ Bundang Hosp, Seongnam, Korea)
J Am Coll Surg 219:933-943, 2014

Background.—The purpose of this study was to show the feasibility and safety of pure single-port laparoscopic distal gastrectomy (SDG) by comparing its short-term outcomes with those of conventional multiport totally laparoscopic distal gastrectomy (TLDG).

Study Design.—Prospectively collected data of 50 gastric cancer patients who underwent pure SDG from November 2011 through October 2013 were compared with the matched data of 50 TLDG patients.

Results.—Mean operation time (144.5 vs 140.3 minutes; $p = 0.561$) and number of harvested lymph nodes (51.7 ± 16.3 vs 52.4 ± 17.9; $p = 0.836$) were comparable. Estimated blood loss was lower in the SDG patients (50.5 ± 31.5 mL vs 87.5 ± 79.6 mL; $p = 0.007$). Postoperative recovery was faster in the SDG patients in terms of lower maximum pain score on the operative day (6.1 ± 1.4 vs 6.9 ± 1.5; $p = 0.015$) and postoperative day 1 (4.6 ± 1.0 vs 5.5 ± 1.4; $p < 0.001$), less use of parenteral analgesics (0.8 ± 1.0 vs 1.4 ± 1.0; $p = 0.020$), and less increase in C-reactive protein level on postoperative day 5 (4.57 ± 6.26 mg/L vs 8.51 ± 5.25 mg/L; $p = 0.008$). Postoperative morbidity occurred in 6 (12%) and 5 (10%) patients in the SDG and TLDG group, respectively.

Conclusions.—This study showed that pure SDG is both safe and feasible for early gastric cancer, with similar operation time and better short-term outcomes than TLDG in terms of postoperative pain, estimated blood loss, inflammatory reaction, and cosmetic result.

▶ Laparoscopic resection for gastric cancer is now generally accepted, even though the data are not as robust as what is available for colorectal cancer. These procedures clearly require a level of laparoscopic skill that is quite advanced. This group is pushing the envelope even a bit further with the use of a single-port apparatus made by Nelis. One hundred patients with early-stage cancer underwent either standard laparoscopic resection or single-port resection. The outcomes where similar with regard to operative time and numbers of lymph nodes resected. What was different is that the patients who underwent a single-port approach had a bit shorter hospital stay and less need for pain medication. Single-port surgery can be hindered by standard laparoscopic instrumentation, but this group used a flexible camera that helped to improve the camera view and prevent instruments from clashing. No data are included to know whether the oncologic outcomes were similar, but given that these were early-stage tumors and that the nodal harvests where generally more than 50 lymph nodes, it is likely these are good.

J. Hines, MD

Chronic Intestinal Failure After Crohn Disease: When to Perform Transplantation

Gerlach UA, Vrakas G, Reddy S, et al (Charité-Universitätsmedizin Berlin, Germany; Churchill Hosp, Oxford, UK)
JAMA Surg 149:1060-1066, 2014

Importance.—Because of the severity of disease and additional surgery, Crohn disease (CD) may result in intestinal failure (IF) and dependency on home parenteral nutrition (HPN). Defining the indication and timing for intestinal transplantation (ITx) is challenging.

Objectives.—To determine the limitations of conventional surgery and to facilitate the decision making for transplantation.

Design, Setting, and Participants.—Data were collected prospectively and obtained by retrospective review of medical records from all patients with CD who were assessed for ITx in Oxford, United Kingdom, and Berlin, Germany, from October 10, 2003, through July 31, 2013. Patients were considered suitable for ITx if a diagnosis of irreversible IF was established and life-threatening complications under HPN were unresolvable. Twenty patients with CD and IF, established on HPN, were evaluated for ITx. The mean (SD) age at CD onset was 17.8 (9.8) years. On first diagnosis, most patients had a stricturing CD. By the time of referral, most had a combination of stricturing and fistulizing disease.

Interventions.—New scoring system: a modification of the American Gastroenterology Association guidelines for ITx. Modifications are related to CD-specific issues that potentially lead to a poorer outcome and are based on the findings of the study to determine the expected benefit from ITx.

Main Outcomes and Measures.—A scoring system that would alert the physician to the severity of the patient's CD and trigger early referral for ITx. This system may translate into better long-term outcomes for patients with CD. In addition, the Karnofsky performance status score was used to compare pretransplantation and posttransplantation outcomes.

Results.—Ten patients underwent ITx, 4 were on the waiting list, and 4 were unavailable for follow-up. One patient was taken off the waiting list because of severe deterioration. One patient underwent conventional stricturoplasty and did not need transplantation. Among the transplant recipients, 17 (85%) had a stoma or enterocutaneous fistula, and the mean (SD) residual bowel length was 71.5 (38) cm. A total of 80% of transplant recipients had life-threatening catheter infections, and 13 (65%) had a significant decrease in the estimated glomerular filtration rate. At a mean (SD) follow-up of 27.6 (36.1) months for transplant recipients, the patient and graft survival is 80%, and their Karnofsky performance status score increased by a mean of 18.6%.

Conclusions and Relevance.—Intestinal transplantation is a suitable treatment option for patients with CD and IF. It should be considered before any additional attempts at conventional surgery, which may cause eligible patients to miss this opportunity through perioperative complications. The suggested scoring system enables the physician to identify patients who may benefit from transplantation before HPN-associated secondary organ failure.

▶ Crohn disease can be an extraordinarily challenging condition, especially because many patients require surgery despite the advent of new agents with targeted anti-inflammatory properties. If the disease remains active, repeated surgery can result in the development of fistulae and short gut syndrome. The management strategy becomes more complex when patients require intravenous parenteral nutrition and the complications that come with it. Some have advocated intestinal transplantation for these very advanced cases. The American Gastroenterological Association has developed criteria for referral/consideration for transplantation, and using these criteria, a scoring system can be used to categorize patients (Table 1 in the original article). Generally, patients who should be considered for intestinal transplant are those with impending liver failure or dysfunction, a paucity of catheter access, and multiple life-threatening catheter infections. This small series of patients with Crohn disease that underwent transplantation showed an 80% graft survival rate at 3 years. Although it may not be common that we would refer patients with Crohn disease for transplant, it is important to know that it can be a consideration, and knowing the criteria for intestinal transplantation may be important for other patients with intestinal failure for whom we manage. Reaching out to a center that specializes in intestinal transplant can be life saving for this group of patients.

J. Hines, MD

A global consensus on the classification, diagnosis and multidisciplinary treatment of perianal fistulising Crohn's disease

Gecse KB, for the World Gastroenterology Organization, International Organisation for Inflammatory Bowel Diseases IOIBD, European Society of Coloproctology and Robarts Clinical Trials (Academic Med Ctr, Univ of Amsterdam, The Netherlands; et al)
Gut 63:1381-1392, 2014

Objective.—To develop a consensus on the classification, diagnosis and multidisciplinary treatment of perianal fistulising Crohn's disease (pCD), based on best available evidence.

Methods.—Based on a systematic literature review, statements were formed, discussed and approved in multiple rounds by the 20 working group participants. Consensus was defined as at least 80% agreement among voters. Evidence was assessed using the modified GRADE (Grading of Recommendations Assessment, Development, and Evaluation) criteria.

Results.—Highest diagnostic accuracy can only be established if a combination of modalities is used. Drainage of sepsis is always first line therapy before initiating immunosuppressive treatment. Mucosal healing is the goal in the presence of proctitis. Whereas antibiotics and thiopurines

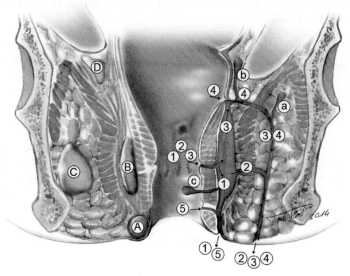

FIGURE 1.—Disease characteristics relevant for fistula management. A fistula is a tract of pus and/or granulation tissue between two epithelial surfaces lined with a fibrous wall.[10] Primary tracts are connections between the internal and external openings (1 5), while secondary tracts are blind extensions (a–c). A tract is defined 'low' when it runs through the lower one third of the external anal sphincter.[6] The *course of the fistula tracts* is described by the Parks classification. The external sphincter complex, defined by the external sphincter and the puborectal muscle, serves as reference: (1) intersphincteric: the tract penetrates the internal sphincter and runs through the intersphincteric space to the perianal skin; (2) transsphincteric: the tract penetrates both the internal and the external sphincter or the puborectal muscle; (3) suprasphincteric: tract runs first upwards in the intersphincteric space, then downwards crossing the levator ani muscle and then reaching the perianal skin; (4) extrasphincteric: tract originates from the rectal wall and runs down through the levator ani muscle, without penetrating the external sphincter or the puborectal muscle.[6] Later a fifth category was added for superficial tracts (5) that did not involve the sphincter complex. *Secondary tracts* and their relationship to the levator plate (a) infralevator or (b) supralevator and (c) horizontal extension, also known as 'horseshoes', are distinguished. Furthermore *proctitis* and the presence of *abscesses* with regard to their localisation (A, perianal; B, intersphincteric; C, ischiorectal; D, suprasphincteric) are also noted. *Editor's Note*: Please refer to original journal article for full references. (Reprinted from Gecse KB, for the World Gastroenterology Organization, International Organisation for Inflammatory Bowel Diseases IOIBD, European Society of Coloproctology and Robarts Clinical Trials. A global consensus on the classification, diagnosis and multidisciplinary treatment of perianal fistulising Crohn's disease. *Gut*. 2014;63:1381-1392, with permission from the BMJ Publishing Group Ltd.)

have a role as adjunctive treatments in pCD, anti-tumour necrosis factor (anti-TNF) is the current gold standard. The efficacy of infliximab is best documented although adalimumab and certolizumab pegol are moderately effective. Oral tacrolimus could be used in patients failing anti-TNF therapy. Definite surgical repair is only of consideration in the absence of luminal inflammation.

Conclusions.—Based on a multidisciplinary approach, items relevant for fistula management were identified and algorithms on diagnosis and treatment of pCD were developed (Figs 1-3 and 5).

▶ The management of anal fistula can be complex, especially in the setting of Crohn disease. Patients who present with multiple or recurrent anal fistula should

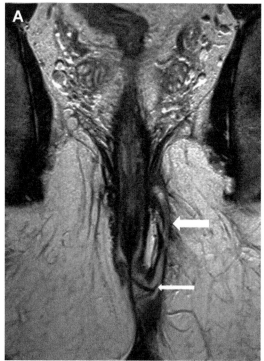

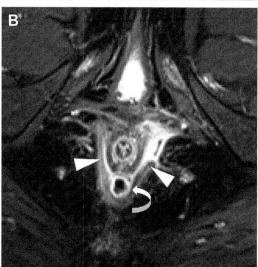

FIGURE 2.—Representative MR image of a male patient with perianal fistulising Crohn's disease. (A) Coronal oblique T2 weighted turbo spin-echo sequence and (B) axial oblique fat saturated T1 weighted turbo spin-echo sequence demonstrate a transsphincteric fistula (arrow) with a seton in place (thin arrow), an intersphincteric abscess (curved arrow) with bilateral granulation tissue filled extensions (arrowheads) in the puborectal muscle. (Reprinted from Gecse KB, for the World Gastroenterology Organization, International Organisation for Inflammatory Bowel Diseases IOIBD, European Society of Coloproctology and Robarts Clinical Trials. A global consensus on the classification, diagnosis and multidisciplinary treatment of perianal fistulising Crohn's disease. *Gut*. 2014;63:1381-1392, with permission from the BMJ Publishing Group Ltd.)

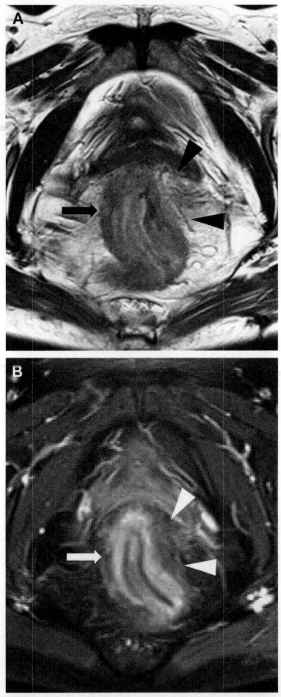

FIGURE 3.—Representative MR image of a female patient with perianal fistulising Crohn's disease and proctitis. (A) Axial oblique T2 weighted turbo spin-echo sequence and (B) axial oblique fat saturated T1 weighted turbo spin-echo sequence show a thickened rectal wall (arrow), with increased enhancement and surrounding infiltrate (arrowheads). (Reprinted from Gecse KB, for the World Gastroenterology Organization, International Organisation for Inflammatory Bowel Diseases IOIBD, European Society of Coloproctology and Robarts Clinical Trials. A global consensus on the classification, diagnosis and multidisciplinary treatment of perianal fistulising Crohn's disease. *Gut.* 2014;63:1381-1392, with permission from the BMJ Publishing Group Ltd.)

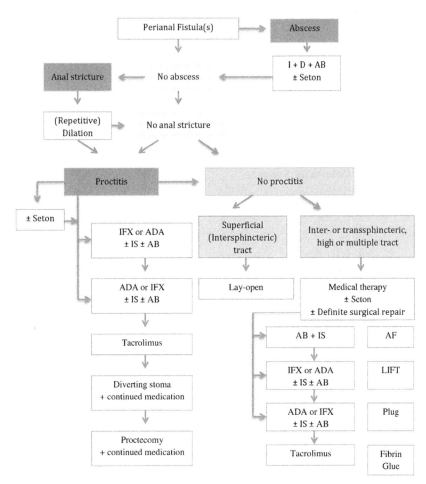

FIGURE 5.—Treatment algorithm for perianal fistulising Crohn's disease. AB, antibiotics; ADA, adalimumab; AF, advancement flap; D, drainage; I, incision; IFX, infliximab; IS, immunosuppressants; LIFT, ligation of the intersphincteric fistula tract. (Reprinted from Gecse KB, for the World Gastroenterology Organization, International Organisation for Inflammatory Bowel Diseases IOIBD, European Society of Coloproctology and Robarts Clinical Trials. A global consensus on the classification, diagnosis and multidisciplinary treatment of perianal fistulising Crohn's disease. *Gut.* 2014;63:1381-1392, with permission from the BMJ Publishing Group Ltd.)

be considered for an evaluation for Crohn disease. The approach for these patients is not always clear, and the data from the literature is uncertain. With these limitations, this group developed a series of consensus statements based on literature and expert opinion. The take-home points are that abscesses should be drained and treated with antibiotics, proctitis must be identified and treated if present, magnetic resonance imaging is the best imaging modality to document complex disease, definitive surgical therapy can include many approaches but should never use a cutting Seton, and medical management of the Crohn disease should include anti-tumor necrosis factor drugs. When deciding how to address anal fistulae surgically, it is critically important to understand the anatomy of the tract and its relationship to the surrounding musculature (Fig 1). To define the extent of disease, both physical exam and imaging can be important (Fig 2). Multiple modalities and surgical approaches may be required to heal this often recalcitrant condition (Fig 5).

J. Hines, MD

The HARM Score: A Novel, Easy Measure to Evaluate Quality and Outcomes in Colorectal Surgery

Keller DS, Chien H-L, Hashemi L, et al (Univ Hosps—Case Med Ctr, Cleveland, OH; Healthcare Economics and Outcomes Res, Mansfield, MA; et al)
Ann Surg 259:1119-1125, 2014

Objective.—To develop a measurement tool based on HospitAl stay, Readmission, and Mortality rates (HARM) score, which is easily calculated from routine administrative data. Secondary goals were to validate the HARM score on a national inpatient sample.

Background.—Concerns about patient safety, quality, and health care costs have increased demand for outcome measurement. Performance metrics such as Surgical Care Improvement Project and National Surgical Quality Improvement Program have been described, but they require significant personnel and expenses to maintain.

Methods.—A national inpatient database was reviewed for all colectomy discharges from 2010 to 2011. Cases were stratified into emergent and elective. For each discharge, a 1 to 10 score was calculated on the basis of length of stay, vital status, and 30-day readmissions. The HARM score was correlated to the complication rate to test validity, and bootstrapping was used to test reliability.

Results.—A total of 81,622 colectomy discharges were evaluated: 44% emergent and 56% elective. The mean HARM score was 3.04 (SD = 0.57) for emergent and 2.64 (SD = 0.65) for elective cases. For hospitals with a HARM score of less than 2, 2 to 3, 3 to 4, and 4+, the mean complication rates were 30.3%, 41.9%, 49.3%, and 56.6% (emergent) and 15.2%, 18.2%, 24.0%, and 35.6% (elective), respectively. Pearson correlation coefficients for the mean score and the complication rate were 0.45 ($P < 0.01$) for elective and emergent cases. Bootstrapping correlation demonstrated reliability for emergent and elective cases.

Conclusions.—The HARM score is easy, reliable, and valid for assessing quality in colorectal surgery. It may provide a low-cost solution for comparative quality assessment in surgery focused on true outlier performance rather than process or clinical outcome metrics alone.

▶ Almost certainly you or the facilities in which you operate are engaged in some type of quality improvement. Hundreds of groups are looking at analytics and process improvements to improve patient care, especially in the field of surgery. This group has created a simple measurement for quality in the field of colon and rectal surgery called the HARM (HospitAl stay, Readmission rate, and Mortality rate) score. Using these simple administrative data points, the group was able to reliably categorize facilities regarding complication rates for both elective and emergent colorectal procedures. Facilities with the highest score found complication rates of 70.5% in emergent cases. This type of scoring will be used more often to judge our results and drive change at all levels. The name *HARM* is an unfortunate choice in my opinion, as it assigns blame and shame—something in quality improvement that we should avoid. Nonetheless, if you have not bought into the quality improvement movement yet, you should—you do not want to be left behind.

J. Hines, MD

Early Use of Low Residue Diet Is Superior to Clear Liquid Diet After Elective Colorectal Surgery: A Randomized Controlled Trial

Lau C, Phillips E, Bresee C, et al (Cedars-Sinai Med Ctr, Los Angeles, CA)
Ann Surg 260:641-649, 2014

Objective.—Compare the feasibility and patient tolerance to either a clear fluid (CF) or low residue diet (LRD) started on postoperative day (POD) 1 after elective colorectal surgery.

Background.—Diet advancement after surgery traditionally starts gradually with liquids, on the basis of fears that early solid intake may increase nausea, vomiting, and overall complications. A randomized controlled trial comparing LRD and CF on POD 1 was performed.

Methods.—111 elective colorectal surgery patients were randomized to CF (n = 57) or LRD (n = 54). The primary end point was vomiting on POD 2. Secondary endpoints included nausea score, days to flatus, length of hospital stay (LOS), and postoperative morbidity.

Results.—Patient characteristics, surgical technique, intraoperative characteristics, and postoperative opioid use were similar between study arms. CF versus LRD results were as follows: POD2 vomiting (28% vs 14%; $P = 0.09$), and significant increase in mean nausea score (4.7 vs 3.5; $P = 0.01$), days to flatus (4.8 vs 3.7 days; $P = 0.04$), and LOS (7.0 vs 5.0 days; $P = 0.01$). LOS remained significantly shorter even after adjusting for significant covariates (laparoscopic technique, surgical site, postoperative comorbidity, stoma, and nasogastric tube) with LRD patients having an adjusted 1.4-day decrease in LOS ($P < 0.01$). There was no significant difference in postoperative morbidity between study arms. Multivariate analysis of all secondary endpoints confirmed an overall significant improvement in outcomes for LRD vs CF ($P < 0.01$).

TABLE 3.—Postoperative Gastrointestinal Outcomes

Variable	Study Cohort (n = 104)	CFs (n = 54)	Low Residue (n = 50)	P
Vomiting				
POD1	26 (25)	18 (33)	8 (16)	0.04
POD2	22 (21)	15 (28)	7 (14)	0.09
Nausea (Likert score)				
POD2	4.1 (2.5)	4.7 (2.7)	3.5 (2.0)	0.01
Discharge date	1.3 (1.1)	1.5 (1.2)	1.1 (1.0)	0.07
Pain (Likert score)				
POD2	6.74 (1.42)	6.93 (1.44)	6.54 (1.39)	0.17
Discharge date	2.80 (0.82)	2.98 (0.81)	2.56 (0.73)	0.006
Oral intake (cc/d)				
POD1	543.4 (367.8)	491.1 (306.1)	613.8 (412.7)	0.09
POD2	767.9 (434.9)	739.3 (409.2)	798.9 (463.1)	0.49
Time to passage of flatus (d)	4.2 (2.4)	4.8 (2.6)	3.7 (2.0)	0.04
Time to tolerance of LRD (d)	3.1 (3.3)	4.1 (3.8)	2.0 (2.2)	0.001
Postoperative ileus	21 (20)	14 (26)	7 (14)	0.13
Nasogastric tube required	14 (13)	8 (15)	6 (12)	0.67
TPN required	10 (10)	8 (15)	2 (4)	0.08
Intravenous antiemetic use (d)	4.0 (3.1)	4.8 (3.6)	3.1 (2.1)	0.004

All values in parentheses denote % except nausea score, oral intake, time to passage of flatus, time to tolerance of LRD, and number of days of intravenous antiemetic use (mean ± standard deviation).

Reprinted from Lau C, Phillips E, Bresee C, et al. Early Use of Low Residue Diet Is Superior to Clear Liquid Diet After Elective Colorectal Surgery: A Randomized Controlled Trial. *Ann Surg.* 2014;260:641-649, © 2014, Southeastern Surgical Congress.

Conclusions.—LRD, rather than CF, on POD1 after colorectal surgery is associated with less nausea, faster return of bowel function, and a shorter hospital stay without increasing postoperative morbidity (Table 3).

▶ Worried about early feeding for patients undergoing colorectal surgery? You should not be, as this randomized study found that a low-residue diet commencing on postoperative day 1 resulted in better outcomes than starting a clear liquid diet on day 1. A low-residue diet consisted of refined bread and pastas, white rice, mashed potatoes, and ground fish and eggs. Patients experienced less nausea, half the frequency of vomiting, flatus 1 day earlier, and a 2-day shorter hospital stay (Table 3). There was no difference in the complications between the 2 groups. How could this be? Colonic motility is the main determinant of clinical recovery after these procedures, and fat in the diet is a stimulant of ileal contractility. Edema and inflammation in the postsurgical intestines could potentially affect contractile forces and absorptive capacity, and early feedings have been found to decrease intestinal inflammation and improve nutrient permeability.[1] So maybe it is time to change your practice and place a tray of food in front of your patients the first day after surgery.

J. Hines, MD

Reference

1. Peuhkuri K, Vapaatalo H, Korpela R. Even low-grade inflammation impacts on small intestinal function. *World J Gastroenterol.* 2010;16:1057-1062.

The Preventive Surgical Site Infection Bundle in Colorectal Surgery: An Effective Approach to Surgical Site Infection Reduction and Health Care Cost Savings

Keenan JE, Speicher PJ, Thacker JK, et al (Duke Univ Med Ctr, Durham, NC; et al)
JAMA Surg 149:1045-1052, 2014

Importance.—Surgical site infections (SSIs) in colorectal surgery are associated with increased morbidity and health care costs.

Objective.—To determine the effect of a preventive SSI bundle (hereafter bundle) on SSI rates and costs in colorectal surgery.

Design.—Retrospective study of institutional clinical and cost data. The study period was January 1, 2008, to December 31, 2012, and outcomes were assessed and compared before and after implementation of the bundle on July 1, 2011.

Setting and Participants.—Academic tertiary referral center among 559 patients who underwent major elective colorectal surgery.

Main Outcomes and Measures.—The primary outcome was the rate of superficial SSIs before and after implementation of the bundle. Secondary outcomes included deep SSIs, organ-space SSIs, wound disruption, postoperative sepsis, length of stay, 30-day readmission, and variable direct costs of the index admission.

Results.—Of 559 patients in the study, 346 (61.9%) and 213 (38.1%) underwent their operation before and after implementation of the bundle, respectively. Groups were matched on their propensity to be treated with the bundle to account for significant differences in the preimplementation and postimplementation characteristics. Comparison of the matched groups revealed that implementation of the bundle was associated with reduced superficial SSIs (19.3% vs 5.7%, *P* < .001) and postoperative sepsis (8.5% vs 2.4%, *P* =.009). No significant difference was observed in deep SSIs, organ-space SSIs, wound disruption, length of stay, 30-day readmission, or variable direct costs between the matched groups. However, in a subgroup analysis of the postbundle period, superficial SSI occurrence was associated with a 35.5% increase in variable direct costs ($13 253 vs $9779, *P* =.001) and a 71.7% increase in length of stay (7.9 vs 4.6 days, *P* < .001).

Conclusions and Relevance.—The preventive SSI bundle was associated with a substantial reduction in SSIs after colorectal surgery. The increased costs associated with SSIs support that the bundle represents an effective approach to reduce health care costs.

▶ You may now be aware of your own surgical site infection rate or at least the rates in the hospital(s) where you practice. All too often these are quite high, but many have now adopted programs to substantially decrease these complications. The group from Duke presents their work that decreased surgical site infections from 19.3% to 5.7%. How did they do it? The effort was multidisciplinary and included surgeons, anesthesiologists, clinic nurses, operating room staff, unit nurses, house staff, and hospital midlevel providers. They created a bundled of interventions (Fig 1 in the original article) that included chlorhexidine showers, mechanical bowel preparation with antibiotics, a dedicated wound closure tray, and daily washing of the incision with chlorhexidine among others. The outcome not only impacted wound infection rates but also deep space infections, length of stay, and readmission. This work cut costs in half and created a working group that was invested in making a change and impact on patient outcome—maybe the most important factor.

J. Hines, MD

Short-Term Surgical Outcomes From a Randomized Controlled Trial to Evaluate Laparoscopic and Open D3 Dissection for Stage II/III Colon Cancer: Japan Clinical Oncology Group Study JCOG 0404

Yamamoto S, Clinical Oncology Group Colorectal Cancer Study Group (Natl Cancer Ctr Hosp, Tokyo, Japan; et al)

Ann Surg 260:23-30, 2014

Objective.—A randomized controlled trial to confirm the noninferiority of laparoscopic surgery to open surgery in terms of overall survival was conducted, and short-term surgical outcomes are demonstrated.

Background.—The efficacy and safety outcome of laparoscopic surgery for clinical stages II/III colon cancer undergoing Japanese D3 dissection are still unclear.

Methods.—Eligibility criteria included colon cancer; tumor located in the cecum, ascending, sigmoid, or rectosigmoid colon; T3 or T4 without involvement of other organs; N0—2; and M0. Patients were randomized preoperatively and underwent tumor resection with D3 dissection. Safety analyses were conducted by per-protocol set.

Results.—A total of 1057 patients were randomized between October 2004 and March 2009. By per-protocol set, 524 patients who underwent open surgery and 533 patients who underwent laparoscopic surgery were analyzed. D3 dissection was performed in 521 (99.4%) patients in the open surgery arm and 529 (99.2%) patients in the laparoscopic surgery arm. Conversion to open surgery was needed for 29 (5.4%) patients. Patients assigned to laparoscopic surgery had less blood loss ($P < 0.001$), although laparoscopic surgery lasted 52 minutes longer ($P < 0.001$). Laparoscopic surgery was associated with a shorter time to pass first flatus, decreased use of analgesics after 5 postoperative days, and a shorter hospital stay. Morbidity [14.3% (76/533) vs 22.3% (117/524), $P < 0.001$] was lower in the laparoscopic surgery arm.

Conclusions.—Short-term surgical safety and clinical benefits of laparoscopic D3 dissection were demonstrated. The primary endpoint will be reported after the primary analysis, planned for 2014 (Fig 3B).

▶ This large randomized trial from Japan adds further evidence that laparoscopic surgery for colorectal cancer is at least as good as open and may provide some advantages. Several randomized trials have confirmed the same, but this trial examined the use of a D3 resection. D3 implies that the draining vessels

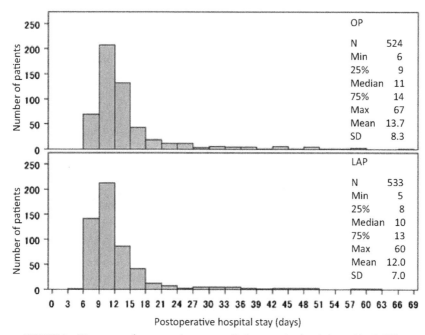

FIGURE 3.—Histograms of postoperative recovery. B, Postoperative hospital stay (days); Wilcoxon rank sum test *P* < 0.0001. (Reprinted from Yamamoto S, Clinical Oncology Group Colorectal Cancer Study Group. Short-term surgical outcomes from a randomized controlled trial to evaluate laparoscopic and open D3 dissection for stage II/III colon cancer: Japan clinical oncology group study JCOG 0404. *Ann Surg.* 2014;260:23-30, © 2014, Southeastern Surgical Congress.)

to the named area of the colon to be resected are taken at their origin. This, in theory, would provide a more extensive nodal harvest. The value of this technique can be argued, as many studies have found equivalency with more extensive node resections for several gastrointestinal malignancies. One must resect a certain threshold of nodes (12—15) to properly stage the disease, but a more extensive resection does not seem to lead to better survival outcomes. There were fewer wound infections and a shorter hospital stays in the laparoscopic group (Fig 3B). This study group showed feasibility for a more extensive resection laparoscopically, but the survival outcomes have not been reported yet, and the utility of a D3 resection is not detailed in this report.

J. Hines, MD

Analgesia After Open Abdominal Surgery in the Setting of Enhanced Recovery Surgery: A Systematic Review and Meta-Analysis

Hughes MJ, Ventham NT, McNally S, et al (Royal Infirmary of Edinburgh, Scotland)
JAMA Surg 149:1224-1230, 2014

Importance.—The optimal analgesic technique following open abdominal surgery within an enhanced recovery protocol remains controversial.

Thoracic epidural is often recommended; however, its role is increasingly being challenged and alternative techniques are being suggested as suitable replacements.

Objective.—To determine by meta-analysis whether epidurals are superior to alternative analgesic techniques following open abdominal surgery within an enhanced recovery setting in terms of postoperative morbidity and other markers of recovery.

Data Sources.—A literature search was performed of EMBASE, Medline, PubMed, and the Cochrane databases from 1966 through May 2013.

Study Selection.—All randomized clinical trials comparing epidurals with an alternative analgesic technique following open abdominal surgery within an enhanced recovery protocol were included.

Data Extraction and Synthesis.—All studies were assessed by 2 independent reviewers. Study quality was assessed using the Cochrane bias assessment tool and the Jadad and Chalmers modified bias risk assessment tools. Dichotomous data were analyzed by random or fixed-effects odds ratios. Qualitative analysis was performed where appropriate.

Results.—Seven trials with a total of 378 patients were identified. No significant difference in complication rate was detected between epidurals and alternative analgesic methods (odds ratio, 1.14; 95% CI, 0.49-2.64; $P = .76$). Subgroup analysis showed fewer complications in the patient-controlled analgesia group compared with epidural analgesia (odds ratio, 1.97; 95% CI, 1.10-3.53; $P = .02$). Following qualitative assessment, epidural analgesia was associated with faster return of gut function and reduced pain scores; however, no difference was observed in length of stay.

Conclusions and Relevance.—Epidurals may be associated with superior pain control but this does not translate into improved recovery or reduced morbidity when compared with alternative analgesic techniques when used within an enhanced recovery protocol.

▶ Perioperative pain management is an important issue for patients undergoing open operation and impacts physical recovery and patient satisfaction. Oral, intravenous, patient-controlled, local, and epidural analgesia all offer individual advantages and drawbacks. These issues are coupled with the efforts for early recovery and discharge, and many facilities now offer continuous epidural to improve pain control and shorten hospital stay. This systematic review and meta-analysis compared epidural with alternative strategies. Overall, there were no differences when comparing complications (Fig 2 in the original article), but subgroup analysis found patient-controlled analgesia was safer than epidural. However, epidural analgesia was associated with a faster return of gut function and lower pain scores. These results did not translate into a short hospital stay, however. The institution of an in-house pain team at our place that is responsive and staffed by the anesthesia group has improved pain scores overall and may have helped reduced stay; this is probably the right approach for open abdominal surgery.

J. Hines, MD

Unique risks for mortality in patients with end-stage renal disease undergoing nonemergent colorectal surgery

Liu JJ, Kohut AY, Stein DE, et al (Drexel Univ College of Medicine, Philadelphia, PA)
Am J Surg 208:41-44, 2014

Background.—The aim of this study was to identify unique risk factors for mortality in patients with end-stage renal disease undergoing nonemergent colorectal surgery.

Methods.—A multivariate logistic regression model predicting 30-day mortality was constructed for patients with end-stage renal disease undergoing nonemergent colorectal procedures. Data were obtained from the National Surgical Quality Improvement Program (2005−2010).

Results.—Among the 394 patients analyzed, those with serum creatinine levels >7.5 mg/dL had .07 times the adjusted mortality risk of those with levels <3.5 mg/dL. For colorectal surgery patients, the average serum creatinine level was 5.52 ± 2.6 mg/dL, and mortality was 13% (n = 50).

Conclusions.—High serum creatinine was associated with a lower risk for mortality in patients with end-stage renal disease, even though creatinine is often considered a risk factor for surgery. These results show how variables from a patient-centered subpopulation can differ in meaning from the general population (Table 3).

▶ Whenever we evaluate a patient for elective surgery and know that they have end-stage renal disease requiring dialysis, we worry about the risk for complications and death from the operation. It is clear that these patients do realize worse

TABLE 3.—Odds Ratios, 95% Confidence Intervals, and *P* Values for Variables Predicting Mortality in Patients with End-Stage Renal Disease (n = 394)

Predictor	Adjusted Odds Ratio (95% Confidence Interval)	*P*	Case Mortality (% of All Mortality)
Creatinine (mg/dL)			
<3.5	1	—	31 (62%)
3.5−5.3	.23 (.09−.54)	<.001	9 (18%)
5.3−7.2	.22 (.09−.54)	.001	8 (16%)
>7.2	.07 (.02−.34)	<.001	2 (4%)
Functional status (totally dependent)	3.46 (1.49−8.05)	.004	16 (32%)
Bleeding disorders	2.56 (1.19−5.52)	.016	17 (34%)
Dyspnea	2.51 (1.22−5.16)	.013	22 (44%)
Age (y)			
55	1	—	5 (10%)
55−65	1.84 (.54−6.32)	.332	10 (20%)
65−75	2.76 (.87−8.77)	.086	16 (32%)
>75	2.55 (.81−8.07)	.111	19 (38%)

Hosmer-Lemeshow statistic = 8.017 (*P* = .432, *df* = 8); C-statistic = .822.

outcomes compared with those without renal failure. But how do patients with renal failure compare among themselves—are there groups of these patients that fare even worse? This article provides an interesting data point: patients with end-stage renal disease and a higher creatinine have a lower mortality than those with a lower creatinine. This concept on first pass makes no sense; higher creatinine means worse outcomes, right? It turns out that patients on chronic dialysis who have higher creatinines are probably in better shape. In this state, creatinine is a surrogate for muscle mass and nutrition.[1] Without muscle mass, serum creatinine levels are low. So a patient with a creatinine of 7.5 is better nourished, has more muscle mass, and lower mortality than a patient with a creatinine of 2.5 (Table 3). We all know that better nourished patients with improved functional status have lower risk. So when your patient is on chronic dialysis, you can worry a bit less about those patients with a higher creatinine.

J. Hines, MD

Reference

1. Kalantar-Zadeh K, Streja E, Kovesdy CP, et al. The obesity paradox and mortality associated with surrogates of body size and muscle mass in patients receiving hemodialysis. *Mayo Clin Proc.* 2010;85:991-1001.

Addressing the Appropriateness of Elective Colon Resection for Diverticulitis: A Report from the SCOAP CERTAIN Collaborative
Simianu VV, Bastawrous AL, Billingham RP, et al (Univ of Washington, Seattle; Swedish Med Ctr, Seattle, WA; et al)
Ann Surg 260:533-539, 2014

Objective.—To assess the reported indications for elective colon resection for diverticulitis and concordance with professional guidelines.

Background.—Despite modern professional guidelines recommending delay in elective colon resection beyond 2 episodes of uncomplicated diverticulitis, the incidence of elective colectomy has increased dramatically in the last 2 decades. Whether surgeons have changed their threshold for recommending a surgical intervention is unknown. In 2010, Washington State's Surgical Care and Outcomes Assessment Program initiated a benchmarking and education initiative related to the indications for colon resection.

Methods.—Prospective cohort study evaluating indications from chronic complications (fistula, stricture, bleeding) or the number of previously treated diverticulitis episodes for patients undergoing elective colectomy at 1 of 49 participating hospitals (2010—2013).

Results.—Among 2724 patients (58.7 ± 13 years; 46% men), 29.4% had a chronic complication indication (15.6% fistula, 7.4% stricture, 3.0% bleeding, 5.8% other). For the 70.5% with an episode-based indication, 39.4% had 2 or fewer episodes, 56.5% had 3 to 10 episodes, and 4.1% had more than 10 episodes. Thirty-one percent of patients failed to meet indications for either a chronic complication or 3 or more episodes. Over the 4 years, the proportion of patients with an indication of 3 or more episodes increased from 36.6% to 52.7% ($P < 0.001$) whereas the proportion of those who failed to meet either clinical or episode-based indications decreased from 38.4% to 26.4% ($P < 0.001$). The annual rate of emergency resections did not increase significantly, varying from 5.6 to 5.9 per year ($P = 0.81$).

Conclusions.—Adherence to a guideline based on 3 or more episodes for elective colectomy increased concurrently with a benchmarking and peer-to-peer messaging initiative. Improving adherence to professional guidelines related to appropriate care is critical and can be facilitated by quality improvement collaboratives.

▶ The indications for surgery for diverticulitis have rapidly evolved because of a better understanding of the disease process and the quite limited risk of recurrence requiring emergent operation. The American Society of Colon and Rectal Surgeons (ASCRS) advises against elective resection for uncomplicated diverticulitis and consider multiple episodes as an indication only for those with complicated disease.[1] Complicated diverticulitis includes those episodes associated with free perforation, abscess, fistula, obstruction, or stricture. This group examined the current trends of surgery for diverticulitis in the state of Washington over a recent 3-year period. More than 2700 patients were evaluated. About 30% of patients failed to meet the indications as outlined by the ASCRS. It did appear, however, that over the study period, a higher percentage of patients more regularly met criteria for resection. We need to remember that routine elective resection based on young age (< 50 years) is no longer recommended. Despite previous emphasis on the number of attacks dictating the need for surgery, the literature demonstrates that patients with more than 2 episodes are not at an increased risk for morbidity and mortality compared with patients who have had fewer episodes, indicating that diverticulitis is not a progressive disease.

J. Hines, MD

Reference

1. Feingold D, Steele SR, Lee S, et al. Practice parameters for the treatment of sigmoid diverticulitis. *Dis Colon Rectum*. 2014;57:284-294.

The effect of race on outcomes for appendicitis in children: a nationwide analysis
Zwintscher NP, Steele SR, Martin MJ, et al (Madigan Army Med Ctr, Tacoma, WA; et al)
Am J Surg 207:748-753, 2014

Background.—We sought to examine the impact of race on the management and outcomes of appendicitis in children aged 20 years or younger.

Methods.—We studied 96,865 inpatient admissions for children undergoing an appendectomy for acute appendicitis in 2009 using the Kids' Inpatient Database.

Results.—Perforation at presentation was more common among African-Americans and Hispanics than Caucasians (27.5% and 32.5%, respectively, vs 23.9%, $P < .001$). African-Americans were less likely to have a laparoscopic procedure (odds ratio [OR]: .839, $P < .001$) and more likely to experience a complication (OR: 1.753, $P < .001$). Hispanics were also more likely to have a complication (OR: 1.123, $P = .001$). African-Americans and Hispanics remained in the hospital for .73 more days than Caucasians (3.07 vs 2.34 days, $P < .001$).

Conclusions.—African-American and Hispanic children present more often with perforation. Adjusting for perforation, they were more likely to have a complication and longer hospital stays. Access to care and delayed presentations may be potential explanations.

▶ Disparity in care among surgical patients based on ethnicity is well documented. The reasons for these differences are complex and include access to care and bias across the health care continuum. This article examines outcomes of children with appendicitis among white, African-American, and Hispanic populations. The data include a large number of patients—nearly 100 000—and are well controlled. African-American and Hispanic patients were more likely to present with a perforation (27% and 31%, respectively) and have a complication. This was the case even when there was control for the issue of advanced presentation/perforation. These patients were more likely to be operated on the next day and experience almost an entire day longer of hospitalization. The African-American patients were less likely to receive a laparoscopic procedure. With regard to economic disparity, those in the lowest income quartile were more likely to experience a complication compared with those in the highest quartile. Finally, children in the Midwest, South, and West were more likely to experience a complication than patients in the Northwest. The reasons for findings like this are complex, but awareness and acknowledgment is an important first step.

J. Hines, MD

The effect of appendectomy in future tubal infertility and ectopic pregnancy: a systematic review and meta-analysis

Elraiyah T, Hashim Y, Elamin M, et al (Mayo Clinic, Rochester, MN; Washington Univ School of Medicine, St Louis, MO; Texas Tech Univ Health Science Ctr at Amarillo)
J Surg Res 192:368-374, 2014

Background.—Ruptured appendicitis has been implicated in causing scarring, which can lead to infertility and/or ectopic pregnancy. To assess the degree of association and the quality of evidence supporting the relation among appendectomy, female fertility outcomes, and ectopic pregnancy.

Study name	Odds ratio	Lower limit	Upper limit	P-value	Odds ratio and 95% CI
Coste, 1991	1.60	1.04	2.46	0.03	
Hanyu Ni 1990 **	1.80	0.59	5.45	0.30	
Hanyu Ni 1990 ***	1.20	0.67	2.14	0.54	
Michalas 1992	1.80	1.30	2.50	0.00	
Nordenskjold 1991	2.16	1.52	3.06	0.00	
Pooled estimate	**1.78**	**1.46**	**2.16**	**0.00**	

$I^2 = 0.0\%$

0.1 0.2 0.5 1 2 5 10

Decrease ectopic   Increase ectopic

- ** **Perforated appendix**
- ***Non-perforated appendix**

FIGURE 3.—Appendectomy versus control—the risk of ectopic pregnancy. (Reprinted from The Journal of Surgical Research. Elraiyah T, Hashim Y, Elamin M, et al. The effect of appendectomy in future tubal infertility and ectopic pregnancy: a systematic review and meta-analysis. *J Surg Res.* 2014;192:368-374, Copyright 2014, with permission from Elsevier.)

Methods.—We systematically searched multiple electronic databases from inception through May 2013 for randomized trials and observational studies. Reviewers working independently and in duplicate extracted the study characteristics, the quality of the included studies, and the outcomes of interest. Random effects meta-analysis was used to pool the odds ratio (OR) from the included studies.

Results.—Our meta-analysis based on seven observational studies provided evidence that previous appendectomy is not associated with increased incidence of infertility in women (OR = 1.03, 0.86–1.24, $P = 0.71$). This finding was further augmented by several noncomparative cohorts that discussed the same issue and reported nearly the same conclusion; however, these studies pointed toward putative negative impact of surgery for complicated appendicitis on fertility. Our second meta-analysis revealed the effect of appendectomy on ectopic pregnancy was found to be significant based on a pooled estimate from four studies (OR = 1.78, 95% confidence interval = 1.46–2.16, $P < 0.0001$).

Conclusions.—Appendectomy is significantly associated with an increased risk of ectopic pregnancy but not significantly associated with future infertility in women (Fig 3).

▶ Can I still get pregnant, doctor? This is a classic and common concern of women with surgical disease who want to have children. For a long time, there has been discussion on the impact of appendicitis on infertility, and many have felt or advised that this could be the case—a lower chance of pregnancy after appendicitis. This statement makes some teleological sense because the appendix is located in close proximity to the adnexa in most women. Inflammation, abscess, and scarring might impact the function of the ovaries and obstruction of the fallopian tubes. This large meta-analysis shows that a history of appendicitis does not impact fertility. It does, however, seem to increase the risk of ectopic pregnancy (Fig 3) by about 78%. So it is true that appendicitis can impact this issue, and your patient may want to be fully informed of this possibility when considering treatment and potential outcomes.

J. Hines, MD

Time to Appendectomy and Risk of Perforation in Acute Appendicitis

Drake FT, Mottey NE, Farrokhi ET, et al (Univ of Washington Med Ctr, Seattle; Univ of Washington Surgical Outcomes Res Ctr, Seattle; et al)
JAMA Surg 149:837-844, 2014

Importance.—In the traditional model of acute appendicitis, time is the major driver of disease progression; luminal obstruction leads inexorably to perforation without timely intervention. This perceived association has long guided clinical behavior related to the timing of appendectomy.

Objective.—To evaluate whether there is an association between time and perforation after patients present to the hospital.

Design, Setting, and Participants.—Using data from the Washington State Surgical Care and Outcomes Assessment Program (SCOAP), we evaluated patterns of perforation among patients (≥18 years) who underwent appendectomy from January 1, 2010, to December 31, 2011. Patients were treated at 52 diverse hospitals including urban tertiary centers, a university hospital, small community and rural hospitals, and hospitals within multi-institutional organizations.

Main Outcomes and Measures.—The main outcome of interest was perforation as diagnosed on final pathology reports. The main predictor of interest was elapsed time as measured between presentation to the hospital and operating room (OR) start time. The relationship between in-hospital time and perforation was adjusted for potential confounding using multivariate logistic regression. Additional predictors of interest included sex, age, number of comorbid conditions, race and/or ethnicity, insurance status, and hospital characteristics such as community type and appendectomy volume.

Results.—A total of 9048 adults underwent appendectomy (15.8% perforated). Mean time from presentation to OR was the same (8.6 hours) for patients with perforated and nonperforated appendicitis. In multivariate analysis, increasing time to OR was not a predictor of perforation, either as a continuous variable (odds ratio = 1.0 [95% CI, 0.99-1.01]) or when considered as a categorical variable (patients ordered by elapsed time and divided into deciles). Factors associated with perforation were male sex, increasing age, 3 or more comorbid conditions, and lack of insurance.

Conclusions and Relevance.—There was no association between perforation and in-hospital time prior to surgery among adults treated with appendectomy. These findings may reflect selection of those at higher risk of perforation for earlier intervention or the effect of antibiotics begun at diagnosis but they are also consistent with the hypothesis that perforation is most often a prehospital occurrence and/or not strictly a time-dependent phenomenon. These findings may also guide decisions regarding personnel and resource allocation when considering timing of nonelective appendectomy. Copyright 2014 American Medical Association.

▶ We have always thought that appendicitis is an emergency and requires expeditious care and surgery. Many have felt that this approach is best and works toward limiting progression of disease leading to perforation. This study calls that concept into question. The authors evaluated the time to operation in more than 9000 patients and found no difference in perforation rates. Overall, men were more likely to have perforation (17.3%) as were elderly patients (36.1%). With regard to race and ethnicity, African-American patients had the longest wait times to surgery but the second lowest perforation rate. Overall, the time from admission to the operating room was the same for patients who experienced perforation and those that did not (Table 2 in the original article). Time to imaging and time from imaging to the operating room were also similar between the 2 groups. These results, that perforation occurs in most patients before presentation (if they are going to do so) and rushing to the operating room, will not change this outcome.

J. Hines, MD

The NOTA study (Non Operative Treatment for Acute Appendicitis): Prospective Study on the Efficacy and Safety of Antibiotics (Amoxicillin and Clavulanic Acid) for Treating Patients With Right Lower Quadrant Abdominal Pain and Long-Term Follow-up of Conservatively Treated Suspected Appendicitis

Di Saverio S, Sibilio A, Giorgini E, et al (Maggiore Hosp Regional Trauma Ctr, Bologna, Italy; et al)
Ann Surg 260:109-117, 2014

Objectives.—To assess the safety and efficacy of antibiotics treatment for suspected acute uncomplicated appendicitis and to monitor the long term follow-up of non-operated patients.

Background.—Right lower quadrant abdominal pain is a common cause of emergency department admission. The natural history of acute appendicitis nonoperatively treated with antibiotics remains unclear.

Methods.—In 2010, a total of 159 patients [mean AIR (Appendicitis Inflammatory Response) score = 4.9 and mean Alvarado score = 5.2] with suspected appendicitis were enrolled and underwent nonoperative management (NOM) with amoxicillin/clavulanate. The follow-up period was 2 years.

Results.—Short-term (7 days) NOM failure rate was 11.9%. All patients with initial failures were operated within 7 days. At 15 days, no recurrences were recorded. After 2 years, the overall recurrence rate was 13.8% (22/159); 14 of 22 patients were successfully treated with further cycle of amoxicillin/clavulanate. No major side effects occurred. Abdominal pain assessed by the Numeric Rating Scale and the visual analog scale; median Numeric Rating Scale score was 3 at 5 days and 2 after 7 days. Mean length of stay of nonoperatively managed patients was 0.4 days, and mean sick leave period was 5.8 days. Long-term efficacy of NOM treatment was 83% (118 patients recurrence free and 14 patients with recurrence nonoperatively managed). None of the single factors forming the Alvarado or AIR score were independent predictors of failure of NOM or long-term recurrence. Alvarado and AIR scores were the only independent predictive factors of NOM failure after multivariate analysis, but both did not correlate with recurrences. Overall costs of NOM and antibiotics were €316.20 per patient.

Conclusions.—Antibiotics for suspected acute appendicitis are safe and effective and may avoid unnecessary appendectomy, reducing operation rate, surgical risks, and overall costs. After 2 years of follow-up, recurrences of nonoperatively treated right lower quadrant abdominal pain are less than 14% and may be safely and effectively treated with further antibiotics.

▶ The management of acute appendicitis is certainly in evolution. With imaging, the diagnosis can be reliably established, and for decades now, the management has been surgery. Growing evidence suggests, though, that appendicitis can be managed nonoperatively. The interest to change to nonoperative management is so significant now that the National Institutes of Health is funding studies to examine this option. This study details the evidence to date and enrolls more than 100 patients with appendicitis to antibiotic treatment. The failure rate or need for operation was 11.9% during the first week, and long-term recurrence rate within 2 years was 13.8%. The authors argue that these are acceptable numbers given the risks of surgery and the required anesthetic, need for reoperation or second procedure for abscess, other perioperative complications, and long-term risk of bowel obstruction after operation. As the authors point out, this is not a new concept. In 1908, Alfred Stengel wrote: "Treated in a purely medical or tentative manner, the great majority of patients with appendicitis recover."[1]

J. Hines, MD

Reference

1. Stengel A. Appendicitis. In: Osler W, McCrae T, eds. *Modern Medicine, Volume V: Diseases of the Alimentary Tract.* Philadelphia: Lea & Febiger; 1908.

The Use of Magnetic Resonance Imaging in the Diagnosis of Suspected Appendicitis in Pregnancy: Shortened Length of Stay Without Increase in Hospital Charges

Fonseca AL, Schuster KM, Kaplan LJ, et al (Yale Univ, New Haven, CT)
JAMA Surg 149:687-693, 2014

Importance.—Making an accurate diagnosis of appendicitis in pregnancy is critical for maternal and fetal outcomes.

Objective.—To determine whether magnetic resonance (MR) imaging in pregnant patients with suspected appendicitis improves outcomes, minimizes length of stay (LOS), and lowers hospital charges.

Design, Setting, and Participants.—Retrospective review at a university tertiary referral center of all pregnant patients seen with abdominal pain and suspected appendicitis who were followed up through delivery during an 11-year period.

Main Outcomes and Measures.—Time to operation, LOS, complications, nontherapeutic exploration, fetal outcomes, and hospital charges.

Results.—Seventy-nine patients were included in this study, 34 of whom had pathology-confirmed appendicitis. Thirty-one patients underwent MR imaging. A trend toward fewer operations (odds ratio [OR], 0.45; 95% CI, 0.18-1.16; $P = .07$) was observed in the MR imaging group. Seven nontherapeutic explorations were performed in the non—MR imaging group and 1 nontherapeutic exploration in the MR imaging group (OR, 0.44; 95% CI, 0.08-2.32; $P = .13$). Patients in the MR imaging group were more frequently discharged from the emergency department (OR, 0.35; 95% CI, 0.13-0.94; $P = .04$) and had shorter LOS (33.7 vs 64.8 hours, $P < .001$). Gestational age, time to operation, and the presence of perforated appendicitis were similar between groups. No patient discharged without operation returned with appendicitis in either group. On multivariable analysis, the receipt of MR imaging ($P < .001$) and the absence of operative intervention ($P = .001$) were associated with shorter LOS. The mean hospital charges were similar in those with vs without appendicitis. One fetal loss occurred in the non—MR imaging group.

Conclusions and Relevance.—Magnetic resonance imaging in pregnant patients with suspected appendicitis does not affect clinical outcomes or hospital charges. It allows safe discharge from the emergency department and improves resource use.

▶ Pregnant patients who present for evaluation of abdominal pain are a clinical and diagnostic challenge. Pregnancy itself can be responsible for pain, and these patients often have an elevated white blood cell count without any pathology. The examination of a patient with suspected appendicitis is confounded by the expanded uterus and often repositioned appendix during mid- to late-term pregnancy. Traditional imaging with CT scan may expose the fetus to the untoward effect of radiation in the first trimester. Fetal loss from both appendicitis and nontherapeutic exploration is a real concern for this population.[1] This study examined the efficacy of MRI for pregnant patients with a suspected appendicitis. MRI was very good at diagnosing appendicitis (Table 1 in original article), and for those patients who underwent an MRI, there was a trend toward fewer operations and ability to discharge from the emergency room rather than admitting patients for observation. Including MRI did not save on hospital charges, however. Everyone would agree that these patients deserve special consideration. If available and feasibly accessed, pregnant patients being considered for appendicitis may be advantaged by MRI.

J. Hines, MD

Reference

1. McGory ML, Zingmond DS, Tillou A, Hiatt JR, Ko CY, Cryer HM. Negative appendectomy in pregnant women is associated with a substantial risk of fetal loss. *J Am Coll Surg.* 2007;205:534-540.

Incidental Gallbladder Cancer at Cholecystectomy: When Should the Surgeon be Suspicious?
Pitt SC, Jin LX, Hall BL, et al (Washington Univ, School of Medicine in St Louis, MO; et al)
Ann Surg 260:128-133, 2014

Background.—Preoperative predictors of incidental gallbladder cancer (iGBC) have been poorly defined despite the frequency with which cholecystectomy is performed. The objective of this study was to define the incidence of and consider risk factors for iGBC at cholecystectomy.

Methods.—The American College of Surgeons-National Surgical Quality Improvement Program (ACS-NSQIP) database (2005-2009) was used to identify all patients who underwent cholecystectomy (N = 91,260). Patients with an *International Classification of Diseases, Ninth Revision,* diagnosis of gallbladder malignancy who underwent a laparoscopic cholecystectomy (LC; n = 80,924) or open cholecystectomy (OC; n = 10,336) alone were included.

Results.—The incidence of iGBC was 0.19% (n = 170) for all cholecystectomy cases, but 0.05% at LC, 0.60% at LC converted to OC (*P* < 0.001 vs LC), and 1.13% at OC (*P* < 0.001 vs others). Patients undergoing OC were 17.3 times more likely to have iGBC than LC patients. Age

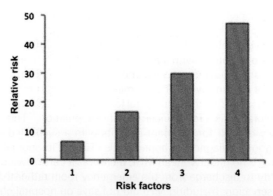

FIGURE 2.—Risk factors for iGBC include OC, age 65 years or older, Asian or African American race, an elevated alkaline phosphatase level, and female sex. The figure demonstrates that average relative risk of iGBC increases dramatically with the number of risk factors observed in a patient. The zero risk factor referent (male, <65 years, non-Asian or African American, with a normal alkaline phosphatase level undergoing an LC) had a 0.03% incidence of iGBC. (Reprinted from Pitt SC, Jin LX, Hall BL, et al. Incidental gallbladder cancer at cholecystectomy: when should the surgeon be suspicious? *Ann Surg.* 2014;260:128-133, © 2014, Southeastern Surgical Congress.)

TABLE 3.—Multivariable Predictors of iGBC in Patients Undergoing Cholecystectomy

Risk Factor	Odds Ratio	95% CI	P
OC	12.0	8.5–16.7	<0.001
Age ≥65 yr	5.3	3.7–7.4	<0.001
Race			
Asian	2.2	1.1–4.4	0.02
African American	1.7	1.1–2.6	0.02
Alk phos ≥120 units/L	1.7	1.3–2.3	0.001
Female sex	1.6	1.1–2.2	0.006

Alk phos indicates alkaline phosphatase; CI, confidence interval.
Reprinted from Pitt SC, Jin LX, Hall BL, et al. Incidental gallbladder cancer at cholecystectomy: when should the surgeon be suspicious? *Ann Surg.* 2014;260:128-133. © 2014, Southeastern Surgical Congress.

65 years or older, Asian or African American race, ASA (American Society of Anesthesiologists) class 3 or more, diabetes mellitus, hypertension, weight loss more than 10%, alkaline phosphatase levels 120 units/L or more, and albumin levels 3.6 g/dL or less were associated with iGBC. Multiple logistic regression identified having an OC, age 65 years or older, Asian or African American race, an elevated alkaline phosphatase level, and female sex as independent risk factors. Patients with 1, 2, 3, and 4 of these factors had a 6.3-, 16.7-, 30.0-, and 47.4-fold risk of iGBC, respectively, from a zero-risk factor baseline of 0.03%.

Conclusions.—Surgeons' suspicion for GBC should be heightened when they are performing or converting from LC to OC and when patients are older, Asian or African American, female, and have an elevated alkaline phosphatase level (Fig 2, Table 3).

► An estimated 900 000 cholecystectomies are performed each year in the United States, and most of these are performed with a laparoscope. The most common indication is biliary colic, but it has been a tenant for all general surgeons that we must be mindful of potential cancer. Traditionally, we have been taught that 1% of all gallbladders removed harbor a cancer. This study shows that this estimate is 10-fold higher and is instead 0.19%. The trick with these procedures is to have a high index of suspicion when the cancer is present. Once the gallbladder has been removed and the wall violated, we compromise the potential of a complete resection. According to this National Surgical Quality Improvement Program-based analysis, we should have the increased suspicion of an occult cancer in cases in which an open operation is required in older patients who are Asian or African-American women with an elevated alkaline phosphatase level (Table 3 and Fig 2). When we are suspicious and the diagnosis is made intraoperatively by frozen section, operative management can be appropriately altered by considering partial liver resection or portal lymphadenectomy if indicated, and complete excision of the gallbladder without bile spillage.

J. Hines, MD

The timing of complications impacts risk of readmission after hepatopancreatobiliary surgery

Lucas DJ, Sweeney JF, Pawlik TM (Walter Reed Natl Military Med Ctr, Bethesda, MD; Emory Univ Hosp, Atlanta, GA; The Johns Hopkins Hosp, Baltimore, MD)
Surgery 155:945-953, 2014

Background.—Readmission is frequent in hepatopancreatobiliary (HPB) surgery. Medicare began penalizing hospitals recently for excess readmission for specific diagnoses, including some operative procedures. We sought to define the incidence and risk factors for readmission after HPB surgery.

Study Design.—Elective HPB resections were selected from the 2011 American College of Surgeons National Surgical Quality Improvement Program (NSQIP) dataset. Risk factors associated with readmission were assessed using modified Poisson univariate and adjusted regression models.

Results.—We identified 5,081 patients; 2,980 underwent pancreatic resection and 2,101 had a hepatectomy. Median age was 62 (interquartile range, 52–70), 53% of patients were women; 74% were non-Hispanic white; and 31% were American Society of Anesthesiologists (ASA) class 2, and 64% were ASA class 3. About 75% of cases had a malignant diagnosis on final pathology. Of all these patients, 16.2% were readmitted within 30 days of operation. The strongest risk factors for readmission on multivariable analysis were minor (risk ratio [RR], 3.13, 95% confidence interval [CI], 2.47–3.97; $P < .001$) and major (RR, 8.45; 95% CI, 7.59–9.40; $P < .001$) complications after discharge; in contrast, major inpatient complications only had a modest effect on the risk of readmission (RR, 1.29; 95% CI, 1.05–1.58; $P < .014$). Among all patients who were readmitted, 40% experienced a major complication after discharge, and 83% of patients who had a major outpatient complication were readmitted.

Conclusion.—Outpatient complications were by far the strongest risk factor for readmission. Decreasing complications as well as improving outpatient case management to prevent and treat postdischarge complications hold considerable promise in the efforts to decrease readmission (Table 2).

▶ Readmissions are a challenge, and the need to decrease the current rates is not only for good patient care but also to improve throughput and remuneration. This report examines the readmission rates of patients undergoing hepatic and pancreatic surgery using National Surgical Quality Improvement Program (NSQIP) data. Approximately 5000 patients experienced a 16.2% rate of readmission. These readmissions were most commonly for wound complications, sepsis, urinary tract infection, pulmonary complications, and venous thromboembolism (Table 2). To decrease readmissions, surgeons should focus on programs to decrease surgical site infection, catheter-related blood stream infections, pneumonia, and venous thromboembolism. Some reasons for readmissions for the patients in this study were not captured by the NSQIP database and the new hepatopancreatobiliary NSQIP is currently being piloted to help with this issue.

TABLE 2.—Complication Type and Setting

Complication Type	Overall, n (%)	Inpatient, n (%)	Outpatient, n (%)	P Value
Total	5,081	5,081	5,081	
Any complication	1,062 (20.9)	558 (11.0)	565 (11.1)	.843
Minor	324 (6.4)	168 (3.3)	189 (3.7)	.275
Major	738 (14.5)	390 (7.7)	376 (7.4)	.626
Any wound complication	636 (12.5)	235 (4.6)	410 (8.1)	<.001
Superficial SSI	311 (6.1)	143 (2.8)	166 (3.3)	.197
Deep SSI	63 (1.2)	16 (0.3)	45 (0.9)	<.001
Organ space SSI	279 (5.5)	83 (1.6)	195 (3.8)	<.001
Dehiscence	25 (0.5)	4 (0.1)	21 (0.4)	.001
Sepsis	291 (5.7)	133 (2.6)	157 (3.1)	.165
Urinary tract infection	160 (3.1)	102 (2.0)	57 (1.1)	<.001
Respiratory	148 (2.9)	124 (2.4)	23 (0.5)	<.001
Venous thromboembolism	113 (2.2)	57 (1.1)	54 (1.1)	.777
Reoperative bleeding	38 (0.7)	38 (0.7)	0 (0.0)	<.001*
Cardiac	32 (0.6)	24 (0.5)	8 (0.2)	.007*
Renal	26 (0.5)	14 (0.3)	12 (0.2)	.845*
CVA or coma	11 (0.2)	8 (0.2)	3 (0.1)	.226*

P values represent Chi-square tests.
CVA, Cerebrovascular accident; SSI, surgical site infection.
*Fisher's exact test used due to low number of events.
Reprinted from Surgery. Lucas DJ, Sweeney JF, Pawlik TM. The timing of complications impacts risk of readmission after hepatopancreatobiliary surgery. Surgery. 2014;155:945-953, Copyright 2014, with permission from Elsevier.

Resources in the outpatient setting may also help decrease readmission rates, allowing for the prevention of complications, early identification of complications before more serious progression, and the mechanisms to address complications as an outpatient.

J. Hines, MD

Natural Course vs Interventions to Clear Common Bile Duct Stones: Data From the Swedish Registry for Gallstone Surgery and Endoscopic Retrograde Cholangiopancreatography (GallRiks)

Möller M, Gustafsson U, Rasmussen F, et al (Ersta Hosp, Stockholm, Sweden; Karolinska Institutet, Stockholm, Sweden; et al)
JAMA Surg 149:1008-1014, 2014

Importance.—The optimal strategy for common bile duct stones (CBDSs) encountered during cholecystectomy is yet to be determined.

Objective.—To evaluate the outcomes after various interventional techniques to clear the bile ducts and the natural course of CBDSs found during intraoperative cholangiography.

Design, Setting, and Participants.—In a large retrospective cohort analysis, we analyzed data from the Swedish Registry for Gallstone Surgery and Endoscopic Retrograde Cholangiopancreatography (GallRiks). We included all patients with CBDSs found on intraoperative cholangiography during cholecystectomy from May 1, 2005, through December 31, 2009.

Exposures.—Presence of CBDSs on intraoperative cholangiography.

Main Outcomes and Measures.—Relation between strategies for handling CBDSs in terms of complication rates and/or incomplete clearance with need of intervention (ie, unfavorable outcomes).

Results.—In 38 864 cholecystectomies, CBDSs were found in 3969 patients, of whom 3828 underwent analysis. Earlier or ongoing symptoms were more common with increasing stone size ($P < .001$). In total, postoperative unfavorable outcomes were found in 14.9% but less frequently for patients with smaller stones ($P < .01$). Among patients in whom no intraoperative measures were taken (representing natural course), the risk for unfavorable outcomes was 25.3%. This risk was significantly lower in patients in whom any measure was taken to clear the ducts (12.7%; odds ratio, 0.44 [95% CI, 0.35-0.55]). The same was found when small (<4 mm) and medium (4-8 mm) stones were analyzed separately (odds ratio, 0.52 [95% CI, 0.34-0.79] and 0.24 [95% CI, 0.17-0.32], respectively).

Conclusions and Relevance.—The high rates of unfavorable outcomes associated with taking no measures when CBDSs are found during cholecystectomy suggest that the natural course might not be as favorable as earlier suggested. This finding implies that, in general, efforts should be made to clear the bile ducts.

▶ What is the plan when a common bile duct stone is identified at the time of cholecystectomy? The choices are vast and include observation, intraoperative or postoperative endoscopic retrograde cholangiopancreatography and stone extraction, laparoscopic or open choledocotomy, laparoscopic transcystic stone extraction, and flushing of the common bile duct. Recently, many have advocated observation with the thought that the stone will pass without the need for intervention. Large stones or multiple stones probably need some type of intervention, however. This group found a surprisingly high percentage of patients who underwent cholecystectomy that found common bile duct stones, and as high as 25% had unfavorable outcomes when this path was taken (Table 4 in the original article). The size of the stone did not matter; even when stones were smaller than 4 mm there was still a 16% rate of complications from the stone. Most surgeons still use judgment at the time of surgery, based on the local expertise, individual technical ability, and resources, to assess the need for immediate intervention.

J. Hines, MD

Low-pressure versus standard-pressure pneumoperitoneum for laparoscopic cholecystectomy: a systematic review and meta-analysis
Hua J, Gong J, Yao L, et al (Tongji Univ of Medicine, Shanghai, China)
Am J Surg 208:143-150, 2014

Background.—The feasibility and safety of low-pressure pneumoperitoneum in laparoscopic cholecystectomy remain unclear.

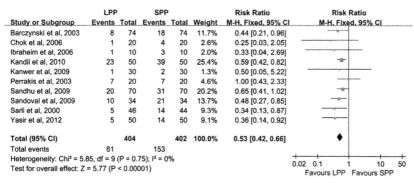

Study or Subgroup	LPP Events	Total	SPP Events	Total	Weight	Risk Ratio M-H, Fixed, 95% CI
Barczynski et al, 2003	8	74	18	74	11.7%	0.44 [0.21, 0.96]
Chok et al, 2006	1	20	4	20	2.6%	0.25 [0.03, 2.05]
Ibraheim et al, 2006	1	10	3	10	2.0%	0.33 [0.04, 2.69]
Kandil et al, 2010	23	50	39	50	25.4%	0.59 [0.42, 0.82]
Kanwer et al, 2009	1	30	2	30	1.3%	0.50 [0.05, 5.22]
Perrakis et al, 2003	7	20	7	20	4.6%	1.00 [0.43, 2.33]
Sandhu et al, 2009	20	70	31	70	20.2%	0.65 [0.41, 1.02]
Sandoval et al, 2009	10	34	21	34	13.7%	0.48 [0.27, 0.85]
Sarli et al, 2000	5	46	14	44	9.3%	0.34 [0.13, 0.87]
Yasir et al, 2012	5	50	14	50	9.1%	0.36 [0.14, 0.92]
Total (95% CI)		**404**		**402**	**100.0%**	**0.53 [0.42, 0.66]**
Total events	81		153			

Heterogeneity: Chi² = 5.85, df = 9 (P = 0.75); I² = 0%
Test for overall effect: Z = 5.77 (P < 0.00001)

Favours LPP   Favours SPP

FIGURE 4.—RR of incidence of shoulder pain in low-pressure versus standard-pressure pneumoperitoneum groups. Low-pressure pneumoperitoneum was associated with a significantly lower incidence of shoulder pain compared with standard-pressure pneumoperitoneum. LPP = low-pressure pneumoperitoneum; M-H = Mantel—Haenszel method; SPP = standard-pressure pneumoperitoneum. (Reprinted from The American Journal of Surgery. Hua J, Gong J, Yao L, et al. Low-pressure versus standard-pressure pneumoperitoneum for laparoscopic cholecystectomy: a systematic review and meta-analysis. Am J Surg. 2014;208:143-150, Copyright 2014, with permission from Elsevier.)

Methods.—A meta-analysis of randomized controlled trials comparing low-pressure with standard-pressure pneumoperitoneum was performed.

Results.—A total of 1,263 patients were included. Low-pressure pneumoperitoneum was associated with significantly decreased postoperative pain. The requirement for increased pressure was significantly greater in the low-pressure group (risk ratio = 6.16; $P < .001$). Operative time was similar, with only a slight statistical significance (weighted mean difference = 2.07; $P < .001$). Length of hospital stay was shorter in the low-pressure group (weighted mean difference = $-.27$; $P = .01$). No significant differences were found in surgical complications or conversion to open surgery.

Conclusions.—Low-pressure pneumoperitoneum is feasible and safe and results in reduced postoperative pain and near-equal operative time compared with standard-pressure pneumoperitoneum. More studies are required to investigate the potential benefits of the reduced length of hospital stay (Fig 4).

▶ The impact of CO_2 insufflation for laparoscopy on physiology is known and included diminished cardiac output, decreased pulmonary compliance, less kidney and liver perfusion, and potentially increased postoperative pain. Most commonly, we insufflate to a pressure of 12 to 15 mm Hg to adequately visualize the field of interest. This systematic review and meta-analysis examined the efficacy of low-pressure pneumoperitoneum on laparoscopic cholecystectomy. Overall postoperative pain scores, which were half the reported incidence of shoulder pain (Fig 4), showed lower pain medication usage, and no difference in intraoperative complications or rate of conversion to an open operation. In this time of increased financial pressure, an interesting finding was that the length of hospital stay was shorter in the low-pressure group—about a 6-hour advantage. Operating time was 2 minutes longer in the low-pressure group, but this was significantly longer because of the large number of patients included. This finding is not likely to convert to any practical significance. Generally, low pressure refers to pressures of 7 to 10 mm Hg.

J. Hines, MD

Is Nighttime the Right Time? Risk of Complications after Laparoscopic Cholecystectomy at Night

Phatak UR, Chan WM, Lew DF et al (Univ of Texas Health Science Ctr at Houston)

J Am Coll Surg 219:718-724, 2014

Background.—Laparoscopic cholecystectomies can be performed at night in high-volume acute care hospitals. We hypothesized that nonelective nighttime laparoscopic cholecystectomies are associated with increased postoperative complications.

Study Design.—We conducted a single-center retrospective review of consecutive laparoscopic cholecystectomy patients between October 2010 and May 2011 at a safety-net hospital in Houston, Texas. Data were collected on demographics, operative time, time of incision, length of stay, 30-day postoperative complications (ie, bile leak/biloma, common bile duct injury, retained stone, superficial surgical site infection, organ space abscess, and bleeding) and death. Statistical analyses were performed using STATA software (version 12; Stata Corp).

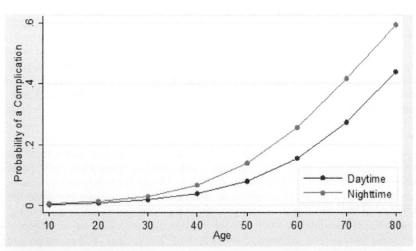

FIGURE 2.—Predicted probability of a complication by age after laparoscopic cholecystectomy at nighttime vs daytime. (Reprinted from the Journal of the American College of Surgeons. Phatak UR, Chan WM, Lew DF, et al. Is nighttime the right time? Risk of complications after laparoscopic cholecystectomy at night. *J Am Coll Surg.* 2014;219:718-724, Copyright 2014, with permission from the American College of Surgeons.)

Results.—During 8 months, 356 patients had nonelective laparoscopic cholecystectomies. A majority were female (n = 289 [81.1%]) and Hispanic (n = 299 [84%]). There were 108 (30%) nighttime operations. There were 29 complications in 18 patients; there were fewer daytime than nighttime patients who had at least 1 complication (4.0% vs 7.4%; $p = 0.18$). On multivariate analysis, age (odds ratio = 1.06 per year; 95% CI, 1.02—1.10; $p = 0.002$), case duration (odds ratio = 1.02 per minute; 95% CI, 1.01—1.02; $p = 0.001$), and nighttime surgery (odds ratio = 3.33; 95% CI, 1.14—9.74; $p = 0.001$) were associated with an increased risk of 30-day surgical complications. Length of stay was significantly longer for daytime than nighttime patients (median 3 vs 2 days; $p < 0.001$).

Conclusions.—Age, case duration, and nighttime laparoscopic cholecystectomy were predictive of increased 30-day surgical complications at a high-volume safety-net hospital. The small but increased risk of complications with nighttime laparoscopic cholecystectomy must be balanced against improved efficiency at a high-volume, resource-poor hospital (Fig 2).

▶ Who wants to operate at night? For those of us who are so busy, this may be the only option for urgent cases that come into the emergency room. And one of the most common procedures is cholecystectomy. There is a fair amount of evidence to show that operations performed at night will result in higher complication rates. This study examines the issue of day or night operations and whether patients' outcomes differ. Age, length of operation, and night time operation were associated with increased 30-day surgical complication rate. Having the surgery at night increases the odds of a complication by 333% (Fig 2). This was the case even when the difficulty of the procedures was evenly distributed throughout the day and night. So what is the solution? You can ask the facility to dedicate a room for urgent cases that can be completed during the daytime when all of the personnel and expertise are available. This activity will help decrease length of stay, decrease complications, and increase revenue for the facility. The added bonus will be that you can sleep at night and provided a higher level of care for your patients.

J. Hines, MD

Long-Term Health-Related Quality of Life after Iatrogenic Bile Duct Injury Repair

Ejaz A, Spolverato G, Kim Y, et al (Johns Hopkins Hosp, Baltimore, MD)
J Am Coll Surg 219:923-932, 2014

Background.—Data on the effect of bile duct injuries (BDI) on health-related quality of life (HRQOL) are not well defined. We sought to assess long-term HRQOL after BDI repair in a large cohort of patients spanning a 23-year period.

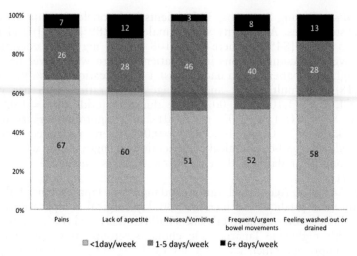

FIGURE 4.—Current incidence of commonly reported symptoms. (Reprinted from the Journal of the American College of Surgeons. Ejaz A, Spolverato G, Kim Y, et al. Long-term health-related quality of life after iatrogenic bile duct injury repair. *J Am Coll Surg.* 2014;219:923-932, Copyright 2014, with permission from American College of Surgeons.)

Study Design.—We identified and mailed HRQOL questionnaires to all patients treated for major BDI after laparoscopic cholecystectomy between January 1, 1990 and December 31, 2012 at Johns Hopkins Hospital.

Results.—We identified 167 patients alive at the time of the study who met the inclusion criteria. Median age at BDI was 42 years (interquartile range 31 to 54 years); the majority of patients were female (n = 131 [78.4%]) and of white race (n = 137 [83.0%]). Most patients had Bismuth level 2 (n = 56 [33.7%]) or Bismuth level 3 (n = 40 [24.1%]) BDI. Surgical repair most commonly involved a Roux-en-Y hepaticojejunostomy (n = 142 [86.1%]). Sixty-two patients (37.1%) responded to the HRQOL questionnaire. Median follow-up was 169 months (interquartile range 125 to 222 months). At the time of BDI, mental health was most affected, with patients commonly reporting a depressed mood (49.2%) or low energy level (40.0%). These symptoms improved significantly after definitive repair (both $p < 0.05$). Limitations in physical activity and general health remained unchanged before and after surgical repair (both $p > 0.05$).

Conclusions.—Mental health concerns were more commonplace vs physical or general health issues among patients with BDI followed long term. Optimal multidisciplinary management of BDI can help restore HRQOL to preinjury levels (Fig 4).

▶ Most have experienced the very unfortunate situation of a common bile duct injury during cholecystectomy. The algorithm to address this injury is fairly standard and the outcomes for the patients reasonable. This study examined the long-term impact of common bile duct injury on patients' well-being. Most of these patients experienced a Bismuth level 2 or 3 injury (mid to high common duct injury).[1] Before definitive repair, many patients reported that the biliary tubes were embarrassing and impacted their relationships negatively. The long-term outcomes specific to the repair were particularly favorable with nearly 90% of patients receiving a Roux-en-Y hepaticojejunostomy. A fair number of patients, however, continued to experience pain, lack of appetite, nausea, frequent bowel movements and fatigue (Fig 4). Seventy percent of patients sought litigation, and most stated that they had won the suit. These patients had no better long-term outcomes, however, than those who did not sue or lost. Overall, this group reported that multidisciplinary management of bile duct injuries can restore health-related quality of life to preinjury levels.

J. Hines, MD

Reference

1. Bismuth H, Majno PE. Biliary strictures: classification based on the principles of surgical treatment. *World J Surg.* 2001;25:1241-1244.

Laparoscopic Transgastric Necrosectomy for the Management of Pancreatic Necrosis
Worhunsky DJ, Qadan M, Dua MM, et al (Stanford Univ Med Ctr, CA)
J Am Coll Surg 219:735-743, 2014

Background.—Traditional open necrosectomy for pancreatic necrosis is associated with significant morbidity and mortality. Although minimally invasive techniques have been described and offer some promise, each has considerable limitations. This study assesses the safety and effectiveness of laparoscopic transgastric necrosectomy (LTN), a novel technique for the management of necrotizing pancreatitis.

Study Design.—Between 2009 and 2013, patients with retrogastric pancreatic necrosis requiring debridement were evaluated for LTN. Debridement was performed via a laparoscopic transgastric approach using 2 to 3 ports and the wide cystgastrostomy left open. Patient demographics, disease severity, operative characteristics, and outcomes were collected and analyzed.

Results.—Twenty-one patients (13 men, median age 54 years; interquartile range [IQR] 46 to 62 years) underwent LTN during the study period. The duration between pancreatitis onset and debridement was 65 days (IQR 53 to 124 years). Indications for operation included infection (7 patients) and persistent unwellness (14 patients). Median duration of LTN was 170 minutes (IQR 136 to 199 minutes); there were no conversions. Control of the necrosis was achieved via the single procedure in 19 of 21 patients. Median postoperative hospital stay was 5 days (IQR 3 to 14 days) and the majority (71%) of patients experienced no (n = 9) or only minor postoperative complications (n = 6) by Clavien-Dindo grade.

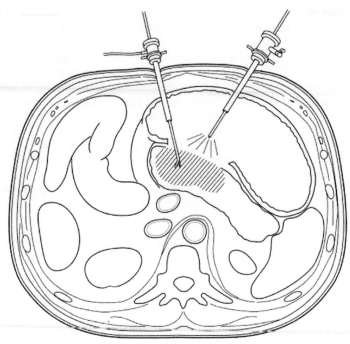

FIGURE 1.—Laparoscopic transgastric necrosectomy. (B) Schematic showing port placement and approach to necrosum. (Reprinted from the Journal of the American College of Surgeons. Worhunsky DJ, Qadan M, Dua MM, et al. Laparoscopic transgastric necrosectomy for the management of pancreatic necrosis. *J Am Coll Surg*. 2014;219:735-743, Copyright 2014, with permission from the American College of Surgeons.)

Complications of Clavien-Dindo grade 3 or higher developed in 6 patients, including 1 death (5%). With a median follow-up of 11 months (IQR 7 to 22 months), none of the patients required additional operative debridement or had pancreatic/enteric fistulae or wound complications develop.

Conclusions.—Laparoscopic transgastric necrosectomy is a novel, minimally invasive technique for the management of pancreatic necrosis that allows for debridement in a single operation. When feasible, LTN can reduce the morbidity associated with traditional open necrosectomy and avoid the limitations of other minimally invasive approaches (Fig 1B).

▶ The management of severe acute pancreatitis has evolved substantially over the last 10 years. If you are still treating patients with this entity the same way that you did during training, it is probably time to update your practice. You learned over the last decade that early operation leads to worse outcomes. Patients with sterile necrosis should be generally treated nonoperatively. Those with infected necrosis should be first treated with percutaneous drainage, and then a consideration for debridement can be made. This study out of Stanford details the use of a laparoscopic transgastric approach to debride infected necrosis (Fig 1B). In the hands of this group, this approach was highly effective.

There was one death caused by bleeding and a much lower rate of complications compared with that of standard open techniques. Newer techniques, including percutaneous drainage and lavage, endoscopic transgastric drainage, laparoscopic-assisted debridement, and at the minimally invasive retroperitoneal debridement, are all acceptable approaches with excellent outcomes and fewer complications. Going forward, some type of step-up approach should be part of your treatment for severe acute necrotizing pancreatitis.

J. Hines, MD

Natural resolution or intervention for fluid collections in acute severe pancreatitis
Sarathi Patra P, Das K, Bhattacharyya A, et al (Inst of Post-Graduate Med Education and Res, Kolkata, India)
Br J Surg 101:1721-1728, 2014

Background.—Revisions in terminology of fluid collections in acute pancreatitis have necessitated reanalysis of their evolution and outcome. The course of fluid collections in patients with acute pancreatitis was evaluated prospectively.

Methods.—Consecutive adults with acute pancreatitis, who had contrast-enhanced CT (CECT) within $5-7$ days of symptom onset, were enrolled in a prospective cohort study in a tertiary-care centre. Patients were treated according to standard guidelines. Follow-up transabdominal ultrasonography was done at 4-week intervals for at least 6 months. CECT was repeated at $6-10$ weeks, or at any time if there were new or persistent symptoms. Asymptomatic collections were followed until spontaneous resolution. Risk factors for pancreatic pseudocysts or walled-off necrosis (WON) were assessed in multivariable analyses.

Results.—Of 122 patients with acute pancreatitis, 109 were analysed. Some 91 patients (83·5 per cent) had fluid collections at baseline. Eleven of 29 with interstitial oedematous pancreatitis had acute peripancreatic fluid collections, none of which evolved into pseudocysts. All 80 patients with acute necrotizing pancreatitis had at least one acute necrotizing collection (ANC); of these, five patients died (2 after drainage), three underwent successful drainage within 5 weeks, and collections resolved spontaneously in 33 and evolved into WON in 39. By 6 months' follow-up, WON had required drainage in eight patients, resolved spontaneously in 23 and was persistent but asymptomatic in seven. Factors associated with increased risk of WON were blood urea nitrogen 20 mg/dl or more (odds ratio (OR) 10·96, 95 per cent c.i. 2·57 to 46·73; $P = 0·001$) and baseline ANC diameter greater than 6 cm (OR 14·57, 1·60 to 132·35; $P - 0·017$). Baseline ANC diameter over 6 cm was the only independent predictor of either the need for drainage or persistence of such collections beyond 6 months (hazard ratio 6·61, 1·77 to 24·59; $P = 0·005$).

Conclusion.—Pancreatic pseudocysts develop infrequently in oedematous acute pancreatitis. Only one-quarter of ANCs either require intervention or persist beyond 6 months, whereas more than one-half of WONs resolve without any intervention within 6 months of onset. Baseline diameter of ANC(s) is an important predictor of outcome.

▶ Understanding the natural history of severe acute pancreatitis and the various intra-abdominal fluid collections that accompany this entity helps the surgeon make clinical decisions and determine the need for intervention. In this series of patients, most of whom had fluid collection, none developed a pseudocyst. Many of the patients had pancreatic necrosis, and most never required intervention, the pancreatitis resolving with observation. When intervention was required for infection, these were generally managed with a mixture of percutaneous drainage and surgical debridement. Most patients with severe necrotizing pancreatitis do not require operative debridement, and the group found that a significant change in blood urea nitrogen or a collection greater than 6 cm predicted a higher chance of required intervention. As long as patients remain asymptomatic and without signs of infection, it is safe to observe these collections until resolution. It makes sense to document resolution with a CT scan after discharge.

J. Hines, MD

Meta-analysis of randomized controlled trials comparing Lichtenstein and totally extraperitoneal laparoscopic hernioplasty in treatment of inguinal hernias
Bobo Z, Nan W, Qin Q, et al (Fourth Military Med Univ, Xi'an, China)
J Surg Res 192:409-420, 2014

Background.—Finding the optimal approach to repair an inguinal hernia is controversial. Therefore, for the scientific evaluation of the total extraperitoneal (TEP) and Lichtenstein mesh techniques for the repair of inguinal hernia, meta-analyses of randomized controlled trials are necessary.

Methods.—A complete literature search was conducted in the Cochrane Controlled Trials Register Databases, Pubmed, Embase, International Scientific Institute databases, and Chinese Biomedical Literature Database in various languages.

Results.—Randomized controlled trials (13), including 3279 patients, were retrieved from the electronic databases. The Lichtenstein group was associated with a shorter operating time; however, results show that TEP repair enabled patients a shorter time to return to work, less chronic pain compared with Lichtenstein operation. There was no significant difference in seromas, wound infections, or neuralgia. There are no statistically significant difference in terms of hernia recurrence when the follow-up time is ≤3 y. When follow-up time is >3 y, TEP repair shows a higher recurrence rate compared with Lichtenstein repairs.

Conclusions.—There was insufficient evidence to determine the greater effectiveness between TEP and Lichtenstein mesh techniques. In future

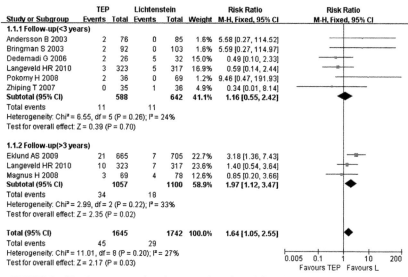

Study or Subgroup	TEP Events	Total	Lichtenstein Events	Total	Weight	Risk Ratio M-H, Fixed, 95% CI
1.1.1 Follow-up(<3 years)						
Andersson B 2003	2	76	0	85	1.6%	5.58 [0.27, 114.52]
Bringman S 2003	2	92	0	103	1.6%	5.59 [0.27, 114.97]
Dedemadi G 2006	2	26	5	32	15.0%	0.49 [0.10, 2.33]
Langeveld HR 2010	3	323	5	317	16.9%	0.59 [0.14, 2.44]
Pokorny H 2008	2	36	0	69	1.2%	9.46 [0.47, 191.93]
Zhiping T 2007	0	35	1	36	4.9%	0.34 [0.01, 8.14]
Subtotal (95% CI)		**588**		**642**	**41.1%**	**1.16 [0.55, 2.42]**
Total events	11		11			
Heterogeneity: Chi² = 6.55, df = 5 (P = 0.26); I² = 24%						
Test for overall effect: Z = 0.39 (P = 0.70)						
1.1.2 Follow-up(>3 years)						
Eklund AS 2009	21	665	7	705	22.7%	3.18 [1.36, 7.43]
Langeveld HR 2010	10	323	7	317	23.6%	1.40 [0.54, 3.64]
Magnus H 2008	3	69	4	78	12.6%	0.85 [0.20, 3.66]
Subtotal (95% CI)		**1057**		**1100**	**58.9%**	**1.97 [1.12, 3.47]**
Total events	34		18			
Heterogeneity: Chi² = 2.99, df = 2 (P = 0.22); I² = 33%						
Test for overall effect: Z = 2.35 (P = 0.02)						
Total (95% CI)		**1645**		**1742**	**100.0%**	**1.64 [1.05, 2.55]**
Total events	45		29			
Heterogeneity: Chi² = 11.01, df = 8 (P = 0.20); I² = 27%						
Test for overall effect: Z = 2.17 (P = 0.03)						

Favours TEP   Favours L

FIGURE 2.—Hernia recurrence: the subgroup analysis showed that there was no significant difference between TEP and Lichtenstein when follow-up time is ≤3 y. However, when follow-up time is >3 y, the subgroup analysis demonstrated a significant difference between the two groups. (Color version of figure is available online.) (Reprinted from The Journal of Surgical Research. Bobo Z, Nan W, Qin Q, et al. Meta-analysis of randomized controlled trials comparing Lichtenstein and totally extraperitoneal laparoscopic hernioplasty in treatment of inguinal hernias. *J Surg Res.* 2014;192:409-420, Copyright 2014, with permission from Elsevier.)

research, it is necessary for subgroup analyses of unilateral primary hernias, recurrent hernias, and simultaneous bilateral repair to be conducted to define the indications for the TEP approach (Fig 2).

▶ Are you an open or laparoscopic surgeon when it comes to inguinal hernia repair? Maybe you are both depending on the circumstances of the patient's condition. This large meta-analysis of more than 3000 patients compared Lichtenstein with laparoscopic extraperitoneal repair of inguinal hernias. Overall, return to work and activities was faster for the laparoscopic group, but the long-term recurrence rate was higher in this group (Fig 2). These patients also experience less chronic pain. Lichtenstein patients enjoyed shorter operations and less testicular pain postoperatively. Good advice for your patients might go something like this: If you have a single-sided hernia, an open repair probably makes sense because the anesthetic risk is slightly lower, the recovery almost equal, and the recurrence slightly less. If you have a bilateral hernia and are a good anesthetic risk, then a laparoscopic approach is best. For patients with recurrent inguinal hernias, it probably makes sense to take an alternate approach to the problem using a laparoscope. This series of recommendations covers most situations, but you will need to keep nimble with several techniques available to assure the best outcome for your patient.

J. Hines, MD

Incidence of and risk factors for incisional hernia after abdominal surgery

Itatsu K, Yokoyama Y, Sugawara G, et al (Nagoya Univ Graduate School of Medicine, Japan; Social Insurance Chukyo Hosp, Japan; et al)
Br J Surg 101:1439-1447, 2014

Background.—Few larger studies have estimated the incidence of incisional hernia (IH) after abdominal surgery.

Methods.—Patients who had abdominal surgery between November 2009 and February 2011 were included in the study. The incidence rate and risk factors for IH were monitored for at least 180 days.

Results.—A total of 4305 consecutive patients were registered. Of these, 378 were excluded because of failure to complete follow-up and 3927 patients were analysed. IH was diagnosed in 318 patients. The estimated incidence rates for IH were 5·2 per cent at 12 months and 10·3 per cent at 24 months. In multivariable analysis, wound classification III and IV (hazard ratio (HR) 2·26, 95 per cent confidence interval 1·52 to 3·35), body mass index of 25 kg/m² or higher (HR 1·76, 1·35 to 2·30), midline incision (HR 1·74, 1·28 to 2·38), incisional surgical-site infection (I-SSI) (HR 1·68, 1·24 to 2·28), preoperative chemotherapy (HR 1·61, 1·08 to 2·37), blood transfusion (HR 1·46, 1·04 to 2·05), increasing age by 10-year interval (HR 1·30, 1·16 to 1·45), female sex (HR 1·26, 1·01 to 1·59) and thickness of subcutaneous tissue for every 1-cm increase (HR 1·18, 1·03 to 1·35) were identified as independent risk factors. Compared with superficial I-SSI, deep I-SSI was more strongly associated with the development of IH.

Conclusion.—Although there are several risk factors for IH, reducing I-SSI is an important step in the prevention of IH. Registration number: UMIN000004723 (University Hospital Medical Information Network, http://www.umin.ac.jp/ctr/index.htm) (Fig 2, Table 3).

▶ Incisional hernias are common and often a source of consternation for our patients. We all know that avoiding wound infections and optimizing patient factors can help, but the true incidence of this problem is not truly known. This large-scale study that included 4000 patients found an incisional hernia rate of 5.2% at 12 months and 10.3% at 2 years. Risk factors included wound infections (Fig 2), obesity, a midline incision, blood transfusion, female sex, and preoperative chemotherapy (Table 3). Interestingly, for every 1 cm increase in abdominal wall fat there was an 18% increase in risk for the development of a hernia. The type of closure was not assessed by this study but was largely performed with interrupted braided suture. Others have suggested that running monofilament sutures work best.[1] I find these types of problems to be a real nuisance. We have the surgeon who focuses on this and all the nuances and techniques required for the repair of complex abdominal wall hernias. I am grateful for his expertise. Who

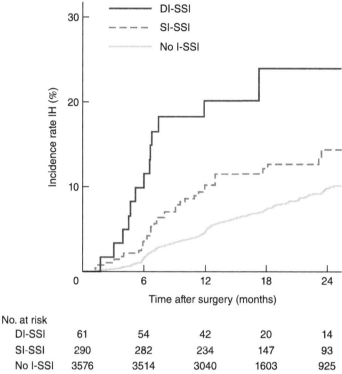

FIGURE 2.—Kaplan—Meier analysis of incisional hernia (IH) in relation to depth of incisional surgical-site infection (I-SSI). DI-SSI, deep incisional surgical-site infection; SI-SSI, superficial incisional surgical-site infection. $P = 0.001$ (DI-SSI versus SI-SSI), $P < 0.001$ (DI-SSI versus no I-SSI) (log rank test). (Reprinted from Itatsu K, Yokoyama Y, Sugawara G, et al. Incidence of and risk factors for incisional hernia after abdominal surgery. *Br J Surg.* 2014;101:1439-1447, © British Journal of Surgery Society Ltd. Reproduced with permission. Permission is granted by John Wiley & Sons Ltd on behalf of the BJSS Ltd.)

TABLE 3.—Multivariable Cox Regression Analysis of Independent Risk Factors for Incisional Hernia

	Hazard Ratio	P
Age (for every 10-year increase)	1·30 (1·16, 1·45)	< 0·001
Sex (F *versus* M)	1·26 (1·01, 1·59)	0·042
Body mass index (≥ 25 *versus* < 25 kg/m^2)	1·76 (1·35, 2·30)	< 0·001
Preoperative chemotherapy	1·61 (1·08, 2·37)	0·017
Thickness of subcutaneous fat based on CT (for every 1-cm increase)	1·18 (1·03, 1·35)	0·017
Wound classification (III/IV *versus* I/II)	2·26 (1·52, 3·35)	< 0·001
Intraoperative blood transfusion	1·46 (1·04, 2·05)	0·028
Type of incision (midline *versus* non-midline)	1·74 (1·28, 2·38)	< 0·001
Incisional surgical-site infection	1·68 (1·24, 2·28)	< 0·001

Values in parentheses are 95 per cent confidence intervals. CT, computed tomography.

Reprinted from Itatsu K, Yokoyama Y, Sugawara G, et al. Incidence of and risk factors for incisional hernia after abdominal surgery. *Br J Surg.* 2014;101:1439-1447. © British Journal of Surgery Society Ltd. Reproduced with permission. Permission is granted by John Wiley & Sons Ltd on behalf of the BJSS Ltd.

knew that the risk of a hernia after an abdominal surgery was as high as 10% at 2 years?

J. Hines, MD

Reference

1. van't Riet M, Steyerberg EW, Nellensteyn J, Bonjer HJ, Jeekel J. Meta-analysis of techniques for closure of midline abdominal incisions. *Br J Surg.* 2002;89: 1350-1356.

Hernia repair in the presence of ascites
Ecker BL, Bartlett EK, Hoffman RL, et al (Univ of Pennsylvania, Philadelphia)
J Surg Res 190:471-477, 2014

Background.—The model for end-stage liver disease (MELD) has been validated as a prediction tool for postoperative mortality, but its role in predicting morbidity has not been well studied. We sought to determine the role of MELD, among other factors, in predicting morbidity and mortality in patients with nonmalignant ascites undergoing hernia repair.

Methods.—All patients undergoing hernia repair in the American College of Surgeons National Surgical Quality Improvement database (2009—11) were identified. Those with nonmalignant ascites were compared with patients without ascites. A subset analysis of patients with nonmalignant ascites was performed to evaluate the association between MELD and morbidity and mortality with adjustment for potential confounders. The association of significant factors with the rate of morbidity was displayed using a best-fit polynomial regression.

Results.—Of 138,366 hernia repairs, 778 (0.56%) were performed on patients with nonmalignant ascites. Thirty-day morbidity (4% versus 19%) and mortality (0.2% versus 5.3%) were significantly more frequent in patients with ascites ($P < 0.001$). In univariate analysis of the 636 patients with a calculable MELD, MELD was associated with both morbidity and mortality ($P < 0.001$ each). In multivariate analysis, MELD remained significantly associated with morbidity (odds ratio [OR] = 1.11). Ventral hernia repair (OR = 2.9), dependent functional status (OR = 2.3), alcohol use (OR = 2.3), emergent operation (OR = 2.0) white blood count (OR = 1.1), and age (OR = 1.02) were also significantly associated with morbidity ($P < 0.05$).

Conclusions.—Before hernia repair, the MELD score can be used to risk-stratify patients with nonmalignant ascites not only for mortality but also morbidity. Morbidity rates increase rapidly with MELD above 15, but other factors should additionally be accounted for when counseling patients on their perioperative risk.

▶ We all have been asked to perform a hernia repair in a patient with ascites. This is generally a difficult decision but mostly discouraged given the issues of complications and recurrence. This study examined the use of model for end-staged liver disease (MELD) score to predict outcome for these patients. This has a 3-month mortality after transjugular intrahepatic portosystemic shunt procedure. This score incorporates serum creatinine, total bilirubin, and international normalized ratio. Some important findings from this study suggest that MELD is quite predictive of outcome for this group. For patients with a MELD < 10, the morbidity rate was 15%; for MELD 10-19, morbidity was 20%; for MELD 20-29, morbidity was 42%; and for those with a MELD of ≥30, morbidity was 100%. For every point increase above a MELD of 15, the morbidity increases 3%. This is an easy way to make an assessment for these patients, and the data can help inform the patient about the final decision.

J. Hines, MD

10 Oncology

Breast

Anastrozole for prevention of breast cancer in high-risk postmenopausal women (IBIS-II): an international, double-blind, randomised placebo-controlled trial
Cuzick J, on behalf of the IBIS-II investigators (Queen Mary Univ of London, UK; et al)
Lancet 383:1041-1048, 2014

Background.—Aromatase inhibitors effectively prevent breast cancer recurrence and development of new contralateral tumours in postmenopausal women. We assessed the efficacy and safety of the aromatase inhibitor anastrozole for prevention of breast cancer in postmenopausal women who are at high risk of the disease.

Methods.—Between Feb 2, 2003, and Jan 31, 2012, we recruited postmenopausal women aged 40–70 years from 18 countries into an international, double-blind, randomised placebo-controlled trial. To be eligible, women had to be at increased risk of breast cancer (judged on the basis of specific criteria). Eligible women were randomly assigned (1:1) by central computer allocation to receive 1 mg oral anastrozole or matching placebo every day for 5 years. Randomisation was stratified by country and was done with blocks (size six, eight, or ten). All trial personnel, participants, and clinicians were masked to treatment allocation; only the trial statistician was unmasked. The primary endpoint was histologically confirmed breast cancer (invasive cancers or non-invasive ductal carcinoma in situ). Analyses were done by intention to treat. This trial is registered, number ISRCTN31488319.

Findings.—1920 women were randomly assigned to receive anastrozole and 1944 to placebo. After a median follow-up of 5·0 years (IQR 3·0–7·1), 40 women in the anastrozole group (2%) and 85 in the placebo group (4%) had developed breast cancer (hazard ratio 0·47, 95% CI 0·32–0·68, $p < 0·0001$). The predicted cumulative incidence of all breast cancers after 7 years was 5·6% in the placebo group and 2·8% in the anastrozole group. 18 deaths were reported in the anastrozole group and 17 in the placebo group, and no specific causes were more common in one group than the other ($p = 0·836$).

307

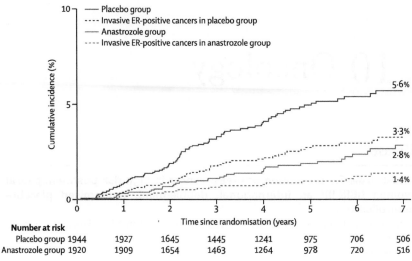

FIGURE 3.—Cumulative incidence of all breast cancers and of invasive ER-positive breast cancers. ER = oestrogen receptor. (Reprinted from The Lancet. Cuzick J, on behalf of the IBIS-II investigators. Anastrozole for prevention of breast cancer in high-risk postmenopausal women (IBIS-II): an international, double-blind, randomised placebo-controlled trial. *Lancet.* 2014;383:1041-1048 Copyright 2014, with permission from Elsevier.)

Interpretation.—Anastrozole effectively reduces incidence of breast cancer in high-risk postmenopausal women. This finding, along with the fact that most of the side-effects associated with oestrogen deprivation were not attributable to treatment, provides support for the use of anastrozole in postmenopausal women at high risk of breast cancer (Fig 3).

▶ Estrogen receptor modulators such as tamoxifen, and aromatase inhibitors, which inhibit the conversion of androgens to estrogens, have been found useful in the prevention of recurrence and development of contralateral breast cancers in the adjuvant setting. The adjuvant utility of the aromatase inhibitor, exemestane, has been found to be significant, with more than 50% reduction in breast cancers. In this trial (MAP.3), the follow-up was only a median of 3 years. The objective of this study (IBIS-II) was to study the efficacy of a different aromatase inhibitor, anastrozole, in the prevention of breast cancers with longer follow-up. Patients selected for this study needed to be considered at high risk for breast cancer development and generally postmenopausal. In younger age groups, such as 40 to 44 year olds, the calculated risk of breast cancer would need to be 4 times higher than that of the normal population; in ages 45 to 60, the risk would need to be 2-fold higher; in ages 60 to 70, it would have to 1.5 times higher than their the normal counterparts. Premenopausal patients, those with a previous diagnosis of breast cancer (not including ductal carcinoma in situ [DCIS]), and those with severe osteoporosis, were excluded. A total of 1920 patients were randomly assigned to receive 5 years of anastrozole and 1944 to receive 5 years of placebo. The compliance was approximately 70% over the duration of these 5 years, and patients were followed up annually and mammograms were done at least every other year. The median follow-up was 5.0 years, and 32 patients (1.7%) in the anastrozole group had subsequent invasive breast cancer, and 64 (3.2%) of the patients in the placebo group had subsequent invasive breast cancer (Fig 3). These differences were statistically significantly different as was the incidence of DCIS, which developed in 6 patients in the anastrozole group and 20 in the placebo group. The greatest risk reduction was in estrogen receptor-positive cancers, and there was no significant difference in *estrogen receptor*-negative cancers. These benefits were seen across all groups regardless of age, body mass index, previous presence of DCIS, or previous use of hormone therapy. There was an increased prevention of high-grade invasive cancers in the anastrozole group. Side effects of the treatment were minimal and did not involve cardiovascular effects as seen with other agents, but there was an increased frequency in musculoskeletal events, especially moderate arthralgia, carpal tunnel symptoms, joint stiffness, increased vasomotor symptoms, and hypertension. There was no overall difference in other types of tumors, although there was a statistically significant decrease in nonmelanoma skin cancer and colorectal cancer in the anastrozole group. This study once again confirmed the utility of aromatase inhibitors in the prevention of breast cancer in women at high risk, with minimal side effects. This study did not address the utility of this agent in the adjuvant role for patients with breast cancer or its usefulness in premenopausal patients at high risk for breast cancer.

J. R. Howe, MD

Sector Resection With or Without Postoperative Radiotherapy for Stage I Breast Cancer: 20-Year Results of a Randomized Trial

Wickberg Å, Holmberg L, Adami H-O, et al (Örebro Univ Hosp, Sweden; Uppsala Univ, Sweden; Karolinska Institutet, Stockholm, Sweden; et al)
J Clin Oncol 32:791-797, 2014

Purpose.—To investigate how radiotherapy (XRT) adds to tumor control using a standardized surgical technique with meticulous control of surgical margins in a randomized trial with 20 years of follow-up.

Patients and Methods.—Three hundred eighty-one women with pT1N0 breast cancer were randomly assigned to sector resection with (XRT group) or without (non-XRT group) postoperative radiotherapy to the breast. With follow-up through 2010, we estimated cumulative proportion of recurrence, breast cancer death, and all-cause mortality.

Results.—The cumulative probability of a first breast cancer event of any type after 20 years was 30.9% in the XRT group and 45.1% in the non-XRT group (hazard ratio [HR], 0.58; 95% CI, 0.41 to 0.82). The benefit of radiotherapy was achieved within the first 5 years. After 20 years, 50.4% of the women in the XRT group died compared with 54.0% in the non-XRT group (HR, 0.92; 95% CI, 0.71 to 1.19). The cumulative probability of contralateral cancer or death as a result of cancer other than breast cancer was 27.1% in the XRT group and 24.9% in the non-XRT group (HR, 1.17; 95% CI, 0.77 to 1.77). In an anticipated low-risk group, the cumulative incidence of first breast cancer of any type was 24.8% in the XRT group and 36.1% in the non-XRT group (HR, 0.61; 95% CI, 0.35 to 1.07).

Conclusion.—Radiotherapy protects against recurrences during the first 5 years of follow-up, indicating that XRT mainly eradicates undetected cancer foci present at primary treatment. The similar rate of recurrences beyond 5 years in the two groups indicates that late recurrences are new tumors. There are subgroups with clinically relevant differences in risk.

▶ Multiple trials have found that the addition of radiation therapy to breast conservation surgery reduces local recurrence rates. A recent meta-analysis showed that not only was there a reduction in breast cancer-specific death and recurrence in patients treated with radiation, but that this effect was partially negated by increased risk of cardiovascular disease and lung cancer, likely as a consequence of the radiation. These effects were seen mostly in the second decade. The current study is a 20-year follow-up of a trial in which patients with stage 1 breast cancer had resection of the sector and ipsilateral level 1 and 2 axillary dissection followed by random assignment to either postoperative radiation therapy or no radiation therapy. No patients received adjuvant therapy. After 20 years of follow-up, they found that there was an absolute decrease in recurrent breast cancer by 14% in the group receiving radiation. Furthermore, the effect of radiation was seen within the first 5 years (Fig 2a in the original article). Other factors, such as the development of contralateral breast cancer, death from breast cancer, and death from other causes were not significantly different in the 2 groups. In this trial, there was not an increased risk of cardiovascular events after radiation therapy. The final conclusions were that radiation therapy protects against local recurrence within the first 5 years, but after therapy does not protect against breast cancer death or other causes of death. The treatment received by patients in this trial is significantly different from the treatment that these patients might receive today, because all had axillary dissections, and none were treated with adjuvant chemotherapy or tamoxifen. However, this study effectively showed (once again) that radiation reduces local recurrence and did not find an increased risk of lung tumors or cardiac events associated with this treatment.

J. R. Howe, MD

Breast-Conserving Treatment With or Without Radiotherapy in Ductal Carcinoma In Situ: 15-Year Recurrence Rates and Outcome After a Recurrence, From the EORTC 10853 Randomized Phase III Trial
Donker M, Litière S, Werutsky G, et al (The Netherlands Cancer Inst, Amsterdam; European Organisation for Research and Treatment of Cancer (EORTC), Brussels, Belgium; et al)
J Clin Oncol 31:4054-4059, 2013

Purpose.—Adjuvant radiotherapy (RT) after a local excision (LE) for ductal carcinoma in situ (DCIS) aims at reduction of the incidence of a local recurrence (LR). We analyzed the long-term risk on developing LR and its impact on survival after local treatment for DCIS.

Patients and Methods.—Between 1986 and 1996, 1,010 women with complete LE of DCIS less than 5 cm were randomly assigned to no further treatment (LE group, n = 503) or RT (LE+RT group, n = 507). The median follow-up time was 15.8 years.

Results.—Radiotherapy reduced the risk of any LR by 48% (hazard ratio [HR], 0.52; 95% CI, 0.40 to 0.68; $P < .001$). The 15-year LR-free rate was 69% in the LE group, which was increased to 82% in the LE+RT group. The 15-year invasive LR-free rate was 84% in the LE group and 90% in the LE+RT group (HR, 0.61; 95% CI, 0.42 to 0.87). The differences in LR in both arms did not lead to differences in breast cancer—specific survival (BCSS; HR, 1.07; 95% CI, 0.60 to 1.91) or overall survival (OS; HR, 1.02; 95% CI, 0.71 to 1.44). Patients with invasive LR had a significantly worse BCSS (HR, 17.66; 95% CI, 8.86 to 35.18) and OS (HR, 5.17; 95% CI, 3.09 to 8.66) compared with those who did not experience recurrence. A lower overall salvage mastectomy rate after LR was observed in the LE+RT group than in the LE group (13% v 19%, respectively).

Conclusion.—At 15 years, almost one in three nonirradiated women developed an LR after LE for DCIS. RT reduced this risk by a factor of 2. Although women who developed an invasive recurrence had worse survival, the long-term prognosis was good and independent of the given treatment.

▶ Multiple studies have shown the advantages of local excision and radiation therapy on the reduction of local recurrence in ductal carcinoma in situ (DCIS). These include the National Surgical Adjuvant Breast and Bowel Project B-17 trial, the SweDCIS trial, and the UK/ANZ DCIS trial. This study is a 15-year follow-up on the European Organization for Research and Treatment of Cancer 10853 DCIS trial, where women with unilateral DCIS > 5 cm in size were randomized to local excision (LE) alone or local excision with radiation therapy (LERT) to 50 Gy. The trial included 1110 women with a median follow-up of 15.8 years; over this period, 23% of patients developed local recurrence, 30% of those in the LE group versus 17% in the LERT group (Fig 2 in the original article). Approximately 50% of recurrences were DCIS and 50% were invasive carcinomas. Interestingly, the presence of recurrent DCIS did not affect breast cancer-specific survival or overall survival, but if they had an invasive recurrence occur, there was a 5-fold increased risk of death. There was no increased risk of contralateral breast cancer in either group, but there was an increased risk of regional recurrence in patients just having local excision. There was no difference in distant metastases in the 2 groups. There was a trend toward increasing risk from secondary cancers in patients receiving radiation therapy. This well-conducted randomized trial confirmed that LE plus radiation therapy confers a decreased risk of local recurrence of both DCIS and invasive carcinoma versus LE alone by about one-half. The majority of these benefits were seen within the first 5 years. The second observation from this trial was that, despite the risk reduction in local recurrence, this did not translate into survival benefit in either breast cancer-specific survival or overall survival. Patients who recurred after radiation therapy had a higher percentage of salvage mastectomy then the LE only group. Although radiation therapy did reduce local recurrence rates, it did not translate into a survival benefit, and it remains to be seen whether these results will change the thinking on the role of radiation therapy in the treatment of DCIS in the future.

J. R. Howe, MD

Twenty five year follow-up for breast cancer incidence and mortality of the Canadian National Breast Screening Study: randomised screening trial
Miller AB, Wall C, Baines CJ, et al (Univ of Toronto, Ontario, Canada; et al)
BMJ 348:g366, 2014

Objective.—To compare breast cancer incidence and mortality up to 25 years in women aged 40-59 who did or did not undergo mammography screening.

Design.—Follow-up of randomised screening trial by centre coordinators, the study's central office, and linkage to cancer registries and vital statistics databases.

Setting.—15 screening centres in six Canadian provinces, 1980-85 (Nova Scotia, Quebec, Ontario, Manitoba, Alberta, and British Columbia).

Participants.—89 835 women, aged 40-59, randomly assigned to mammography (five annual mammography screens) or control (no mammography).

Interventions.—Women aged 40-49 in the mammography arm and all women aged 50-59 in both arms received annual physical breast examinations. Women aged 40-49 in the control arm received a single examination followed by usual care in the community.

Main Outcome Measure.—Deaths from breast cancer.

Results.—During the five year screening period, 666 invasive breast cancers were diagnosed in the mammography arm (n = 44 925 participants) and 524 in the controls (n = 44 910), and of these, 180 women in the mammography arm and 171 women in the control arm died of breast cancer during the 25 year follow-up period. The overall hazard ratio for death from breast cancer diagnosed during the screening period associated with mammography was 1.05 (95% confidence interval 0.85 to 1.30). The findings for women aged 40-49 and 50-59 were almost identical. During the entire study period, 3250 women in the mammography arm and 3133 in the control arm had a diagnosis of breast cancer, and 500 and 505, respectively, died of breast cancer. Thus the cumulative mortality from breast cancer was similar between women in the mammography arm and in the control arm (hazard ratio 0.99, 95% confidence interval 0.88 to 1.12). After 15 years of follow-up a residual excess of 106 cancers was observed in the mammography arm, attributable to over-diagnosis.

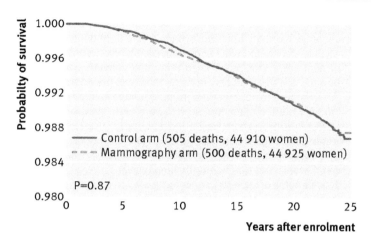

FIGURE 3.—Breast cancer specific mortality, by assignment to mammography or control arms (all participants). (Reprinted from Miller AB, Wall C, Baines CJ, et al. Twenty five year follow-up for breast cancer incidence and mortality of the Canadian national breast screening study: randomised screening trial. *BMJ.* 2014;348:g366, with permission from the BMJ Publishing Group Ltd.)

Conclusion.—Annual mammography in women aged 40-59 does not reduce mortality from breast cancer beyond that of physical examination or usual care when adjuvant therapy for breast cancer is freely available. Overall, 22% (106/484) of screen detected invasive breast cancers were over-diagnosed, representing one over-diagnosed breast cancer for every 424 women who received mammography screening in the trial (Fig 3).

▶ Screening mammography is a widely accepted practice in developed nations for reduction of mortality from breast cancer. Long-term follow-up studies are necessary to prove the value of screening programs, and this study reviewed results from the Canadian National Breast Screening study with 25-year follow-up data. The trial began in 1980, where women aged 40 to 59 who had not had mammography done in the previous 1 year and had no history of breast cancer; all had breast examination done and were taught self-breast examination. They were then randomized to receive either annual mammograms for 5 years or alternatively no mammography and were just followed by their local physicians. In total, 89 835 women were randomized, and 666 breast cancers were diagnosed in the mammography group vs 524 in the controls in the first 5 years of the program. In the 25-year follow-up interval, 2584 cancers were identified in the mammography group vs 2609 in the control group. Looking specifically at the 666 cancers diagnosed within 5 years in the mammography group, 212 or roughly one-third were nonpalpable and were identified by screening, whereas the remainder were palpable. The mean sizes of the tumors were 1.91 cm in the mammography group vs 2.1 cm in controls, which were statistically significantly different. In the mammography group 30.6% of cancers were node positive vs 32.4% in controls ($P = $ NS). During the follow-up period, 1.1% or 1005 died of breast cancer, including 351 diagnosed in the screening period. The 25-year survival for women with breast cancer detected in the mammography group was

70.6% vs 62.8% in the control group, which was significantly better; however, the 25-year cumulative mortality from breast cancer (Fig 3) and the cumulative mortality from all causes of death were similar in the mammography versus the control arm. Furthermore, it was determined that in the mammography group there were 142 excess cases of breast cancer diagnosed (calculated by the number difference in the screening vs no screening groups), and after this 5-year point, there were no significant differences in cancer diagnosis in the 2 groups. This suggested that 22% of the breast cancers in the screening group were overdiagnosed. There was a statistically significant difference in survival between the one-third of breast cancers diagnosed by mammography and those by physical examination, but it was felt that this was due to length-time bias and overdiagnosis. This trial questioned the benefits of screening mammography in patients 40 to 59 years of age, and the authors recommended that a reassessment of annual mammography should be undertaken because it did not reduce breast cancer-specific mortality of women in this age group.

J. R. Howe, MD

Margins for Breast-Conserving Surgery With Whole-Breast Irradiation in Stage I and II Invasive Breast Cancer: American Society of Clinical Oncology Endorsement of the Society of Surgical Oncology/American Society for Radiation Oncology Consensus Guideline
Buchholz TA, Somerfield MR, Griggs JJ, et al (Texas MD Anderson Cancer Ctr, Houston; American Society of Clinical Oncology, Alexandria, VA; Univ of Michigan, Ann Arbor; et al)
J Clin Oncol 32:1502-1506, 2014

Purpose.—The Society of Surgical Oncology (SSO)/American Society for Radiation Oncology (ASTRO) guideline on surgical margins for breast-conserving surgery with whole-breast irradiation in stage I and II invasive breast cancer was considered for endorsement.

Methods.—The American Society of Clinical Oncology (ASCO) has a policy and set of procedures for endorsing practice guidelines developed by other organizations. ASCO staff reviewed the SSO/ASTRO guideline for developmental rigor; an ASCO ad hoc review panel of experts reviewed the guideline content.

Results.—The ASCO ad hoc guideline review panel concurred that the recommendations are clear, thorough, and based on the most relevant scientific evidence in this content area and that they present options acceptable to patients. According to the SSO/ASTRO guideline, the use of no ink on tumor (ie, no cancer cells adjacent to any inked edge/surface of specimen) as the standard for an adequate margin in invasive cancer in the era of multidisciplinary therapy is associated with low rates of ipsilateral breast tumor recurrence and has the potential to decrease re-excision rates, improve cosmetic outcomes, and decrease health care costs.

Conclusion.—The ASCO review panel endorses the SSO/ASTRO recommendations with qualifications, as follows. The panel reinforces and amplifies the guideline authors' call for the monitoring of outcomes of the guideline at the institutional level, as institutions transition to adopting the SSO/ASTRO recommendations; would place greater emphasis on the importance of postlumpectomy mammography for cases involving microcalcifications; and calls for flexibility in the application of the guideline in light of the generally weak evidence supporting the recommendations.

▶ The Society of Surgical Oncology and American Society for Radiation Oncology released a practice guideline early this year (*Annals of Surgical Oncology* 21:704, 2014) for what constitutes an adequate margin in patients having breast-conserving surgery and whole breast irradiation. This article is from the American Society of Clinical Oncology's review of these guidelines. The reason these societies establish these guidelines is that it is currently unclear what constitutes an adequate margin of excision in patients with invasive breast cancer (particularly in stage 1 and 2) who will undergo breast conservation therapy followed by whole breast radiation. As many as one-quarter of women will have reexcision performed in current practice, which leads to cosmetic issues and may not significantly decrease the risk of recurrence within the ipsilateral breast. These groups reviewed the available literature to come up with these guidelines; in this article, this included 33 studies, all but 2 of which were retrospective, and no randomized trial has addressed this particular issue. Several questions were examined. One was what the risk of having a positive margin is on ipsilateral recurrence; the answer is a 2-fold increase, which is not negated by radiation or systemic therapy. The next question was whether wider margins reduced the risk of recurrence, and there was no evidence for this. Another question was whether more biologically aggressive subtypes of breast cancer (such as triple negative breast cancer) need wider margins, and the conclusion was that wider margins are not indicated. It was concluded that lobular carcinoma in situ at the margins is not an indication for reexcision and that wider margins were not necessary for invasive lobular cancer. It is also concluded that there was no evidence that a wider margin is necessary in patients < 40 years of age or those with an extensive intraductal component. The final recommendations from these groups are that an adequate margin consists of no ink on tumor; in other words, there is no evidence of cancer cells being present on any edge of the ink in patients with stage 1 and 2 invasive breast cancer who will be having breast irradiation. It is furthermore recommended that postlumpectomy mammography is important in patients with microcalcifications to be sure of the adequacy of their removal before undergoing radiation. These recommendations helped to clarify for general surgeons and surgical oncologists acceptable practice patterns with the best available evidence. However, they still leave room for practitioners to take wider margins in specific cases where they feel the patient may be at higher risk.

J. R. Howe, MD

Axillary Lymph Node Dissection Versus No Dissection in Patients With T1N0 Breast Cancer: A Randomized Clinical Trial (INT09/98)

Agresti R, Martelli G, Sandri M, et al (Fondazione IRCCS Istituto Nazionale dei Tumori, Milan, Italy)
Cancer 120:885-893, 2014

Background.—Although axillary surgery is still considered to be a fundamental part of the management of early breast cancer, it may no longer be necessary either as treatment or as a guide to adjuvant treatment. The authors conducted a single-center randomized trial (INT09/98) to determine the impact of avoiding axillary surgery in patients with T1N0 breast cancer and planning chemotherapy based on biological factors of the primary tumor on long-term disease control.

Methods.—From June 1998 to June 2003, 565 patients aged 30 years to 65 years with T1N0 breast cancer were randomized to either quadrantectomy with (QUAD) or without (QU) axillary lymph node dissection; a total of 517 patients finally were evaluated. All patients received radiotherapy to the residual breast only. Chemotherapy for patients in the QUAD treatment arm was determined based on lymph node status, estrogen receptor status, and tumor grade. Chemotherapy for patients in the QU treatment arm was based on estrogen receptor status, tumor grade, and human epidermal growth factor receptor 2 and laminin receptor status. Overall survival (OS) was the primary endpoint. Disease-free survival (DFS) and rate and time of axillary lymph node recurrence in the QU treatment arm were the secondary endpoints.

Results.—After a median follow-up of >10 years, the estimated adjusted hazards ratio of the QUAD versus QU treatment arms for OS was 1.09 (95% confidence interval, 0.59-2.00; $P = .783$) and was 1.04 (95% confidence interval, 0.56-1.94; $P = .898$) for DFS. Of the 245 patients in the QU treatment arm, 22 (9.0%) experienced axillary lymph node recurrence. The median time to axillary lymph node recurrence from breast surgery was 30.0 months (interquartile range, 24.2 months-73.4 months).

Conclusions.—Patients with T1N0 breast cancer did not appear to benefit in terms of DFS and OS from immediate axillary lymph node dissection in the current randomized trial. The biological characteristics of the primary tumor appear adequate for guiding adjuvant treatment (Fig 3).

▶ The surgical treatment of breast cancer has evolved significantly over the past decades. This includes breast conservation therapy, replacing mastectomy with lumpectomy and radiation, and sentinel lymph node biopsy of the axilla rather than axillary dissection. The ACOSOG Z0011 trial randomized patients with T1N0 or T2N0 breast cancers who were found to have 1 or 2 sentinel lymph nodes involved to be randomized to axillary dissection versus sentinel lymph node alone; this revealed that there was no difference in overall survival or disease-free survival. This study from a single cancer center in Milan, Italy, looked at a slightly different question, where patients with T1N0 breast cancer presenting to their center between 1998 and 2003 were treated by quadrantectomy and

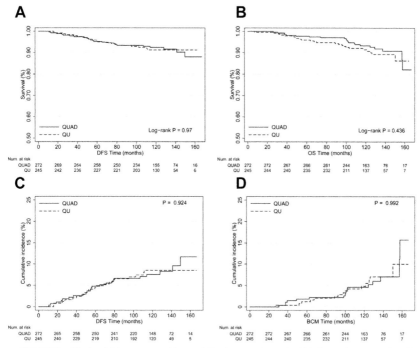

FIGURE 3.—Kaplan-Meier curves and log-rank P values are shown for (A) disease-free survival (DFS) and (B) overall survival (OS) in the quadrantectomy without axillary lymph node dissection (QU) and quadrantectomy with axillary lymph node dissection (QUAD) treatment arms. Cumulative incidence functions and Gray test P values are shown for (C) DFS and (D) breast cancer mortality (BCM) in the QU and QUAD treatment arms. (Reprinted from Cancer. Agresti R, Martelli G, Sandri M, et al. Axillary lymph node dissection versus no dissection in patients with T1N0 breast cancer: a randomized clinical trial (INT09/98). *Cancer*. 2014;120:885-893, Copyright 2014, American Cancer Society. This material is reproduced with permission of Wiley-Liss, Inc., a subsidiary of John Wiley & Sons, Inc., www.interscience.wiley.com.)

radiation then randomized to either complete level 1—3 axillary dissection or no axillary dissection. The radiation therapy did not cover the axilla, internal mammary, or supraclavicular lymph nodes. Patients were then evaluated postoperatively to determine whether they had good prognostic factors or poor prognostic factors, and based on this, they received chemotherapy (epirubicin, cyclophosphamide, methotrexate, 5-fluorouracil) or not. Patients receiving chemotherapy also received tamoxifen for 5 years. When lymph nodes were dissected, the good prognostic factors were considered: node negative disease, ER-positivity, and grade 1 or 2 tumors. However, if the lymph nodes were positive or the estrogen receptors were negative, or if they had grade 3 tumors, then those patient received adjuvant chemotherapy after quadrantectomy and axillary dissection. In the group undergoing quadrantectomy alone, the factors that were considered were estrogen receptor status, grade, HER2, and laminin receptor status. Patients received chemotherapy if they had at least 1 or more of the following: grade 3, HER2 positivity, or laminin receptor positivity. Patients were followed for a median of more than 10 years, and the interesting finding was that there was no difference in disease-free survival or overall survival in patients with respect to having axillary node dissection. A similar number of patients developed distant metastases in each group (which was 8.3% overall), and a similar number died of breast cancer in each group (which was 6.2% overall). Of those undergoing axillary dissection, a median of 20 lymph nodes were harvested, and 29% had positive lymph nodes. Of those with positive lymph nodes, 54% had 1 involved lymph node, with more than half having just micrometastases and the other half having more gross nodal involvement. In the group with positive lymph nodes, 46% had more than 1 lymph node and 31% had greater than 3 lymph nodes involved. None of the patients having axillary dissection had nodal recurrence in the axilla. On the other hand, those patients who did not have axillary lymph node dissection had an axillary recurrence rate of 10%. These patients then underwent axillary node dissection, with a median time to axillary recurrence of 30 months. Five percent of patients in both groups developed local disease recurrence, and all of these patients underwent wide excision, and those patients had no axillary dissection then also had axillary dissection performed. Five percent in each group developed contralateral breast cancer. This trial (INT09/98) revealed that in patients with T1N0 breast cancer, there was no significant survival benefit when performing axillary nodal dissection in patients treated with quadrantectomy and radiation and selective chemotherapy based on prognostic factors in the tumors. Patients with axillary recurrence were salvaged, and of interest was that the pathologic nodal involvement rate in patients undergoing axillary dissection was 29%; however, the axillary recurrence rate was only 10%, which was similar to the findings in NSABP B04 trial, suggesting that not all patients with axillary disease develop clinically significant axillary recurrence. In this study, patients who underwent axillary dissection were more likely to receive chemotherapy than patients stratified by tumor-specific factors, likely because of the inclusion of all patients with lymph node-positive disease. Despite a significantly higher degree of chemotherapy to the quadrantectomy and axillary dissection group, there was no improvement of survival (Fig 3). The final conclusion from this article was that because survival did not differ between these groups, it was reasonable to use tumor factors such as tumor grade, HER2, laminin receptor, and estrogen receptor status over lymph node involvement to predict patients that might benefit from chemotherapy, and therefore axillary dissection may no longer be needed as a staging tool. The authors also commented that with improved molecular testing a more precise stratification model will likely be developed to further reinforce that axillary dissection is unnecessary in early-stage breast cancer.

J. R. Howe, MD

Melanoma

Intensity of Follow-Up After Melanoma Surgery

Scally CP, Wong SL (Univ of Michigan, Ann Arbor)
Ann Surg Oncol 21:752-757, 2014

This contemporary review of melanoma surveillance strategies seeks to help practitioners examine and improve their surveillance protocols based on the currently available data. In general, there is no definitive benefit from increased screening or more aggressive use of interval imaging. Low-intensity surveillance strategies do not appear to adversely affect patient outcomes and should be the preferred approach compared with high-intensity strategies for most melanoma patients. All surveillance programs should emphasize education in order to maximize the effectiveness of patient-based detection of recurrent disease (Table 1).

▶ The appropriate follow-up for melanoma patients is not clear, and there are many differences in practice patterns (Table 1). Even the National Comprehensive Cancer Network guidelines give a lot of latitude, such as physical examination every 3 to 12 months for 5 years in stage 1 and 2 melanomas. For stage 2B to stage 4 patients, surveillance may range anywhere from 3 to 6 months for the first 2 years, and chest radiographs, CT scans, or PET CT scans every 6 to 12 months as well as annual brain MRI may be recommended in higher risk patients,. The essential question addressed by this report is whether early detection of nodal metastases, local recurrence, or distant metastases will improve outcomes. It defines strategies as low intensity or high intensity, with the low intensity strategies focusing on examination of the skin and the regional nodal basins without laboratory or imaging studies. Higher intensity strategies might include routine laboratory tests and imaging and more frequent follow-up. Important facts highlighted in the article are that 20% of recurrences are local, 50% are in the regional nodal basins, and 30% are distant metastases. Most recurrences will occur within the first 2 years, but it is not uncommon to see recurrence even after 10 years. Some have recommended annual surveillance for stage 1 patients, every 6 month visits for patients with stage 2 lesions for the first 2 years, and every 3 months for patients with stage 3 disease for the first year, being spread out over time after this. Not all agree with this surveillance, and some have pointed out that few relapses are detected with intense surveillance and that even in stage 3 patients the risk of local or regional relapse is less than 5%. Furthermore, most recurrences are detected by the patients themselves, questioning the need for close follow-up and laboratory and imaging tests by physicians. This review suggests that high-intensity surveillance is not beneficial for patients with early-stage disease and that chest radiographs, abdominal ultrasonography and blood work have little utility. They conclude that low-intensity surveillance is preferred over high-intensity surveillance and does not adversely affect patient survival. High-intensity surveillance can be expensive, with a high incidence of false-positive results requiring even further evaluation. The authors suggest that early-stage melanoma patients should probably not have imaging done, or it should

TABLE 1.—Summary of Published Work on Melanoma Surveillance

Reference	Study Population	Tumor Stage	Modality of Follow-up	Duration of Follow-up	Recurrences	Recommendations for Follow-up	Notes
Basseres et al.[21]	528	Stage I	Clinical exam, US, X-ray, CT	NR	115 (22 %)	Follow-up intensity determined by tumor stage; clinical exam is the only cost-effective surveillance for stage I	Review of state registry data
Shumate et al.[22]	1,475	Stage I–II	Clinical exam, X-ray, lab studies	6.5 years (median)	195 (15 %)	Reduction in frequency of follow-up; limited use of imaging/labs	
Weiss et al.[23]	261	>1.69 mm thick or regional nodal metastasis	Clinical exam, X-ray, lab studies	4 years (minimum)	161 (60 %)	Frequent follow-up exams for high-risk patients; no routine imaging/labs	
Moloney et al.[24]	602	Stage I	NR	5 years (minimum)	24 (4 %)	Reduction in frequency of follow-up	
Sylaidis et al.[25]	244	>4.0 mm thick	NR	10 years (minimum, unless patient died)	176 (72 %)	High-intensity initial follow-up for thick melanomas	
Mooney et al.[26]	1,004	Stage I–II	Clinical exam, X-ray, lab studies	6 years (median)	174 (17 %)	Limited use of imaging in select patients; no routine labs	
Dicker et al.[27]	961	Stage I	NR	5 years (minimum)	242 (25 %)	More frequent follow-up for thick melanomas; no follow-up after 5 years	Review of national registry data
Johnson et al.[28]	306	<1.5 mm thick	Clinical exam only	4 years (mean)	20 (7 %)	No follow-up needed for melanomas <0.75 mm thick	
Poo-Hwu et al.[10]	373	Stage I–III	Clinical exam, X-ray, lab studies	2 years (minimum)	78 (21 %)	Reduction in frequency of follow-up, stratified by tumor stage	
Kitler et al.[29]	513	Stage I	Clinical exam, US, X-ray, lab studies	4 years (minimum)	20 (4 %)	Regular follow-up exams only, no routine labs or imaging	

Study	N	Stage	Modality	Follow-up duration	Recurrences	Conclusion	Study type
Hofmann et al.[30]	661	Stage I–IV	Clinical exam, US, X-ray, lab studies	4 years (stage IV), 2 years (other stages)	127/630 (20 %)	Emphasized importance of clinical exam, limited to no use for labs/imaging	
Garbe[11]	2,008	Stage I–IV	Clinical exam, US, X-ray, lab studies	2 years (median)	112 (6 %)	High-intensity follow-up may aid in early detection; follow-up schedule can be reduced in early-stage disease	
Kalady et al.[31]	1,563	<1.0 mm thick	Clinical exam, X-ray	11 years (median)	140 (12 %)	Prolonged surveillance needed	
Schmidt-Wendtner et al.[32]	2,302	Stage Ia	Clinical exam	62 months (median)	77 (3 %)	In thin melanoma, certain sites and histologic types higher risk and benefit from intense surveillance	
Einwachter-Thompson and MacKie[15]	430	<0.5 mm thick	NR	5 years (minimum)	NR	Follow-up for thin melanomas is low yield	
Francken et al.[33]	4,726	Stage I–II	NR	6 years (median)	895 (19 %)	Follow-up for thin melanomas can be reduced or eliminated; more frequent early follow-up for high-risk patients	
Moore Dalal et al.[34]	1,062	Stage I–II	Clinical exam, X-ray, lab studies	17 months (median)	203 (19 %)	Emphasis on patient self-education and clinical exam	Prospective database review
Meyers et al.[35]	118	Stage II–III	NR	44 months (median)	43 (36 %)	Scheduled surveillance exams should be mainstay of surveillance; X-rays may have some benefit in stage II–III	Prospective database review
Romano et al.[12]	340	Stage III	Clinical exam, CT, lab studies	77 months (median)	N/A (study population included only patients with recurrence) 229/1,000	Follow-up visits and imaging have decreased utility over time	
Turner et al.[16]	2,998	Stage I–II	NR	2.7 years (median)		Less frequent follow-up visits likely lead to only minimal delay in diagnosis	

Editor's Note: Please refer to original journal article for full references.
With kind permission from Springer Science+Business Media: Scally CP, Wong SL. Intensity of Follow-Up After Melanoma Surgery. *Ann Surg Oncol.* 2014;21:752-757.

be carefully considered, and that perhaps the most important aspect of surveillance is education of the patient for the signs of local, regional, or distant recurrence. Furthermore, there is no clear consensus between groups, and the National Comprehensive Cancer Network guidelines remain somewhat vague.

J. R. Howe, MD

Observation After a Positive Sentinel Lymph Node Biopsy in Patients with Melanoma

Bamboat ZM, Konstantinidis IT, Kuk D, et al (Memorial Sloan-Kettering Cancer Ctr, NY)
Ann Surg Oncol 21:3117-3123, 2014

Background.—The benefit of completion lymph node dissection (CLND) in melanoma patients with a positive sentinel lymph node (SLN) remains unknown.

Methods.—We identified patients with a positive SLN from 1994 to 2012. Patient and tumor characteristics, reasons for not undergoing CLND, patterns of recurrence, and melanoma-specific survival data were analyzed.

Results.—Of 4,310 patients undergoing SLN biopsy (SLNB), 495 (11 %) had a positive SLN—167 (34 %) patients underwent nodal observation and 328 (66 %) had immediate CLND. Patients in the no-CLND group were older (66 vs. 56 years; $p < 0.001$) and more likely to have lower extremity lesions (57 vs. 42 %; $p = 0.006$). There were no differences in tumor thickness, Clark level of invasion, ulceration, or SLN tumor burden. Median follow-up was 23 and 80 months for the no-CLND and CLND groups, respectively, and median time to recurrence was similar at 9 and 12 months, respectively ($p = 0.48$). There was no difference in local and in transit recurrence rates between groups (16 %, no CLND, and 18 %, CLND; $p = 0.48$). Nodal disease as a site of first recurrence occurred in 15 % of patients in the no-CLND group and 6 % of CLND patients ($p = 0.002$). In contrast, systemic recurrences occurred in 8 % of no-CLND patients compared with 27 % of CLND patients ($p < 0.001$). While median recurrence-free survival was higher after CLND (34.5 vs. 20.9 months; $p = 0.02$), melanoma-specific survival was similar (not reached, no CLND vs. 110 months, CLND; $p = 0.09$).

Conclusions.—Immediate CLND after a positive SLNB is associated with fewer initial nodal basin recurrences but similar melanoma-specific survival. These results support ongoing equipoise in the Multicenter Selective Lymphadenectomy Trial II (MSLT-II) (Fig 1a).

▶ In patients found to have a positive sentinel lymph node during wide excision of melanoma, the standard of care has been to perform completion lymph node dissection (CLND) of the involved nodal basins. However, in most cases of positive sentinel lymph nodes, the remainder of the excised lymph nodes will be negative. A recent multi-institutional study found that

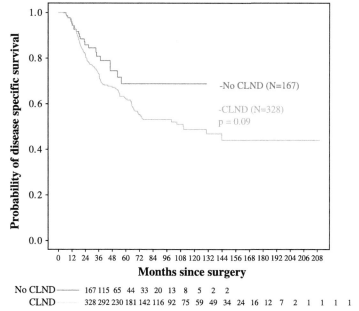

No CLND——— 167 115 65 44 33 20 13 8 5 2 2
CLND——— 328 292 230 181 142 116 92 75 59 49 34 24 16 12 7 2 1 1 1 1

FIGURE 1.—Outcome in melanoma patients with a positive SLN selected for nodal basin observation; (a) Disease-specific survival of patients selected for nodal basin observation (N–Ã = –Ã 167) vs. those who underwent CLND (N–Ã = –Ã 328). (With kind permission from Springer Science+Business Media. Bamboat ZM, Konstantinidis IT, Kuk D, et al. Observation after a positive sentinel lymph node biopsy in patients with melanoma. *Ann Surg Oncol*. 2014;21:3117-3123, with permission from Society of Surgical Oncology.)

patients being observed rather than having completion nodal dissection had similar disease-specific survivals to patients who had CLND. Arguments for performing CLND are to excise additional lymph nodes that may be positive, to reduce the risk of nodal basin recurrence, and to potentially improve survival. Reasons to not perform a CLND are the increased risk of complications, decreased quality of life, and the fact that most patients do not have additional involved nodes. This study was a retrospective single institutional study that looked at the population of patients that had a positive sentinel lymph node that did not undergo CLND compared with patients who did undergo CLND. Four hundred ninety-five patients (11%) had a positive sentinel lymph node, of which 167 (34%) underwent observation, whereas 328 (66%) had CLND. The median follow-up was 23 months for the observation group and 80 months for the CLND group. There were some differences between the 2 groups, with the observation group being a mean of 10 years older and more commonly having lower extremity lesions (this may have been because of the increased morbidity of inguinal relative to axillary nodal dissection). In two thirds of cases it was the patient's decision to not undergo CLND, in 22% it was the physician's decision, and patient comorbidity accounted for another 4% of patients not having CLND. In patients undergoing observation, 49% had recurrence at a median of 9 months, and in the CLND group, 55% patients had recurrence at a median of 12 months. There was no difference in local or in-transit recurrences (16% observation, 18% CLND). However, there was a significant difference in nodal recurrence, which was 15% in the observation group and 6% in the CLND group, and in systemic recurrence, which was 8% in the observation and 27% in the CLND group. With respect to survival, the median disease-specific survival was very similar, and this difference was not statistically significant (Fig 1a). Recurrence-free survival was higher in the CLND group vs observation, which was statistically significant. Patients in the observation group who had nodal recurrence generally had node dissection performed at that time in 72% of cases, and the median disease-free survival in this group was surprisingly significantly higher than that in the CLND group. Conclusions reached from this study were that although CLND is currently the standard of care, the lack of a difference in disease-specific survival between observation in patients with a positive sentinel node and CLND raises questions as to whether CLND is the correct approach. The fact that patients who had recurrence in the observation group had better survival after salvage lymphadenectomy than those undergoing CLND should be interpreted with caution, because there were only 18 patients in this group, and these numbers may be skewed. This study is also limited because it is retrospective, and the MSLT-2 trial will hopefully help answer this question more definitively in the near future.

J. R. Howe, MD

Final Trial Report of Sentinel-Node Biopsy versus Nodal Observation in Melanoma

Morton DL, Thompson JF, Cochran AJ, et al (John Wayne Cancer Inst, Santa Monica, CA; Univ of Sydney, Australia; Univ of California, Los Angeles; et al)
N Engl J Med 370:599-609, 2014

Background.—Sentinel-node biopsy, a minimally invasive procedure for regional melanoma staging, was evaluated in a phase 3 trial.

Methods.—We evaluated outcomes in 2001 patients with primary cutaneous melanomas randomly assigned to undergo wide excision and nodal observation, with lymphadenectomy for nodal relapse (observation group), or wide excision and sentinel-node biopsy, with immediate lymphadenectomy for nodal metastases detected on biopsy (biopsy group).

Results.—No significant treatment-related difference in the 10-year melanoma-specific survival rate was seen in the overall study population (20.8% with and 79.2% without nodal metastases). Mean ($\pm$ SE) 10-year disease-free survival rates were significantly improved in the biopsy group, as compared with the observation group, among patients with intermediate-thickness melanomas, defined as 1.20 to 3.50 mm (71.3 $\pm$ 1.8% vs. 64.7 $\pm$ 2.3%; hazard ratio for recurrence or metastasis, 0.76; $P = 0.01$), and those with thick melanomas, defined as >3.50 mm (50.7 $\pm$ 4.0% vs. 40.5 $\pm$ 4.7%; hazard ratio, 0.70; $P = 0.03$). Among patients with intermediate-thickness melanomas, the 10-year melanoma-specific survival rate was 62.1 $\pm$ 4.8% among those with metastasis versus

85.1 ± 1.5% for those without metastasis (hazard ratio for death from melanoma, 3.09; $P < 0.001$); among patients with thick melanomas, the respective rates were 48.0 ± 7.0% and 64.6 ± 4.9% (hazard ratio, 1.75; $P = 0.03$). Biopsy-based management improved the 10-year rate of distant disease—free survival (hazard ratio for distant metastasis, 0.62; $P = 0.02$) and the 10-year rate of melanoma-specific survival (hazard ratio for death from melanoma, 0.56; $P = 0.006$) for patients with intermediate-thickness melanomas and nodal metastases. Accelerated-failure-time latent-subgroup analysis was performed to account for the fact that nodal status was initially known only in the biopsy group, and a significant treatment benefit persisted.

Conclusions.—Biopsy-based staging of intermediate-thickness or thick primary melanomas provides important prognostic information and identifies patients with nodal metastases who may benefit from immediate complete lymphadenectomy. Biopsy-based management prolongs disease-free survival for all patients and prolongs distant disease—free survival and melanoma-specific survival for patients with nodal metastases from intermediate-thickness melanomas. (Funded by the National Cancer Institute, National Institutes of Health, and the Australia and New Zealand Melanoma Trials Group; ClinicalTrials.gov number, NCT00275496.)

▶ Morton introduced the concept of sentinel lymph node (SLN) mapping in the early 1990s as a way of determining whether regional lymph nodes were involved with malignant melanoma, which would allow for better stratification of who should receive elective nodal dissection vs observation in this disease. It was hoped that this procedure would not only give prognostic information for patients but might also translate into a survival benefit. Therefore, in 1994, the Multicenter Selective Lymphadenectomy Trial (MSLT-1) began accrual of patients with intermediate and thick melanomas where patients were randomly assigned to undergo wide local excision with 2- to 3-cm margins with or without SNL biopsy. In patients assigned to the SLN biopsy group, if the SLN was positive, patients would undergo completion lymphadenectomy. In the non-SLN group, lymphadenectomy was performed if clinically involved nodes developed over the observation period. There were 1270 evaluable patients in the intermediate thickness group and 290 in the thick melanoma group in this 10-year follow-up study of MSLT-1. Important findings were that there was no difference in melanoma-specific survival between the SLN biopsy and observation groups in either intermediate or thick melanomas. However, there was a difference in disease-free survival in these 2 groups (which was 71% in intermediate-thickness melanomas having SLN biopsies vs 65% in those being observed; Fig 3 C in the original article). There was a significant difference in 10-year melanoma-specific survival in those with positive sentinel nodes (62.1% in positive vs 85.1% in negative SLNs with intermediate thickness melanomas); this was also seen in patients with thick melanomas (48% with positive 65% with negative SLNs). Overall, 21% of patients had positive sentinel lymph nodes. In the observation group, 17% of patients with intermediate-thickness melanomas developed nodal metastases at a median of 19 months after randomization. Five percent of patients with negative SLNs later developed enlarged lymph nodes in the nodal basin requiring delayed lymphadenectomy. Interestingly, distant disease-free survival was improved when patients had nodal metastases detected by SLN biopsy and had immediate lymphadenectomy as opposed to delayed lymphadenectomy. The overall conclusions of this 10-year follow-up study were that there was not a significant survival advantage of SLN biopsy in patients with intermediate thickness melanomas. Patients who do not have nodal metastases do not benefit from SLN biopsy, although this procedure does give valuable staging information. In patients found to have clinically occult disease in sentinel lymph nodes with intermediate thickness melanoma, however, the early intervention appeared to decrease the risk of nodal recurrence and of distant metastases and death from melanoma. This was not seen in patients with thick melanomas. One of the more interesting results was that patients who had positive sentinel lymph nodes and underwent lymphadenectomy had a survival advantage over patients who were observed and had lymphadenectomy after developing clinically evident nodes. The observation group had more positive lymph nodes and reduced survival. The long-term results of the MSLT-1 trial therefore demonstrated that SLN biopsy is an accurate staging procedure that gives important prognostic information, has a low complication rate, and may improve the survival of patients who have microscopic nodal disease, but it did not improve overall survival.

J. R. Howe, MD

Oncologic Outcomes of Patients Undergoing Videoscopic Inguinal Lymphadenectomy for Metastatic Melanoma

Martin BM, Etra JW, Russell MC, et al (Winship Cancer Inst-Emory Univ, Atlanta, GA)
J Am Coll Surg 218:620-627, 2014

Background.—Open inguinal lymphadenectomy for regionally metastatic melanoma is associated with a high wound-related morbidity. Videoscopic inguinal lymphadenectomy (VIL) is a minimally invasive approach with fewer wound-related complications, yet its adoption has been hindered by a lack of oncologic outcomes data.

Study Design.—Data were prospectively collected on all VILs performed for melanoma from 2008 to 2012 (n = 40) and compared with a retrospective cohort of open superficial inguinal lymphadenectomies from 2005 to 2012 (n = 40). Continuous variables were analyzed with Student's t-test, binomial variables with chi-square, and survival curves using log-rank comparison.

Results.—Median follow-up for patients undergoing VIL was 19.1 months compared with 33.9 months in the open inguinal lymphadenectomy group. There were no statistical differences in demographics (age, sex, body mass index, smoking status, Charlson comorbidity index) or clinicopathologic features (primary site, stage, Breslow depth, ulceration).

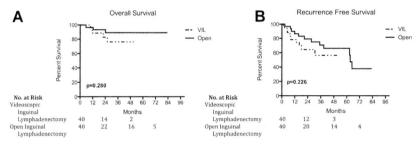

FIGURE 1.—Overall and recurrence free survival after videoscopic inguinal lymphadenectomy (VIL) or open superficial inguinal lymphadenectomy for patients with metastatic melanoma to the inguinal lymph node basin (panels A and B). (Reprinted from the Journal of the American College of Surgeons. Martin BM, Etra JW, Russell MC, et al. Oncologic outcomes of patients undergoing videoscopic inguinal lymphadenectomy for metastatic melanoma. *J Am Coll Surg.* 2014;218:620-627, Copyright 2014, with permission from the American College of Surgeons.)

Lymph node yield was similar (VIL, 12.6; open, 14.2; $p = 0.131$). Overall recurrence rates were also similar: 27.5% in the VIL group and 30.0% in the open group ($p = 0.805$). One patient in the VIL group and 2 in the open group suffered recurrence in the nodal basin. Although median survival was not reached in the VIL group, Kaplan-Meier estimates of disease-free survival ($p = 0.226$) and overall survival ($p = 0.308$) were similar. In a comprehensive analysis of wound complications including infection, skin necrosis, and seroma, patients undergoing VIL had markedly less morbidity (VIL, 47.5%; open, 80.0%; $p = 0.002$).

Conclusions.—Videoscopic inguinal lymphadenectomy is associated with similar oncologic outcomes and markedly reduced wound complications when compared with open inguinal lymphadenectomy. The minimally invasive procedure may be the preferred method for inguinal lymphadenectomy in melanoma (Fig 1).

▶ Inguinal lymph node dissection for patients with melanoma involving the regional lymph nodes has a significant morbidity. There is an approximately 50% risk of wound dehiscence, skin necrosis, and lymphedema. The wound complications may be due to thin skin flaps and the length of the incision in the groin, which is at higher risk for infection than other regions. Videoscopic inguinal lymphadenectomy (VIL) was originally developed in 2003 for the treatment of penile cancer but more recently has been applied by this group for the treatment of patients with melanoma. In this operation, patients are placed on a split-leg table with the leg flexed and externally rotated, and then 3 trocars are placed in a triangulated fashion; the incision from sentinel lymph node biopsy is left intact. Sartorius flaps are not created, and a drain is left exiting 1 of the trocar sites. Patients generally stay overnight and are discharged the day after surgery with the drain in place. This study compared 40 VIL to 40 open inguinal lymphadenectomy procedures done at a single institution by a single surgeon. The 2 groups were relatively well matched for demographics and comorbidities; there were 4 patients with clinically palpable lymph nodes in the VIL group and 3 in the open group. Significant findings from this study were that there were few differences in operative or oncologic measures. The mean operative time was 25 minutes longer for the VIL procedure, and 4 procedures needed to be converted to open (2 for the sentinel node site dehiscing, another for hypercarbia, and another due to uncertain anatomy). The lymph node retrieval was 12.6 nodes in the VIL group vs 14.2 in the open group, and the length of stay and duration of the drain were similar between both groups. The biggest difference was in the rate of complications, which was 47.5% in the VIL group and 80% in the open group. The biggest differences were seen in rates of infection (40% VIL vs 65% open), and rates of flap necrosis or dehiscence (2.5 vs 15%). There was a similar rate of seroma in both groups, but curiously, the endpoint of lymphedema was not evaluated in this study. There were no differences in overall survival or recurrence-free survival (Fig 1A, B), and the follow-up was 19 months for the VIL group and 34 months for the open group. Recurrence rates were similar, at 28% in the VIL group and 30% in the open group. Of 11 patients with recurrence in the VIL group, 8 were in-transit, 1 was in the groin, and 2 were distant. In the open group there were 12 recurrences, 4 were in-transit disease, 2 in the groin, and 6 to distant sites. This study showed that VIL can be performed with equivalent outcomes as for open inguinal lymphadenectomy, with a reduced rate of complications. The rate of complication seen appeared to be somewhat higher than most studies of open lymphadenectomy at 80%, although the study used a more liberal definition of infection, which included any patient treated with antibiotics. Another concern raised regarding the technique is that insufflation could lead to subcutaneous dissemination of tumor cells up through the trunk. No distant subcutaneous recurrences were noted in the follow-up period suggestive of this, but 1 of the limitations was that the follow-up was shorter in the VIL group. The authors conclude from their results that it is reasonable to offer patients this procedure for those who wish to have a minimally invasive approach because the oncologic outcomes appear equivalent.

J. R. Howe, MD

Gastric

Prospective, Randomized, Multicenter, Phase III Study of Fluorouracil, Leucovorin, and Irinotecan Versus Epirubicin, Cisplatin, and Capecitabine in Advanced Gastric Adenocarcinoma: A French Intergroup (Fédération Francophone de Cancérologie Digestive, Fédération Nationale des Centres de Lutte Contre le Cancer, and Groupe Coopérateur Multidisciplinaire en Oncologie) Study

Guimbaud R, Louvet C, Ries P, et al (Centre Hospitalier Universitaire Toulouse, Toulouse, France; Hôpital Saint Antoine, France; Institut Paoli Calmettes, Marseille, France; et al)
J Clin Oncol 32:3520-3526, 2014

Purpose.—To compare epirubicin, cisplatin, and capecitabine (ECX) with fluorouracil, leucovorin, and irinotecan (FOLFIRI) as first-line treatments in patients with advanced gastric or esophagogastric junction (EGJ) adenocarcinoma.

Patients and Methods.—This open, randomized, phase III study was carried out in 71 centers. Patients with locally advanced or metastatic gastric or EGJ cancer were randomly assigned to receive either ECX as first-line treatment (ECX arm) or FOLFIRI (FOLFIRI arm). Second-line treatment was predefined (FOLFIRI for the ECX arm and ECX for the FOLFIRI arm). The primary criterion was time-to-treatment failure (TTF) of the first-line therapy. Secondary criteria were progression-free survival (PFS), overall survival (OS), toxicity, and quality of life.

Results.—In all, 416 patients were included (median age, 61.4 years; 74% male). After a median follow-up of 31 months, median TTF was significantly longer with FOLFIRI than with ECX (5.1 *v* 4.2 months; *P* =.008). There was no significant difference between the two groups in median PFS (5.3 *v* 5.8 months; *P* =.96), median OS (9.5 *v* 9.7 months; *P* =.95), or response rate (39.2% *v* 37.8%). First-line FOLFIRI was better tolerated (overall rate of grade 3 to 4 toxicity, 69% *v* 84%; *P* < .001; hematologic adverse events [AEs], 38% *v* 64.5%; *P* < .001; nonhematologic AEs: 53% *v* 53.5%; *P* =.81).

Conclusion.—FOLFIRI as first-line treatment for advanced gastric and EGJ cancer demonstrated significantly better TTF than did ECX. Other outcome results indicate that FOLFIRI is an acceptable first-line regimen in this setting and should be explored as a backbone regimen for targeted agents.

▶ Patients with advanced or metastatic gastric cancer have poor survival, which is often in the range of 3 to 6 months. Chemotherapy has been used in these patients, and multiple regimens have been tried. One popular regimen is epirubicin, cisplatin, and 5-fluorouracil (ECF), and the substitution of oral capecitabine for 5-fluorouracil (5-FU) has been shown to be roughly equivalent (ECX). One problem with these regimens is their toxicity, and some have advocated the efficacy of irinotecan regimens in advanced gastric cancer. Therefore, this French randomized controlled trial involving 71 centers recruited 416 patients with histologically confirmed but unresectable (or locally advanced or metastatic) gastric or gastroesophageal junction adenocarcinoma to receive either ECX or FOLFIRI (5-FU, leucovorin, irinotecan). In this study, patients were given these drugs as first-line treatment, but when disease progressed, there was unacceptable toxicity, or the patient requested stopping the treatment, then second-line treatment with the other regimen was given after 3 weeks of recovery. In the patients recruited, 65% had gastric cancer and 33% had gastroesophageal junction tumors; in 25% of cases, the primary had been resected; 24% had linitis plastica; 84% had metastatic disease. This study used the unusual end point of time to treatment failure as a primary end point, which could be due to disease progression, toxicity, death, or a request to stop the regimen. There was a significantly shorter time to treatment failure in the ECX arm (Fig 2 in the original article) at 4.24 months vs the FOLFIRI arm at 5.08 months. There was no difference in either progression-free survival or overall survival in the 2 groups. The objective response rates were similar in both arms, at 39% for ECX and 38% for FOLFIRI. There was a higher rate of grade 3–4 toxicity with ECX (84%) vs

FOLFIRI (69%), and the majority of these toxicities were hematologic. This study concluded that FOLFIRI had a favorable time to treatment failure and a toxicity profile that supports its use in patients with advanced gastric cancer. Problems with this study were using time to treatment failure as its primary end point and also giving the alternative chemotherapy regimen as second-line therapy. Approximately one-half of the patients in each group had the second-line therapy, and patients were evaluated in the intent-to-treat arm. These factors do confuse the analyses, but it is reasonable to conclude that FOLFIRI has similar activity to the more toxic regimen of ECF and should be considered in patients with advanced gastric cancer.

J. R. Howe, MD

Optimal Management of Gastric Cancer Results From an International RAND/UCLA Expert Panel

Coburn N, Seevaratnam R, Paszat L, et al (Univ of Toronto, ON, Canada; Sunnybrook Research Inst, Toronto, ON, Canada)

Ann Surg 259:102-108, 2014

Objective.—Defining processes of care, which are appropriate and necessary for management of gastric cancer (GC), is an important step toward improving outcomes.

Methods.—Using a RAND/UCLA Appropriateness Method, an international multidisciplinary expert panel created 22 statements reflecting optimal management. All statements were scored for appropriateness and necessity.

Results.—The following tenets were scored appropriate and necessary: (1) preoperative staging by computed tomography of abdomen/pelvis; (2) positron-emission tomographic scans not routinely indicated; (3) consideration for adjuvant therapy; (4) further clinical trials; (5) multidisciplinary decision making; (6) sufficient support at hospitals; (7) assessment of 16 or more lymph nodes (LNs); (8) in metastatic disease, surgery only for palliation of major symptoms; (9) surgeons experienced in GC management; (10) and surgeons experienced in both GC management and advanced laparoscopic surgery for laparoscopic resection. The following were scored appropriate, but of indeterminate necessity: (1) diagnostic laparoscopy before treatment; (2) a multidisciplinary approach to linitis plastica; (3) genetic assessment for diffuse GC and family history, or age less than 45 years; (4) endoscopic removal of select T1aN0 lesions; (5) D2 LN dissection in curative intent cases; (6) D1 LN dissection for early GC or patients with comorbidities; (7) frozen section analysis of margins; (8) nonemergent cases performed in a hospital with a volume of more than 15 resections per year; and (9) by a surgeon with more than 6 resection per year.

Conclusions.—The expert panel has created 22 statements for the perioperative management of GC patients, to provide guidance to clinicians and improve the care received by patients.

▶ Although there are guidelines for the treatment of patients with gastric cancer, there is not widespread agreement, and there may be differences in opinion between surgeons in the Eastern and Western worlds, and between different specialties. With this in mind, a group of 16 international experts (weighted toward surgical oncologists) were assembled, and the RAND/UCLA appropriateness methodology was applied to a variety of aspects of care for patients with gastric cancer. The group reviewed the literature on a variety of important topics and then met to decide which aspects of care were necessary, appropriate, and gave scores for each. At the conclusion of these meetings, 22 summary statements were issued for what was deemed to be appropriate care and 12 as being necessary. Recommendations from the panel included that a CT scan of the abdomen and pelvis should be performed for preoperative staging; however, positron emission tomography is not necessary for staging. Laparoscopy is an important method for determining whether patients have metastatic disease (except in cases of early cancer or known metastases), and the group recommended performing this before initiating treatment for patients. The panel made the point that with the complexity of management with neoadjuvant chemotherapy, adjuvant chemoradiation, and adjuvant chemotherapy, patients with gastric cancer should be managed by a multidisciplinary team. Furthermore, because 10% of cases may have a familial basis, those patients with diffuse gastric cancer and a family history of diffuse gastric cancer or those diagnosed at < 45 years of age should be referred to a genetic counselor for further evaluation. Hereditary nonpolyposis colorectal cancer, familial adenomatous polyposis, Peutz-Jeghers syndrome, and hereditary diffuse gastric cancer should be tested for in these cases. In patients with early gastric cancer (such as T1aN0 lesions), these tumors may be removed through the endoscope. In patients with metastatic disease, surgery should only be considered when needed for palliation; asymptomatic patients should have nonsurgical options pursued. With respect to the operation of choice, a D2 lymph node dissection should be performed for patients with advanced cancer and no metastases, although a D1 dissection may be appropriate for patients with early cancer or significant comorbidities. There should be pathologic examination of at least 16 lymph nodes, which is often not reached in the United States. When patients have a total gastrectomy, the panel recommended a Roux-en-Y reconstruction. The panel recommended that nonemergent cases should be managed by surgeons with experience in gastric cancer management, and preferably by surgeons who have a volume of at least 6 cases per year. The laparoscopic approach is deemed to be appropriate, but only by those with significant expertise in these techniques and oncologic surgery. These recommendations are helpful for summarizing the optimal management of gastric cancer patients in our practices. Limitations of this study are that most data were derived from retrospective studies, and there was a heavy emphasis of input from surgical oncologists relative to other specialties.

J. R. Howe, MD

Colon

A Randomized Study on 1-Week Versus 4-Week Prophylaxis for Venous Thromboembolism After Laparoscopic Surgery for Colorectal Cancer

Vedovati MC, Becattini C, Rondelli F, et al (Univ of Perugia, Italy; et al)
Ann Surg 259:665-669, 2014

Objective.—To compare the efficacy and safety of antithrombotic prophylaxis given for 1 week or 4 weeks in patients undergoing laparoscopic surgery for colorectal cancer.

Background.—Extending antithrombotic prophylaxis beyond 1 week reduces the incidence of venous thromboembolism (VTE) after open abdominal surgery for cancer.

Methods.—In consecutive patients who underwent laparoscopic surgery for colorectal cancer, complete compression ultrasonography of the lower limbs was performed after 8 ± 2 days of antithrombotic prophylaxis. Patients with no evidence of VTE were randomized to short (heparin withdrawal) or to extended (heparin continued for 3 additional weeks) prophylaxis. Complete compression ultrasonography was repeated at day 28 ± 2 after surgery by investigators blinded to treatment allocation. The primary outcome of the study was the composite of symptomatic and ultrasonography-detected VTE at day 28 ± 2 after surgery.

Results.—Overall, 301 patients were evaluated for inclusion in the study and 225 were randomized. VTE occurred in 11 of 113 patients randomized to short (9.7%) and in none of the 112 patients randomized to extended heparin prophylaxis ($P = 0.001$). The incidence of VTE at 3 months was 9.7% and 0.9% in patients randomized to short or to extended heparin prophylaxis, respectively (relative risk reduction: 91%, 95% confidence interval: 30%−99%; $P = 0.005$). The rate of bleeding was similar in the 2 treatment groups. Two patients died during the study period, 1 in each treatment group.

Conclusions.—After laparoscopic surgery for colorectal cancer, extended antithrombotic prophylaxis is safe and reduces the risk for VTE as compared with 1-week prophylaxis (NCT01589146) (Fig 2).

▶ Studies of venous thromboembolism (VTE) after major abdominal/pelvic surgery indicate that low-molecular-weight heparin (LMWH) can reduce the risk by 60% in patients who receive prolonged prophylaxis as outpatients compared with those who are just treated during their hospital stay. Other studies have found that the incidence of VTE is higher in open vs laparoscopic cases. However, it is unclear whether patients undergoing laparoscopic surgery have additional risks for VTE, including pneumoperitoneum and use of Trendelenburg position. The aim of this study was to determine the role of prolonged vs in hospital prophylaxis with LMWH in patients undergoing laparoscopic colorectal cancer surgery. All patients were given LMWH, which consisted of enoxaparin in 37%, dalteparin in 18%, and nadroparin in 45% of patients. These were given beginning 1 night preoperatively and continued for 8 days, at which point a complete

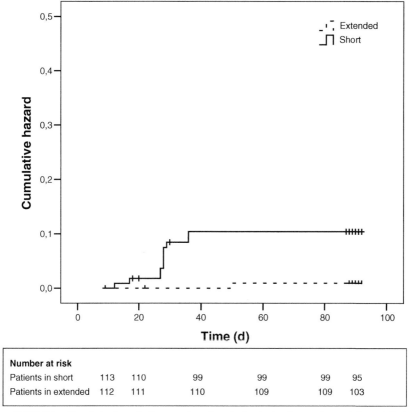

FIGURE 2.—Cumulative hazard of venous thromboembolism in the short and extended prophylaxis groups. (Reprinted from Vedovati MC, Becattini C, Rondelli F, et al. A randomized study on 1-week versus 4-week prophylaxis for venous thromboembolism after laparoscopic surgery for colorectal cancer. *Ann Surg.* 2014;259:665-669, © 2014, Southeastern Surgical Congress.)

compression ultrasound scan of the venous system of the lower limbs was performed. When patients had no evidence of VTE, they were then randomly assigned to no further LMWH or 3 additional weeks of LMWH. All patients were then tested by repeat ultrasonography at day 28, and the rates of VTE were compared. Prior to randomization, 17% of patients were found to have deep vein thrombosis (DVT) at the time of the first ultrasound scan and were excluded from the analyses. In all, 113 patients were randomly assigned to the short prophylaxis group versus 112 assigned to the extended prophylaxis group; VTE developed in 11 patients in the short prophylaxis group, whereas VTE developed in none of those receiving extended prophylaxis (9.7% vs 0%; $P = .0001$, Fig 2). In those 11 patients who had VTE, 2 had symptomatic and proximal DVTs whereas the other 9 were asymptomatic, and DVTs were more distal. No patients suffered pulmonary embolism. Patients were followed up for 3 months, and 1 additional patient in the extended prophylaxis group subsequently had a VTE. There was no significant difference in major bleeding episodes, with 1 patient in each group having one. The only independent risk factor for VTE was age less than 70 years, and a trend toward increased VTE in patients with stage 4 disease. One potential criticism of this study is that 3 LMWHs were used; however, in the extended group, most received enoxaparin after 8 days. Results of this trial suggest that we should consider extended prophylaxis in our patients undergoing laparoscopic colorectal cancer surgery, and, by extension, perhaps even other major abdominal procedures.

J. R. Howe, MD

Anastomotic Leak Increases Distant Recurrence and Long-Term Mortality After Curative Resection for Colonic Cancer: A Nationwide Cohort Study
Krarup P-M, on behalf of the Danish Colorectal Cancer Group (Univ of Copenhagen, Denmark)
Ann Surg 259:930-938, 2014

Objective.—To investigate the impact of anastomotic leak (AL) on disease recurrence and long-term mortality in patients alive 120 days after curative resection for colonic cancer.

Background.—There is no solid data as to whether AL after colonic cancer surgery increases the risk of disease recurrence.

Methods.—This was a nationwide cohort study of 9333 patients, prospectively registered in the database of the Danish Colorectal Cancer Group and merged with data from the Danish Pathology Registry and the National Patient Registry. Multivariable Cox regression analysis was used to adjust for confounding.

Results.—The incidence of AL was 6.4%, 744 patients died within 120 days. Of the remaining 8589 patients, 861 (10.0%) developed local recurrence with no association to AL [adjusted hazard ratio (HR) = 0.78; 95% confidence interval (CI): $0.55-1.12$; $P = 0.184$]. Distant recurrence developed in 1281 (14.9%) patients and more frequently after AL (adjusted HR = 1.42; 95% CI: $1.13-1.78$; $P = 0.003$). AL was also associated with increased long-term mortality (adjusted HR = 1.20; 95% CI: $1.01-1.44$; $P = 0.042$). In 2841 patients with stage III cancer, AL was associated with both decreased likelihood of receiving adjuvant chemotherapy (adjusted HR = 0.58; 95% CI: $0.45-0.74$; $P < 0.001$) and a delay to initial administration (16 days; 95% CI: $12-20$ days; $P < 0.001$).

Conclusions.—AL was significantly associated with increased rates of distant recurrence and long-term all-cause mortality. Cancelled or delayed administration of adjuvant chemotherapy may partly account for these findings (Fig 2).

▶ One of the most significant complications after colon surgery is anastomotic leak (AL). The incidence is 3% to 12%, and after rectal cancer surgery it is found to cause increased local recurrence and mortality but does not affect distant recurrence. In previous studies in colon resection, the risk of AL has not shown an increased incidence of either local or distant recurrence but may impact

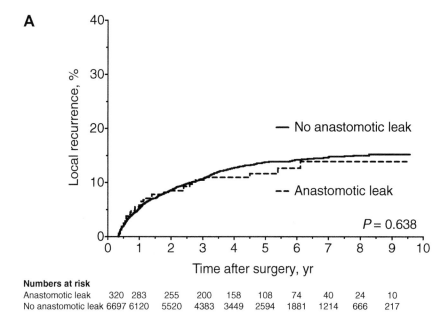

Numbers at risk
Anastomotic leak   320 283   255   200   158   108   74   40   24   10
No anastomotic leak 6697 6120   5520   4383   3449   2594   1881 1214   666   217

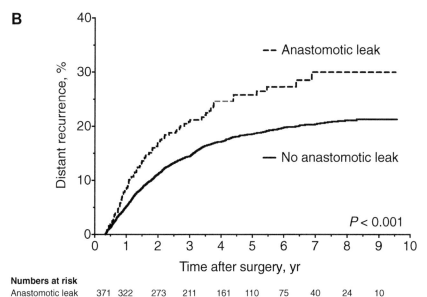

Numbers at risk
Anastomotic leak   371 322   273   211   161   110   75   40   24   10
No anastomotic leak 7066 6473   5692   4470   3499   2626   1889 1219   666   217

FIGURE 2.—Kaplan-Meier plots illustrating the association between AL and the rates of local (A) and distant (B) recurrence in patients alive 120 days after curative colonic cancer surgery. (Reprinted from Krarup P-M, on behalf of the Danish Colorectal Cancer Group. Anastomotic leak increases distant recurrence and long-term mortality after curative resection for colonic cancer: a nationwide cohort study. *Ann Surg.* 2014;259:930-938, © 2014, Southeastern Surgical Congress.)

overall survival. This study set out to look at these relationships more carefully in a group of patients from Denmark who underwent colorectal surgery between 2001 and 2008. This study included more than 9000 patients, capturing approximately 95% of all patients in the country of Denmark during this period. They excluded patients who died within the first 120 days of surgery, so as not to confound it with operative mortality. The overall rate of AL was 6.4% in this study, and the rate of 120-day mortality was 7.9%. The median follow-up was 5.3 years. Local recurrence occurred in 10% of patients, and 15% experienced distant recurrence. Unlike in rectal cancer, AL was not correlated with increased risk of local recurrence. There was a significant correlation with distant recurrence, however, and this held up on a multivariate analysis with a hazard ratio of 1.42 (Fig 2). Local recurrences were seen at a median of 1.2 years after surgery, and distant recurrences at 1.5 years. AL was also a significant contributor to overall mortality, as was distant recurrence. One-third of patients had stage III disease, and patients with AL received chemotherapy a median of 16 days later relative to those without AL, and patients with AL were less likely to receive adjuvant chemotherapy. This study establishes that an AL is a significant risk factor for mortality after colon surgery. This mortality is not caused by increased local recurrence but rather by increased distant recurrence, which is different from AL in rectal cancer surgery. The authors believe that contributing factors to an increased rate of distant metastases from AL may be caused by reduced administration of adjuvant chemotherapy and potentially the intense inflammatory reaction. Overall, this was a well-done, population-based, retrospective study, the findings of which supersede those of a recent meta-analysis, which did not show an association of AL with distant recurrence (but included data from both colon and rectal studies). Inclusion of these findings with this meta-analysis confirms this association of AL with distant recurrence.

J. R. Howe, MD

Effect of 3 to 5 Years of Scheduled CEA and CT Follow-up to Detect Recurrence of Colorectal Cancer: The FACS Randomized Clinical Trial

Primrose JN, Perera R, Gray A, et al (Univ of Southampton, England; Univ of Oxford, England)
JAMA 311:263-270, 2014

Importance.—Intensive follow-up after surgery for colorectal cancer is common practice but is based on limited evidence.

Objective.—To assess the effect of scheduled blood measurement of carcinoembryonic antigen (CEA) and computed tomography (CT) as follow-up to detect recurrent colorectal cancer treatable with curative intent.

Design, Setting, and Participants.—Randomized clinical trial in 39 National Health Service hospitals in the United Kingdom; 1202 eligible participants were recruited between January 2003 and August 2009 who had undergone curative surgery for primary colorectal cancer, including adjuvant treatment if indicated, with no evidence of residual disease on investigation.

Interventions.—Participants were randomly assigned to 1 of 4 groups: CEA only (n = 300), CT only (n = 299), CEA+CT (n = 302), or minimum follow-up (n = 301). Blood CEA was measured every 3 months for 2 years, then every 6 months for 3 years; CT scans of the chest, abdomen, and pelvis were performed every 6 months for 2 years, then annually for 3 years; and the minimum follow-up group received follow-up if symptoms occurred.

Main Outcomes and Measures.—The primary outcome was surgical treatment of recurrence with curative intent; secondary outcomes were mortality (total and colorectal cancer), time to detection of recurrence, and survival after treatment of recurrence with curative intent.

Results.—After a mean 4.4 (SD, 0.8) years of observation, cancer recurrence was detected in 199 participants (16.6%; 95% CI, 14.5%-18.7%) overall; 71 of 1202 participants (5.9%; 95% CI, 4.6%-7.2%) were treated for recurrence with curative intent, with little difference according to Dukes staging (stage A, 5.1% [13/254]; stage B, 6.1% [34/553]; stage C, 6.2% [22/354]). Surgical treatment of recurrence with curative intent was 2.3% (7/301) in the minimum follow-up group, 6.7% (20/300) in the CEA group, 8% (24/299) in the CT group, and 6.6% (20/302) in the CEA+CT group. Compared with minimum follow-up, the absolute difference in the percentage of patients treated with curative intent in the CEA group was 4.4% (95% CI, 1.0%-7.9%; adjusted odds ratio [OR], 3.00; 95% CI, 1.23-7.33), in the CT group was 5.7% (95% CI, 2.2%-9.5%; adjusted OR, 3.63; 95% CI, 1.51-8.69), and in the CEA+CT group was 4.3% (95% CI, 1.0%-7.9%; adjusted OR, 3.10; 95% CI, 1.10-8.71). The number of deaths was not significantly different in the combined intensive monitoring groups (CEA, CT, and CEA+CT; 18.2% [164/901]) vs the minimum follow-up group (15.9% [48/301]; difference, 2.3%; 95% CI, −2.6% to 7.1%).

Conclusions and Relevance.—Among patients who had undergone curative surgery for primary colorectal cancer, intensive imaging or CEA screening each provided an increased rate of surgical treatment of recurrence with curative intent compared with minimal follow-up; there was no advantage in combining CEA and CT. If there is a survival advantage to any strategy, it is likely to be small.

Trial Registration.—isrctn.org Identifier: 41458548.

▶ In patients undergoing potentially curative surgery for colorectal cancer, the detection of early recurrences could improve survival. Five-year survival of patients with metastatic disease is estimated to approach 40% for those who can have liver or lung metastases successfully resected. The optimal strategy for detecting these recurrences is not known, but meta-analyses have found that serum carcinoembryonic antigen (CEA) levels and CT scanning are the modalities most likely to detect potentially curative recurrences. This study by Primrose et al set out to assess the survival differences in patients followed up with by these modalities after potentially curative surgery. This was a randomized trial in which participants were allocated into 4 separate groups: (1) CEA levels were followed up every 3 months for 2 years then every 6 months for the following 3 years with all patients receiving a CT scan of the chest, abdomen, and pelvis at somewhere between 12 and 18 months; (2) patients had CT of the chest, abdomen, and pelvis every 6 months for 2 years, then once a year every 3 years; (3) patients had both CEA and CT follow-up as described; and (4) patients had just minimum follow-up, which included a CT scan of the chest, abdomen, and pelvis at 12 to 18 months if requested by the clinician. All patients entered into these groups had stages 1–3 colon colorectal cancer with no residual disease, negative margins, and postoperative CEA levels less than 10 μg/L. All patients had a colonoscopy done at the time of trial entry to make sure there was no residual disease, and patients having CT screening had an additional colonoscopy at 2 years. A total of 1211 patients were randomly assigned to each of these 4 groups and then were followed up for a mean of 4.4 years. Patients were fairly evenly balanced between the 4 groups; 40.5% had adjuvant chemotherapy, and 11.6% had radiation therapy for rectal cancer. A total of 16.6% of all patients experienced recurrence (Fig 2 in the original article), of which, 3.4% of all patients had locoregional recurrence and 8.4% had metastatic disease limited to the liver or lung. Two-thirds of the recurrences were detected by CEA or CT scanning, and the other one-third were patients who presented with symptoms or were undergoing workup for another malady. Six percent of all patients had surgical treatment for their recurrences (of the total 16.6% of patients having recurrence, and the frequency of recurrence was similar in stages 1–3). Patients monitored by CEA or CT scanning or a combination had a 3-fold higher rate of surgical treatment for recurrence, and those patients who were treated surgically had a 2- to 3-fold increased chance of still being alive. Interestingly, the overall rate of death and colorectal cancer-specific death was slightly lower in the patients undergoing minimum follow-up vs the other 3 groups, but this number was not statistically significant. Important conclusions from this study were that patients who undergo screening with CEA or CT scanning are more likely to have recurrences detected at an earlier time and are more likely to be treated by surgery. No patients in the minimal follow-up group who presented with recurrence after 2 years underwent surgery. There appeared to be no advantage in doing both CEA and CT scanning versus either alone. Finally, it does not appear that there was a survival advantage to using CT or CEA screening over minimal follow-up; however, this study was underpowered to show that there was truly no difference. This finding certainly raises questions as to the appropriate follow-up for patients with colorectal cancer, and one might argue that in the setting of limited health care resources, few lives are saved by the more intensive follow-up.

J. R. Howe, MD

Multitarget Stool DNA Testing for Colorectal-Cancer Screening

Imperiale TF, Ransohoff DF, Itzkowitz SH, et al (Indiana Univ School of Medicine, Indianapolis; Univ of North Carolina at Chapel Hill; Icahn School of Medicine at Mount Sinai, NY; et al)
N Engl J Med 370:1287-1297, 2014

Background.—An accurate, noninvasive test could improve the effectiveness of colorectal-cancer screening.

Methods.—We compared a noninvasive, multitarget stool DNA test with a fecal immunochemical test (FIT) in persons at average risk for colorectal cancer. The DNA test includes quantitative molecular assays for KRAS mutations, aberrant NDRG4 and BMP3 methylation, and β-actin, plus a hemoglobin immunoassay. Results were generated with the use of a logistic-regression algorithm, with values of 183 or more considered to be positive. FIT values of more than 100 ng of hemoglobin per milliliter of buffer were considered to be positive. Tests were processed independently of colonoscopic findings.

Results.—Of the 9989 participants who could be evaluated, 65 (0.7%) had colorectal cancer and 757 (7.6%) had advanced precancerous lesions (advanced adenomas or sessile serrated polyps measuring ≥ 1 cm in the greatest dimension) on colonoscopy. The sensitivity for detecting colorectal cancer was 92.3% with DNA testing and 73.8% with FIT ($P = 0.002$). The sensitivity for detecting advanced precancerous lesions was 42.4% with DNA testing and 23.8% with FIT ($P < 0.001$). The rate of detection of polyps with high-grade dysplasia was 69.2% with DNA testing and 46.2% with FIT ($P = 0.004$); the rates of detection of serrated sessile polyps measuring 1 cm or more were 42.4% and 5.1%, respectively ($P < 0.001$). Specificities with DNA testing and FIT were 86.6% and 94.9%, respectively, among participants with nonadvanced or negative findings ($P < 0.001$) and 89.8% and 96.4%, respectively, among those with negative results on colonoscopy ($P < 0.001$). The numbers of persons who would need to be screened to detect one cancer were 154 with colonoscopy, 166 with DNA testing, and 208 with FIT.

Conclusions.—In asymptomatic persons at average risk for colorectal cancer, multitarget stool DNA testing detected significantly more cancers than did FIT but had more false positive results. (Funded by Exact Sciences; ClinicalTrials.gov number, NCT01397747.)

▶ Screening for colorectal cancer in the United States relies predominantly on testing for fecal occult blood and colonoscopy. Recently, new tests have been devised that are less invasive than colonoscopy, which include a fecal immuno-histochemical test (FIT) for human hemoglobin as well as DNA testing of the stool. This study compared the results of the gold standard, colonoscopy, with the FIT test and DNA tests. The patient population was those who were asymptomatic, aged 50 to 84 years, and at average risk for colorectal cancer who had screening colonoscopy scheduled. Patients with previous gastrointestinal or colon cancers who had undergone screening in the past 9 years or had positive fecal occult blood testing were excluded. Patients had stool samples taken ahead of their bowel preparation for colonoscopy, and these samples were frozen in appropriate buffer for the DNA test and refrigerated for the FIT test. The DNA test looked specifically at aberrant methylation of the promoters of BMP3 and NDRG4, mutant KRAS, an immunochemical assay for hemoglobin, and beta actin as a control. In all, 9989 patients participated in this study, and of this group, 65 were found on colonoscopy to have colorectal cancer (0.7%). Sixty of 65 patients had stage I—III cancer. Another 757 patients (7.6%) had advanced precancerous lesions (which included adenomas with high grade dysplasia, greater than 25% villous features, measuring more than 1 cm, or serrated polyps over 1 cm). The DNA stool test identified 60 of 65 cancers (92%) and 321 (42%) of the advanced precancerous lesions. In comparison, the FIT test identified 48 of 65 colon cancers (74%) and 180 (24%) advanced precancerous lesions. In patients who had no lesions found on colonoscopy, 10.2% had false-positive results by stool testing, as did 13.4% of patients who had either no lesions or no advanced adenomas. For the FIT test, 3.6% with no lesions found had a false-positive test, and 5.1% with no lesions or no advanced adenomas. This study calculated that to identify 1 colorectal cancer, 154 patients would require colonoscopy, 166 by the DNA stool test, and 208 by the FIT test. This study demonstrated the superiority of this DNA stool test over FIT for identification of colorectal cancers in asymptomatic, average risk patients. It did fairly well with identifying advanced pre-cancerous lesions as well, and exceeded that of FIT. However, it did have a higher rate of false-positives and therefore reduced specificity as compared to FIT. This study shows that these tests could be useful in determining which patients will benefit most from colonoscopy, with few cancers being missed by the DNA stool test. But many precancerous lesions would be missed, which could be treated at an earlier stage if they were found by colonoscopy, and there were many false positives. It is therefore not clear at this time what the role of this DNA stool test should be, although the simplicity of this test with examination of just 3 genes raises questions as to whether it could be improved using additional ones.

J. R. Howe, MD

Hepatic Colorectal

Prognostic Impact of Primary Tumor Resection and Lymph Node Dissection in Stage IV Colorectal Cancer with Unresectable Metastasis: A Propensity Score Analysis in a Multicenter Retrospective Study
Ishihara S, Hayama T, Yamada H, et al (Univ of Tokyo Hosp, Japan; Teikyo Univ, Tokyo, Japan; et al)
Ann Surg Oncol 21:2949-2955, 2014

Background.—Retrospective studies have shown that primary tumor resection improves the prognosis of patients with colorectal cancer with unresectable metastasis (mCRC). Prognostic significance of lymph node dissection (LND) in mCRC has not been examined previously. The aim of this study was to investigate the prognostic impact of primary tumor resection and LND in mCRC.

Methods.—A total of 1,982 patients with mCRC from January 1997 to December 2007 were retrospectively studied. The impact of primary tumor resection and LND on overall survival (OS) was analyzed using Cox proportional hazards model and propensity score analysis to mitigate the selection bias. Covariates in the models for propensity scores included treatment period, institution, age, sex, carcinoembryonic antigen, tumor location, histology, depth, lymph node metastasis, lymphovascular invasion, and number of metastatic organs.

Results.—In a multivariate analysis, primary tumor resection and treatment in the latter period were associated with an improved OS, and age over 70 years, female sex, lymph node metastasis, and multiple organ metastasis were associated with a decreased OS. In the propensity-matched cohort, patients treated with primary tumor resection showed a significantly better OS than those without tumor resection (median OS 13.8 vs. 6.3 months; $p = 0.0001$). Furthermore, among patients treated with primary tumor resection, patients treated with D3 LND showed a significantly better OS than those with less extensive LND (median OS 17.2 vs. 13.7 months; $p < 0.0001$).

Conclusions.—It was suggested that primary tumor resection with D3 LND improves the survival of patients with mCRC.

▶ When patients with colorectal cancer have distant metastases that appear to be unresectable at presentation, the indications for going in to remove the primary tumor are generally when patients have symptoms, such as obstruction, bleeding, or perforation. This study examined the question of whether patients who have unresectable distant metastases benefit from having their primary tumors resected, and furthermore, whether extended lymph node dissection might also be of benefit. They performed a retrospective study of 17 institutions in Japan in patients with stage 4 colorectal cancer between 1997 and 2007. Patients who had resection of both the primary and metastatic disease were excluded, which left them with 1982 patients who had a median follow-up of 13.3 months. Of these patients, a surprising 90% had their primary tumors resected, whereas only 10% did not. They then compared a variety of clinicopathologic factors between patients who had resection vs no resection, and did a propensity score analysis to try to control for some of these variables. They also divided the group into 2 time periods, the first being 1997–2003 and second 2003–2007. Eighty-two percent of patients died within the follow-up period. They performed a multivariate analysis to determine factors associated with improved survival and found that resection of the primary tumor, being treated in the second time interval, age > 70, absence of clinical nodal metastases, and absence of metastases to multiple organs were significantly associated with improved survival. Median survival with resection was 13.8 vs 6.3 months without resection ($P = .0001$). Examination of patients who had D3 nodal dissection (dissection of nodes up to the origin of the feeding artery) revealed that they had improved survival compared with those having D0-D2 resections. This finding seemed somewhat counterintuitive given that these patients had unresected distant metastases. One potential hypothesis for this, given in the article, was reduced tolerance of the immune system with resection of these lymph nodes, although this could merely be selection bias. They did do a propensity analysis, and this continued to hold up as being significant. This study concluded that there appeared to be a survival benefit to resecting the primary tumor even in asymptomatic patients with unresectable metastatic disease and that a D3 lymph node dissection was associated with further improvement in survival. Despite the fact that they performed a propensity analysis, the fact that only 10% of patients did not have resection of the primary raises questions about selection bias and cultural differences from practice patterns more commonly seen in the United States. Patients had resection of their primary at a median of 12 days after diagnosis of their stage 4 disease, before the initiation of chemotherapy in most cases. The fact that patients did better in the second half of the study reflects the possibility that this might have been related to the improved chemotherapy; however, it was unclear from the data presented how many patients were actually treated with chemotherapy, for how long, and with what agents. It should also be noted that chemotherapy is often given by the surgeon in Japan. This study raises several interesting questions about whether we should be resecting primaries in asymptomatic patients with metastatic disease. The trend in the United States has been to treat these patients with chemotherapy while leaving the primary tumor in place; this was affirmed by the National Surgical Adjuvant Breast and Bowel Project (NSABP) C10 trial in which patients with asymptomatic colon tumors with unresectable metastases were treated with FOLFOX6 and bevacizumab. Only 14% had significant morbidity due to leaving the tumor in place (12% required surgery, 2% died). The median survival in NSABP C10 study was 19.9 months, which is better than that seen in the current study for surgical resection. Japanese patients during that era were likely to have been treated with 5-fluorouracil and leucovorin alone, and therefore these results are not directly comparable.

J. R. Howe, MD

Cause of Death from Liver Metastases in Colorectal Cancer

Helling TS, Martin M (Univ of Mississippi Med Ctr, Jackson)
Ann Surg Oncol 21:501-506, 2014

Background.—Surgically directed therapy for liver metastases from colorectal cancer (CRC) has received substantial attention in the literature as a major focus of treatment for metastatic CRC. It is presumed, but not proven, that liver metastases are a major threat to life. This study examined the course of a cohort of consecutive patients who died with CRC to determine the role played by the presence of liver metastases.

Methods.—This is single-institution retrospective observational study involved all patients who died of CRC. Records were examined and imaging studies reviewed to determine the extent of liver and extrahepatic metastases in these patients. Overall survival in patients with and without liver metastases and those in whom liver metastases were thought to contribute to death was determined.

Results.—After patient exclusions, the study population totaled 121 patients. There were 75 patients (62 %) with liver metastases at death. In 40 of 75 (53 %) patients, the liver metastases contributed to the patients' death. In 46 of 121 patients (38 %), metastatic disease did not include liver metastases. Overall survival in patients with and without liver metastases (median survival 12 vs. 8.5 months, $p = 0.089$) and in those whose liver metastases did or did not contribute to death (median survival 11.5 vs. 14 months, $p = 0.361$) was not significant.

Conclusions.—The presence of liver metastases seemed to contribute to death in approximately half of the study patients, although there did not appear to be a survival disadvantage in these patients.

▶ It has long been thought that the major cause of death from colorectal cancer was due to liver metastases. However, this has not been definitively shown, and therefore this study was intended to review a single institutional experience of all patients who died of colorectal cancer to try to determine the actual causes of death. The authors performed a retrospective review and identified 147 patients dying of colorectal cancer over 10 years at their center, although it was unclear how they determined whether patients actually died of colorectal cancer vs other causes. They systematically reviewed the charts for evidence of whether the patients had liver metastases, what the distribution of extrahepatic metastases was, the length of survival of patients, what they died of, and finally whether it appeared as if the liver metastases were involved in causing the death of the patient. Criteria for this latter category were having greater than 50% involvement of the liver, involvement of the main portal vein, or biliary obstruction. From the group of 147, 26 were excluded either because of insufficient data or (in 13 cases) due to postoperative deaths; 41% of patients had liver metastases present at the time of diagnosis, 51% had liver metastases present at their death, and 61% developed extrahepatic metastases by the time of death. In 40 of 75 patients who had liver metastases present at death (53%), the liver metastases were thought to contribute to the patient's death. The leading cause of death in just under half of these patients was inanition, followed by multisystem organ failure in 18%, liver failure in 8%, cirrhotic liver tumor in 5%, portal vein obstruction in 5%, and biliary obstruction in 10%. Interestingly, in 35 of 75 patients with liver metastases (47%), liver involvement by tumor was not thought to be a major contributor to the death of the patients. Of 92 total patients with extrahepatic disease at death, 69 (75%) also had liver metastases. Survival curves were generated looking at median survival of patients with no liver metastases vs liver metastases at death and those with massive liver disease vs more limited liver disease, but these differences were not statistically significant. This study revealed that 62% of patients who died of colorectal cancer had liver metastases, and in more than half of these patients, the liver metastases were a major contributor to the patient's death, but it came up short in helping us to understand how these patients die of metastatic colorectal cancer. It did not enumerate the most common sites of extrahepatic metastases, which would also have also been of interest. So this study provided some insight into the question at hand but was subject to the limitations of a retrospective review and insufficient information on how the cause of death was actually determined.

J. R. Howe, MD

Pancreatic

A Randomized Prospective Multicenter Trial of Pancreaticoduodenectomy With and Without Routine Intraperitoneal Drainage

Van Buren G, II, Bloomston M, Hughes SJ, et al (The Dan L. Duncan Cancer Ctr, Houston, TX; The Ohio State Univ, Columbus, OH; Univ of Florida, Gainesville; et al)
Ann Surg 259:605-612, 2014

Objective.—To test by randomized prospective multicenter trial the hypothesis that pancreaticoduodenectomy (PD) without the use of intraperitoneal drainage does not increase the frequency or severity of complications.

Background.—Some surgeons have abandoned the use of drains placed during pancreas resection.

Methods.—We randomized 137 patients to PD with (n = 68, drain group) and without (n = 69, no-drain group) the use of intraperitoneal drainage and compared the safety of this approach and spectrum of complications between the 2 groups.

Results.—There were no differences between drain and no-drain cohorts in demographics, comorbidities, pathology, pancreatic duct size, pancreas texture, baseline quality of life, or operative technique. PD without intraperitoneal drainage was associated with an increase in the number of complications per patient [1 (0-2) vs 2 (1-4), $P = 0.029$]; an increase in the number of patients who had at least 1 ≥grade 2 complication [35 (52%) vs 47 (68%), $P = 0.047$]; and a higher average complication severity [2 (0-2) vs 2 (1-3), $P = 0.027$]. PD without intraperitoneal drainage was associated with a higher incidence of gastroparesis, intra-abdominal fluid collection, intra-abdominal abscess (10% vs 25%, $P = 0.027$), severe (≥grade 2) diarrhea, need for a postoperative percutaneous drain, and a prolonged length of stay. The Data Safety Monitoring Board stopped the study early because of an increase in mortality from 3% to 12% in the patients undergoing PD without intraperitoneal drainage.

Conclusions.—This study provides level 1 data, suggesting that elimination of intraperitoneal drainage in all cases of PD increases the frequency and severity of complications (Table 3).

▶ An area of continuing controversy has been the need for drainage after pancreaticoduodenectomy. The placement of drains near a pancreaticojejunostomy or bile duct anastomosis was relatively routine until retrospective studies found that there was no difference in complication rates between patients with and without drains. A randomized trial from Memorial Sloan Kettering Cancer Center

TABLE 3.—. Morbidity 30 and 60 Days After Pancreaticoduodenectomy

N (%) or Median (Interquartile Range)	30 d Drain (68)	No Drain (69)	P	60 d Drain (68)	No Drain (69)	P
Any complication	50 (74)	52 (75)	0.8057	50 (74)	55 (80)	0.393
Any ≥grade 2 complication (primary endpoint)	32 (47)	44 (64)	0.049	35 (52)	47 (68)	0.047
Any ≥grade 3 complication	19 (28)	28 (41)	0.119	21 (31)	28 (41)	0.236
Median number of complications per patient (any grade)	1 (0-2)	2 (1-3)	0.123	1 (0-2)	2 (1-4)	0.029*
Mean complication grade (all subjects)	1 (0-2)	2 (1-3)	0.059	2 (0-2)	2 (1-3)	0.027[†]
Mean complication grade (subjects with ≥ 1 Comp.)	2 (1-2)	2 (2-3)	0.007	2 (1-3)	2 (2-3)	0.017[†]
Complications with a significant difference						
Gastroparesis	16 (24)	26 (38)	0.075	16 (24)	29 (42)	0.021
Intra-abdominal abscess	7 (10)	17 (25)	0.027*	8 (12)	18 (26)	0.033
Diarrhea (grade 1 excluded)	2 (3)	9 (13)	0.030	2 (3)	12 (17)	0.005
Abdominal fluid collection	1 (2)	8 (12)	0.033*	1 (2)	8 (12)	0.033*
Complications without a significant difference						
Fistulas						
Pancreatic fistula	21 (31)	14 (20)	0.155	21 (31)	14 (20)	0.155
Pancreatic fistula (grade A excluded)	7 (10)	14 (20)	0.104	8 (12)	14 (20)	0.174
Biliary fistula	3 (4)	1 (1)	0.366*	3 (4)	2 (3)	0.681*
Enteric fistula	—	1 (2)	1*	—	1 (2)	1*
Chyle fistula	1 (2)		0.496*	1 (2)	—	0.495*
Infection and wound healing						
Pneumonia	3 (4)	6 (9)	0.493*	3 (4)	7 (10)	0.325*
Wound infection	6 (9)	10 (15)	0.302	7 (10)	10 (15)	0.456
Wound seroma	3 (4)	5 (7)	0.718*	3 (4)	6 (9)	0.493*
Wound dehiscence	2 (3)	4 (6)	0.681*	2 (3)	5 (7)	0.441*
Urinary tract infection	3 (4)	3 (4)	1*	4 (6)	5 (7)	1*
Bacteremia/sepsis	2 (3)	4 (6)	0.681*	4 (6)	5 (7)	1*
Cardiovascular complications						
Central venous catheter infection	2 (3)	1 (2)	0.620*	2 (3)	1 (2)	0.620*
Intra-abdominal hemorrhage	4 (6)	4 (6)	1*	4 (6)	6 (9)	0.745*
Gastrointestinal hemorrhage	2 (3)	6 (9)	0.274*	2 (3)	7 (10)	0.165*
Thromboembolic event	4 (6)	1 (2)	0.208*	5 (7)	1 (2)	0.115*
Arrhythmia	9 (13)	6 (9)	0.395	9 (13)	6 (9)	0.395
Myocardial infarction	1 (2)	—	0.496*	1 (2)	1 (2)	1*
Organ failure						
Acute respiratory distress syndrome/respiratory failure	2 (3)	4 (6)	0.681*	2 (3)	6 (9)	0.274*
Hepatic failure	—	1 (2)	1*	1 (2)	1 (2)	1*
Renal failure/insufficiency	1 (2)	7 (10)	0.062*	3 (4)	9 (13)	0.074
Neurologic complications						
Transient ischemic attack	1 (2)	—	0.496*	1 (2)	—	0.497*
Cerebral infarct/hemorrhage (stroke)	1 (2)	—	0.496*	1 (2)	—	0.497*
Altered mental status	1 (2)	5 (7)	0.208*	1 (2)	7 (10)	0.062*
Miscellaneous complications						
Urinary retention	5 (7)	3 (4)	0.493*	5 (7)	4 (6)	0.745*
Diarrhea (all grades)	9 (13)	13 (19)	0.372	10 (15)	19 (28)	0.066
Other	5 (7)	5 (7)	1*	5 (7)	9 (13)	0.272

*Fisher exact test.
[†]Wilcoxon rank sum test; others: χ^2 test.

found no difference in mortality or complication rates after pancreaticoduodenectomy or distal pancreatectomy with or without drains.[1] Arguments against drainage include the possibility of causing fistulas, the fact that fistulas do not develop in most patients, and if fistula does occur, a percutaneous drain can be placed later. This study was a randomized, prospective, multicenter trial to evaluate the need for drainage after pancreaticoduodenectomy. A total of 137 patients were randomly assigned, 68 of whom had drains and 69 of whom had no drains. Drain amylase was measured on postoperative day 3, and drains were left in place until the amylase concentration was less than 3 times normal or the output was less than 20 mL/d for 2 consecutive days. The authors carefully recorded complications up to 60 days and mortality up to 90 days. Both groups were similar in terms of comorbidities, two-thirds of the patients receiving drains had 2 drains, and one-third had 1 drain placed. The data safety monitoring board stopped the study early because of the finding of increased mortality in patients without drains, with a 12% death rate in the no-drain group and 3% in the drain group; however, this difference was not statistically significant ($P = .097$). Five of the 10 deaths were caused by intra-abdominal hemorrhage, and 2 were related to recurrent pancreatic cancer. Interestingly, 4 of the 8 deaths in the no-drain group occurred within 30 days, whereas the remaining 4 occurred between 30 and 90 days. Neither of the 2 deaths in the drain group occurred in the first 30 days. There was a higher incidence of grade 2 complications in the no-drain group—a higher rate of intra-abdominal abscess, diarrhea, and abdominal fluid collections, all of which were statistically significant. At 60 days, there was an increased incidence of gastroparesis in the no-drain group as well. Seventy percent of the deaths were associated with pancreatic fistula, sepsis, multisystem organ failure, or hemorrhage. This study found that not draining pancreaticoduodenectomy patients resulted in an increase in death and morbidity and increased readmission rate. The authors concluded that the practice of not draining pancreaticoduodenectomy patients was not safe in all patients. Unique to this study was that it followed up with patients for up to 90 days for complications and deaths, which is not characteristic of other series. It was also randomized, and the 2 groups were well matched. Sixty percent of deaths occurred after 30 days, and 6 of the 8 patients who died in the no-drain group died of sepsis and multisystem organ failure caused by pancreatic fistula. This is a very well-performed study, which should be required reading for all pancreatic surgeons.

J. R. Howe, MD

Reference

1. Conlon KC, Labow D, Leung D, et al. Prospective randomized clinical trial of the value of intraperitoneal drainage after pancreatic resection. *Ann Surg.* 2001;234: 487-493.

Minimally-Invasive vs Open Pancreaticoduodenectomy: Systematic Review and Meta-Analysis

Correa-Gallego C, Dinkelspiel HE, Sulimanoff I, et al (Memorial Sloan-Kettering Cancer Ctr; New York Presbyterian Hosp; Emory Univ Hosp, Atlanta, GA)

J Am Coll Surg 218:129-139, 2014

Background.—Minimally invasive surgery (MIS) is an established approach for many procedures, but pancreaticoduodenectomy (PD) poses special challenges. However, MIS PD approaches have been used for over 20 years, providing retrospective reports that allow a comparison between the surgical and oncologic outcomes of patients undergoing the MIS or traditional open approach.

Methods.—Comprehensive literature searches were performed of the PubMed, EMBASE, and Cochrane Library databases covering 1994 through January 2013. The six studies selected documented the cases of 542 patients, with 169 having MIS and 373 having open procedures. None of these studies reported randomized controlled trials. Most operations were performed for malignancy, but all indications were considered. The operative and perioperative outcomes were compared between the two approaches.

Results.—MIS PD was associated with less intraoperative blood loss but longer operative times than the traditional open approach. However, the MIS patients had a significantly higher retrieval of lymph nodes (3 nodes higher) compared to those having the open approach, and the likelihood that these patients would require a resection for a microscopically positive margin (R1) was significantly lower than with the open surgery. The open group patients had significantly larger tumors than those in the MIS group. Twenty-one percent of the MIS group and 17% of the open group developed pancreatic fistula; these were clinically relevant in 8% and 7%, respectively, of the cases. Comparable outcomes were noted for morbidity, need for reoperation, and certain complications, including delayed gastric emptying, postpancreatectomy hemorrhage, and wound infection. The MIS group spent approximately 3.7 days less time in the hospital than the open group, which was a significant difference. Seventeen patients in the MIS group required conversion to an open procedure, with most in response to a hemorrhage or an inability to obtain adequate vascular control laparoscopically. The perioperative death of one patient was directly related to surgical bleeding.

Conclusions.—The conclusions of the meta-analysis are influenced by the fact that the experiences documented occurred early in the course of using a complex minimally invasive technique and do not consider the learning curve that develops over time. However, MIS PD appears to be a feasible procedure in highly selected patients cared for in specific centers. Its advantages include a shorter hospital stay and possibly higher lymph node retrieval. However, randomized controlled trials or prospective cohort

Study name Events / Total Statistics for each study   **Odds ratio and 95% CI**

	MIS	Open	Odds ratio	Lower limit	Upper limit	p-Value
Buchs	3 / 33	5 / 27	0,4	0,1	2,0	0,294
Zhou	0 / 8	1 / 6	0,2	0,0	6,3	0,373
Zureikat	0 / 12	1 / 12	0,3	0,0	8,3	0,483
Asbun	2 / 39	24 / 141	0,3	0,1	1,2	0,079
Chalikonda	0 / 14	4 / 14	0,1	0,0	1,7	0,103
Lai	4 / 15	21 / 53	0,6	0,2	2,0	0,362
	9 / 121	56 / 253	0,4	0,2	0,8	0,007

0,1 0,2 0,5 1 2 5 10

Favours MIS   Favours Open

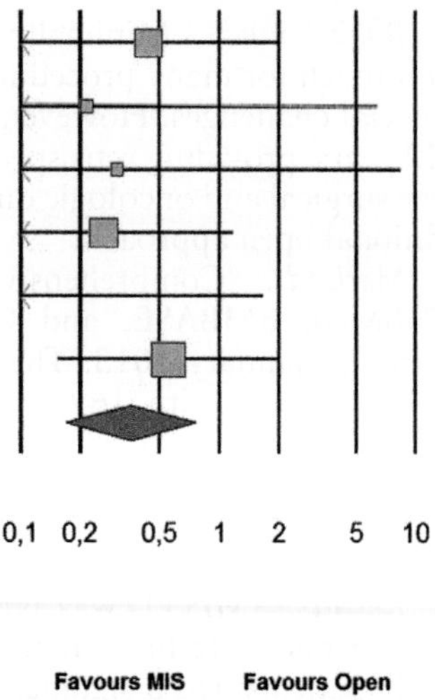

FIGURE 5.—Pooled estimate of rate of R0 resections for minimally invasive surgery (MIS) vs open pancreaticoduodenectomy. (Reprinted from Correa-Gallego C, Dinkelspiel HE, Sulimanoff I, et al. Minimally-invasive vs open pancreaticoduodenectomy: systematic review and meta-analysis. *J Am Coll Surg.* 2014;218:129-139, with permission from the American College of Surgeons.)

studies are required to substantiate the occurrence of these improved outcomes (Fig 5).

▶ The first laparoscopic pancreaticoduodenectomy was described by Gagner in 1994, and since then, various surgeons and centers have gradually been accumulating experience with this procedure. An important question is whether this minimally invasive procedure results in improved outcomes in terms of length of stay and complications and comparable oncologic outcomes, such as lymph node harvest, completeness of resection, and long-term survival. Because there have been no randomized, controlled trials to assess open vs minimally invasive pancreaticoduodenectomy (PD), this report attempted to compare these groups by performing a meta-analysis of published studies. After identifying 527 references for minimally invasive PD, 6 met the criteria of comparing open with minimally invasive techniques, having greater than 8 cases and reporting at least 1 outcome variable. These 6 studies totaled 542 patients, 169 of whom underwent minimally invasive PD and 373 of whom had open PD. The significant findings from pooling these studies were that there was a reduction of intraoperative blood loss and longer operating times but improved retrieval of lymph nodes (> 3 nodes higher) and higher likelihood of an R0 resection in the minimally invasive group (Fig 5). The size of tumors was smaller in the minimally invasive group, but the complication rates of pancreatic fistula, wound infection, a need for reoperation, delayed gastric emptying, and pancreatic fistula were not significantly different between the open and laparoscopic groups. Ten percent of minimally invasive procedures required conversion to an open procedure, and many of these patients were then included in the open arms of their respective studies, introducing bias into the open group. Conclusions to be drawn from this study were that minimally invasive techniques are feasible, with several centers showing expertise and good outcomes. The minimally invasive approach allowed for reduced blood loss, perhaps due to better magnification, shorter length of stay by 3 days, improved lymph node retrieval, and more R0 resections. None of these studies had long-term follow-up and, therefore, the effect on survival was not available. It does appear that complication rates are similar for these 2 techniques; therefore, minimally invasive PD does appear to be a reasonable alternative to the open procedure. There was potential for bias because these reports were limited to centers shown to have expertise in the technique, but, conversely, many of these cases would have been performed during the learning curve of the operation with bias toward reduced efficacy. Whether this operation will replace the open procedure in the future because of these benefits or surgeons conclude that the results are not great enough to warrant training future generations of surgeons to do these complex cases, remains to be seen. A randomized, controlled trial reporting long-term oncologic outcomes would clearly be the best way to determine this, as has been done for laparoscopic colorectal surgery in colon cancer.

J. R. Howe, MD

Parenchyma-Sparing Pancreatectomy for Presumed Noninvasive Intraductal Papillary Mucinous Neoplasms of the Pancreas
Sauvanet A, Gaujoux S, Blanc B, et al (Beaujon Hosp, Clichy, France; et al)
Ann Surg 260:364-371, 2014

Objective.—To assess the feasibility and outcomes of parenchyma-sparing pancreatectomy (PSP), including enucleation (EN), resection of uncinate process (RUP), and central pancreatectomy (CP), as an alternative to standard pancreatectomy for presumed noninvasive intraductal papillary and mucinous neoplasms (IPMNs).

Background.—Pancreaticoduodenectomy and distal pancreatectomy are associated with significant perioperative morbidity, a substantial risk of pancreatic insufficiency, and may overtreat noninvasive IPMNs.

Methods.—From 1999 to 2011, PSP was attempted in 91 patients with presumed noninvasive IPMNs, after complete preoperative work-up including computed tomography, magnetic resonance imaging, and endoscopic ultrasonography. Intraoperative frozen section examination was routinely performed to assess surgical margins and rule out invasive malignancy. Follow-up included clinical, biochemical, and radiological assessments.

Results.—Overall PSP was achieved with a feasibility rate of 89% (n = 81), including 44 ENs, 5 RUPs, and 32 CPs. Postoperative mortality rate was 1.3% (n = 1), and overall morbidity was noteworthy (61%; n = 47). Definitive pathological examination confirmed IPMN diagnosis in 95% of patients (n = 77), all except 2 (3%), without invasive component. After a median follow-up of 50 months, both pancreatic endocrine/exocrine functions were preserved in 92% of patients. Ten-year progression-free survival was 76%, and reoperation for recurrence was required in 4% of patients (n = 3).

Conclusions. In selected patients, PSP for presumed noninvasive IPMN in experienced hands is highly feasible and avoids inappropriate standard resections for IPMN-mimicking lesions. Early morbidity is greater than that after standard resections but counterbalanced by preservation of pancreatic endocrine/exocrine functions and a low rate of reoperation for tumor recurrence (Fig 1).

▶ Intraductal papillary mucinous neoplasms (IPMNs) of the pancreas are challenging tumors in that they can be multifocal, may be invasive, and may involve the main duct. Patients can have symptoms of pancreatitis or epigastric pain, and these tumors can progress to adenocarcinoma. The standard practice for these lesions has been adequate preoperative evaluation to categorize them into low- and high-risk groups for malignancy. The finding of a mural nodule greater than 5 mm in size, main ductal dilatation greater than 10–15 mm, and an infiltrating mass are indications for standard pancreatic resections with procedures such as pancreaticoduodenectomy or distal pancreatectomy. However, when these features are not seen, patients may be eligible for procedures that will preserve more pancreatic parenchyma, improving the likelihood of better long-term endocrine and exocrine function. This report reviewed one center's experience with performing pancreatic enucleation, resection of the uncinate process, and central pancreatectomy for patients suspected of having IPMNs deemed at low risk for invasive components. Of 413 patients seen with a presumptive diagnosis of IPMN after undergoing pancreatic protocol CT, MRI with cholangio-pancreatography, or endoscopic ultrasound scan, the authors excluded all patients with main duct IPMNs, tumor size greater than 3 cm, tumors that increased in size over successive follow-up imaging, those with mural nodules, and those with symptoms attributable to IPMN. When patients had lesions deemed to be amenable to these lesser procedures, patients underwent laparotomy, and intraoperative ultrasound scan was performed. When enucleation was performed, they tried to dissect the dilated duct and ligate it; when central pancreatectomy was carried out, pancreaticogastrostomy was carried out for the distal segment; and in resection of the uncinate process, they tried to ligate branch ducts, keeping parallel to the main duct, and preserve the pancreaticoduodenal arcade. Frozen sections were used liberally to rule out the presence of invasive carcinoma. Patients were treated with octreotide, 100 μg 3 times a day, and drains were generally removed when the output was less than 25 mL/d. Out of their initial 413 patients, they attempted parenchyma-sparing surgery in 91 patients, but in 10 patients, a standard pancreatectomy was instead performed

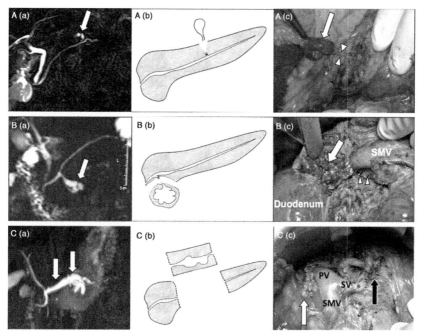

FIGURE 1.—Parenchyma-sparing pancreatic resections for presumed noninvasive IPMNs of the pancreas: A, EN of a branch-duct IPMN of the pancreas: MRI with cholangiopancreatography (a); schematic representation (b); and intraoperative view (c) (large arrow: enucleated branch duct; arrowheads: communicating duct). B, RUP for a branch-duct IPMN of the pancreas: MRI with cholangiopancreatography (a); schematic representation (b); and intraoperative view (c) (large arrow: communicating duct on the pancreatic cut surface; arrowheads: superior mesenteric artery). SMV indicates superior mesenteric vein. C, CP for a main-duct IPMN of the pancreas: MRI with cholangiopancreatography (a); schematic representation (b); and intraoperative view (c) (white arrow: cephalic remnant; black arrow: distal remnant to be anastomosed to the stomach). PV indicates portal vein; SMV, superior mesenteric vein; SV, splenic vein. (Reprinted from Sauvanet A, Gaujoux S, Blanc B, et al. Parenchyma-sparing pancreatectomy for presumed noninvasive intraductal papillary mucinous neoplasms of the pancreas. *Ann Surg.* 2014;260:364-371, © 2014, Southeastern Surgical Congress.)

(in 7 cases because of frozen section results, and in 3 severe inflammation precluded performing a lesser procedure). Of the 81 parenchymal-sparing procedures, 77 were IPMNs on pathologic examination, whereas 2 others were simple cysts, another was a serous cystadenoma, and one other was a pseudocyst. Forty-two (55%) patients had enucleation, 5 (6%) had resection of the uncinate process, and 30 (39%) had central pancreatectomy. The general features of these operations are shown in Fig 1. There was 1 mortality in this series, and the overall morbidity rate was high, at 61% (major morbidity, 27%). There were no significant differences in complications between central pancreatectomy, enucleation, or uncinate process resection. Fifty-one percent of the group had pancreatic fistula with 30% of the entire group having grade A and 21% grade B or C. Six percent of patients required reoperation, and 10% had interventional radiology or endoscopic procedures performed. The mean length of stay was fairly long at 25 days, but readmission rates were low (1 patient).

The accuracy of frozen section was approximately 95%, and only 2 patients ended up having invasive cancer, both of which were less than 5 mm in size. Follow-up was an impressive 50 months in this series, and the 5-year progression-free survival rate was 92%. Only 4 (5%) patients had endocrine function deterioration, and 4 (5%) had exocrine insufficiency. This report shows that parenchymal-preserving pancreas surgery may be beneficial in patients with noninvasive IPMNs in terms of preservation of pancreatic endocrine and exocrine function with a low risk for needing reoperation for recurrent disease (3 patients). However, these procedures come at a high price of postoperative complications in more than one-half of the patients, with a high risk of pancreatic fistula.

J. R. Howe, MD

Prognostic Impact of CA 19-9 on Outcome after Neoadjuvant Chemoradiation in Patients with Locally Advanced Pancreatic Cancer
Combs SE, Habermehl D, Kessel KA, et al (Univ Hosp of Heidelberg, Germany; Technische Universität München (TUM), Munich, Germany)
Ann Surg Oncol 21:2801-2807, 2014

Background.—To assess the impact of CA 19-9 and weight loss/gain on outcome after neoadjuvant chemoradiation (CRT) in patients with locally advanced pancreatic cancer (LAPC).

Methods.—We analyzed 289 patients with LAPC treated with CRT for LAPC. All patients received concomitant chemotherapy parallel to radiotherapy and adjuvant treatments. CA 19-9 and body weight were collected as prognostic and predictive markers. All patients were included into a regular follow-up with reassessment of resectability.

Results.—Median overall survival in all patients was 14 months. Actuarial overall survival was 37% at 12 months, 12% at 24 months, and 4% at 36 months. Secondary resectability was achieved in 35% of the patients. R0/R1 resection was significantly associated with increase in overall survival ($p = 0.04$). Intraoperative radiotherapy was applied in 50 patients, but it did not influence overall survival ($p = 0.05$). Pretreatment CA 19-9 significantly influenced overall survival using different cutoff values. With increase in CA 19-9 levels, the possibility of secondary surgical resection decreased from 46% in patients with CA 19-9 levels below 90 U/ml to 31% in the group with CA 19-9 levels higher than 269 U/ml.

Discussion.—This large group of patients with LAPC treated with neoadjuvant CRT confirms that CA 19-9 and body weight are strong predictive and prognostic factors of outcome. In the future, individual patient factors should be taken into account to tailor treatment (Fig 2).

▶ Patients with locally advanced pancreatic cancer are now commonly treated with neoadjuvant chemotherapy or chemoradiation. It would be helpful to have clinical indicators that might suggest which patients will be resectable or might have improved survival after receiving this treatment. This study focused

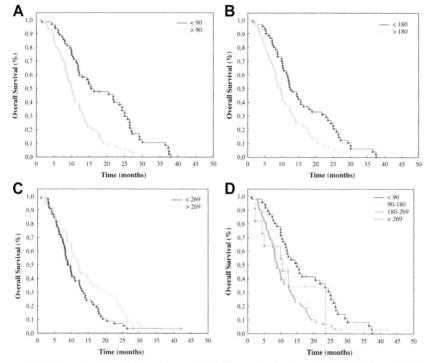

FIGURE 2.—Overall survival according to CA 19-9 levels. Cutoff values of 90 (**a**), 180 (**b**), and 269 U/ml (**c**) had significant impact on outcome. Subclassification into 4 CA 19-9 levels following 3 cutoff values also showed significant influence on outcome. (With kind permission from Springer Science+Business Media. Combs SE, Habermehl D, Kessel KA, et al. Prognostic impact of CA 19-9 on outcome after neoadjuvant chemoradiation in patients with locally advanced pancreatic cancer. *Ann Surg Oncol.* 2014;21:2801-2807, with permission from Society of Surgical Oncology.)

on looking at CA 19-9 levels and weight loss in patients undergoing neoadjuvant chemoradiation to determine whether these were significantly associated with resectability or survival. They looked at 289 patients with locally advanced pancreatic cancer, as defined by >180 degrees encasement of the superior mesenteric artery, infiltration of the celiac axis, occlusion of the superior mesenteric vein or portal vein, or aortic involvement. These patients received radiation therapy, generally 50 to 54 Gy, the vast majority with concurrent gemcitabine. Fifty patients received intraoperative radiation therapy, usually in cases deemed to be unresectable. Patients had CA 19-9 levels checked preoperatively and after treatment, and weight was determined before chemoradiation and then 4 to 6 weeks after completion. Overall, the patients treated in this manner had a median survival of 14 months (37% at 12 months, 12% at 24 months, and 4% at 36 months). With this strategy, 35% of patients became resectable, with significantly improved survival in those having R0/R1 resections vs R2 resections or unresectability. With respect to weight loss, the median weight loss was 2.3 kg, but there was no correlation with overall survival noted between patients with weight loss above or below the median. There were significant differences in survival based upon CA 19-9 levels, which were seen whether the cutoff levels were set at 90 (as used in the CONKO-001 trial; Fig 2), 180 (as suggested by Montgomery et al[1]), or below the median value in this cohort, which was 269 U/mL. There was also a correlation with CA 19-9 levels and resectability, with 46% of patients having a CA 19-9 level < 90 U/mL decreasing down to 31% in those with levels > 269 U/mL. This study demonstrated the potential prognostic value for CA 19-9 levels; however, the ideal cutoff value that should be used to determine prognosis remains unclear. Certainly patients should not be excluded from resection due only to high CA 19-9 levels, but it is clear that patients with levels < 90 U/mL do better than those with more elevated levels. There was no correlation with weight loss in the study. Another limitation of this study is that it used chemoradiation, which is being replaced in many centers by neoadjuvant FOLFIRINOX or gemcitabine with Abraxane.

J. R. Howe, MD

Reference

1. Montgomery RC, Hoffman JP, Riley LB, Rogatko A, Ridge JA, Eisenberg BL. Prediction of recurrence and survival by post-resection CA 19-9 values in patients with adenocarcinoma of the pancreas. *Ann Surg Oncol.* 1997;4:551-556.

A Prospective Randomized Controlled Study Comparing Outcomes of Standard Resection and Extended Resection, Including Dissection of the Nerve Plexus and Various Lymph Nodes, in Patients With Pancreatic Head Cancer

Jang J-Y, Kang MJ, Heo JS, et al (Seoul Natl Univ College of Medicine, South Korea; Sungkyunkwan Univ School of Medicine, Seoul, South Korea; et al)

Ann Surg 259:656-664, 2014

Objective.—To prospectively evaluate the survival benefit of dissection of the nerve plexus and lymphadenectomy in patients with pancreatic head cancer.

Background.—Despite randomized controlled trials on the extent of surgery in pancreatic cancer, attempts have been made to perform more extended resections.

Methods.—A total of 244 patients were enrolled; of these, 200 were randomized to undergo standard resection or extended resection, with the latter including the dissection of additional lymph nodes and the right half of the nerve plexus around the superior mesenteric artery and celiac axis. We evaluated 167 patients from 7 centers who fulfilled all of the required criteria.

Result.—Operation time was longer and estimated blood loss was higher in the extended resection group than in the standard resection group, but the R0 resection rate was comparable. The mean number of lymph nodes retrieved per patient was higher in the extended resection group than in the standard resection group (33.7 vs 17.3; $P < 0.001$). The morbidity rate was slightly higher in the extended resection group than in the standard resection group. Two patients in the extended resection group died in hospital. Median survival after R0 resection was similar in the extended resection and standard resection groups (18.0 vs 19.0 months; $P = 0.239$) regardless of lymph node metastasis. Adjuvant chemoradiation had a positive impact on overall survival.

Conclusions.—This study suggests that extended lymphadenectomy with dissection of the nerve plexus does not provide a significant survival benefit compared with standard resection in pancreatic head cancer. Standard resection can be performed safely and efficiently, without negatively affecting oncologic efficacy or long-term survival, when compared with extended pancreaticoduodenal resection. (NCT00679913)?

▶ Long-term outcomes for patients with pancreatic adenocarcinoma remain dismal. Four randomized controlled trials have evaluated whether there are advantages to extended resections over standard pancreaticoduodenectomy to gain increased lymph node clearance in areas that might be invaded or involved with perineural invasion (such as the plexus around the celiac or superior mesenteric artery [SMA]). These randomized trials have not revealed a survival benefit, and in fact, when circumferential dissection of the neural plexus has been carried out, patients have developed intractable diarrhea. Some of the limitations of these trials were low numbers, inclusion of patients who did not have pancreatic adenocarcinoma, and variabilities in the operative procedures. For this reason, this Korean trial set out to prospectively randomize patients to standard pancreaticoduodenectomy vs extended resection to include lymph nodes around the hepatic artery, celiac axis, skeletonization of the hepatoduodenal ligament, the area around the SMA, the periaortic region between the celiac axis, and the inferior mesenteric artery, and resection of the right side of the nerve plexus along the celiac axis and SMA. Patients were randomized from 7 tertiary hospitals in Korea, and ultimately 83 patients were randomized to receive standard pancreaticoduodenectomy and 86 for the extended resection. Interesting findings from this study included a mean operative time 64 minutes longer in the extended group (420 minutes vs 356 minutes, $P = .001$) and increased blood loss in the extended group (563 mL vs 372 mL, $P = .02$). There were 2 postoperative deaths in the extended group and none in the standard group, and morbidity was similar. Patients who had the right side of the celiac or SMA plexus removed did not have a significant increase in postoperative diarrhea. Pathologically there was an increased rate of lymph node clearance in the extended group (mean of 34 lymph nodes vs 17 lymph nodes, $P > .001$), but the total number of positive lymph nodes was similar, suggesting that improved lymph node clearance did not result in improved harvest of involved lymph nodes. With respect to disease-free and overall survival, there were no significant differences between these 2 groups. The 2-year overall survival was 44.5% in the standard resection group and 35.7% in the extended group, which was not significantly different. Also, there was no difference in survival between patients who had positive lymph nodes or negative lymph nodes in all patients. However, there was a difference in survival in patients who received adjuvant chemoradiation (most commonly 45 Gy of radiation and 5-fluorouracil chemotherapy), with a median overall survival of 20.8 vs 14 months ($P = .016$). With respect to other prognostic factors combining both groups, the type of operation did not result in significant change in survival, but poorly differentiated tumors, endovascular tumor emboli, and adjuvant treatment were all independent factors contributing to survival. The factors of portal vein resection and R1 resection approached but did not reach statistical significance. The takeaway message from this study is that extended resection for pancreatic adenocarcinoma does not result in improved survival, despite improved clearance of lymph nodes. It does appear that treatment with chemoradiation did improve survival, but patients were not randomized to receive these treatments, and this was not a variable that was controlled. Although the morbidity was similar between the 2 procedures, results were not improved, and therefore the extended procedure does not appear to be justified.

J. R. Howe, MD

Intensity of Follow-up after Pancreatic Cancer Resection
Castellanos JA, Merchant NB (Vanderbilt Univ Med Ctr, Nashville, TN)
Ann Surg Oncol 21:747-751, 2014

The prognosis of patients diagnosed with pancreatic adenocarcinoma remains dismal. Of the 15–20% of patients who are candidates for potentially curative resection, 66–92% will develop recurrent disease. Although guidelines for surveillance in the postoperative setting exist, they are not evidence based, and there is wide variability of strategies utilized. Current surveillance guidelines as suggested by the National Comprehensive Cancer Network (NCCN) include routine history and physical, measurement of serum cancer-associated antigen 19-9 (CA19-9) levels, and computed tomographic imaging at 3- to 6-month intervals for the first 2 years, and annually thereafter. However, the lack of prospective clinical data examining the efficacy of different surveillance strategies has led to a variability of the intensity of follow-up and a lack of consensus on its necessity and efficacy. Recent therapeutic advances may have the potential to significantly alter survival after recurrence, but a careful consideration of current surveillance strategies should be undertaken to optimize existing approaches in the face of high recurrence and low survival rates.

▶ Despite intensive efforts on many fronts, the survival of patients with pancreatic ductal adenocarcinoma (PDA) has not improved significantly over the past several decades. In the favorable subset of patients who have resectable disease (15%–20%), this article quotes a 66%–92% risk of recurrence within the first 2 years. If there were effective therapies for treating recurrent or metastatic PDA, then surveillance would be important. However, there are no good guidelines for following these patients after resection based on solid clinical trial data. The National Comprehensive Cancer Network (NCCN) recommends physical examination, CA 19-9 testing, and CT scanning every 3 to 6 months for the first 2 years then annually thereafter, but this is based solely on expert opinion.

The European Society of Medical Oncology leaves this more open, with the follow-up schedule being discussed with the patient. They recommended that if the CA 19-9 is elevated before surgery, then this should be followed every 3 months for the first 2 years, and abdominal CT scans should be performed every 6 months. This again is based on expert opinion. This article reviews the rationale for surveillance of patients with PDA. It cites the modest improvements that have been made in chemotherapy in patients with recurrence or metastases. In patients with advanced disease, it has been shown that gemcitabine improved survival over 5-fluorouracil by 1 month, with decreased toxicity, and this has become the standard regimen for these patients. Recent trials comparing FOLFIRINOX with gemcitabine demonstrated an increase in survival by 4.7 months in patients with metastatic PDA (11.1 vs 6.4 months, $P < .001$). Improvement in survival was also seen with the regimen of nab-paclitaxel with gemcitabine vs gemcitabine alone, increasing survival to 8.5 months from 6.7 months. Both of these regimens have significant toxicity, and therefore not all patients will tolerate them.

Some patients with recurrent disease can benefit from repeat resection if this is identified during surveillance, but this is only possible in a small subset of patients. Chemoradiation has been applied to patients with local recurrence, which in retrospective studies has been shown to improve survival, but this was only demonstrated in a small group of patients. Previous studies have shown that celiac plexus block alone may improve survival in patients with recurrent disease. In most cases, however, it is not clear how much patients will benefit from these interventions after identification of recurrence. Studies looking at surveillance regimens have shown that cost is increased with more intensive surveillance without adding survival benefit. Some studies suggest that CA 19-9 and clinical evaluation alone may be a reasonable strategy. Elevations of this tumor marker may predict for clinical or radiologic recurrence within the next 2 to 6 months, but clinicians are hesitant to initiate treatment based on this number. When patients have preoperative levels greater than 50, they have a higher risk for recurrence, and normalization after surgery predicts for improved survival. However, 5%–10% of patients do not manifest increased CA 19-9 because it depends on expression of a Lewis blood group antigen. The addition of CT scanning to surveillance may result in more patients being detected when they are asymptomatic and have better performance status and therefore are more likely to receive treatment than those who develop symptoms. However, this is not a strong direct argument for the value of surveillance. The authors conclude that we currently lack evidence-based surveillance guidelines, and therefore a less intense regimen, as suggested by the Europeans Society of Medical Oncology, may be preferable to that suggested by the NCCN.

J. R. Howe, MD

Other

A Retrospective Review of 126 High-Grade Neuroendocrine Carcinomas of the Colon and Rectum

Smith JD, Reidy DL, Goodman KA, et al (Memorial Sloan Kettering Cancer Ctr, NY)

Ann Surg Oncol 21:2956-2962, 2014

Background.—High-grade neuroendocrine carcinomas (HGNECs) of the colon and rectum are rare, constituting less than 1 % of colorectal cancers. The purpose of this study was to identify the natural history and oncologic outcomes of this disease, describe the use of surgery, and determine the clinical and pathological factors associated with outcomes.

Methods.—Following Institutional Review Board approval, patients with HGNEC were identified from our institutional database. Patient charts and pathology reports were analyzed retrospectively for clinical and pathological factors.

Results.—A total of 126 patients with a median follow-up of 9 months were identified. Median survival was 13.2 months, and 85 (67 %) patients had metastatic disease at diagnosis. Three-year overall survival (OS) was 5 and 18 % for patients with and without metastatic disease, respectively. Factors associated with improved OS on multivariable analysis were

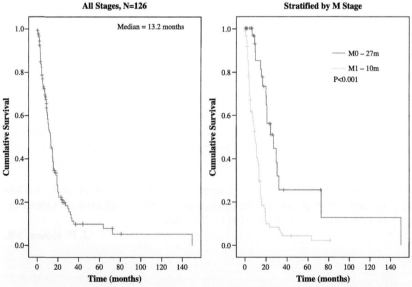

FIGURE 1.—Kaplan—Meier curves demonstrating overall survival and overall survival stratified for the presence of metastatic disease at presentation. (With kind permission from Springer Science+Business Media: Smith JD, Reidy DL, Goodman KA, et al. A retrospective review of 126 high-grade neuroendocrine carcinomas of the colon and rectum. *Ann Surg Oncol.* 2014;21:2956-2962, with permission from Society of Surgical Oncology.)

absence of metastatic disease and presence of an adenocarcinoma component within the tumor. In patients with metastatic disease, response to chemotherapy was the only factor associated with survival. In patients with localized disease, an adenocarcinoma component within the tumor was the only factor associated with survival. Resection of tumor was not associated with survival in either localized or metastatic disease.

Conclusion.—High-grade colorectal NECs are extremely aggressive tumors with poor prognosis. Patients appear to have a marginally better prognosis if they present without metastatic disease, have an adenocarcinoma component within their tumor, or respond to chemotherapy. Surgery, particularly in the presence of metastatic disease, may not offer a survival benefit for the majority of patients (Fig 1).

▶ High-grade neuroendocrine carcinomas (HGNEC) are rare and aggressive tumors that behave like small-cell carcinomas of the lung. They constitute only a small fraction of colorectal neoplasms, and their biologic behavior is distinctly different. For these tumors, chemotherapy is the mainstay of treatment, which may involve surgery. This is the largest series of patients with HGNEC of the colorectum and was a single institutional review of 126 patients treated between 1991 and 2010. The definition of high grade is generally made by greater than 10 mitotic figures per 10 high-powered fields or Ki-67 index of greater than 20%. However, not all tumors were graded in this fashion from this study, as it spanned 2 decades, with most occurring before the institution of the World Health Organization classification system (which incorporates mitoses and Ki-67). A total of 47% of patients had anorectal tumors, 53% had colonic primaries, 67% had metastatic disease, and the remainder had localized disease. Localized disease was more common with anorectal primaries (seen in 61%), whereas those with colonic primaries had a 62% risk of metastatic disease. Patients received several different chemotherapy treatments, including fluorouracil-based regimens, but more commonly platinum-based regimens. Surgical resection was defined as resection of the primary tumor with associated lymph nodes; therefore, transanal or endoscopic removal did not qualify. The median follow-up was 9.4 months, 3-year overall survival rate was a dismal 8.7%, and the median survival was 13.2 months (Fig 1). On multivariate analysis, factors associated with significantly decreased survival included metastatic disease at presentation and lack of an adenocarcinoma component to the HGNEC. Interestingly, surgical resection and the presence of inflammatory bowel disease were associated with improved survival on univariate analyses but did not hold up on multivariate analyses. In patients with localized disease, the presence of an adenocarcinoma component was the only feature that was significantly associated with improved survival. In those with metastatic disease, the only factor on multivariate analysis that was associated with improved survival was response to chemotherapy. The conclusions of this study were that most of these patients had a poor prognosis that was not improved by surgery; therefore, surgical resection of the primary tumor or metastatic disease does not appear to be indicated if the diagnosis of colorectal HGNEC can be made. There may be exceptions if there is an adenocarcinoma component in a colon HGNEC or if they are symptomatic (which is rare). Although there may be benefits to resection in cases of very early disease, such as in small-cell carcinoma of the lung, the authors recommend that when the surgical procedure is associated with significant morbidity such as an APR or LAR, these patients should be treated with chemoradiation, which will give similar survival rates. They also recommended that HGNECs be treated with a platinum-based regimen; however, if there is an adenocarcinoma component, fluorouracil combinations also had reasonable response rates. Bevacizumab was given in a small subset of patients, which did not appear to benefit.

J. R. Howe, MD

Intraperitoneal Chemotherapy for Peritoneal Surface Malignancy: Experience with 1,000 Patients
Levine EA, Stewart JH IV, Shen P, et al (Wake Forest Univ School of Medicine, Winston-Salem, NC)
J Am Coll Surg 218:573-585, 2014

Background.—Peritoneal dissemination of abdominal malignancy (carcinomatosis) has a clinical course marked by bowel obstruction and death; it traditionally does not respond well to systemic therapy and has been approached with nihilism. To treat carcinomatosis, we use cytoreductive surgery (CS) with hyperthermic intraperitoneal chemotherapy (HIPEC).

Methods.—A prospective database of patients has been maintained since 1992. Patients with biopsy-proven peritoneal surface disease were uniformly evaluated for, and treated with, CS and HIPEC. Patient demographics, performance status (Eastern Cooperative Oncology Group), resection status, and peritoneal surface disease were classified according to primary site. Univariate and multivariate analyses were performed. The experience was divided into quintiles and outcomes compared.

Results.—Between 1991 and 2013, a total of 1,000 patients underwent 1,097 HIPEC procedures. Mean age was 52.9 years and 53.1% were female. Primary tumor site was appendix in 472 (47.2%), colorectal in 248 (24.8%), mesothelioma in 72 (7.2%), ovary in 69 (6.9%), gastric in 46 (4.6%), and other in 97 (9.7%). Thirty-day mortality rate was 3.8% and median hospital stay was 8 days. Median overall survival was 29.4 months, with a 5-year survival rate of 32.5%. Factors correlating with improved survival on univariate and multivariate analysis ($p \leq 0.0001$ for each) were preoperative performance status, primary tumor type, resection status, and experience quintile ($p = 0.04$). For the 5 quintiles, the 1- and 5-year survival rates, as well as the complete cytoreduction score (R0, R1, R2a) have increased, and transfusions, stoma creations, and complications have all decreased significantly ($p < .001$ for all).

Conclusions.—This largest reported single-center experience with CS and HIPEC demonstrates that prognostic factors include primary site, performance status, completeness of resection, and institutional experience. The data show that outcomes have improved over time, with more complete cytoreduction and fewer serious complications, transfusions, and

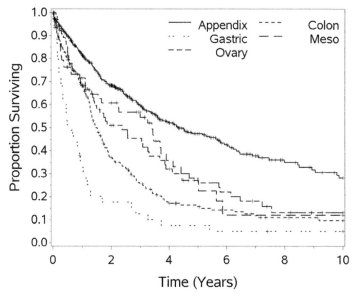

FIGURE 3.—Overall survival by primary tumor site, differences significant (p < 0.0001). (Reprinted from the Journal of the American College of Surgeons. Levine EA, Stewart JH IV, Shen P, et al. Intraperitoneal chemotherapy for peritoneal surface malignancy: experience with 1,000 patients. *J Am Coll Surg.* 2014;218:573-585, Copyright 2014, with permission from the American College of Surgeons.)

stomas. This was due to better patient selection and increased operative experience. Cytoreductive surgery with HIPEC represents a substantial improvement in outcomes compared with historical series, and shows that meaningful long-term survival is possible for selected carcinomatosis patients. Multi-institutional cooperative trials are needed to refine the use of CS and HIPEC (Fig 3).

▶ When cancer disseminates within the peritoneal cavity, the natural history is one of bowel obstruction and usually death within 1 year. Several centers have developed significant expertise with debulking of intraperitoneal malignancy and in administration of hyperthermic intraperitoneal chemotherapy (HIPEC), which appears to significantly improve survival for patients with these malignancies. This report chronicles 1000 patients treated at 1 center between 1991 and 2013. They looked at the results for different types of tumors, their complication rates over time, and overall survivals. The operative approach involves aggressive cytoreduction of tumor, with the removal of all gross disease when at all possible, with lysis of all adhesions and peritoneotomy only in areas of disease. Patients selected for these procedures had to have absence of extra-abdominal disease, decent performance status, and organ function. After cytoreductive surgery, patients were given heated intraperitoneal chemotherapy, usually 30 mg of mitomycin C in 3 L of ringers lactate heated to a mean temperature of 40° C for approximately 120 minutes. The authors show that with this approach they had a mean hospital stay of 14 days, usually with 1 to 2 days in the intensive care unit. During these procedures, approximately 50% of patients had colonic resection, 32% had small bowel resection, 42% had spleens removed, 72% had their omentum removed, and 10% had liver tumors removed. The average time was just under 10 hours for these procedures; The 30-day morbidity was 42%, and mortality was 3.8%. The most common histology was appendiceal cancer, which accounted for nearly half of cases, followed by colorectal cancer, mesothelioma, ovarian, gastric, and then other primaries. Over 5 successive time quintiles, the surgeons were able to reduce their rate of colostomy and ileostomy, improve their rates of complete resection, and decrease their rate of class 4 and 5 complications. Although there was a learning curve, which they estimate to be approximately 50 to 200 cases, the improvement in their results they felt was due to improved patient selection rather than technique. With this, there were increasing numbers of patients with appendiceal malignancies and decreasing numbers with gastric cancer and sarcoma. They had a median follow-up of 54.1 months, and the median overall survival was 29.4 months for all patients. Median survival was best in patients with appendiceal malignances at 63.5 months; it was 16.4 months for colorectal, 27.1 months for mesothelioma, 28.5 months for ovarian, 28.1 for sarcoma, and 6.1 months for gastric cancer (Fig 3). This study demonstrates the significant progress that has been made in patients who previously had a dismal prognosis, through the efforts of dedicated surgeons willing to put in significant time in the operating room to cytoreduce tumors to improve the delivery of chemotherapy. This strategy allows for much higher concentrations of the chemotherapeutic agent to get to the peritoneal surfaces, and potentially have an impact on residual microscopic disease that is likely present. These types of doses cannot be delivered systemically without significant toxicities. A multivariate analysis of factors associated with improved survival included complete resection, good performance status, tumor histology, those without complications, and the time quintile of experience of the surgeons. Patients with appendiceal, colorectal, and mesothelioma appeared to benefit from these procedures the most. The success from this and other centers of excellence has led to the dissemination of this experience nationally, giving these challenging patients an opportunity for long-term survival, where before there was none.

J. R. Howe, MD

Radiofrequency Ablation of Hepatic Metastases: Factors Influencing Local Tumor Progression

Liu C-H, Yu C-Y, Chang W-C, et al (Tri-Service General Hosp and Natl Defense Med Ctr, Taipei, Taiwan, R.O.C; et al)
Ann Surg Oncol 21:3090-3095, 2014

Background.—Although radiofrequency ablation (RFA) of nonresectable hepatic metastases has gained wide acceptance by showing survival benefit in selected patients, scattered reports are available regarding risk factors of local control of percutaneous RFA. The purpose of this study

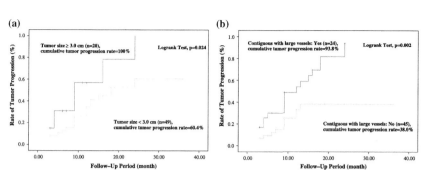

FIGURE 1.—Curves of local tumor progression showing log-rank test results, calculated by Kaplan—Meier method, according to risk factors of local tumor progression and time. a Presence of tumor ≥3.0 cm in size was associated with significantly high rate of local tumor progression in hepatic metastases ($p = 0.024$). b Presence of a tumor contiguous with large vessels was associated with significantly high rate of local tumor progression in hepatic metastases ($p = 0.002$). (With kind permission from Springer Science+Business Media: Liu C-H, Yu C-Y, Chang W-C, et al. Radiofrequency ablation of hepatic metastases: factors influencing local tumor progression. *Ann Surg Oncol.* 2014;21:3090-3095, with permission from Society of Surgical Oncology.)

was to prospectively evaluate the factors influencing local tumor progression after percutaneous RFA of hepatic metastases.

Methods.—Sixty-nine hepatic metastatic lesions in 54 patients were treated by percutaneous RFA. Efficacy was evaluated by contrast-enhanced computed tomography or magnetic resonance imaging at 1 month after ablation, then at 3-month intervals for the first year and biannually thereafter.

Results.—The results of the log-rank test showed that tumor size of <3 cm ($p = 0.024$) and the absence of tumor contiguous with large vessels ($p = 0.002$) significantly correlated with local control for hepatic metastases. Cox regression analysis showed that the tumor size <3 cm and the absence of tumor contiguous with large vessels were independent factors ($p = 0.055$ and 0.009, respectively). The results of the log-rank test showed that neither the threshold post-ablation margin of 1.8 cm ($p = 0.064$) nor the presence of a tumor with subcapsular location ($p = 0.134$) correlated with the success of local control.

Conclusions.—Percutaneous RFA is more effective in achieving local control in patients with hepatic metastases when the tumor size is <3 cm and not contiguous with large vessels (Fig 1a, b).

▶ The liver is one of the most common sites of metastatic disease, but not all patients can have resection of their liver metastases. For some patients, percutaneous radiofrequency ablation is an option for treating these tumors. Ablation is associated with higher recurrence rates than resection, and this study set out to look at what factors were correlated with increased risk of local recurrence or progression at the sites of percutaneous ablation. The authors used 2 radiologists with significant experience with these procedures and treated 54 patients for a total of 69 separate lesions (1 tumor in 45 patients, 2 tumors in 5 patients, 3 tumors in 2 patients, and 4 tumors in 2 patients). They included patients with several different primary tumor sites, including 20 colorectal cancers, 10 breast cancers, 4 pancreatic cancers, 4 cholangiocarcinomas, 3 lung cancers, 3 gallbladder cancers, 2 ovarian cancers, 2 esophageal cancers, 2 renal cell cancers, 2 leiomyosarcomas, 1 gastric cancer, and 1 melanoma. Patients had to have fewer than 5 nodules and tumors less than 8 cm in size to be included in the study. The mean ablation zone was 4.3 cm, and 4 ablations were done on average per tumor. The mean tumor size was 2.4 cm. The factors they specifically examined were whether the tumors were larger or smaller than 3 cm in size, whether margins postablation were 1.8 cm or less, whether the tumors were contiguous with large vessels (defined as a tumor within 5 mm of a 3-mm size vessel or larger), and whether the tumor was subcapsular. Univariate analysis found that tumor size greater than 3 cm and those contiguous with large blood vessels had a significantly higher rate of recurrence. They found that all tumors greater than 3 cm recurred within 24 months, whereas only 60% of those less than 3 cm recurred by this interval (Fig 1a). In tumors that were contiguous with large vessels, 94% recurred as opposed to 38% of those that were not contiguous (Fig 1b). Having a postablation margin of less than 1.8 cm or being in a subcapsular location was correlated with an increased incidence of recurrence. In multivariate analysis, proximity to a large blood vessel remained significant and size greater than 3 cm closely approached significance for increased recurrence. No patients had major complications or death from these procedures. This study shows what had already been shown previously, that larger tumors and those adjacent to blood vessels are much more likely to recur. Limitations of the study were the small number of patients and the fact that multiple disease sites were included in the analyses, some likely with higher risk of progression than others. The increased rate of recurrence along blood vessels is caused by the heat sync effect, which is most pronounced with radiofrequency ablation, but is less of a problem when using microwave ablation or electroporation.

J. R. Howe, MD

Expanded criteria for carcinoid liver debulking: Maintaining survival and increasing the number of eligible patients
Graff-Baker AN, Sauer DA, Pommier SJ, et al (Oregon Health & Science Univ, Portland)
Surgery 156:1369-1377, 2014

Background.—Cytoreduction of carcinoid liver metastases typically aims for ≥90% debulking in patients without extrahepatic disease. Data on the impact of less-restrictive resection criteria and other clinical and tumor-specific factors on outcomes are limited.

Methods.—Records of carcinoid patients undergoing liver debulking from 2007 to 2011 were reviewed. Debulking threshold was 70%, extrahepatic disease did not preclude cytoreduction, and positive margins were allowed. Kaplan-Meier liver progression-free (PFS) and disease-specific (DSS) survival were calculated and compared by log-rank analysis and

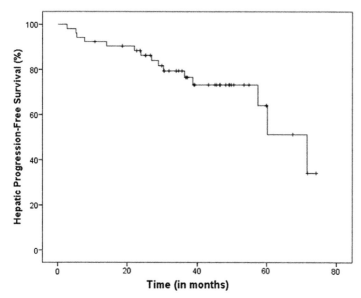

FIGURE 2.—Kaplan-Meier curve of liver progression-free survival rates from the time of liver resection for patients with carcinoid liver metastases. Overall, 15 patients (28.8%) had liver progression. Median liver progression-free survival was 71.6 months, with a 5-year liver progression-free rate of 64%. (Reprinted from Surgery. Graff-Baker AN, Sauer DA, Pommier SJ, et al. Expanded criteria for carcinoid liver debulking: maintaining survival and increasing the number of eligible patients. *Surgery.* 2014;156:1369-1377, Copyright 2014, with permission from Elsevier.)

statistical significance of differences in distributions of factors between patient groups was determined by chi-squared analysis.

Results.—Fifty-two patients were identified. Complete resection of intrahepatic and extrahepatic gross disease was achieved in 12 patients. All primaries reviewed were low grade, but one third of patients had at least one intermediate-grade metastasis. Fifteen patients (29%) had liver progression; median PFS was 72 months. Five-year DSS was 90%, with all deaths from liver failure. Only age was an important prognostic factor for PFS and DSS. Five-year DSS for patients <50 years was 73% and was 97% for patients 50 or older ($P = .03$).

Conclusion.—The use of expanded criteria for debulking resulted in 90% 5-year DSS. Although younger age portends a poorer prognosis, the favorable PFS and DSS justify also using expanded criteria in this subgroup (Fig 2).

▶ Patients with neuroendocrine tumors (NETs) frequently present with metastatic disease. Retrospective data has shown the potential benefit of resecting the primaries in these patients even in the face of metastases. Other studies have shown that compared with historical controls, resection or debulking of the liver metastases can improve long-term survival. One problem with NET patients is that there is an approximately 95% recurrence rate at 10 years after removing liver tumors, and therefore the role of resection versus ablative therapies, and the degree of debulking that should be achieved has not been well defined. Many believe that 90% or greater debulking of metastases is the objective that should be sought out, based on an article by Sarmiento et al.[1] The current article challenges that assessment, and furthermore suggests that the threshold for significant debulking could potentially be lowered to 70%. To come up with this conclusion, they studied patients with gastrointestinal NETs metastatic to the liver where it was felt that < 70% debulking could be carried out. All tumors were classified as low-grade, and they went on to group the patients into degree of resection (70%–89%, 90%–99%, and 100% debulking). The majority of procedures were wedge resections and enucleations, as well as segmental resections and lobectomies. They had 52 patients in the series, the majority of whom were on long-acting octreotide injections. They then compared various clinicopathologic factors in patients who developed progression within the liver relative to those who had stable disease. The type of resection, whether a primary was resected simultaneously (which was done in 44% of cases), the mean number of liver tumors treated, the presence of extrahepatic disease, the location of the primary tumor (small bowel, colon, or appendix) were all not correlated with progression. The only significant factor associated with liver progression was age < 50 years. Median follow-up in this study was 37.4 months, and all patients who died of disease died of liver failure. Another finding from this study was that one-third of liver metastases had an intermediate grade, rather than the low grade seen in the primary tumor. All 3 groups of debulking (70%–89%, 90%–99%, and 100%) had similar risks of liver progression, which was approximately 30%. The median progression-free survival in the whole group was 71.6 months (Fig 2), 5-year disease-specific survival was 90%, and the 5-year overall survival was 88%. This study raised the question of whether 90% debulking is really the appropriate threshold value for effective debulking. This study, albeit small, showed no difference in survival or disease-free progression if the threshold was lowered to 70 than if it was 90% or even 100%. They therefore recommend that the threshold for liver debulking was lowered to 70%. Furthermore, they found no association with progression whether there was extrahepatic disease or not, and in this study, 65% had extrahepatic disease. Therefore, they also recommend that patients with extrahepatic disease should not be excluded from potential debulking. The limitations of this study were low numbers, and therefore their ability to find differences in progression-free survival between groups might have been limited. However, their survival results were very good, which helps affirm their provocative conclusion that debulking may be indicated if a threshold of as low as 70% can be achieved.

J. R. Howe, MD

Reference

1. Sarmiento JM, Heywood G, Rubin J, et al. Surgical treatment of neuroendocrine metastases to the liver: a plea for resection to increase survival. *J Am Coll Surg.* 2003;197:29-37.

Pancreastatin Predicts Survival in Neuroendocrine Tumors

Sherman SK, Maxwell JE, O'Dorisio MS, et al (Univ of Iowa Carver College of Medicine)
Ann Surg Oncol 21:2971-2980, 2014

Background.—Serum neurokinin A, chromogranin A, serotonin, and pancreastatin reflect tumor burden in neuroendocrine tumors. We sought to determine whether their levels correlate with survival in surgically managed small bowel (SBNETs) and pancreatic neuroendocrine tumors (PNETs).

Methods.—Clinical data were collected with Institutional Review Board approval for patients undergoing surgery at one center. Progression-free (PFS) and overall (OS) survival were from the time of surgery. Event times were estimated by the Kaplan—Meier method. Preoperative and postoperative laboratory values were tested for correlation with outcomes. A multivariate Cox model adjusted for confounders.

Results.—Included were 98 SBNETs and 78 PNETs. Median follow-up was 3.8 years; 62 % had metastatic disease. SBNETs had lower median PFS than PNETs (2.0 vs. 5.6 years; $p < 0.01$). Median OS was 10.5 years for PNETs and was not reached for SBNETs. Preoperative neurokinin A did not correlate with PFS or OS. Preoperative serotonin correlated with PFS but not OS. Higher levels of preoperative chromogranin A and pancreastatin showed significant correlation with worse PFS and OS ($p < 0.05$). After multivariate adjustment for confounders, preoperative and postoperative pancreastatin remained independently predictive of worse PFS and OS ($p < 0.05$). Whether pancreastatin normalized postoperatively further discriminated outcomes. Median PFS was 1.7 years in patients with elevated preoperative pancreastatin versus 6.5 years in patients with normal levels ($p < 0.001$).

Conclusions.—Higher pancreastatin levels are significantly associated with worse PFS and OS in SBNETs and PNETs. This effect is independent of age, primary tumor site, and presence of nodal or metastatic disease. Pancreastatin provides valuable prognostic information and identifies surgical patients at high risk of recurrence who could benefit most from novel therapies (Fig 2).

▶ Patients with small bowel neuroendocrine tumors (SBNETs) and pancreatic neuroendocrine tumors (PNETs) can have prolonged survival despite advanced disease. Serum markers of protein secreted by these tumors have been used to determine the extent of disease and for follow-up and generally include chromogranin A (CGA), neurokinin A (NKA), and serotonin. CGA is recommended by the European Neuroendocrine Tumor Society as the marker of choice in follow-up for patients with NETs. Recently, however, the marker, pancreastatin, which is a 52-amino acid fragment of CGA, has been found to have certain advantages. It is not affected by proton pump inhibitors as is CGA, and it has greater sensitivity and specificity for measuring disease burden. In this study, the authors looked at 176 patients with SBNETs and PNETs treated surgically at a single institution.

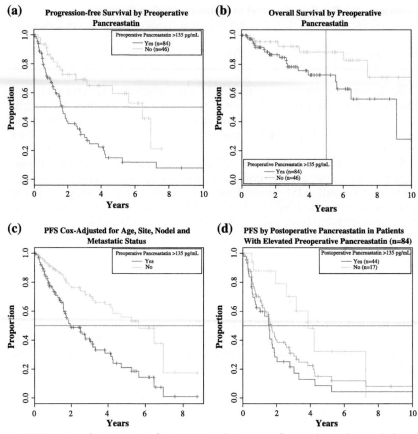

(a) Progression-free Survival by Preoperative Pancreastatin

(b) Overall Survival by Preoperative Pancreastatin

(c) PFS Cox-Adjusted for Age, Site, Nodel and Metastatic Status

(d) PFS by Postoperative Pancreastatin in Patients With Elevated Preoperative Pancreastatin (n=84)

FIGURE 2.—Median progression-free (PFS) (a) and 5-year overall survival (OS) (b) were higher in patients with normal (*upper lighter line*, *n* = 46) versus elevated preoperative pancreastatin (*lower darker line*, *n* = 84; median PFS, 6.5 vs. 1.7 years; 5-year OS, 88 vs. 73 %). c Multivariate Cox model-adjusted PFS. Estimated median PFS was significantly longer in patients with normal preoperative pancreastatin (*upper lighter line*) compared with elevated (*lower darker line*) even after adjustment for confounding factors. d PFS by postoperative pancreastatin in patients with elevated preoperative pancreastatin levels. Patients with elevated preoperative pancreastatin (*middle line*; same as the *darker line* in a; *n* = 84) can be further stratified by elevated (*lower darker line*, *n* = 44) versus normalized (*upper lighter line*, *n* = 17) postoperative pancreastatin levels. (With kind permission from Springer Science+Business Media. Sherman SK, Maxwell JE, O'Dorisio MS, et al. Pancreastatin predicts survival in neuroendocrine tumors. *Ann Surg Oncol.* 2014;21:2971-2980, © The Society of Thoracic Surgeons 2014.)

They measured preoperative and postoperative levels of serotonin, CGA, NKA, and pancreastatin and tried to make correlations with progression-free survival (PFS) and overall survival. Serotonin was found neither particularly useful nor was NKA (which had been previously suggested to be prognostic in SBNET patients). There was a significant difference in PFS in patients with preoperative elevation of CGA or pancreastatin compared with those who had normal levels, and preoperative pancreastatin also correlated with overall survival. The median PFS for patients with elevated preoperative pancreastatin was 1.7 years versus

6.5 years for those with normal levels (Fig 2). For CGA, patients with elevated levels preoperatively had a median PFS of 2.0 years versus 3.2 years for those with normal levels. Overall, survival was a median of 9.1 years for patients with high levels of preoperative pancreastatin, and the median was not reached in patients with normal preoperative levels. Furthermore, if pancreastatin levels could be normalized by surgery, the median PFS improved to 3.9 years from 1.7 years for all those with preoperative elevation; in those in whom pancreastatin remained elevated after surgery, the 5-year PFS was only 8.6%. Multivariate analyses found that factors independently associated with worse PFS were tumor site, age at surgery, the presence of positive nodes or metastases, and higher preoperative pancreastatin (but not preoperative CGA). These findings suggest that pancreastatin is a valuable marker in predicting outcomes in patients with SBNETs and PNETs and in their response to surgery. Patients at higher risk (ie, those with elevation of preoperative pancreastatin and especially when this does not normalize postoperatively) should be considered for clinical trials. Of these 4 commonly used markers, it appears that pancreastatin has the highest discriminatory capability. Limitations of this study are its retrospective nature and combining patients with SBNETs and PNETs. However, these primary sites were examined separately in the report, and the utility of the marker appeared to be good for both sites.

J. R. Howe, MD

Regional lymphadenectomy is indicated in the surgical treatment of pancreatic neuroendocrine tumors (PNETs)
Hashim YM, Trinkaus KM, Linehan DC, et al (Washington Univ School of Medicine, St Louis, MO; et al)
Ann Surg 259:197-203, 2014

Objective.—To explore the prognostic importance and preoperative predictors of lymph node metastasis in an effort to guide surgical decision making in patients with pancreatic neuroendocrine tumors (PNETs).

Background.—PNETs are uncommon, and the natural history of the disease is not well described. As a result, there remains controversy regarding the optimal management of regional lymph nodes during resection of the primary tumor.

Methods.—A retrospective review of a prospectively maintained database of patients who underwent surgery for locoregional PNET between 1994 and 2012 was performed. Logistic regression was used to identify predictors of nodal metastasis. Overall survival (OS) and disease-free survival (DFS) were calculated using Kaplan Meier method. Results were expressed as *p*-values and odds ratio estimates with 95% confidence intervals.

Results.—One-hundred thirty six patients were identified, of whom 50 (38%) patients had nodal metastasis. The frequency of lymph node metastasis was higher for: larger tumors (> 1.5 cm (OR = 4.7), tumors of the head as compared to body-tail of the pancreas (OR = 2.8), tumors with Ki-67 > 20% (OR = 6.7), and tumors with lymph vascular invasion

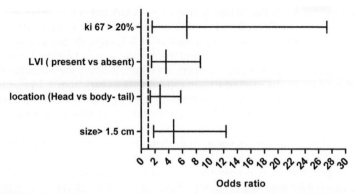

FIGURE 1.—Logistic regression, probability of lymph node metastasis Ki-67 > 20, LVI, tumor in the head vs. body-tail and size > 1.5 cm, were found to be associated with increase in probability of lymph node metastasis (*P* values = 0.008, 0.008, 0.004 and 0.002 respectively). (Reprinted from Hashim YM, Trinkaus KM, Linehan DC, et al. Regional lymphadenectomy is indicated in the surgical treatment of pancreatic neuroendocrine tumors (PNETs). *Ann Surg.* 2014;259:197-203, © 2014, Southeastern Surgical Congress.)

(OR = 3.6), (*p* value <0.05). Median DFS was lower for patients with nodal metastases (4.5 v 14.6 years, *p* < 0.0001).

Conclusions.—Lymph node metastasis is predictive of poor outcomes in patients with PNETs. Preoperative variables are not able to reliably predict patients where the probability of lymph node involvement was less than 12%. These data support inclusion of regional lymphadenectmy in patients undergoing pancreatic resections for PNET (Fig 1).

▶ Pancreatic neuroendocrine tumors (PNETs) have increased 5-fold in incidence over the last 3 decades. These tumors can be indolent, and they can be aggressive, and many patients will have prolonged long-term survival. One area of controversy has been the importance of nodal metastases to the survival of patients with PNETs. Some studies have found that lymph node status does not correlate with survival, whereas others have found that it does. The aim of this study was to see which clinicopathologic features correlated with the presence of lymph node metastases and to see whether nodal metastases correlate with survival in PNETs. To do this, the authors retrospectively reviewed a prospectively collected database from 1994 to 2012 in a single institution. They identified 175 patients who had PNETs resected during that period, of whom, 25 were excluded because they presented with distant metastases and 14 because of incomplete information. The remaining 136 patients had various clinicopathologic features evaluated for their relationship to nodal status. They found that 98% of patients had lymph nodes removed, with 62% of patients being node negative and 38% node positive (the mean number of nodes removed was 14). There were no mortalities in these operations, and the complication rate was 39%. Of these patients, 13 (10%) had MEN1, and 6% were functional. Factors that were found to be significantly correlated with positive lymph nodes were tumor location in the head of the gland (as opposed to the body and tail), larger tumor size, lymphovascular invasion, and elevated Ki-67 index (Fig 1). With respect to tumor size, when lesions were greater than 1.5 cm there was a 4.7-fold increased risk of nodal metastases, but interestingly, even in patients with tumors less than 1 cm in size, 12% of patients had positive nodes. Location of the tumor in the pancreatic head resulted in a 2.8-fold increased risk of lymph node metastases relative to the body and tail, and Ki-67 greater than 20 resulted in a 6.7-fold increase in nodal metastases relative to Ki-67 less than 2%. With respect to survival, lymph node metastasis was significantly correlated with worse disease-free survival (median of 4.5 years with positive nodes vs 14.6 years with negative nodes) but not with overall survival (5-year survival of 77% with positive nodes, 91% with negative nodes). Another factor correlated with survival was margin status, where patients with R1 resections had a median of overall survival of 7.6 years versus 11.7 years in those with R0 resections. Tumor grade was also significantly correlated with overall survival, with 5-year survival rate of 89% for well-differentiated tumors vs 64% for poorly differentiated tumors. Ki-67 was also correlated with overall survival, which decreased with increasing Ki-67. In multivariate analysis, the 2 factors that were correlated with disease-free survival were nodal status and Ki-67, and for overall survival positive surgical margins and Ki-67 were independently associated with overall survival (but not nodal status). This study found that involved lymph nodes resulted in significantly shorter disease-free survival, but the differences in overall survival were not significant, and factors such as tumor size, tumor location, Ki-67, and lymphovascular invasion were all related to the development of nodal metastases. Even small tumors (< 1 cm) may occasionally have lymph node metastases, so the ideal treatment of pancreatic neuroendocrine tumors is still unclear. Certainly, many believe that smaller lesions that are not located near the main duct may be amenable to enucleation, whereas larger lesions should have a more oncologic resection. This study would argue that tumors located in the head of the gland more often are node positive, and perhaps these should be treated more aggressively. The incidence of positive nodes was 53% in tumors greater than 2 cm, and, therefore, these should also be more aggressively treated.

J. R. Howe, MD

Lanreotide in Metastatic Enteropancreatic Neuroendocrine Tumors
Caplin ME, for the CLARINET Investigators (Royal Free Hosp, London; et al)
N Engl J Med 371:224-233, 2014

Background.—Somatostatin analogues are commonly used to treat symptoms associated with hormone hypersecretion in neuroendocrine tumors; however, data on their antitumor effects are limited.

Methods.—We conducted a randomized, double-blind, placebo-controlled, multinational study of the somatostatin analogue lanreotide in patients with advanced, well-differentiated or moderately differentiated, nonfunctioning, somatostatin receptor—positive neuroendocrine tumors of grade 1 or 2 (a tumor proliferation index [on staining for the Ki-67 antigen] of (<10%) and documented disease-progression status. The tumors originated in the pancreas, midgut, or hindgut or were of unknown origin. Patients were randomly assigned to receive an extended-release aqueous-gel formulation of lanreotide (Autogel [known in the United States as Depot], Ipsen) at a dose of 120 mg (101 patients) or placebo (103 patients) once every 28 days for 96 weeks. The primary end point was progression-free survival, defined as the time to disease progression (according to the Response Evaluation Criteria in Solid Tumors, version 1.0) or death. Secondary end points included overall survival, quality of life (assessed with the European Organization for Research and Treatment of Cancer questionnaires QLQ-C30 and QLQ-GI.NET21), and safety.

Results.—Most patients (96%) had no tumor progression in the 3 to 6 months before randomization, and 33% had hepatic tumor volumes greater than 25%. Lanreotide, as compared with placebo, was associated with significantly prolonged progression-free survival (median not reached vs. median of 18.0 months, $P < 0.001$ by the stratified log-rank test; hazard ratio for progression or death, 0.47; 95% confidence interval [CI], 0.30 to 0.73). The estimated rates of progression-free survival at 24 months were 65.1% (95% CI, 54.0 to 74.1) in the lanreotide group and 33.0% (95% CI, 23.0 to 43.3) in the placebo group. The therapeutic effect in predefined subgroups was generally consistent with that in the overall population, with the exception of small subgroups in which confidence intervals were wide. There were no significant between group differences in quality of life or overall survival. The most common treatment-related adverse event was diarrhea (in 26% of the patients in the lanreotide group and 9% of those in the placebo group).

Conclusions.—Lanreotide was associated with significantly prolonged progression-free survival among patients with metastatic enteropancreatic neuroendocrine tumors of grade 1 or 2 (Ki-67 <10%). (Funded by Ipsen; CLARINET ClinicalTrials.gov number, NCT00353496; EudraCT 2005-004904-35.)

▶ Gastroenteropancreatic (GEP) neuroendocrine tumors (NETs) may affect approximately 2 in 100 000 persons and have been increasing in incidence. Patients with these tumors can have significant long-term survival. Most these tumors have somatostatin receptors on their cell surfaces, and treatment with somatostatin analogs can hypothetically limit tumor growth and promote stable disease. One previous randomized, controlled trial, the PROMID study, randomly assigned patients with well-differentiated midgut NETs to receive long-acting octreotide or placebo and found a benefit in progression-free survival in the treatment group. This study was limited to midgut tumors, and all these tumors were of low grade. The current study, the CLARINET study, randomly assigned patients with GEP NETs to receive a different somatostatin analog, lanreotide, at 120 mg per month, or placebo. Inclusion criteria were patients with well or moderately differentiated tumors originating in the pancreas, midgut, or hindgut with locally unresectable tumors, metastatic disease, and tumors that were shown to have at least grade 2 uptake on OctreoScan. Patients previously receiving chemotherapy, interferon, or chemoembolization and having metastatic enteropancreatic neuro-endocrine type 1 or surgery within 3 months were excluded from the study. The objective of the study was to follow up with patients closely in the 2 arms to see if there was a difference in progression-free survival. Patients had baseline CT scan performed and then a CT scan within 3 to 6 months to measure the target lesions. Patients were then randomly assigned. Patients were followed up and CT scans were performed at intervals of 3, 6, 9, 12, 18, and 24 months from random-ization, and patients were evaluated for progression, adverse events, and overall survival. The study found that there were fewer events of progression or death in the Lanreotide-treated group (52% had no events) vs the placebo group (25% had no events) and that the median progression-free survival was not reached in the Lanreotide group, whereas it was 18 months in the placebo group (Fig 1 in the original article). It should be noted that 96% of the patients did not have progression in the 3- to 6-month interval prior to randomization, so this study selected for patients with relatively stable disease and it might be pre-dicted to show fewer progression events than were seen in the PROMID study. The 101 patients receiving Lanreotide vs the 103 receiving placebo were well matched for various demographic and clinical features, although there was a slightly increased incidence of pancreatic and midgut NETs in the placebo group versus hindgut and unknown in the Lanreotide group. The Ki-67 grades were similar in the 2 groups, and approximately 40% of patients in each group had undergone surgical resection previously. There were relatively few deaths (2 patients in each group), and because of these few events and the relatively indolent course of these tumors, there was no difference seen in overall survival in the 2 groups. The progression-free survival at 24 months was 65% in the Lan-reotide group versus 33% in the placebo group. There were no significant differ-ences in the quality of life in the 2 groups, but patients in the Lanreotide group experienced diarrhea in 26% of cases, and there was also higher incidences of hyperglycemia and cholelithiasis. Overall, one-half of the patients in the Lanreo-tide group had adverse events related to Lanreotide vs 28% in the placebo group. This is a very important study and gives further insights into the value of somatos-tatin analogs in patients with neuroendocrine tumors. Compared with the PROMID study, the CLARINET study also included patients with neuroendocrine tumors from other gastrointestinal sites including the pancreas, which is of value. This study found that there was improvement in progression-free survival and that most adverse events were quite tolerable, showing the potential efficacy of this agent at delaying disease progression, which was estimated to be a 53% decrease over placebo during the 96 weeks of the study. It should be noted that this study selected for patients with minimal progression, and it allowed for crossover if pro-gression was noted. Therefore, the finding of no difference in overall survival is complicated by the indolent course of the disease, the low rate of progression, and the ability to cross over to the study drug if progression was witnessed. This study extended not only to other tumor sites relative to the PROMID study but it also included patients with grade 2 lesions. From these 2 randomized, con-trol trials, we can conclude that somatostatin analogs improve progression-free survival in patients with GEP NETs when they are low to intermediate grade, which had already become standard clinical practice prior to the completion of these studies. This study confirms the rationale of this approach.

J. R. Howe, MD

Pathologic and Molecular Features Correlate With Long-Term Outcome After Adjuvant Therapy of Resected Primary GI Stromal Tumor: The ACOSOG Z9001 Trial

Corless CL, Ballman KV, Antonescu CR, et al (Oregon Health and Science Univ, Portland; Mayo Clinic, Rochester, MN; Memorial Sloan-Kettering Cancer Ctr, NY; et al)
J Clin Oncol 32:1563-1570, 2014

Purpose.—The ACOSOG (American College of Surgeons Oncology Group) Z9001 (Alliance) study, a randomized, placebo-controlled trial, demonstrated that 1 year of adjuvant imatinib prolonged recurrence-free survival (RFS) after resection of primary GI stromal tumor (GIST). We sought to determine the pathologic and molecular factors associated with patient outcome.

Patients and Methods.—There were 328 patients assigned to the placebo arm and 317 to the imatinib arm. Median patient follow-up was 74 months. There were 645 tumor specimens available for mitotic rate or mutation analysis.

Results.—RFS remained superior in the imatinib arm (hazard ratio, 0.6; 95% CI, 0.43 to 0.75; Cox model–adjusted *P* < .001). On multivariable analysis of patients in the placebo arm, large tumor size, small bowel location, and high mitotic rate were associated with lower RFS, whereas tumor genotype was not significantly associated with RFS. Multivariable analysis of patients in the imatinib arm yielded similar findings. When comparing the two arms, imatinib therapy was associated with higher RFS in patients with a KIT exon 11 deletion of any type, but not a KIT exon 11 insertion or point mutation, KIT exon 9 mutation, PDGFRA mutation, or wild-type tumor, although some of these patient groups were small. Adjuvant imatinib did not seem to alter overall survival.

Conclusion.—Our findings show that tumor size, location, and mitotic rate, but not tumor genotype, are associated with the natural history of GIST. Patients with KIT exon 11 deletions assigned to 1 year of adjuvant imatinib had a longer RFS.

▶ The American College of Surgeons Oncology Group Z9001 trial was a landmark study that showed that treating gastrointestinal stromal tumors (GIST) with imatinib for 1 year improved recurrence-free survival. The initial publication had a median follow-up of 20 months, and therefore this study reports the long-term survival data (with a median of 74-month follow-up), and also the identification of factors that correlate with improved survival, with special attention to tumor genotype. This study randomized patients who had resection of a GISTs of > 3 cm that were positive by immunohistochemistry for KIT to 1 year of imatinib at 400 mg per day or placebo for 1 year. Patients in the placebo arm could receive imatinib if they developed recurrence, and patients in the imatinib arm could resume treatment if they recurred after 1 year. Various clinicopathologic factors were evaluated against recurrence-free survival and overall survival, and genotyping of KIT and PDGFRA were performed. Three hundred and seventeen patients were randomized to receive imatinib and 328 to the placebo arm. They found that recurrence-free survival was improved for those receiving imatinib, but overall survival was not (Fig 2 in the original article). Classic pathologic variables such as tumor size > 10 cm, small intestinal location, and mitotic rate > 5 per 50 high-power fields remained significantly associated with reduced recurrence-free survival in univariate and multivariate analyses in both groups. Evaluation by mutation status revealed that recurrence-free survival were not statistically significantly different in patients having KIT exon 9 mutations, exon 11 mutations, PDGFRA mutations, or wild-type tumors. However, in subtype analysis, patients with KIT exon 11 deletion treated with placebo seemed to have worse outcome on univariate analysis, but this did not hold up on multivariate analysis. This report is significant in that it shows that recurrence-free survival remained improved in patients treated with imatinib, but on closer inspection of survival curves, the recurrence-free survival curves approached one another at approximately 6 years, and the overall survival was not significantly different. This may have been complicated by allowing placebo treated patients to start imatinib, and therefore the full effect on survival may not be evident from this trial. Genotype may be an important factor to determine which patients will respond to imatinib, but differences in survival between genotypes observed here did not hold up. The authors felt, however, that KIT wild-type patients benefit less from imatinib, whereas those with exon 11 deletion (as opposed to insertions or point mutation) were most likely to benefit. The absence of convincing differences in survival by multivariate analysis suggest that there may be more complexity to the genetic makeup of these tumors and that perhaps other genes may also play an important role.

J. R. Howe, MD

A Single Institution's Experience with Surgical Cytoreduction of Stage IV, Well-Differentiated, Small Bowel Neuroendocrine Tumors

Boudreaux JP, Wang Y-Z, Diebold AE, et al (Univ Med Ctr, New Orleans, LA; et al)
J Am Coll Surg 218:837-845, 2014

Background.—Well-differentiated neuroendocrine tumors (NETs) of the gastrointestinal tract are rare, slow-growing neoplasms. Clinical outcomes in a group of stage IV, well-differentiated patients with NETs with small bowel primaries undergoing cytoreductive surgery and multidisciplinary management at a single center were evaluated.

Study Design.—The charts of 189 consecutive patients who underwent surgical cytoreduction for their small bowel NETs were reviewed.

Information on the extent of disease, complications, and Kaplan-Meier survival were collected from the patient records.

Results.—A total of 189 patients underwent 229 cytoreductive operations. Ten percent of patients required an intraoperative blood transfusion and 3% (6 of 229) had other intraoperative complications. For all 229 procedures performed, mean (± SD) stay in the ICU was 4 ± 3 days and in the hospital was 9 ± 10 days. Before discharge, 51% of patients had no postoperative complications and 39% of patients had only minor complications. In a 30-day follow-up period from discharge, 85% of patients had no additional complications and 13% had only minor complications. The 30-day postoperative death rate was 3% (5 of 189). Mean survival from histologic diagnosis of NET was 236 months. The 5-, 10-, and 20-year Kaplan-Meier survival rates from diagnosis were 87%, 77%, and 41%, respectively.

Conclusions.—Cytoreductive surgery in patients with well-differentiated midgut NETs has low mortality and complication rates and is associated with prolonged survival. We believe that cytoreductive surgery is a key component in the care of patients with NETs (Fig 3).

▶ Small bowel neuroendocrine tumors (SBNETs) have been increasing in incidence over the past several decades, but the prognosis has not improved significantly over this period. This study represents a large, single-institutional study following the natural history of patients with stage 4 SBNETs undergoing resection of the primary and cytoreduction of metastatic disease. It included 189 patients undergoing 229 operations between 2006 and 2012. They restricted their study to well-differentiated tumors and those in which the primaries were resected. In these 229 operations, 72% had liver resection, 56% had mesenteric masses resected, 52% had the primary tumor removed at the same procedure (the others had been removed at outside hospitals previously). Other lymph nodes were removed in 52% of cases, cholecystectomy was performed in 42% of cases, oophorectomy in 14% of cases, and 31% of patients had radiofrequency ablation of the liver. The extent of liver resections, number of ablations performed, or the number of lesions treated were not enumerated in this study. They followed the patients for complications and mortality as well as survival. The mean hospital stay was 9 days with a mean of 4 days in the intensive care unit. The mean operating time was 380 minutes. They had a 3% mortality rate within 30 days of surgery, and overall, 7% died due to surgical complications. One hundred and ten patients had no complications, whereas 34 had grade 1 complications, 51 grade 2, and 21 had grade 3 or 4 complications. They measured survival from the time of diagnosis (not surgery), and this was 87% at 5 years and 77% at 10 years (20-year survival was 41%). Twenty-three of patients underwent 2 or more cytoreductive surgeries. Conclusions from this article were that in these patients with SBNETs with stage 4 disease, that the survival achieved with cytoreduction was much better than historical controls (Surveillance, Epidemiology, and End Results Program 5-year survival is 54% vs 87% in this series; Fig 3). This was achieved with relatively low mortality, an acceptable number of complications, and with the benefit of significant

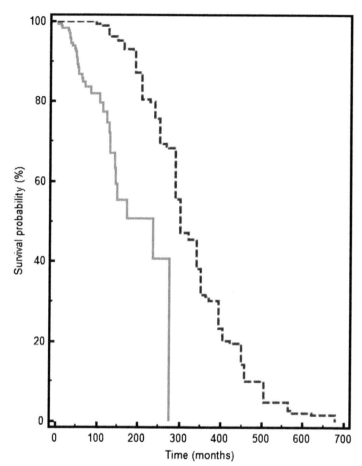

FIGURE 3.—Actuarial survival for patients in this study with stage IV, midgut neuroendocrine tumors compared with expected survival without a neuroendocrine tumor diagnosis (n = 189). Gray line, survival in our clinic of patients with stage IV small bowel neuroendocrine tumors; dashed line, expected survival, general population. (Reprinted from the Journal of the American College of Surgeons. Boudreaux JP, Wang Y-Z, Diebold AE, et al. A single institution's experience with surgical cytoreduction of stage IV, well-differentiated, small bowel neuroendocrine tumors. *J Am Coll Surg.* 2014;218:837-845, Copyright 2014, with permission from the American College of Surgeons.)

long-term survival. This is one of the largest series of stage 4 SBNETs reported with surgical cytoreduction, from a single center with expertise in these tumors. The authors suggest that these tumors should be treated aggressively to obtain this benefit for patients

J. R. Howe, MD

Progress Against GI Cancer During the American Society of Clinical Oncology's First 50 Years
Mayer RJ, Venook AP, Schilsky RL (Harvard Med School, Boston, MA; Univ of California, San Francisco; American Society of Clinical Oncology, Alexandria, VA)
J Clin Oncol 32:1521-1530, 2014

Background.—Gastrointestinal (GI) tract cancers remain among the most frequent causes of cancer-related death even after 50 years of research and advances in techniques and treatments. In 2008, GI cancers caused more than 2.3 million deaths–far more than deaths from any other malignant conditions. Advances in specific GI cancers were noted.

Specific Cancers.—Esophageal cancer includes squamous cell carcinomas and adenocarcinomas. The incidence of squamous cell carcinomas has decreased in the United States, but that of adenomas has increased sevenfold, now accounting for 75% of all esophageal tumors. Minimally invasive surgical techniques reduce perioperative morbidity, and preoperative radiation therapy or platinum-based chemotherapy or their combination improves outcomes. Positron emission tomography (PET) scans can assess responsiveness. Five-year survival is 19%, fourfold greater than 30 years ago.

Both the incidence and the mortality of gastric cancer have had a dramatic but poorly explained decrease over the past 50 years. Gastric cancer causes just 1.9% of anticipated cancer-related deaths, but it is the second most frequent cause of cancer mortality worldwide. Research has identified an intestinal type and a diffuse type of disease, with the latter having a worse prognosis. Environmental exposure early in life is suspected to contribute to these cancers, and the intestinal type appears to be related to *Helicobacter pylori* infection. Computed tomography (CT) scanning and esophagogastroscopy have improved the evaluation of symptomatic patients. Subtotal gastrectomy is the surgery of choice for distal intestinal-type carcinoma, but diffuse carcinomas respond better to preoperative chemotherapy or chemoradiotherapy. Patients with advanced disease have a median survival of less than 12 months, although adding trastuzumab to chemotherapy may increase median survival by nearly 3 months in selected patients. The likelihood of 5-year survival of US patients with gastric adenocarcinoma is up from 15% 30 years ago to 29% currently.

Small improvements have occurred in pancreatic cancer outcomes. Advances in imaging and endoscopic aids in screening facilitate earlier diagnosis. Surgical techniques and postoperative care have also improved, especially when delivered at high-volume centers. Aggressive management of symptoms plus endoluminal stent placement to relieve biliary tree or gastric outlet obstruction provide better palliative care. Five-year survival rates are now 6%, up from 2% 30 years ago.

Development of a vaccine against hepatitis B has proved the causative relationship between hepatocellular carcinoma and hepatitis B. High rates of carcinoma related to hepatitis C continue. Orthotopic liver transplants provide a cure for some patients, and the liberalization of eligibility criteria for transplants opened this option to more patients. Those who undergo standard cytotoxic chemotherapy have poor results, but transhepatic arterial chemoembolization has proved effective and possibly able to prolong survival. Effective systemic treatments are lacking. Biliary tract cancers are not as uncommon as previously thought but are difficult to study and treat. Combining gemcitabine and cisplatin is the treatment of choice for these cancers. The probability of survival for 5 years with hepatobiliary cancer is up from 3% 30 years ago to 18%.

Significant improvements in GI neuroendocrine cancer have transformed pancreatic neuroendocrine tumors (PNET) and intestinal carcinoid tumors into manageable, chronic diseases. Octreotide diminishes symptoms of these tumors. Abdominal imaging that permits the biopsy of lesions deep in the abdomen has increased the diagnostic frequency, and the cellular proliferative index may reliably predict prognosis. New treatment options include targeting the metabolic and angiogenesis pathways with oral tyrosine kinase inhibitors and everolimus.

Substantial progress has been made in the early detection, prevention, and treatment of colorectal cancer. Screening the general population for colorectal polyps and cancer through sigmoidoscopy or colonoscopy has reduced both the incidence and mortality associated with these cancers. The molecular pathways leading to colorectal cancer have been identified, which should help early detection, prevention, and treatment approaches. Surgical resection is the primary treatment, but laparoscopic colectomy is yielding outcomes similar to those with open colectomy with reduced morbidity. Adjustments to postoperative adjuvant chemotherapy formulations have also improved treatment. Total mesorectal excision of the rectum after combined chemotherapy plus pelvic radiation and adjuvant systemic treatment are used to manage rectal cancers. Metastatic colorectal cancer remains incurable, but the median survival is now greater than 2 years. Surgical resection may cure up to 25% of patients who have limited metastatic lesions. Newer therapeutic regimens include fluorouracil (FU), leucovorin, and irinotecan (IFL) plus bevacizumab, anti-n-epidermal growth factor receptor (EGFR) monoclonal antibodies, and ziv-aflibercept and regorafenib. Therapy is adjusted based on the presence of mutations in the *KRAS* and *NRAS* genes.

Anal cancer is now known to be caused by human papillomavirus (HPV) infection transmitted via sexual activity. Cancer risk is increased in homosexual males and men and women with AIDS. Vaccination against HPV may reduce the likelihood of developing anal cancer. The Nigro regimen has proved curative in about 70% of patients without surgery and without a colostomy, but its use is confined to cases where the primary cancer is less than 3 cm in size. About 87% of patients anticipated to develop the disease are projected to be cured.

Conclusions.—GI cancers are a leading cause of cancer-related death globally. Over the past 50 years, progress has been made in their early detection, improved understanding of their molecular origins, and better targeting of treatment regimens.

▶ The American Society of Clinical Oncology was founded in 1964, and at that time more deaths occurred from gastrointestinal (GI) cancer than any other type of cancer. This article summarizes the progress over this 5-decade span for the more common GI cancers. This reminiscence focuses on different sites of cancer, beginning with esophageal cancer, where they note that squamous cell carcinoma was the most common type of esophageal cancer, but over the past 50 years, adenocarcinoma has increased 7-fold and now accounts for 75% of all esophageal cancers. Changes in treatment have shifted from surgery only to preoperative chemotherapy and radiation therapy, and in cases of squamous cell carcinoma, sometimes just chemoradiotherapy without surgery. The survival for esophageal cancer has increased overall from 5% to 19% over this period. For gastric cancer, its contribution to US cancer-related deaths has continued to fall from 5.7% to 1.9%, but it remains the second leading cause of cancer death worldwide. It has been learned over this time that *Helicobacter pylori* and carcinogens in our diet contribute to gastric cancer. Gastric cancer has also been characterized as 2 separate types, intestinal and diffuse, with the diffuse type having a poorer prognosis and frequently requiring preoperative chemotherapy or chemoradiation. It has been demonstrated that there is a survival benefit in some populations by more aggressive surgery with D2 and D3 resections, but these come at a price of increased morbidity, and the benefits in the Western population has not been as great. Advances have been made in chemoradiotherapy for gastric cancer, and the regimen of epirubicin, cisplatin, and 5-fluorouracil (FU) in the neoadjuvant and adjuvant setting. Over the 50-year period, 5-year survival has increased from 15% to 29%. For pancreatic cancer, the improvements have come mostly from improvements in imaging, endoscopic retrograde cholangiopancreatography, endoscopic ultrasound with biopsy, and the marker CA 19-9 for earlier diagnosis. Palliation has improved with endoscopic stenting procedures, and risk factors have been identified, including obesity, diabetes, and cigarette smoking. Several familial syndromes such as Peutz-Jeghers, hereditary nonpolyposis colorectal cancer, and *BRCA2* also predispose to the cancer. Clinical trials have not yielded effective chemotherapy regimens since the initial trials of 5-FU in 1985 and gemcitabine in 1997, but more recently, the regimens of FOLFIRINOX and gemcitabine/NAB-paclitaxel have shown significant responses in metastatic pancreatic cancer and is now being used in the neoadjuvant setting. Unfortunately, 5-year survival has only increased from 2 to 6% in the past decades. With respect to hepatocellular carcinoma, the old notion that most of these were related to alcoholic cirrhosis has been replaced by the knowledge that hepatitis B and C infection are the primary causes throughout the world of this cancer. Liver transplantation has emerged as a useful treatment option for patients with hepatocellular carcinoma, especially if the disease is limited to 3 or fewer lesions, there is limited blood vessel involvement, and no extrahepatic metastases. Chemotherapy has not been particularly useful, and embolization and ablation are used for some tumors. Sorafenib has shown promise in the treatment of some patients as well. Survival has increased from 3% to 18% over these decades. For neuroendocrine tumors of the pancreas and small bowel, the increasing use of octreotide since the 1990s has been helpful for palliating symptoms, and it may also have some antitumor effects. The incidence of these tumors has increased significantly, which may be due in part to improved imaging techniques.

In colorectal cancer, we have learned that obesity, limited physical activity, and red meat help predispose to colon cancer, whereas aspirin is a useful preventative agent. Widespread screening programs, including colonoscopy, have been instituted, allowing for earlier diagnosis and improvements in cancer-related mortality. We have learned that 6 months of postoperative chemotherapy improved survival in stage 3 colon cancer and, recently, we have learned that the regimen of 5-FU, leucovorin, and oxaliplatin (FOLFOX) is perhaps the most active combination in the adjuvant setting. In the metastatic setting, FOLFOX and FOLFIRI with bevacizumab show the best efficacy. Randomized trials have revealed that laparoscopic colectomy can be performed leading with equivalent oncologic outcomes and reduced length of stay over open procedures. CEA is a useful antigen to screen patients for recurrence, and when metastases develop in the liver, surgical resection can cure up to 30% of patients. The antibodies cetuximab and panitumumab may be useful in patients with wild-type *KRAS* genes, and patients with microsatellite instability are less likely to respond to chemotherapy and generally have a better prognosis. The 5-year survival in colorectal cancer has improved from 50% to 66%. Rectal cancer results have improved with pre- or postoperative chemoradiation and total mesorectal excision. For anal cancer, the most important development was the Nigro regimen of infusional 5-FU, mitomycin, and radiation therapy without surgery, where 70% of patients are cured with this combination. This article is an excellent overview of the progress that has been made over these decades in GI cancer but also makes it clear that much progress still needs to be made.

J. R. Howe, MD

Sentinel Lymph Node Biopsy is Associated with Improved Survival in Merkel Cell Carcinoma

Kachare SD, Wong JH, Vohra NA, et al (East Carolina Univ, Greenville, NC)
Ann Surg Oncol 21:1624-1630, 2014

Background.—Although sentinel lymph node biopsy (SNB) has become a standard for Merkel cell carcinoma (MCC), the impact on survival is unclear. To better define the staging and therapeutic value of SNB, we compared SNB with nodal observation.

Methods.—Patients with clinical stage I and II MCC in the Surveillance, Epidemiology, and End Results (SEER) registry undergoing surgery between 2003 and 2009 were identified and divided into two groups—SNB and observation.

Results.—A total of 1,193 patients met the inclusion criteria (SNB 474 and Observation 719). The median age was 78 years, and the majority were White (95.3 %), male (58.8 %), received radiation therapy (52.9

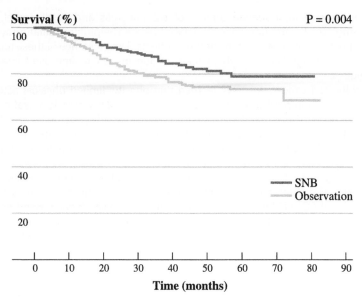

FIGURE 1.—Merkel cell carcinoma-specific survival sentinel lymph node biopsy (SNB) versus observation, SEER tumor registry. (With kind permission from Springer Science+Business Media. Kachare SD, Wong JH, Vohra NA, et al. Sentinel lymph node biopsy is associated with improved survival in merkel cell carcinoma. *Ann Surg Oncol.* 2014;21:1624-1630, with permission from Society of Surgical Oncology.)

%) and had T1 tumors (65.3 %). Twenty-four percent had a positive SNB. SNB patients were younger (73 vs. 81 years; $p < 0.0001$), had T1 tumors (69.6 vs. 62.5 %; $p = 0.04$) and received radiotherapy (57.8 vs. 40 %; $p < 0.0001$). Among biopsy patients, a negative SNB was associated with improved 5-year MCC-specific survival (84.5 vs. 64.6 %; $p < 0.0001$). Univariate analysis demonstrated an increased 5-year MCC-specific survival for the SNB group versus the Observation group (79.2 vs. 73.8 %; $p = 0.004$), female gender (83.2 vs. 70.4 %; $p = 0.0004$), and lower T stage ($p < 0.0001$). On Cox regression, diminished survival was noted for the Observation group (risk ratio [RR] 1.43; $p = 0.04$), male gender (RR 2.06; $p < 0.0001$), and a higher T stage.

Conclusion.—SNB for MCC provides prognostic information and is associated with a significant survival advantage (Figs 1 and 2).

▶ Merkel cell carcinoma (MCC) of the skin is an uncommon tumor, which derives from neuroendocrine cells and can have an aggressive disease course. In some ways, it behaves like melanoma, with early spread to regional lymph nodes. Therefore, surgeons have been adopting the sentinel lymph node concept and applying it to MCC. What is unclear is whether patients who have a sentinel lymph node biopsy (SNB) have improved survival relative to patients who are merely observed. To attempt to answer this question, the authors reviewed the SEER database for cases of stage 1 and 2 MCC from 2003 to 2009. Patients had to have clinically negative nodes, no evidence of metastatic disease, and

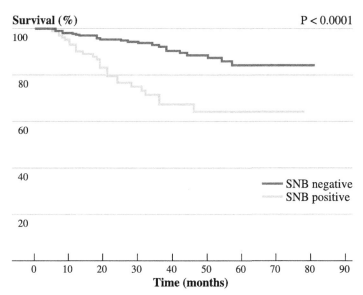

FIGURE 2.—Merkel cell carcinoma-specific survival for positive versus negative sentinel lymph node biopsy (SNB), SEER tumor registry. (With kind permission from Springer Science+Business Media. Kachare SD, Wong JH, Vohra NA, et al. Sentinel lymph node biopsy is associated with improved survival in merkel cell carcinoma. *Ann Surg Oncol.* 2014;21:1624-1630, with permission from Society of Surgical Oncology.)

not lymphadenectomy. There were 1193 patients with a mean age of 78 years, with a preponderance toward males (59%) and white patients (95%). Four hundred and seventy-four patients (40%) underwent SNB, and 719 (60%) were observed. There were some differences between these groups as might be expected in a retrospective study. Patients who had SNB performed were significantly younger (by a mean of 8 years), more likely to have T1 tumors, and to have undergone radiation therapy. Median follow-up was 21 months, and the overall 5-year MCC-specific survival was 76%. They found significantly greater 5-year MCC-specific survival in patients who had SNB versus observation (79 vs 74%; Fig 1). Patients who had a negative node by SNB had significantly higher survival than those with a positive node, as might be expected (85 vs 65%; Fig 2). Female patients did significantly better than males in terms of MCC-specific survival, as did patients with T1 versus T2 tumors. In a multivariate analyses, female gender, T1 lesions, and SNB were independent prognostic factors for improved survival. Of the patients who had positive sentinel lymph nodes, a total of 70% had radiation therapy, and 56% had completion lymph node dissection (35% had both, 10% had neither). The fact that patients who had SNB performed had improved survival suggests that there was a therapeutic benefit gained from this, that is, completion lymphadenectomy or radiation therapy in node positive patients resulted in improved survival. This finding is at odds with 1 large single institutional study that found that the sentinel lymph node status did not predict for survival. However, the findings of this retrospective and much larger Surveillance, Epidemiology, and End Results Program study do suggest a survival benefit, and therefore the authors recommend that patients with local-ized MCC should have SNB performed so that patients with positive nodes could be considered for lymphadenectomy or radiation therapy. One caveat to this conclusion is not knowing to what degree the survival difference was influenced by the selection bias inherent in this study (where younger patients, with more T1 tumors, and more having radiation therapy were in the SNB group).

J. R. Howe, MD

11 Vascular Surgery

Carotid

Predictors of 30-day postoperative stroke or death after carotid endarterectomy using the 2012 carotid endarterectomy-targeted American College of Surgeons National Surgical Quality Improvement Program database

Bennett KM, Scarborough JE, Shortell CK (Duke Univ Med Ctr, Durham, NC)
J Vasc Surg 61:103-111, 2015

Objective.—This study used a recently released procedure-targeted multicenter data source to determine independent predictors of postoperative stroke or death in patients undergoing carotid endarterectomy (CEA) for carotid artery stenosis.

Methods.—The 2012 CEA-targeted American College of Surgeons (ACS) National Surgical Quality Improvement Program (NSQIP) database was used for this study. Patient, disease, and procedure characteristics of patients undergoing CEA were assessed. Multivariate logistic regression analysis was used to determine independent risk factors for 30-day postoperative stroke/death or other major complications.

Results.—The analysis included 3845 patients undergoing CEA (58.1% with asymptomatic and 41.9% with symptomatic carotid disease). The overall 30-day postoperative stroke/death rate was 3.0% (1.9% in asymptomatic patients, 4.6% in symptomatic patients). The variables that maintained an independent association with postoperative stroke/death after adjustment for other known patient-related and procedure-related factors were age ≥80 years, active smoking, contralateral internal carotid artery stenosis of 80% to 99%, emergency procedure status, preoperative stroke, presence of one or more ACS NSQIP-defined high-risk characteristics (including any or all of New York Heart Association class III/IV congestive heart failure, left ventricular ejection fraction <30%, recent unstable angina, or recent myocardial infarction), and operative time ≥150 minutes.

Conclusions.—After adjustment for a comprehensive array of patient-related and procedure-related variables of particular import to patients with carotid artery stenosis, we have identified several factors that are independently associated with early stroke or death after CEA. These factors are generally related to the comorbid condition of CEA patients and to specific characteristics of their carotid disease, and not to technical features of the CEA procedure. Knowledge of these factors will assist surgeons in selecting appropriate patients for this procedure.

▶ The authors have used the carotid endarterectomy (CEA)-targeted American College of Surgeons (ACS) National Surgical Quality Improvement Program (NISQIP) to identify the predictors of 30-day stroke/mortality after carotid endarterectomy (CEA). The CEA-targeted database is similar to the larger ACS NISQIP database but includes additional variables of concerns for patients undergoing CEA, including those that are patient-, disease-, and procedure-specific. Importantly, the data were all collected prospectively by trained, certified clinical reviewers. The authors reported that the combined 30-day stroke/mortality rates were 1.9% and 4.6% for asymptomatic and symptomatic lesions, respectively, both below the acceptable range in the current national guidelines (asymptomatic = 3.0%, symptomatic = 6.0%). These rates are encouraging and likely reflect "real-world" data given the sample size (N = 3845) and the number of contributing centers (N = 78). The presence of a contralateral internal carotid artery stenosis (ie, 80–99%) and American Society of Anesthesiologists classification of 4 of 5 were independent predictors of 30-day stroke/mortality for asymptomatic lesions, whereas a contralateral stenosis, emergent procedure, physiologic high-risk characteristic (class III/IV congestive heart failure, left ventricular EV < 30%, recent unstable angina, recent myocardial infarction), and preoperative stroke were the predictors for symptomatic lesions. Notably, the presence of 1 of these predictors for either asymptomatic or symptomatic patients increased the expected 30-day stroke/mortality rate to a value that exceeded the current guidelines (asymptomatic = 5.3%, symptomatic = 6.2%). It is interesting that the predictors for 30-day stroke/mortality were all patient- and disease-specific and did not include any procedure-specific components. Notably, surgeon specialty, choice of anesthesia, patch angioplasty, carotid shunt, endarterectomy technique, and operative duration were not associated with the stroke/mortality outcome. The findings underscore the importance of patient selection in terms of outcome. However, these data should be used with some caution, remembering that CEA is a prophylactic, stroke prevention operation, the benefit of which is dependent on the longer term risk-to-benefit balance between medical and surgical treatment, not just the perioperative outcomes.

T. S. Huber, MD, PhD

Long-Term Follow-Up Study of Endarterectomy Versus Angioplasty in Patients With Symptomatic Severe Carotid Stenosis Trial
Mas J-L, on behalf of the EVA-3S Investigators (Université Paris-Descartes, France; et al)
Stroke 45:2750-2756, 2014

Background and Purpose.—We aimed at comparing the long-term benefit-risk balance of carotid stenting versus endarterectomy for symptomatic carotid stenosis.

Methods.—Long-term follow-up study of patients included in Endarterectomy Versus Angioplasty in Patients With Symptomatic Severe Carotid Stenosis (EVA-3S), a randomized, controlled trial of carotid stenting versus endarterectomy in 527 patients with recently symptomatic severe carotid stenosis, conducted in 30 centers in France. The main end point was a composite of any ipsilateral stroke after randomization or any procedural stroke or death.

Results.—During a median follow-up of 7.1 years (interquartile range, 5.1—8.8 years; maximum 12.4 years), the primary end point occurred in 30 patients in the stenting group compared with 18 patients in the endarterectomy group. Cumulative probabilities of this outcome were 11.0% (95% confidence interval, 7.9—15.2) versus 6.3% (4.0—9.8) in the endarterectomy group at the 5-year follow-up (hazard ratio, 1.85; 1.00—3.40; $P = 0.04$) and 11.5% (8.2—15.9) versus 7.6% (4.9—11.8; hazard ratio, 1.70; 0.95—3.06; $P = 0.07$) at the 10-year follow-up. No difference was observed between treatment groups in the rates of ipsilateral stroke beyond the procedural period, severe carotid restenosis ($\geq 70\%$) or occlusion, death, myocardial infarction, and revascularization procedures.

Conclusions.—The long-term benefit-risk balance of carotid stenting versus endarterectomy for symptomatic carotid stenosis favored endarterectomy, a difference driven by a lower risk of procedural stroke after endarterectomy. Both techniques were associated with low and similar long-term risks of recurrent ipsilateral stroke beyond the procedural period.

Clinical Trial Registration.—URL: http://www.clinicaltrials.gov. Unique identifier: NCT00190398.

▶ The authors report the longer-term outcomes from the Endarterectomy Versus Angioplasty in Patients with Symptomatic Carotid Stenosis (EVA-3S) trial, one of the seminal trials comparing the 2 modalities for symptomatic lesions. They found that the initial superiority for carotid endarterectomy were sustained at both the 5-year (11.0% vs 6.3%, hazard ratio, 1.85; 1.00—3.40; $P = .04$) and 10-year (11.5% vs 7.6%, hazard ratio, 1.7; 0.95—3.06; $P = .07$) follow-up intervals. Note that the primary endpoint for the trial was the rate of any stroke or death within 30 days after the procedure, and the prespecified endpoint for the longer-term follow-up was a composite of any ipsilateral stroke after randomization or any procedural stroke (including retinal infarct) or death. The rates of ipsilateral stroke after the procedural period were low (4-year cumulative risk 4.8%, 95% CI 2.6—7.0), and there were no significant differences between the groups. The risk of carotid restenosis was also low, and, likewise, there were no differences between the groups. Additionally, the risk of myocardial infarction and revascularization did not differ between the groups. These data suggest that both carotid endarterectomy and stenting are equivocal, effective modalities to prevent ipsilateral postprocedure stroke and that both modalities are associated with a minimal restenosis rate. The reported benefits of carotid endarterectomy were largely due to the increased procedural risk for nondisabling strokes, a finding consistent with the other seminal trials. The factors responsible for the increased procedure risk with stenting remain unresolved but likely include patient anatomy and operator experience. It is conceivable that this increased risk will decrease over time with the widespread adoption of the technique and the continued evolution of the devices, although extending the indications likely requires additional level 1 evidence. The lack of a difference in longer-term mortality from myocardial infarction is somewhat noteworthy given the observation from the other seminal trials that carotid endarterectomy was associated with a higher myocardial infarction rate that was associated with higher late mortality. Although the data are compelling and support my bias regarding the superiority of carotid endarterectomy over stenting for symptomatic lesions, they must be interpreted with some caution given the retrospective nature of the follow-up.

T. S. Huber, MD, PhD

Evaluation of Carotid Angioplasty and Stenting for Radiation-Induced Carotid Stenosis

Yu SCH, Zou WXY, Soo YOY, et al (The Chinese Univ of Hong Kong, China)

Stroke 45:1402-1407, 2014

Background and Purpose.—We aimed to evaluate the procedural safety, clinical, and angiographic outcome of carotid angioplasty and stenting for high-grade ($\geq$70%) radiation-induced carotid stenosis (RIS) using atherosclerotic stenosis (AS) as a control.

Methods.—In this 6-year prospective nonrandomized study, we compared the carotid angioplasty and stenting outcome of 65 consecutive patients (84 vessels) with RIS with that of a control group of 129 consecutive patients (150 vessels) with AS. Study end points were 30-day periprocedural stroke or death, ipsilateral ischemic stroke, technical success, procedural characteristics, instent restenosis (ISR; $\geq$50%) and symptomatic ISR.

Results.—The median follow-up was 47.3 months (95% confidence interval, 26.9-61.6). Imaging assessment was available in 74 vessels (RIS) and 120 vessels (AS) in 2 years. Comparing RIS group with AS group, the rates of periprocedural stroke or death were 1.5% (1/65) versus 1.6% (2/129; $P = 1$); ipsilateral ischemic stroke rates were 4.6% (3/65) versus 4.7% (6/129; $P = 1$); the annual risks of ipsilateral ischemic stroke were 1.2% (3 patient/254.7 patient year) versus 1.2% (6 patient/494.2 patient year; $P = 0.89$); technical success rates were both 100%. Stenting of common carotid artery and the use of multiple stents was more common in the RIS group ($P = 0$ in both cases); ISR rates were 25.7% (19/74) versus 4.2% (5/120; $P < 0.001$); symptomatic ISR rates were 6.8% (5/74) versus 0.8% (1/120; $P = 0.031$).

Conclusions.—The safety, effectiveness, and technical difficulty of carotid angioplasty and stenting for RIS are comparable with that for AS although it is associated with a higher rate of ISR.

Clinical Trial Registration.—This trial was not registered as enrollment started in 2006.

▶ The authors have performed a nice prospective study examining carotid angioplasty and stenting (CAS) for patients with radiation-induced carotid stenosis. The perioperative and long-term outcomes were compared with those of patients with the typical atherosclerotic carotid artery stenosis, and all patients were assessed by certified raters using the National Institute of Health Stroke scale throughout the evaluation period. The overwhelming majority of the procedures (> 95%) in both groups were performed for symptomatic lesions. The perioperative stroke/mortality (1.5% vs 1.6%) and technical success (100%) were comparable between the 2 groups. Similarly, the cumulative risk of ipsilateral stroke beyond 30 days was comparable, as determined by Kaplan-Meir analysis, whereas the annual risk of ischemic stroke (1.2% per year) was also comparable. However, the incidence of restenosis (25.7% vs 4.2%, $P < .001$) and the incidence of symptomatic restenosis were significantly greater in the radiation group. Although the technical and perioperative outcomes were comparable, the disease processes and patient characteristics were distinctly different between groups. The patients in the radiation group were a decade younger (62 vs 73 years) and had a lower prevalence of the traditional atherosclerotic risk factors. The radiation-induced lesions were longer, more likely to affect to common carotid artery, and more commonly associated with a contralateral extra-cranial carotid stenosis or occlusion. Overall, the results are encouraging and establish carotid angioplasty and stenting as an excellent treatment modality for radiation-induced stenosis, particularly given the potential difficulties associated with carotid endarterectomy or replacement. The increased risk of recurrence likely merits increased surveillance, but the low risk of recurrent symptoms suggests that expectant management may be most appropriate.

T. S. Huber, MD, PhD

Miscellaneous

Nonoperative management of hemodynamically unstable abdominal trauma patients with angioembolization and resuscitative endovascular balloon occlusion of the aorta

Ogura T, Lefor AT, Nakano M, et al (Japan Red Cross Maebashi Hosp, Gunma; Jichi Med Univ, Tochigi, Japan)
J Trauma Acute Care Surg 78:132-135, 2015

Background.—Many hemodynamically stable patients with blunt abdominal solid organ injuries are successfully managed nonoperatively, while unstable patients often require urgent laparotomy. Recently, therapeutic angioembolization has been used in the treatment of intra-abdominal hemorrhage in hemodynamically unstable patients. We undertook this study to review a series of hemodynamically unstable patients with abdominal solid organ injuries managed nonoperatively with angioembolization and resuscitative endovascular balloon occlusion of the aorta.

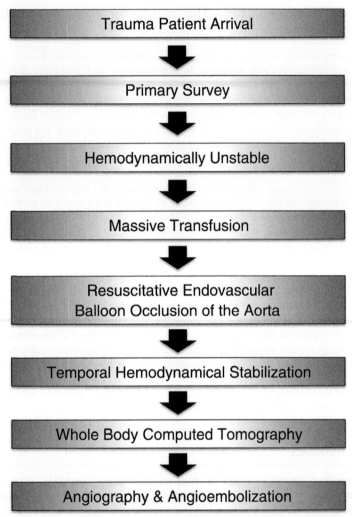

FIGURE 1.—Flow chart of the care provided to patients with abdominal solid organ injuries managed with angioembolization and REBOA. (Reprinted from Ogura T, Lefor AT, Nakano M, et al. Nonoperative management of hemodynamically unstable abdominal trauma patients with angioembolization and resuscitative endovascular balloon occlusion of the aorta. *J Trauma Acute Care Surg*. 2015;78:132-135, with permission from Wolters Kluwer Health, Inc.)

Methods.—The institutional review board approved this study. All patients were appropriately resuscitated with transfusions, and angiography was performed after computed tomography. Resuscitative endovascular balloon occlusion of the aorta was performed before computed tomography in all patients.

Results.—Seven patients underwent resuscitative endovascular balloon occlusion of the aorta following severe blunt abdominal trauma. The

28-day survival rate was 86% (6 of 7). There were no complications related to the procedure.

Conclusion.—We describe the first clinical series of hemodynamically unstable patients with abdominal solid organ injury treated nonoperatively with angioembolization and resuscitative endovascular balloon occlusion of the aorta. Survival rate was 86%, supporting the need for further study of this modality as an adjunct to the nonoperative management of patients with severe traumatic injuries.

Level of Evidence.—Therapeutic study, level V (Fig 1).

▶ The brief report documents the successful nonoperative treatment of unstable trauma patients after blunt, solid organ injury using a combination of resuscitative endovascular balloon occlusion of the aorta (REBOA) and angioembolization. The cornerstone of the treatment algorithm, as shown in Fig 1, is the successful deployment of the occlusion balloon that allows temporary hemodynamic stability, thus permitting additional imaging and definitive endovascular treatment. Although the series was small (*N* = 7), the patient survival was impressive (86%), underscoring the potential for the new technique. The authors report that their overall experience with the REBOA was considerably larger (*N* = 35) and included patients treated both operatively and nonoperatively. The mortality rate in this larger cohort was 46%, with the majority of the deaths result from traumatic brain injuries. Unfortunately, there were not a lot of details provided about the specific endovascular device and/or the insertion technique. Specifically, the authors reported that the "catheter was placed in the routine fashion, through the femoral artery, by an experienced intensive care unit (ICU) or emergency department (ED) physician. Appropriate placement of the balloon was confirmed by sonography." Similarly to the technique used for ruptured aneurysms, the occlusion balloon is usually placed over a stiff wire under fluoroscopic imaging and then inflated until the outer contours of the balloon assume the contour of the aorta. The balloon can be positioned anywhere along the thoracic or abdominal aorta as dictated by the specific injury. A detailed description of the technique has been reported by Stannard et al.[1] Placement of an aortic balloon catheter in an unstable patient in the emergency department sounds like a daunting task but is likely within the skill set of most vascular and trauma surgeons, provided that adequate imaging is available. Fortunately, most trauma patients are young and do not have significant aortoiliac occlusive disease. In our own institution, the trauma surgeons have approached us about participating in our endovascular cases and plan on incorporating a formal rotation on our service for their fellowship training program. It will be interesting to see how the REBOA technique evolves over the next few years. It has a tremendous amount of appeal, particularly considering the futile outcome associated with the alternative emergency department thoracotomy.

T. S. Huber, MD, PhD

Reference

1. Stannard A, Eliason JL, Rasmussen TE. Resuscitative endovascular balloon occlusion of the aorta (REBOA) as an adjunct for hemorrhagic shock. *J Trauma*. 2011; 71:1869-1872.

Evaluation and management of blunt traumatic aortic injury: A practice management guideline from the Eastern Association for the Surgery of Trauma

Fox N, Schwartz D, Salazar JH, et al (Cooper Univ Hosp, Camden, NJ; The Johns Hopkins School of Medicine, Baltimore, MD; et al)
J Trauma Acute Care Surg 78:136-146, 2015

Background.—Blunt traumatic aortic injury (BTAI) is the second most common cause of death in trauma patients. Eighty percent of patients with BTAI will die before reaching a trauma center. The issues of how to diagnose, treat, and manage BTAI were first addressed by the Eastern Association for the Surgery of Trauma (EAST) in the practice management guidelines on this topic published in 2000. Since that time, there have been advances in the management of BTAI. As a result, the EAST guidelines committee decided to develop updated guidelines for this topic using the Grading of Recommendations, Assessment, Development and Evaluation (GRADE) framework recently adopted by EAST.

Methods.—A systematic review of the MEDLINE database using PubMed was performed. The search retrieved English language articles regarding BTAI from 1998 to 2013. Letters to the editor, case reports, book chapters, and review articles were excluded. Topics of investigation included imaging to diagnose BTAI, type of operative repair, and timing of operative repair.

Results.—Sixty articles were identified. Of these, 51 articles were selected to construct the guidelines.

Conclusion.—There have been changes in practice since the publication of the previous guidelines in 2000. Computed tomography of the chest with intravenous contrast is strongly recommended to diagnose clinically significant BTAI. Endovascular repair is strongly recommended for patients without contraindications. Delayed repair of BTAI is suggested, with the stipulation that effective blood pressure control must be used in these patients.

▶ This study details the practice management guidelines for blunt aortic injury from the Eastern Association for the Surgery of Trauma. These represent an update from the 2000 guidelines and were justified by the rapid evolution of CT-based imaging and endovascular therapies. The writing committee performed a systematic review of the literature and employed the Grading of Recommendation, Assessment, Development and Evaluation framework to answer 3 specific questions: diagnostic imaging, type of operative repair, and timing of operation. They strongly recommended that CT scanning was the diagnostic study of choice and that endovascular repair was preferable unless patients had a specific contraindication. These findings are not particularly surprising given the rapid changes in the technologies (both CT and endovascular) over the past 15 years, and the recommendations largely support the current standard of care. However, it is interesting to note that the committee considered the overall quality of the evidence for both recommendations to be low to moderate. The sensitivity and specificity for CT-based diagnosis of blunt aortic injury were both > 90%, whereas the endovascular approach was associated with reduced mortality (relative risk 0.56, 95% confidence interval 0.44–0.73) and paraplegia (relative risk 0.36, 95% confidence interval 0.19–0.71) rates, although there was no difference in the incidence of stroke. The committee suggested delayed repair, stating that effective blood pressure control was critical. The quality of evidence to support the recommendation in terms of the timing of repair was very low (stroke) to high (paraplegia). Unfortunately, this recommendation does not provide a lot of guidance, and the timing of repair remains a critical question. The authors reported that delayed repair is associated with decreased mortality and paraplegia but emphasized that those patients who benefit most have major associated injuries. They stated that the data are not clear as to the timing of repair in patients without associated injury and emphasized that surgeon convenience is not a reason to delay. The committee also stated that "patients at high risk of aortic rupture, based on clinical suspicion, imaging characteristics, and/or grade of injury should not be considered for delayed repair," and they went on to state that these included pseudoaneurysms (grade 3) and active extravasation (grade 4). The anatomic and clinical features that mandate urgent or emergent repair remain an ongoing question. In our own practice, we have felt compelled to repair all the significant pseudoaneurysms urgently (or emergently), but suspect that a more delayed approach is likely safe.

T. S. Huber, MD, PhD

Perioperative management with antiplatelet and statin medication is associated with reduced mortality following vascular surgery

De Martino RR, on behalf of the Vascular Study Group of New England (Dartmouth-Hitchcock Med Ctr, Lebanon, NH; et al)
J Vasc Surg 59:1615-1621.e1, 2014

Objective.—Many patients undergoing vascular surgical procedures are not on appropriate medical therapy. This study sought to examine the variation and impact of antiplatelet (AP) and statin therapy on early and late mortality in patients undergoing vascular surgery in our region.

Methods. We studied all patients (n — 14,489) undergoing elective carotid endarterectomy (n = 6978), carotid stenting (n = 524), and suprainguinal (n = 763) and infrainguinal bypass (n = 3053), as well as patients with known coronary risk factors undergoing open (n = 1044) and endovascular (n = 2127) abdominal aortic aneurysm repair from 2005 to 2012 in the Vascular Study Group of New England. Optimal medical

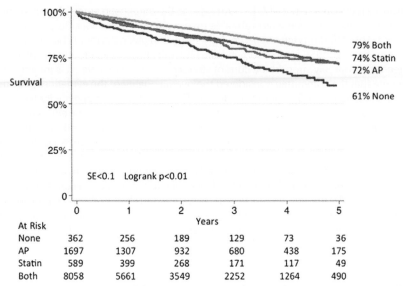

At Risk	0	1	2	3	4	5
None	362	256	189	129	73	36
AP	1697	1307	932	680	438	175
Statin	589	399	268	171	117	49
Both	8058	5661	3549	2252	1264	490

FIGURE 6.—Five-year survival following surgery by discharge medication status. *AP*, Antiplatelet medication. (Reprinted from the Journal of Vascular Surgery. De Martino RR, on behalf of the Vascular Study Group of New England. Perioperative management with antiplatelet and statin medication is associated with reduced mortality following vascular surgery. *J Vasc Surg*. 2014;59:1615-1621.e1, Copyright 2014, with permission from The Society for Vascular Surgery.)

management was defined as treatment with both AP and statin agents, pre-operatively and at discharge. We analyzed temporal, procedural, and center variation of medication use. Multivariable analyses were used to determine the adjusted impact of AP and statin therapy on 30-day mortality and 5-year survival.

Results.—Optimal medical management improved over the study interval (55% in 2005 to 68% in 2012; *P* trend < .01) with carotid interventions having the highest rates of optimal medications use (carotid artery stenting, 78%; carotid endarterectomy, 74%) and abdominal aortic aneurysm repair in patients with known cardiac risk factors having the lowest (open, 57%; endovascular aneurysm repair, 56%). Optimal medication use varied by center as well (range, 40%-86%). Preoperative AP and statin use was associated with reduced 30-day mortality (odds ratio, 0.76; 95% confidence interval [CI], 0.5-1.05; *P* = .09). AP and statin prescription at discharge was additive in survival benefit with improved 5-year survival (hazard ratio, 0.5; 95% CI, 0.4-0.7; *P* < .01) that was consistent across procedure types. Patients prescribed AP and statin at discharge had 5-year survival of 79% (95% CI, 77%-81%) compared with only 61% (95% CI, 52%-68%; *P* < .001) for patients on neither medication.

Conclusions.—AP and statin therapy preoperatively and at discharge was associated with reduced 30-day mortality and an absolute 18% improved 5-year survival after vascular surgery. However, one-third of patients are suboptimally managed in real world practice. This demonstrates an opportunity for quality improvement that can substantially improve survival after vascular surgery (Fig 6).

▶ The authors have performed an insightful analysis of the use of antiplatelet (AP) agents (aspirin or clopidogrel) and statins among patients (N = 14 489) undergoing elective vascular surgical procedures for cerebrovascular, aneurysmal, and aortoiliac/infrainguinal occlusive disease in the Vascular Study Group of New England. They reported that optimal medical therapy (defined by the use of both agents preoperatively and at discharge) improved over the time course of the study (2005—2012) but was achieved in only 68% of the patients during the final year. The use of both agents was associated with a trend (odds ratio 0.75, 95% confidence interval [CI] 0.5—1.05, $P = .09$) toward a reduced 30-day mortality in their multivariate analysis. The 5-year survival rate (Fig 6) was highest among those discharged on both agents, and the multivariate survival analysis demonstrated that being discharged on either agent (hazard ratio [HR] 0.7, 95% CI 0.5—0.9) or both (HR 0.5, 95% CI 0.4—0.7) was associated with improved long-term survival after adjustment for age, procedure type, and comorbidities. These data provide some of the most compelling evidence that we must assume responsibility for ensuring that our patients are on both AP and statins, both preoperatively and postoperatively. Given the relatively simple nature of prescribing these agents, it is somewhat staggering that the survival benefit may be comparable to repairing an abdominal aortic aneurysm, as emphasized by the authors in their discussion. The site-specific data clearly illustrate that it is possible to achieve excellent rates (best center 86%), and cardiology colleagues have consistently had target rates of almost 100% for the use of AP and statins after an acute myocardial infarction. Although many vascular surgeons may feel somewhat uncomfortable starting patients on statins, the treatment is certainly within our expected skill set and expertise and, as one of my partners is fond of saying, "If we can fix an open aneurysm, we can certainly start someone on a statin."

T. S. Huber, MD, PhD

Clinical characteristics associated with readmission among patients undergoing vascular surgery
Engelbert TL, Fernandes-Taylor S, Gupta PK, et al (Univ of Wisconsin Hosps and Clinics, Madison)
J Vasc Surg 59:1349-1355, 2014

Objective.—Readmission after a vascular surgery intervention is frequent, costly, and often considered preventable. Vascular surgery outcomes have recently been scrutinized by Medicare because of the high rates of readmission. We determined patient and clinical characteristics associated with readmission in a cohort of vascular surgery patients.

Methods.—From 2009 to 2013, the medical records of all patients (n = 2505) undergoing interventions by the vascular surgery service at a single tertiary care institution were retrospectively reviewed. Sociodemographic and clinical characteristics were examined for association with 30-day readmission to the same institution.

Results.—The 30-day readmission rate to the same institution was 9.7 % (n = 244). Procedures most likely to result in readmission were below-knee (25%), foot (22%), and toe amputations (19%), as well as lower extremity revascularization (22%). Patients covered by Medicaid (16.8%) and Medicare (10.0%) were most likely to be readmitted, followed by fee-for-service (9.5%), self-pay (8.0%), and health maintenance organizations (5.5%; $P < .05$). Patients urgently admitted were more likely to be readmitted (16.2%) than those electively admitted (9.1%; $P < .01$). Patient severity as rated using the All Patient Refined Diagnosis Related Groups software (3M Health Information Systems, Wallingford, Conn) predicted readmission (16.2% high vs 6.2% low severity; $P < .01$). Initial length of stay was longer for readmitted than nonreadmitted patients (8.5 vs 6.1 days, respectively; $P < .01$). Intensive care unit admission during the initial hospitalization was associated with higher readmission rates in univariable analysis (18.3% with vs 9.5% without intensive care unit stay; $P < .05$). Discharge destination was also a strong predictor of readmission (rehabilitation, 19.2%; skilled nursing facility, 16.2%; home, 6.2%; $P < .01$). The effects of urgent admission, proximity to hospital, length of stay, lower extremity open procedure or amputation, and discharge destination persisted in multivariable logistic regression ($P < .05$).

Conclusions.—To reduce readmission rates effectively, institutions must identify high-risk patients. Efforts should focus on subgroups undergoing selected interventions (amputations, lower extremity revascularization), those with urgent admissions, and patients with extended hospital stays. Patients in need of postacute care upon discharge are especially prone to readmission, requiring special attention to discharge planning and coordination of postdischarge care. By focusing on subgroups at risk for readmission, preventative resources can be efficiently targeted.

▶ The authors have analyzed unplanned hospital readmissions after vascular surgical procedures at their tertiary-care academic center. This analysis is particularly timely given the focus on readmission as a quality improvement metric and the provision in the Affordable Care Act that the Center for Medicare and Medicaid Services will reduce payments to hospitals with higher than expected rates for specific patient populations or diagnoses. These initial penalties have been focused on readmissions for patients with congestive heart failure, pneumonia, and myocardial infarction, although it is conceivable that readmission after vascular surgical procedures may be the next focus given the reported rates of almost 25% in the literature. In the current study, the authors reported a readmission rate of 9.7% with wound complications (37%) and "Other" (19.7%) being the leading readmission diagnoses. Notably, 28% of the readmissions occurred within 7 days of the index hospitalization. On multivariate analysis, the authors identified in-county residence (odds ratio [OR] 1.7), health maintenance organization (HMO) insurance status (OR 0.43), elective procedure (OR 0.72), index length of stay (OR 1.03—rate of readmission increases for each additional hospital day of index admission), open lower extremity procedure/amputation (OR 2.35), and discharge to a skilled nursing facility (OR 1.54) as predictors of readmission. These powerful data ask the important questions as to whether readmission after vascular surgical procedures is really a marker of quality and what strategies can be implemented to further reduce these rates (and avoid any potential financial penalty). However, these data (and the low readmission rate) must be interpreted with some caution given the tertiary-care nature of the institution and the likelihood that many patients were admitted to institutions closer to their primary residence after the index hospitalization. It is not completely clear to me that readmission after vascular surgical procedures is a marker of quality of care but rather a marker of our patient population in terms of disease process (ie, diabetes, critical limb ischemia, emergent presentation, length of index hospitalization) and resources (ie, insurance status, lack of family support). This should not be interpreted that we cannot do better in terms of quality or care and lower readmission rates, but doing highly selected (ie, no amputations/open lower extremity procedures) elective operations on well-insured patients is not a practical solution for most of us. The potential opportunities, albeit all challenging, include improving the preprocedure care and avoiding the need for the procedure itself (eg, diabetic foot infections), reducing the incidence of wound complications, and improving the care delivery system after discharge from the index procedure.

T. S. Huber, MD, PhD

Impact of cumulative intravascular contrast exposure on renal function in patients with occlusive and aneurysmal vascular disease
Kougias P, Sharath S, Barshes NR, et al (Michael E. DeBakey VA Med Ctr, Houston, TX; et al)
J Vasc Surg 59:1644-1650, 2014

Objective.—Patients with occlusive or aneurysmal vascular disease are repeatedly exposed to intravascular (IV) contrast for diagnostic or therapeutic purposes. We sought to determine the long-term impact of cumulative iodinated IV contrast exposure (CIVCE) on renal function; the latter was defined by means of National Kidney Foundation (NKF) criteria.

Methods.—We performed a longitudinal study of consecutive patients without renal insufficiency at baseline (NFK stage I or II) who underwent interventions for arterial occlusive or aneurysmal disease. We collected detailed data on any IV iodinated contrast exposure (including diagnostic or therapeutic angiography, cardiac catheterization, IV pyelography, computed tomography with IV contrast, computed tomographic angiography); medication exposure throughout the observation period; comorbidities; and demographics. The primary end point was the development of renal failure (RF) (defined as NFK stage 4 or 5). Analysis was performed with the use of a shared frailty model with clustering at the patient level.

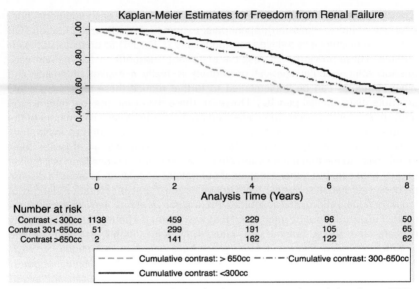

FIGURE 1.—Kaplan-Meier estimates for freedom from stage 4 or 5 chronic kidney disease (CKD). (Reprinted from the Journal of Vascular Surgery. Kougias P, Sharath S, Barshes NR, et al. Impact of cumulative intravascular contrast exposure on renal function in patients with occlusive and aneurysmal vascular disease. *J Vasc Surg*. 2014;59:1644-1650, Copyright 2014, with permission from The Society for Vascular Surgery.)

Results.—Patients (n = 1274) had a mean follow-up of 5.8 (range, 2.2-14) years. In the multivariate model with RF as the dependent variable and after adjusting for the statistically significant covariates of baseline renal function (hazard ratio [HR], 0.95; P < .001), diabetes (HR, 1.8; P = .007), use of an angiotensin-converting enzyme inhibitor (HR, 0.63; P = .03), use of antiplatelets (HR, 0.5; P = .01), cumulative number of open vascular operations performed (HR, 1.2; P = .001), and congestive heart failure (HR, 3.2; P < .001), CIVCE remained an independent predictor for RF development (HR, 1.1; P < .001). In the multivariate survival analysis model and after adjusting for the statistically significant covariates of perioperative myocardial infarction (HR, 3.9; P < .001), age at entry in the cohort (HR, 1.05; P = .035), total number of open operations (HR, 1.51; P < .001), and serum albumin (HR, 0.47; P < .001), CIVCE was an independent predictor of death (HR, 1.07; P < .001).

Conclusions.—Cumulative IV contrast exposure is an independent predictor of RF and death in patients with occlusive and aneurysmal vascular disease (Fig 1).

▶ The authors have attempted to examine retrospectively the cumulative impact of intravascular contrast exposure in our patient population with the primary outcome measure being the development of stage IV or V chronic kidney disease (stage IV—estimated glomerular filtration rate [eGFR] < 30, stage V—end-stage renal disease). They identified a cohort of patients (N = 1274) with minimal renal insufficiency (ie, stage I or II CKD—eGFR > 60) at their Veterans Health Administration center that had undergone some type of vascular surgical procedure (for either aneurysmal or occlusive disease) and tabulated the cumulative contrast exposure from all radiologic and interventional procedures (eg, cardiac catheterization, computed tomographic angiography for aneurysm surveillance) over a 14-year period starting in 1999 (mean follow-up 5.8 years, range 2.2—14 years). Somewhat surprisingly, 9% of the patient population progressed to stage IV or V chronic kidney disease on a permanent basis, whereas 33% progressed to the same end point on a temporary basis. Kaplan-Meier analysis demonstrated that the freedom from the progression to stage IV or V disease was contingent on the cumulative dose of contrast (Fig 1) with 60% of the patients exposed to > 650 mL of contrast developing this end point at 8 years. Multivariate analysis identified that the cumulative dose of contrast (hazard ratio [HR] 1.1), diabetes (HR 1.8), and congestive heart failure (HR 3.2) were all predictive of the major end point, whereas the use of angiotensin converting (HR 0.63) and antiplatelet (HR 0.51) agents were protective. Importantly, the cumulative dose of contrast (HR 1.07) also persisted in their multivariate survival model. These findings underscore the potential adverse effects of contrast administration and, collectively, challenge us all to be extremely judicious in its administration. Indeed, it is somewhat embarrassing to actually quantify the amount of contrast we subject patients to on a routine basis. Furthermore, it challenges us to seek alternative, nonintravascular contrast-based imaging approaches (eg, magnetic resonance angiography, ultrasound) and further push the contrasted-based technologies to obtain comparable (or even better) images with less contrast. Indeed, we have been able to perform fenestrated endovascular aneurysm repairs with our new imaging system using a fraction of the previous contrast requirement.

T. S. Huber, MD, PhD

Vascular and Nerve Injury After Knee Dislocation: A Systematic Review
Medina O, Arom GA, Yeranosian MG, et al (Univ of California-Los Angeles; Rutgers Univ-New Jersey Med School, Newark)
Clin Orthop Relat Res 472:2621-2629, 2014

Background.—Vascular injury is a devastating complication of acute knee dislocation. However, there are wide discrepancies in the reported frequency of vascular injury after knee dislocations, as well as important differences among approaches for diagnosis of this potentially limb-threatening problem.

Questions/Purposes.—We determined (1) the frequency of vascular and neurologic injury after knee dislocation and whether it varied by the type of knee dislocation, (2) the frequency with which surgical intervention was performed for vascular injury in this setting, and (3) the frequency with which each imaging modality was used to detect vascular injury.

Methods.—We searched the MEDLINE® literature database for studies in English that examined the clinical sequelae and diagnostic evaluation after knee dislocation. Vascular and nerve injury incidence after knee dislocation, surgical repair rate within vascular injury, and amputation rate after vascular injury were used to perform a meta-analysis. Other measures such as diagnostic modality used and the vessel injured after knee dislocation were also evaluated.

Results.—We identified 862 patients with knee dislocations, of whom 171 sustained vascular injury, yielding a weighted frequency of 18%. The frequency of nerve injuries after knee dislocation was 25% (75 of 272). We found that 80% (134 of 160) of vascular injuries underwent repair, and 12% (22 of 134) of vascular injuries resulted in amputation. The Schenck and Kennedy knee dislocation classifications with the highest vascular injury prevalence were observed in knees that involved the ACL, PCL, and medial collateral liagment (KDIIIL) (32%) and posterior dislocation (25%), respectively. Selective angiography was the most frequently used diagnostic modality (61%, 14 of 23), followed by nonselective angiography and duplex ultrasonography (22%, five of 23), ankle-brachial index (17%, four of 23), and MR angiography (9%, two of 23).

Conclusions.—This review enhances our understanding of the frequency of vascular injury and repair, amputation, and nerve injuries after knee dislocation. It also illustrates the lack of consensus among practitioners regarding the diagnostic and treatment algorithm for vascular injury. After pooling existing data on this topic, no outcomes-driven conclusions could be drawn regarding the ideal diagnostic modality or indications for surgical repair. In light of these findings and the morbidity associated with a missed diagnosis, clinicians should err on the side of caution in ruling out arterial injury.

▶ The authors have performed a meta-analysis to determine the incidence of vascular and neurologic injury at the time of knee dislocation along with the frequency of surgical intervention and the most commonly used diagnostic study. Notably, vascular injury was defined as occlusion, thrombosis, transection, intimal flap, or intimal tear, and knee dislocation was defined as any gross knee instability with multiligamentous injury. The authors reported that knee dislocations were associated with vascular injuries in 18% (95% confidence interval [CI], 12.8%–22.2%), neurologic injuries in 25% (95% CI, 13.9%–35.7%), surgical repair in 80% (95% CI, 72.8%–87.5%), and amputation in 12% (95% CI, 4.8%–19.3%). The reported incidence of vascular injury is within the range reported in the literature but exceeds the commonly quoted 10% rate associated with posterior knee dislocations, likely reflecting a publication bias. The majority of the vascular injuries were associated with posterior knee locations, although it is important to emphasize that they occurred with all types of dislocations (ie, posterior, anterior, lateral, medial, rotary) and were seen with ultra-low-velocity injuries in obese patients secondary to falls. The significant incidence of amputations underscores the importance of prompt diagnosis and definitive treatment. Indeed, knee dislocations are among the handful of traumatic orthopedic injuries that are associated with a significant incidence of vascular injuries (eg, supracondylar humeral fracture), and their presence should heighten the awareness among providers. Notably, the amputations in the current study resulted from a variety of causes including graft failure, infections, prolonged ischemia, and complete neurovascular disruption. The authors reported that there was no consensus regarding the optimal diagnostic study although catheter-based arteriography was the most commonly used modality (61%). It is interesting that they did not discuss the role of computed tomography (CT) arteriography because it has largely replaced catheter-based arteriography in this setting as advocated by the Eastern Association for the Surgery of Trauma practice guidelines for penetrating extremity trauma.[1] The bias in terms of the role for catheter-based arteriography in the study likely reflects the fact that the majority of the source studies included in the analysis were published before the evolution of CT arteriography. Unfortunately, the current meta-analysis does not provide any insight on the optimal surgical management of these injuries. I have taken a fairly aggressive approach in this setting and have favored open, surgical bypass of the popliteal artery but concede that expectant management (with close follow-up) is probably safe for small intimal injuries.

T. S. Huber, MD, PhD

Reference

1. Fox N, Rajani RR, Bokhari F, et al. Evaluation and management of penetrating lower extremity arterial trauma: an Eastern Association for the Surgery of Trauma practice management guideline. *J Trauma Acute Care Surg.* 2012;73:S315-S320.

Early Primary Care Provider Follow-up and Readmission After High-Risk Surgery

Brooke BS, Stone DH, Cronenwett JL, et al (Univ of Utah School of Medicine, Salt Lake City; Dartmouth-Hitchcock Med Ctr, Lebanon, NH; et al)
JAMA Surg 149:821-828, 2014

Importance.—Follow-up with a primary care provider (PCP) in addition to the surgical team is routinely recommended to patients discharged after major surgery despite no clear evidence that it improves outcomes.

Objective.—To test whether PCP follow-up is associated with lower 30-day readmission rates after open thoracic aortic aneurysm (TAA) repair and ventral hernia repair (VHR), surgical procedures known to have a high and low risk of readmission, respectively.

Design, Setting, and Participants.—In a cohort of Medicare beneficiaries discharged to home after open TAA repair (n = 12 679) and VHR (n = 52 807) between 2003 to 2010, we compared 30-day readmission rates between patients seen and not seen by a PCP within 30 days of discharge and across tertiles of regional primary care use. We stratified our analysis by the presence of complications during the surgical (index) admission.

Main Outcomes and Measures.—Thirty-day readmission rate.

Results.—Overall, 2619 patients (20.6%) undergoing open TAA repair and 4927 patients (9.3%) undergoing VHR were readmitted within

30 days after surgery. Complications occurred in 4649 patients (36.6%) undergoing open TAA repair and 4528 patients (8.6%) undergoing VHR during their surgical admission. Early follow-up with a PCP significantly reduced the risk of readmission among open TAA patients who experienced perioperative complications, from 35.0% (without follow-up) to 20.4% (with follow-up) (*P* < .001). However, PCP follow-up made no significant difference in patients whose hospital course was uncomplicated (19.4% with follow-up vs 21.9% without follow-up; *P* = .31). In comparison, early follow-up with a PCP after VHR did not reduce the risk of readmission, regardless of complications. In adjusted regional analyses, undergoing open TAA repair in regions with high compared with low primary care use was associated with an 18% lower likelihood of 30-day readmission (odds ratio, 0.82; 95% CI, 0.71-0.96; *P* = .02), whereas no significant difference was found among patients after VHR.

Conclusions and Relevance.—Follow-up with a PCP after high-risk surgery (eg, open TAA repair), especially among patients with complications, is associated with a lower risk of hospital readmission. Patients undergoing lower-risk surgery (eg, VHR) do not receive the same benefit from early PCP follow-up. Identifying high-risk surgical patients who will benefit from PCP integration during care transitions may offer a low-cost solution toward limiting readmissions.

▶ The authors have used the Medicare database (both inpatient and outpatient) to examine whether early follow-up (< 30 days) with a primary care provider (ie, primary care physician, nurse practitioner, physician's assistant) reduced early (< 30 days) hospital readmission rates after 2 major surgical procedures. They selected open thoracic aneurysm repair (not thoracoabdominal aortic aneurysm repair) and ventral hernia repair as representative procedures for complex and straightforward procedures, respectively, with the former associated with significant, known complication, and readmission rates. They reported that patients who visited their primary care provider after thoracic aneurysm repair were less likely to be readmitted within the early postoperative period (19.7% vs 28.0%, *P* < .001), although there was no similar benefit for patients after ventral hernia repair (9.4% vs 9.3%, *P* = .77). Among the patients that experienced a postoperative complication after thoracic aneurysm repair, the impact of a primary care visit on the readmission rates was even more impressive (20.4% vs 35%, *P* < .001). Again, no similar benefit was seen for patients experiencing a complication after ventral hernia repair. These findings persisted after correction for patient demographics and complications with the thoracic aneurysm repair patients that experienced a complication and followed up with their primary care provider having a 47% decrease (odds ratio .53; 95% confidence interval 0.37–0.75, *P* < .001) in early readmission rates. These findings confirm the benefit of having patients follow-up with their primary care provider after complex surgical procedures. More important, they identify a potential systemwide solution to reduce early postoperative readmissions. I suspect that we have all experienced pressure from our parent institutions regarding readmission, particularly given that these rates approach 25% after major vascular surgical procedures and the threats from the Affordable Care Act that will reduce reimbursement to hospitals for readmissions for specific patient populations or diagnoses. It seems relatively simple (and beneficial) to schedule an early visit with the patient's primary care provider at the time of hospital discharge. These results must be interpreted with some caution because of several limitations, as highlighted by the authors. Notably, the indication for the readmission was not known, the mechanism through which the primary care visit provided a benefit was unclear, and it is not certain that these findings are relevant to other complex surgical procedures.

T. S. Huber, MD, PhD

Aneurysm

Frailty increases the risk of 30-day mortality, morbidity, and failure to rescue after elective abdominal aortic aneurysm repair independent of age and comorbidities
Arya S, Kim SI, Duwayri Y, et al (Emory Univ School of Medicine, Atlanta, GA; Emory Univ Rollins School of Public Health, Atlanta, GA)
J Vasc Surg 61:324-331, 2015

Background.—Frailty, defined as a biologic syndrome of decreased reserve and resistance to stressors, has been linked to adverse outcomes after surgery. We evaluated the effect of frailty on 30-day mortality, morbidity, and failure to rescue (FTR) in patients undergoing elective abdominal aortic aneurysm (AAA) repair.

Methods.—Patients undergoing elective endovascular AAA repair (EVAR) or open AAA repair (OAR) were identified in the National Surgical Quality Improvement Program database for the years 2005 to 2012. Frailty was assessed using the modified frailty index (mFI) derived from the Canadian Study of Health and Aging (CSHA). The primary outcome was 30-day mortality, and secondary outcomes included 30-day morbidity and FTR. The effect of frailty on outcomes was assessed by multivariate regression analysis, adjusted for age, American Society of Anesthesiology (ASA) class, and significant comorbidities.

Results.—Of 23,207 patients, 339 (1.5% overall; 1.0% EVAR and 3.0% OAR) died ≤30 days of repair. One or more complications occurred in 2567 patients (11.2% overall; 7.8% EVAR and 22.1% OAR). Odds ratios (ORs) for mortality adjusted for age, ASA class, and other comorbidities in the group with the highest frailty score were 1.9 (95% confidence interval [CI], 1.2-3.0) after EVAR and 2.3 (95% CI, 1.4-3.7) after OAR. Similarly, compared with the least frail, the most frail patients were significantly more likely to experience severe (Clavien-Dindo class IV) complications after EVAR (OR, 1.7; 95% CI, 1.3-2.1) and OAR (OR, 1.8; 95%, CI, 1.5-2.1). There was also a higher FTR rate among frail patients, with 1.7-fold higher risk odds of mortality (95% CI, 1.2-2.5) in the highest tertile of frailty compared with the lowest when postoperative complications occurred.

Conclusions.—Higher mFI, independent of other risk factors, is associated with higher mortality and morbidity in patients undergoing elective EVAR and OAR. The mortality in frail patients is further driven by FTR from postoperative complications. Preoperative recognition of frailty may serve as a useful adjunct for risk assessment.

▶ The authors have examined the presence of "frailty" in patients undergoing elective abdominal aortic aneurysm repair, both endovascular and open, in the National Surgical Quality Improvement Program (NSQIP). Frailty is generically defined as "a biological syndrome of decreased reserve and resistance to stressors." Although a variety of frailty scoring systems or indices have been used in the literature, the authors used a modification of the Canadian Study of Health and Aging Frailty Index based on data collected in NISQIP. This included components for comorbidities, cognitive impairment, functional dependence, and living facility. Not surprisingly, the authors found that patient frailty was associated with higher rates of mortality, major morbidity, and failure to rescue for both open and endovascular repair. Furthermore, these findings remained significant in their multivariate models. The impact of patient frailty on outcome has recently been examined after several other major surgical procedures, and thus the current publication is timely. It strikes me that "frailty" index is a quantifiable surrogate for the "eyeball test" or a surgeon's collective judgment as to whether a patient is a suitable candidate for a specific procedure. The comprehensive frailty assessments underscore the limitations of using only patient comorbidities as a preoperative decision tool because a nursing home patient with dementia, coronary artery disease, chronic obstructive pulmonary disease, and chronic kidney disease is dramatically different from a comparably aged patient with the same comorbidities who is independent and physically active. The concept of frailty is particularly relevant for the operative decision making for elective aneurysms because the decision process represents a balance among rupture risk, operative mortality, life expectancy, and patient preference. It is noteworthy that the overall operative mortality rates for the open and endovascular repairs were 3.0% and 1.5%, respectively, among the 23 307 patients undergoing repair. These numbers are impressive and within the range of the randomized clinical trials comparing the 2 approaches. It is interesting that the odds ratios for mortality were higher for elective endovascular abdominal aortic aneurysm repair (EVAR) compared with open repair for the patient variables "admission from a chronic care facility" (4.4 vs 0.3) and "recent, unintended weight loss" (5.0 vs 1.3), suggesting that these patients were more likely offered EVAR and/or precluded from open repair. I am not certain that the scoring system the authors used is clinically practical, but the concepts are good and worth pursing aggressively to enable further refinement of our collective surgical judgment.

T. S. Huber, MD, PhD

Cardiovascular risk in patients with small and medium abdominal aortic aneurysms, and no history of cardiovascular disease
Sohrabi S, Wheatcroft S, Barth JH, et al (Leeds Vascular Inst, UK; Univ of Leeds, UK; Leeds General Infirmary, UK)
Br J Surg 101:1238-1243, 2014

Background.—Cardiovascular disease (CVD) is the main cause of death in people with abdominal aortic aneurysm (AAA). There is little evidence that screening for AAA reduces all-cause or cardiovascular mortality. The aim of the study was to assess whether subjects with a small or medium AAA ($3 \cdot 0 - 5 \cdot 4$ cm), without previous history of clinical CVD, had raised levels of CVD biomarkers or increased total mortality.

Methods.—This prospective study included subjects with a small or medium AAA and controls, all without a history of clinical CVD. CVD biomarkers (high-sensitivity C-reactive protein, hs-CRP; heart-type fatty acid-binding protein, H-FABP) were measured, and survival was recorded.

Results.—Of a total of 815 people, 476 with an AAA and 339 controls, a cohort of 86 with small or medium AAA ($3-5 \cdot 4$ cm) and 158 controls, all with no clinical history of CVD, were identified. The groups were matched for age and sex. The AAA group had higher median (i.q.r.) levels of hs-CRP ($2 \cdot 8$ ($1 \cdot 2 - 6 \cdot 0$) *versus* $1 \cdot 3$ ($0 \cdot 5 - 3 \cdot 5$) mg/l; $P < 0 \cdot 001$) and H-FABP ($4 \cdot 6$ ($3 \cdot 5 - 6 \cdot 0$) *versus* $4 \cdot 0$ ($3 \cdot 3 - 5 \cdot 1$) µg/l; $P = 0 \cdot 011$) than controls. Smoking was more common in the AAA group; however, hs-CRP and H-FABP levels were not related to smoking. Mean survival was lower in the AAA group: $6 \cdot 3$ (95 per cent confidence interval (c.i.) $5 \cdot 6$ to $6 \cdot 9$) years *versus* $8 \cdot 0$ ($7 \cdot 6$ to $8 \cdot 1$) years in controls ($P < 0 \cdot 001$). Adjusted mortality was higher in the AAA group (hazard ratio $3 \cdot 41$, 95 per cent c.i. $2 \cdot 11$ to $9 \cdot 19$; $P < 0 \cdot 001$).

Conclusion.—People with small or medium AAA and no clinical symptoms of CVD have higher levels of hs-CRP and H-FABP, and higher mortality compared with controls. They should continue to receive secondary prevention against CVD (Fig 1).

▶ The authors prospectively analyzed the presence of 2 biomarkers and mortality in patients with small abdominal aortic aneurysms (3.0—5.4 cm) and no history of cardiovascular disease. The biomarkers included high-sensitivity C-reactive protein (hs-CRP) and heart-type fatty acid-binding protein (H-FABP), both known markers for cardiovascular and coronary artery disease. The criteria for cardiovascular disease (or the absence thereof) were fairly inclusive and included the typical presentations of coronary, peripheral, and cerebrovascular disease. Notably, individuals with aneurysms that exceed 5.5 cm at any time during the surveillance period were excluded from the study. The authors reported that the patients with small aneurysms had significantly higher levels of the 2 biomarkers and that the increased levels were not associated with smoking or medications (ie, aspirin, statin, angiotensin-converting enzyme inhibitors). Importantly, the patients with small aneurysms had an increased mortality (Fig 1) with a hazard ratio of 3.42 (95% CI 2.11—9.19; P < .01) after adjustment

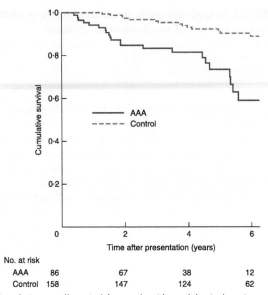

FIGURE 1.—Cumulative overall survival for people with an abdominal aortic aneurysm (AAA) and subjects without cardiovascular disease. $P < 0.001$ (log rank test) (Reprinted from Sohrabi S, Wheatcroft S, Barth JH, et al. Cardiovascular risk in patients with small and medium abdominal aortic aneurysms, and no history of cardiovascular disease. *Br J Surg*. 2014;101:1238-1243, © British Journal of Surgery Society Ltd. Reproduced with permission. Permission is granted by John Wiley & Sons Ltd on behalf of the BJSS Ltd.)

for smoking history, high-density lipoprotein levels, and medication use. The long-term survival was comparable to that reported for patients after abdominal aortic aneurysm repair and particularly noteworthy given that the patients did not have any history of cardiovascular disease. These findings emphasize that the presence of an abdominal aortic aneurysm, regardless of the size, is a marker for increased mortality. Furthermore, they underscore the importance of risk-factor modification and optimal medical therapy in this patient cohort, although it is noteworthy that the findings persisted after correction for several of these factors. These findings support my own bias that an abdominal aortic aneurysm is a disease, similar to either hypertension or diabetes, and that this disease process affects not only the abdominal aorta but the systemic circulation. These findings must be interpreted with some caution because we do not know the causes of death and because the "healthy controls" identified from the outpatient clinics may have been too healthy, and thus not be appropriate controls. However, it suggests that aneurysm screening programs may be helpful to identify patients at increased risk for cardiovascular death rather than just aneurysm rupture.

T. S. Huber, MD, PhD

Critical analysis of results after chimney endovascular aortic aneurysm repair raises cause for concern

Scali ST, Feezor RJ, Chang CK, et al (Univ of Florida, Gainesville)
J Vasc Surg 60:865-875, 2014

Objective.—"Chimney" techniques used to extend landing zones for endovascular aortic repair (chEVAR) have been increasingly reported; however, concerns about durability and patency remain. The purpose of this analysis was to examine midterm outcomes of chEVAR.

Methods.—All patients at the University of Florida treated with chE-VAR were reviewed. Major adverse events (MAEs) were recorded and defined as any chimney stent thrombosis, type Ia endoleak in follow-up, reintervention, 30-day/in-hospital death, or ≥25% decrease in estimated glomerular filtration rate after discharge. Primary end points included chimney stent patency and freedom from MAE. Secondary end points included complications and long-term survival.

Results.—From 2008 to 2012, 41 patients (age ± standard deviation, 73 ± 8 years; male, 66% [n = 27]) were treated with a total of 76 chimney stents (renal, n = 51; superior mesenteric artery, n = 16; celiac artery, n = 9) for a variety of indications: juxtarenal, 42% (n = 17, one rupture), suprarenal, 17% (n = 7), and thoracoabdominal aneurysm, 17% (n = 7); aortic anastomotic pseudoaneurysm, 15% (n = 6; three ruptures); type Ia endoleak after EVAR, 7% (n = 3); and atheromatous disease, 2% (n = 1). Two patients had a single target vessel abandoned because of cannulation failure, and one had a type Ia endoleak at case completion (technical success, 93%). Intraoperative complications occurred in seven patients (17%), including graft maldeployment with unplanned mesenteric chimney (n = 2) and access vessel injury requiring repair (n = 5). Major postoperative complications developed in 20% (n = 8). The 30-day mortality and inhospital mortality were 5% (n = 2) and 7% (n = 3), respectively. At median follow-up of 18.2 months (range, 1.4-41.5 months), 28 of 33 patients (85%) with available postoperative imaging experienced stabilization or reduction of abdominal aortic aneurysm sac diameters. Nine patients (32%) developed endoleak at some point during follow-up (type Ia, 7% [n = 3]; type II, 10% [n = 4]; indeterminate, 7% [n = 3]), and one patient underwent open, surgical conversion. The estimated probability of freedom from reintervention (± standard error mean) was 96% ± 4% at both 1 year and 3 years. Primary patency of all chimney stents was 88% ± 5% and 85% ± 5% at 1 year and 3 years, respectively. Corresponding freedom from MAEs was 83% ± 7% and 57% ± 10% at 1 year and 3 years. The actuarial estimated survival for all patients at 1 year and 5 years was 85% ± 6% and 65% ± 8%, respectively.

Conclusions.—These results demonstrate that chEVAR can be completed with a high degree of success; however, perioperative complications and MAEs during follow-up, including loss of chimney patency and endoleak, may occur at a higher rate than previously reported. Elective use of chEVAR should be performed with caution, and comparison to open and fenestrated EVAR is needed to determine long-term efficacy of this technique.

▶ The authors have retrospectively analyzed the outcomes at their institution with the "chimney" technique (N = 41 patients, N = 76 stents) at the time of endovascular aneurysm repair (chEVAR). The "chimney" technique was defined as the "intentional deployment of a stent/stent graft into visceral aortic branches immediately parallel to the aortic endoprosthesis that covered the target vessel ostia." The authors reported that the 30-day mortality rate was 5% and that 20% of the patients experienced a major postoperative complication. The aortic sac diameters were stable or decreased in 85% of the patients, and only 7% developed a type 1a endoleak. The primary patency rates for the chimney stents was 88% ± 5% and 85% ± 5% at 1 and 3 years, respectively, and freedom from major adverse events was 83% ± 7% and 57% ± 10% at the same time intervals. Based on these results, the authors concluded that the chEVAR technique should not be used in the elective setting and reserved for higher risk patients that are not candidates for other forms of treatment, including fenestrated or branch endografts. I applaud the authors' rigorous, thoughtful analysis of their results but would contend that they could be used to support the alternative view, specifically that the chEVAR technique is effective and may play an important role. Indeed, the stent patency rates were excellent, the incidence of type 1a endoleaks was small, and the overwhelming majority of the aneurysms decreased in size or remained stable. I would concede that the major adverse event rates are significant but would contend that these outcomes may not be different from those associated with the alternative treatment modalities (ie, fenestrated/branch endografts). Clearly, it is difficult to support one therapy over another without the proper control groups. It is not evident what role (if any) the chEVAR technique will play once the fenestrated and branched devices are more widely available. Indeed, the chimney technique never made much sense, but I suspect that it will continue to play a minor role in select situations as defined by the anatomy.

T. S. Huber, MD, PhD

Postapproval outcomes of juxtarenal aortic aneurysms treated with the Zenith fenestrated endovascular graft
Vemuri C, Oderich GS, Lee JT, et al (Washington Univ in St. Louis, MO; Mayo Clinic, Rochester, MN; Stanford Univ, Palo Alto, CA; et al)
J Vasc Surg 60:295-300, 2014

Objective.—The objective of this study was to evaluate postapproval outcomes of patients with juxtarenal aortic aneurysms treated with the Zenith fenestrated endovascular graft (Cook Inc, Bloomington, Ind).

Methods.—We reviewed clinical data of consecutive patients treated with the Zenith fenestrated endovascular graft in the United States at seven institutions with early commercial access from July 2012 to December 2012. Clinical outcomes and compliance to anatomic guidelines were compared with results of the U.S. fenestrated trial (USFT).

Results.—Fifty-seven patients were treated. There were significantly more ($P < .05$) patients with coronary artery disease, myocardial infarction, and preoperative renal insufficiency than in the USFT. Thirty-six patients (63.2%) did not meet the USFT anatomic criteria of a >4-mm infrarenal neck, and there were significantly more mesenteric stents (13 vs 0; $P < .05$) used in this group than in the USFT, reflecting the higher anatomic complexity of these patients. The total operative time was 250.2 ± 14.8 minutes, the fluoroscopy time was 68.9 ± 4.47 minutes, and the average volume of contrast material was 108.6 ± 5.6 mL. Technical success was 100% in regard to aneurysm exclusion, although the left renal fenestration was not able to be aligned in two patients, and one patient had a kinked renal stent that was successfully restented. During this time period, there were a total of 10 endoleaks, of which two were type III and eight were type II.

Conclusions.—Despite higher rates of comorbidities and more challenging anatomy, early 30-day outcomes of juxtarenal aortic aneurysms treated postapproval with the Zenith fenestrated endovascular graft compare well with USFT data. Future studies are needed to assess durability of this treatment modality as the technology diffuses and data mature.

▶ The authors have reported their early outcomes for the Zenith fenestrated endovascular graft (zFEN, Cook Inc, Bloomington, IN), the first commercially available device designed for the treatment of juxtarenal abdominal aortic aneurysms. These data represent the postapproval outcomes (N = 57) from 7 centers of excellence. The inclusion criteria for the device, as outlined in the instructions for use, include access vessels sufficient for a 14- to 22-Fr sheath, an aortic neck angle of < 45, and an infrarenal neck length of < 4 mm. The devices were all custom-made for the individual patient, required up to 6 weeks for construction, and involved some combination of 3 fenestrations or scallops. Successful aneurysm exclusion was achieved in all cases, but the operative time (250.2 ± 14.8 min), fluoroscopy time (68.9 ± 4.47 min), and contrast volume (108.6 ± 5.6 mL) were all significant, underscoring the complexity of the procedure. The perioperative complication rate was low, although there was 1 perioperative death, and 3 left renal arteries were inadvertently covered. Although the postoperative follow-up was brief (mean follow-up 52.7 ± 6.2 days), there were only 2 type I or III endoleaks, and the target vessel patency rates were 97.5%. Overall, these results are encouraging and compare favorably with the manufacturer's U.S. Fenestrated Trial. The device affords an alternative, potentially safer option for patients with juxtarenal abdominal aortic aneurysms. It will be interesting to see whether the device (or variations thereof) replaces open surgery, similar to the scenario for infrarenal repairs. It is important to emphasize that the results are very early and that the utility of the device will be determined by its durability and longer-term results. It strikes me that the technology is an order of magnitude more complicated than the endovascular approach for infrarenal aneurysm repair and associated with new failure modes. The impressive results from the current study must also be interpreted with some caution given the expertise of the various centers and providers. The results are likely not applicable across the country given the requisite skill set and learning curve, begging the question of whether these technologies should be restricted to a limited number of centers.

T. S. Huber, MD, PhD

A propensity-matched comparison of outcomes for fenestrated endovascular aneurysm repair and open surgical repair of complex abdominal aortic aneurysms

Raux M, Patel VI, Cochennec F, et al (Univ of Paris XII, France; Massachusetts General Hosp, Boston)
J Vasc Surg 60:858-864, 2014

Objective.—The benefit of fenestrated endovascular aortic aneurysm repair (FEVAR) compared with open surgical repair (OSR) of complex abdominal aortic aneurysms (CAAAs) is unknown. This study compares 30-day outcomes of these procedures from two high-volume centers where FEVAR was undertaken for high-risk patients.

Methods.—Patients undergoing FEVAR with commercially available devices and OSR of CAAAs (total suprarenal/supravisceral clamp position) were propensity matched by demographic, clinical, and anatomic criteria to identify similar patient cohorts. Perioperative outcomes were evaluated using univariate and multivariate methods.

Results.—From July 2001 to August 2012, 59 FEVAR and 324 OSR patients were identified. After 1:4 propensity matching for age, gender, hypertension, congestive heart failure, coronary disease, chronic obstructive pulmonary disease, stroke, diabetes, preoperative creatinine, and anticipated/actual aortic clamp site, the study cohort consisted of 42 FEVARs and 147 OSRs. The most frequent FEVAR construct was two renal fenestrations, with or without a single mesenteric scallop, in 50% of cases. An average of 2.9 vessels were treated per patient. Univariate analysis demonstrated FEVAR had higher rates of 30-day mortality (9.5% vs 2%; $P = .05$), any complication (41% vs 23%; $P = .01$), procedural complications (24% vs 7%; $P < .01$), and graft complications (30% vs 2%; $P < .01$). Multivariable analysis showed FEVAR was associated with an increased risk of 30-day mortality (odds ratio [OR], 5.1; 95% confidence interval [CI], 1.1-24; $P = .04$), any complication (OR, 2.3; 95% CI, 1.1-4.9; $P = .01$), and graft complications (OR, 24; 95% CI, 4.8-66; $P < .01$).

Conclusions.—FEVAR, in this two-center study, was associated with a significantly higher risk of perioperative mortality and morbidity compared with OSR for management of CAAAs. These data suggest that extension of the paradigm shift comparing EVAR with OSR for routine AAAs to patients with CAAAs is not appropriate. Further study to establish proper patient selection for FEVAR instead of OSR is warranted before widespread use should be considered.

▶ The authors report their impressive series comparing the early results (30-day outcomes) for open surgical (OSAR, $N = 147$) and fenestrated endovascular (FEVAR, $N = 42$) aneurysm repair of complex abdominal aortic aneurysms. Notably, all of the procedures required suprarenal or supravisceral aortic occlusion (or anticipated occlusion in the case of the FEVAR), but type IV thoracoabdominal aortic aneurysms were specifically excluded. Furthermore, all of the FEVAR devices were commercially approved in Europe. The OSAR and FEVAR procedures were performed at separate institutions by separate surgeons, but both centers are recognized as centers of excellence. The FEVAR and OSAR were compared using propensity matching to control for their medical conditions and anticipated clamp location, although the FEVAR patients had been considered "high risk" and not suitable for OSAR based on defined criteria. Somewhat surprisingly, the authors reported that the 30-day mortality rate was greater for FEVAR (2% vs 9.5%, $P = .04$), and multivariate modeling determined that FEVAR was an independent predictor of 30-day mortality (odds ratio [OR] 5.1; 95% confidence interval [CI], $1.1-24$, $P = .04$), any complication (OR, 2.3; 95% CI, $1.1-4.9$; $P = .03$), any procedural complication (OR 4.3; 95% CI, $1.5-12$; $P = .006$), and graft complications (OR 24; 95% CI, $6.5-89$; $P < .0001$). Interestingly, there were 3 deaths in the FEVAR group due to mesenteric ischemia in patients with patent visceral vessels, presumably due to atheroembolic events. The overall findings contradict the general impression about the benefit of FEVAR and multiple other reports in the literature, including pooled results from systematic reviews. Indeed, the morbidity and mortality rates for FEVAR seem too high and those for OSAR seem too low, particularly given the findings from the Vascular Quality Initiative that the complication rate for open surgical repair of infrarenal aortic aneurysms (not necessarily meeting the inclusion criteria of the current study) exceeds 50%. The authors defend their findings in the Discussion, emphasizing that their report represents the first contemporary comparison using rigorous techniques and that there was likely a "learning curve" associated with the FEVARs. These findings should likely be used to temper the enthusiasm for FEVAR, although I suspect that the devices and operator experience will improve over the next few years and eliminate some of the observed discrepancy in the outcomes. However, it is worth repeating the comments in the discussion following the presentation of the article by one of the senior authors that "surgery can give excellent results in experienced hands" and that "FEVAR is not an easy procedure."

T. S. Huber, MD, PhD

Durability of open popliteal artery aneurysm repair

Dorweiler B, Gemechu A, Doemland M, et al (Johannes-Gutenberg Univ, Mainz, Germany)

J Vasc Surg 60:951-957, 2014

Objective.—The objective of this study was to analyze our long-term results after open surgery for popliteal artery aneurysm.

Methods.—Records of patients who received surgery between 1998 and 2010 were retrieved from a computerized database and analyzed retrospectively. End points of the study were perioperative mortality and morbidity and patency and limb salvage rate.

Results.—Two hundred and six popliteal aneurysms (median diameter, 30 mm; interquartile range, 18 mm) were treated (161 elective, 45 emergent) in 154 patients (mean age, 67 ± 11 years) using vein grafts (82%) via the medial approach (92%). Above-knee popliteal artery (45%) and below-knee popliteal artery (65%) were the predominant inflow and outflow vessels. The overall surgical mortality was 2% (2% for elective and 3% for emergent procedures; $P =$ not significant). Primary, assisted primary, and secondary patency rates were 88.1% (73.5%), 92.1% (84.3%), and 96.5% (89.8%) at 5 (at 10) years, respectively, with no significant difference between elective and emergent surgeries. Limb salvage rate was significantly reduced in the emergent group vs the elective group with 91.1% vs 98.6% at 5 and 10 years ($P =.0049$). The rate of freedom from any reintervention was 84.3% at 5 and 69.8% at 10 years, respectively.

Conclusions.—Open surgery for popliteal artery aneurysm is marked by low perioperative mortality and morbidity and provides excellent long-term results.

▶ The authors report their series (N = 206) of open, popliteal artery aneurysm repairs for both elective and emergent indications, allegedly the second largest single-center experience in the literature. Their overall results are excellent in terms of perioperative morbidity (graft occlusion, 4%; hematoma, 8%; major amputation, 2%), perioperative mortality (2%), graft patency (5 year: primary, 88%; secondary, 96%; 10 year: primary, 74%, secondary, 90%), limb salvage (5 and 10 years, 97%), and patient survival (5 year, 64%; 10 year, 41%). Despite the retrospective study design, the results represent a benchmark for the alternative endovascular approach. Indeed, it is reassuring that the results for the open repair are so good. I share the authors' bias that the open repair is the optimal approach for most patients given the limited data supporting the endovascular approach, particularly the long-term outcomes. However, I readily concede that there is a role for the endovascular approach, particularly for older/sicker patients and those with good infrageniculate runoff. I believe that there is clinical equipoise in terms of conducting a randomized controlled trial, although I suspect that it would be difficult to complete given the infrequent nature of the problem. Unfortunately, the current study does not provide any insight on the operative indications for popliteal aneurysm repair. I have used the traditional

2-cm diameter criteria but readily concede that this may be too aggressive. Emergent repairs are clearly associated with inferior outcomes as highlighted in the current publication. However, it is impossible to predict which aneurysms will thrombose or become a source for distal emboli. It is worth noting that no secondary procedures were required because of complications related to a perfused, residual aneurysm, despite the fact that the aneurysms were excluded by ligation. Other authors have reported that endoaneurysmorrhaphy is superior to simple ligation because of this potential adverse outcome, although the added complexity does not seem justified.

T. S. Huber, MD, PhD

Anatomic characteristics and natural history of renal artery aneurysms during longitudinal imaging surveillance
Wayne EJ, Edwards MS, Stafford JM, et al (Wake Forest Univ School of Medicine, Winston-Salem, NC)
J Vasc Surg 60:448-453, 2014

Objective.—Renal artery aneurysms (RAAs) are uncommon, and rates of growth and rupture are unknown. Limited evidence therefore exists to guide clinical management of RAAs, particularly small aneurysms that are asymptomatic. To further characterize the natural history of RAAs, we studied anatomic characteristics and changes in diameter during imaging surveillance.

Methods.—Patients evaluated for native RAAs at a single institution during a 5-year period (July 2008 to July 2013) were identified and analyzed retrospectively. Patients with two or more cross-sectional imaging studies (computed tomography or magnetic resonance imaging) more than 1 month apart were included. Demographic and clinical data were collected from medical records, and anatomic data (including aneurysm diameter, calcification, and location) were obtained from electronic images. Changes in RAA diameters over time were evaluated by plots and Wilcoxon signed rank tests.

Results.—Sixty-eight RAAs in 55 patients were analyzed. Median follow-up was 19.4 months (interquartile range, 11.2-49.0 months). Mean age at presentation was 61.8 6 9.8 years, and 73% of patients were women. Hypertension was prevalent among 73% of patients. Multiple RAAs were present in 18% of patients, and 24% also had arterial aneurysms of other splanchnic or iliac vessels. The majority of RAAs were calcified and located at the main renal artery bifurcation. Mean initial aneurysm diameter was 16.0 ± 6.4 mm. Median annualized growth rate was 0.06 mm (interquartile range, −0.07 to 0.33 mm; $P = .11$). No RAA ruptures or acute symptoms occurred during surveillance, and 10.3% of RAAs were repaired electively.

Conclusions.—Risk of short-term RAA growth or rupture was low. These findings suggest that annual (or less frequent) imaging surveillance is safe in the majority of patients and do not support pre-emptive repair of asymptomatic, small-diameter RAAs.

▶ The authors have documented their recent experience with surveillance for small renal artery aneurysms (N = 68) in an attempt to define their natural history. Notably, surveillance was performed using either computer tomography- or magnetic resonance-based imaging, a significant improvement over historical studies that were based on catheter-based arteriography with its intrinsic limitation that only the lumen of the vessel (or aneurysm) is imaged. The authors report that none of the small aneurysms (mean initial diameter 16.0 ± 6.4 mm) ruptured and that the median annualized growth rate was 0.06 mm (interquartile range, −0.07 to 0.33 mm). Notably, 5 of the 8 aneurysms that were > 25 mm were repaired. These findings confirm the collective impression that small renal artery aneurysms are relatively benign and serve to question the traditional diameter-based criteria (1.5–2.0 cm) that are frequently used to justify repair. Indeed, my criteria include aneurysms > 2 cm, any symptoms, and women of child-bearing age, although I would readily concede that this is likely far too aggressive, and must confess that I have seen only 1 ruptured renal artery aneurysm in my 20-year career at an academic medical center. Similar to abdominal aortic aneurysms, the decision for operative repair represents a balance among rupture risk, operative risk, life expectancy, and patient preference. Unfortunately, the rupture risk component of this decision-making equation has been woefully lacking, and we have largely defined the 2-cm diameter threshold because it "seems" like an appropriate size. The benign "natural history" defined by the current study is certainly reassuring but must be interpreted with some caution given the retrospective nature, the limited follow-up, and the selection bias that the majority of the patients with aneurysms > 2.5 cm underwent repair. The operative risks have been documented, but it is important to emphasize that they are associated with a small but finite risk of losing the kidney. The study highlights that most of the renal artery aneurysms are saccular, calcified, and located at the main renal artery bifurcation. Most of these can be repaired by excising the aneurysmal segment and patching the remaining artery, although it seems like each procedure is different, with the reconstruction dictated by the location and extent of the aneurysm and calcification. Furthermore, the study underscores the fact that many of the renal aneurysms are multifocal and associated with aneurysms in other vessels, justifying additional imaging to exclude synchronous aneurysms.

T. S. Huber, MD, PhD

Early sac shrinkage predicts a low risk of late complications after endovascular aortic aneurysm repair
Bastos Gonçalves F, Baderkhan H, Verhagen HJM, et al (Erasmus Univ Med Centre, Rotterdam, The Netherlands; Uppsala Univ, Sweden)
Br J Surg 101:802-810, 2014

Background.—Aneurysm shrinkage has been proposed as a marker of successful endovascular aneurysm repair (EVAR). Patients with early postoperative shrinkage may experience fewer subsequent complications, and consequently require less intensive surveillance.

Methods.—Patients undergoing EVAR from 2000 to 2011 at three vascular centres (in 2 countries), who had two imaging examinations (postoperative and after 6—18 months), were included. Maximum diameter, complications and secondary interventions during follow-up were registered. Patients were categorized according to early sac dynamics. The primary endpoint was freedom from late complications. Secondary endpoints were freedom from secondary intervention, postimplant rupture and direct (type I/III) endoleaks.

Results.—Some 597 EVARs (71·1 per cent of all EVARs) were included. No shrinkage was observed in 284 patients (47·6 per cent), moderate shrinkage (5—9 mm) in 142 (23·8 per cent) and major shrinkage (at least 10 mm) in 171 patients (28·6 per cent). Four years after the index imaging, the rate of freedom from complications was 84·3 (95 per cent confidence interval 78·7 to 89·8), 88·1 (80·6 to 95·5) and 94·4 (90·1 to 98·7) per cent respectively. No shrinkage was an independent risk factor for late complications compared with major shrinkage (hazard ratio (HR) 3·11; $P < 0·001$). Moderate compared with major shrinkage (HR 2·10; $P = 0·022$), early postoperative complications (HR 3·34; $P < 0·001$) and increasing abdominal aortic aneurysm baseline diameter (HR 1·02; $P = 0·001$) were also risk factors for late complications. Freedom from secondary interventions and direct endoleaks was greater for patients with major sac shrinkage.

Conclusion.—Early change in aneurysm sac diameter is a strong predictor of late complications after EVAR. Patients with major sac shrinkage have a very low risk of complications for up to 5 years. This parameter may be used to tailor postoperative surveillance.

▶ The authors have retrospectively examined the impact of early aneurysm sac shrinkage after endovascular aneurysm repair (EVAR) to determine whether it is associated with longer-term complications (primary end point), secondary interventions, and/or endoleaks. Early aneurysm sac shrinkage was defined as the interval change between the immediate postoperative CT scan (< 30 days) and the consecutive scan performed between 6 and 18 months with the shrinkage quantified as major (> 10 mm), moderate (5—9 mm), or none (< 5 mm). The authors reported that there was no early sac shrinkage in roughly half of the patients (47.6%) with roughly a quarter of the patients demonstrating moderate (23.8%) and major (28.6%) shrinkage. The overall freedom from complications at 4 years was quite good (84.3%) in the whole cohort with no shrinkage (hazard ratio [HR] 3.1), moderate shrinkage (HR 2.1), aneurysm growth (HR 1.0 per mm increase), and complications before baseline CT (HR 3.3) associated with increased complications by multivariable analysis. The secondary outcomes in terms of remedial interventions, late endoleaks, and persistent or lake type II endoleaks were largely consistent with the primary end point in that major shrinkage was associated with better outcomes, whereas no shrinkage was associated with worse ones. Taken together, these findings suggest that early major sac shrinkage is a favorable outcome and a marker for success. The observation that significant sac shrinkage is associated with a better adverse outcome has been reported by other authors, although the significant finding in the current study is the observation that early sac shrinkage appears to be beneficial and/or protective. These observations can potentially be used to refine the postoperative imaging surveillance protocols after EVAR for patients with major sac shrinkage, potentially avoiding the inherent cost, radiation exposure, and contrast-associated complications. Notably, complications developed in only 4.7% of the patients with major sac shrinkage, but the nature of the complications (limb thrombosis—3 of 8; type 1 endoleak—2 of 8; type III endoleak, rupture, infected aneurysm—1 of 8 each) were such that the majority would likely not have been prevented by an aggressive postoperative surveillance protocol. The findings also underscore the fact that some type of surveillance is mandatory given the 15% incidence of remedial procedures, which is potentially increased among patients with the predictors of complications identified here (ie, no sac shrinkage, moderate sac shrinkage, early complications, aneurysm growth). These results should be interpreted with some caution given the retrospective study design, although the data were collected prospectively from 3 separate centers over a prolonged time interval (2000–2011) and involved multiple different endovascular devices. Furthermore, the classification was based on the absolute sac reduction measurement, although the sensitivity analysis demonstrated that the findings were consistent if sac reduction was analyzed using a proportion.

T. S. Huber, MD, PhD

Gaps in preoperative surveillance and rupture of abdominal aortic aneurysms among Medicare beneficiaries
Mell MW, Baker LC, Dalman RL, et al (Stanford Univ School of Medicine, CA)
J Vasc Surg 59:583-588, 2014

Objective.—Screening and surveillance are recommended in the management of small abdominal aortic aneurysms (AAAs). Gaps in surveillance after early diagnosis may lead to unrecognized AAA growth, rupture, and death. This study investigates the frequency and predictors of rupture of previously diagnosed AAAs.

Methods.—Data were extracted from Medicare claims for patients who underwent AAA repair between 2006 and 2009. Relevant preoperative abdominal imaging exams were tabulated up to 5 years prior to AAA repair. Repair for ruptured AAAs was compared with repair for intact AAAs for those with an early diagnosis of an AAA, defined as having received imaging at least 6 months prior to surgery. Gaps in surveillance were defined as no image within 1 year of surgery or no imaging for more than a 2-year time span after the initial image. Logistic regression was used to examine independent predictors of rupture despite early diagnosis.

Results.—A total of 9298 patients had repair after early diagnosis, with rupture occurring in 441 (4.7%). Those with ruptured AAAs were older

(80.2 ± 6.9 vs 77.6 ± 6.2 years; *P* < .001), received fewer images prior to repair (5.7 ± 4.1 vs 6.5 ± 3.5; *P* = .001), were less likely to be treated in a high-volume hospital (45.4% vs 59.5%; *P* < .001), and were more likely to have had gaps in surveillance (47.4% vs 11.8%; *P* < .001) compared with those receiving repair for intact AAAs. After adjusting for medical comorbidities, gaps in surveillance remained the largest predictor of rupture in a multivariate analysis (odds ratio, 5.82; 95% confidence interval, 4.64-7.31; *P* < .001).

Conclusions.—Despite previous diagnosis of AAA, many patients experience rupture prior to repair. Improved mechanisms for surveillance are needed to prevent rupture and ensure timely repair for patients with AAAs.

▶ The authors have attempted to examine the impact of aneurysm surveillance on rupture rates or, more specifically, on the incidence of the operative repair for ruptured aneurysms. In their study design, they identified Medicare patients that had undergone aneurysm repair (for either intact or ruptured aneurysms) and had some type of screening study (ie, abdominal ultrasound, computed tomographic angiography, magnetic resonance angiography) within the preceding 5 years, excluding those who had their initial (ie, only) imaging studies within the 6 months preceding repair. They defined a "gap in surveillance" as no imaging within the year before operative repair or no imaging for a 2-year time span. They identified 9298 patients between 2006 and 2009 who met their criteria with the overwhelming majority (95% vs 5%) undergoing repair for intact aneurysms. The patients who had undergone operative repair for ruptured aneurysms were more likely to be older, female, Medicaid-eligible, and treated at lower-volume hospitals. Gaps in surveillance were identified in 13.5% of the patients and were more likely to occur in older patients and those found to be Medicaid-eligible although they were less likely to be treated at high volume hospitals. Not surprisingly, gaps in surveillance were associated with an increased operative mortality (11.7% vs 3.4%, *P* < .001) and a higher rupture rate (45.6% vs 11.8%, *P* < .001). Multivariate analysis demonstrated that surveillance gaps were the strongest predictor of aneurysm rupture (odds ratio 5.82, confidence interval 4.64–7.31, *P* < .001) and was identified along with patient age and hospital volume as predictors. These findings serve to underscore the importance of aneurysm surveillance before the definitive decision to offer operative repair at the traditional 5.0- to 5.5-cm thresholds. Indeed, these operative thresholds have been well defined by the randomized trials and an elegant meta-analysis included in last year's YEAR BOOK selections defined the most appropriate surveillance intervals for both genders.[1] The findings serve to emphasize that the management of patients with abdominal aortic aneurysms is really a continuum that spans from screening to identify the lesion, appropriate surveillance until a operative threshold is achieved, definitive operative treatment, and then continued postoperative surveillance to identify problems associated with the operative repair (eg, type 1 endoleaks) or additional aneurysmal degeneration. Each of these steps is important and a potential source of problems if not managed appropriately. Appropriate surveillance requires involved patients to ensure that they follow-up with their scheduled appointments and imaging as well as informed providers, both primary care physicians and vascular surgeons, to ensure that the appropriate surveillance studies are performed in a timely fashion. The current data also seem to again provide further support for concentrating aneurysm care in higher-volume centers of excellence given the consistent theme that these centers were associated with better outcomes.

T. S. Huber, MD, PhD

Reference

1. Bown MJ, Sweeting MJ, Brown LC, Powell JT, Thompson SG. Surveillance intervals for small abdominal aortic aneurysms: a meta-analysis. *JAMA*. 2013;309: 806-813.

Epidemiology of aortic aneurysm repair in the United States from 2000 to 2010

Dua A, Kuy S, Lee CJ, et al (Univ of Texas-Houston; Med College of Wisconsin, Milwaukee; et al)
J Vasc Surg 59:1512-1517, 2014

Objective.—Broad application of endovascular aneurysm repair (EVAR) has led to a rapid decline in open aneurysm repair (OAR) and improved patient survival, albeit at a higher overall cost of care. The aim of this report is to evaluate national trends in the incidence of unruptured and ruptured abdominal aortic aneurysms (AAAs), their management by EVAR and OAR, and to compare overall patient characteristics and clinical outcomes between these two approaches.

Methods.—A retrospective analysis of the cross-sectional National Inpatient Sample (2000-2010) was used to evaluate patient characteristics and outcomes related to EVAR and OAR for unruptured and ruptured AAAs. Data were extrapolated to represent population-level statistics through the use of data from the U.S. Census Bureau. Comparisons between groups were made with the use of descriptive statistics.

Results.—There were 101,978 patients in the National Inpatient Sample affected by AAAs over the 11-year span of this study; the average age was 73 years, 21% were women, and 90% were white. Overall in-hospital mortality rate was 7%, with a median length of stay (LOS) of 5 days and median hospital charges of $58,305. In-hospital mortality rate was 13 times greater for ruptured patients, with a median LOS of 9 days and median charges of $84,744. For both unruptured and ruptured patients, EVAR was associated with a lower in-hospital mortality rate (4% vs 1% for unruptured and 41% vs 27% for ruptured; *P* < .001 for each), shorter median LOS (7 vs 2; 9 vs 6; *P* < .001) but a 27%-36% increase in hospital charges.

Conclusions.—The overall use of EVAR has risen sharply in the past 10 years (5.2% to 74% of the total number of AAA repairs) even though the total number of AAAs remains stable at 45,000 cases per year. In-hospital mortality rates for both ruptured and unruptured cases have fallen by more than 50% during this time period. Lower mortality rates and shorter LOS despite a 27%-36% higher cost of care continues to justify the use of EVAR over OAR. For patients with suitable anatomy, EVAR should be the preferred management of both ruptured and unruptured AAAs.

▶ The authors have done a nice job describing the operative treatment for abdominal aortic aneurysms (both intact and ruptured) in the endovascular era using the National Inpatient Sample (2000—2010) and population data from the US Census Bureau. The number of abdominal aortic aneurysm repairs has remained relatively stable (2000 estimate: 45 230; 2010 estimate: 44 005), but there has been a dramatic shift in the breakdown of open and endovascular repairs with the latter accounting for 74% of all repairs (intact: 78%; ruptured: 38%) in 2010. There has been a decrease in the operative mortality associated with endovascular repair for both intact (1.8%—2.1% to 0.9%, $P = .0010$) and ruptured (40.0%—40.8% to 19.8%, $P < .001$) aneurysms and for the mortality rate for open repair of ruptured aneurysms (44.5% to 33.4%, $P < .001$). Not surprisingly, the operative mortality rate and median length of hospital stay was shorter for the endovascular approach despite the fact that the median total charges were greater, both for intact and ruptured aneurysms. Overall, these findings are largely consistent with the early findings from the randomized trials comparing open and endovascular repair and the general clinical impression that the endovascular approach has largely replaced open repair with the relatively rare exception of patients that are not endovascular candidates for anatomic reasons. The mortality trends are reassuring and suggest that we have collectively reduced the overall mortality associated with abdominal aortic aneurysms. The study is limited by the inherent problems with the administrative database that include lack of follow-up data and longer term outcomes. Accordingly, I do not believe that the authors can conclude from their data that the endovascular approach "should be the preferred management of both ruptured and unruptured AAAs" despite the fact that they are probably correct.

T. S. Huber, MD, PhD

Peripheral Arterial Occlusive Disease

Routine use of ultrasound-guided access reduces access site-related complications after lower extremity percutaneous revascularization

Lo RC, Fokkema MTM, Curran T, et al (Beth Israel Deaconess Med Ctr and Harvard Med School, Boston, MA)
J Vasc Surg 61:405-412, 2015

Objective.—We sought to elucidate the risks for access site-related complications (ASCs) after percutaneous lower extremity revascularization and to evaluate the benefit of routine ultrasound-guided access (RUS) in decreasing ASCs.

Methods.—We reviewed all consecutive percutaneous revascularizations (percutaneous transluminal angioplasty or stent) performed for lower extremity atherosclerosis at our institution from 2002 to 2012. RUS began in September 2007. Primary outcome was any ASC (bleeding, groin or retroperitoneal hematoma, vessel rupture, or thrombosis). Multivariable logistic regression was used to determine predictors of ASC.

Results.—A total of 1371 punctures were performed on 877 patients (43% women; median age, 69 [interquartile range, 60-78] years) for claudication (29%), critical limb ischemia (59%), or bypass graft stenosis (12%) with 4F to 8F sheaths. There were 72 ASCs (5%): 52 instances of bleeding or groin hematoma, nine pseudoaneurysms, eight retroperitoneal hematomas, two artery lacerations, and one thrombosis. ASCs were less frequent when RUS was used (4% vs 7%; $P = .02$). Multivariable predictors of ASC were age >75 years (odds ratio [OR], 2.0; 95% confidence interval [CI], 1.1-3.7; $P = .03$), congestive heart failure (OR, 1.9; 95% CI, 1.1-1.3; $P = .02$), preoperative warfarin use (OR, 2.0; 95% CI, 1.1-3.5; $P = .02$), and RUS (OR, 0.4; 95% CI, 0.2-0.7; $P < .01$). Vascular closure devices (VCDs) were not associated with lower rates of ASCs (OR, 1.1; 95% CI, 0.6-1.9; $P = .79$). RUS lowered ASCs in those >75 years (5% vs 12%; $P < .01$) but not in those taking warfarin preoperatively (10% vs 13%; $P = .47$). RUS did not decrease VCD failure (6% vs 4%; $P = .79$).

Conclusions.—We were able to decrease the rate of ASCs during lower extremity revascularization with the implementation of RUS. VCDs did not affect ASCs. Particular care should be taken with patients >75 years old, those with congestive heart failure, and those taking warfarin.

▶ The authors have examined their routine use of ultrasound-guided femoral access for peripheral interventions (ie, not diagnostic studies). The study was a retrospective review of their clinic practice comparing the time periods before and after the universal adoption of the technique. The overwhelming majority of the femoral cannulations were performed in a retrograde approach, and the sheath sizes ranged from 4 to 8 Fr in diameter. They reported a 5% incidence of access-related complications, including hematoma, pseudoaneurysm, retroperitoneal hematoma, vessel laceration, and thrombosis. Notably, the criteria for bleeding and/or hematomas were strict and included the need for transfusion, hemodynamic instability, and increased length of stay. They found that access complications were associated with advanced age (> 75 years), congestive heart failure, and preoperative warfarin use in their multivariate model with the routine use of ultrasound (odds ratio, 0.4; 96% confidence interval, 0.2–0.7) being the only factor that reduced the risk. These findings are interesting and suggest that the only way to reduce the risk of access-related complications is to improve operative technique because patient comorbidities are rarely modifiable. Notably, the predictors of advanced age and congestive heart failure are likely surrogate markers for advanced atherosclerotic occlusive disease. It was somewhat counterintuitive that the use of vascular closure devices did not reduce the incidence of complications, although this has been a consistent observation in other studies as emphasized by the authors in their discussion. The use of ultrasound-based guidance seems like an obvious step to improve quality and one that should be universally incorporated. Although not detailed in the current study, it has been shown to reduce the number of arterial cannulation attempts and reduce to the time to achieve access, and thus it is not only safer but likely faster. The technique has been widely adopted for central venous access and the broader application of ultrasound-based imaging (eg, Focused Assessment with Sonography for Trauma examination) as a diagnostic and therapeutic adjunct has been incorporated into most surgical training programs. Although the current study focused on femoral access, the potential benefit may be even greater for brachial artery cannulations given their intrinsically higher complication rates. A nice description of the authors' technique is provided in the article with detailed steps to ensure cannulation of the common femoral artery.

T. S. Huber, MD, PhD

The LEVANT I (Lutonix Paclitaxel-Coated Balloon for the Prevention of Femoropopliteal Restenosis) Trial for Femoropopliteal Revascularization: First-in-Human Randomized Trial of Low-Dose Drug-Coated Balloon Versus Uncoated Balloon Angioplasty

Scheinert D, Duda S, Zeller T, et al (Heart Ctr Leipzig/Park Hosp, Germany; Jewish Hosp, Berlin, Germany; Herz-Zentrum, Bad Krozingen, Germany; et al)
J Am Coll Cardiol Intv 7:10-19, 2014

Objectives.—This study sought to evaluate the safety and efficacy of the Lutonix drug-coated balloon (DCB) coated with 2 µg/mm^2 paclitaxel and a polysorbate/sorbitol carrier for treatment of femoropopliteal lesions.

Background.—Percutaneous treatment of peripheral vascular disease is associated with a high recurrence. Paclitaxel-coated balloons at 3 µg/mm^2 formulated differently have shown promising results with reduced restenosis.

Methods.—Subjects at 9 centers with Rutherford class 2 to 5 femoropopliteal lesions were randomized between June 2009 and December 2009 to treatment with Lutonix DCB (n = 49) versus uncoated balloons (control group [n = 52]), stratified by whether balloon-only treatment (n = 75) or stenting (n = 26) was intended. The primary endpoint was angiographic late lumen loss at 6 months. Secondary outcomes included adjudicated major adverse events (death, amputation, target lesion thrombosis, reintervention), functional outcomes, and pharmacokinetics.

Results.—Demographic, peripheral vascular disease, and lesion characteristics were matched, with mean lesion length of 8.1 ± 3.8 cm and 42% total occlusions. At 6 months, late lumen loss was 58% lower for the Lutonix DCB group (0.46 ± 1.13 mm) than for the control group (1.09 ± 1.07 mm; $p = 0.016$). Composite 24-month major adverse events were 39% for the DCB group, including 15 target lesion revascularizations, 1 amputation, and 4 deaths versus 46% for uncoated balloon group, with 20 target lesion revascularizations, 1 thrombosis, and 5 deaths. Pharmacokinetics showed biexponential decay with peak

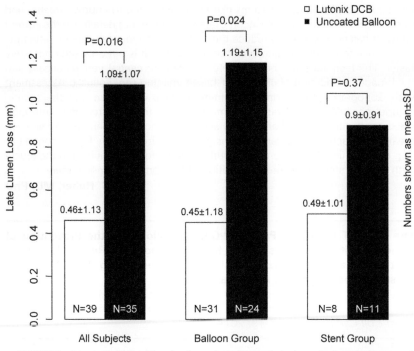

FIGURE 3.—Primary Endpoint. Mean late lumen loss at 6 months is shown for Lutonix drug-coated balloon (DCB) (**open bars**) versus control uncoated balloon percutaneous balloon angioplasty (**solid bars**) in the intention-to-treat population (all subjects in pooled strata) and separately for each stratum (intended balloon or stent groups) with *p* values. Columns are labeled with evaluable sample size (n) at base and mean late lumen loss ± SD (mm) at top. (Reprinted from Scheinert D, Duda S, Zeller T, et al. The LEVANT I (lutonix paclitaxel-coated balloon for the prevention of femoropopliteal restenosis) trial for femoropopliteal revascularization: first-in-human randomized trial of low-dose drug-coated balloon versus uncoated balloon angioplasty. *J Am Coll Cardiol Intv.* 2014;7:10-19, with permission from The American College of Cardiology Foundation.)

concentration (C_{max}) of 59 ng/ml and total observed exposure (AUC_{all}) of 73 ng h/ml. For successful DCB deployment excluding 8 malfunctions, 6-month late lumen loss was 0.39 mm and the 24-month target lesion revascularization rate was 24%.

Conclusions.—Treatment of femoropopliteal lesions with the low-dose Lutonix DCB reduced late lumen loss with safety comparable to that of control angioplasty. (LEVANT I, The Lutonix Paclitaxel-Coated Balloon for the Prevention of Femoropopliteal Restenosis; NCT00930813) (Fig 3).

▶ The authors report the results of the LEVANT 1 trial, a nonblinded, randomized, controlled trial comparing the results of angioplasty with drug-coated (paclitaxel) and standard balloons for femoropopliteal lesions. Notably, the lesions were either single de novo or restenotic ones in the femoropopliteal vessels that had a stenosis > 70% and a lesion length between 4 and 15 cm. Exclusion criteria included severely calcified vessels, the absence of > 1 patent untreated runoff vessel, and significant inflow disease. The study used a novel design such that the patients were stratified into intended stenting and intended balloon angioplasty to balance out the differences in stent use. The primary end point was lumen loss at 6 months as determined by angiography. The authors reported the lumen loss was significantly lower (0.46 + 1.18 mm vs 1.19 + 1.15 mm, $P = .16$) in the drug-coated balloon group (Fig 3) and that this significant difference was also seen in the balloon-only group (but not the stent group). The benefit of the drug-coated balloon appeared to be even more beneficial when restricted to the subset of patients that actually got the drug delivered to the intended target lesion (ie, geographic misses and balloon deployment failures excluded). The drug-coated balloon appears to be safe given that there were no differences in the safety and functional outcomes out to 24 months. Interestingly, the pharmacokinetic studies performed in a small subset of patients ($n = 7$) demonstrated a rapid decay of the serum paclitaxel concentrations with the last measureable concentration at 5.6 + 4.6 hours. These data are encouraging and appear to justify the more widespread use of drug-coated balloons in the periphery, but they should be interpreted with some caution. Notably, the absolute difference in lumen loss was small and may not be clinically relevant. There were no differences in the target lesion revascularizations nor composite major adverse event rates that included amputation, thrombosis, and reintervention. Furthermore, the cost of the device was not factored into the analyses. Not surprisingly, the drug-coated balloons are significantly more expensive and they are "single use" in that the drug is delivered during the initial insufflation such that repeated treatments or additional treatments at a separate site require another balloon. Lastly, the study was funded by the manufacturer, and the majority of the authors disclosed that they received financial support from the sponsor. I am not certain what role drug-coated balloons will play in the treatment of peripheral arterial occlusive lesions but suspect that may have a niche for complex or restenotic lesions; I suspect, however, that our enthusiastic industry partners will lobby for their use as a primary modality.

T. S. Huber, MD, PhD

Cilostazol is associated with improved outcomes after peripheral endovascular interventions
Warner CJ, Greaves SW, Larson RJ, et al (Dartmouth-Hitchcock Med Ctr, Lebanon, NH; et al)
J Vasc Surg 59:1607-1614, 2014

Objective.—Although cilostazol is commonly used as an adjunct after peripheral vascular interventions, its efficacy remains uncertain. We assessed the effect of cilostazol on outcomes after peripheral vascular interventions using meta-analytic techniques.

Methods.—We searched MEDLINE (1946-2012), Cochrane CENTRAL (1996-2012), and trial registries for studies comparing cilostazol in combination with antiplatelet therapy to antiplatelet therapy alone after peripheral vascular interventions. Treatment effects were reported as pooled risk/hazard ratio (HR) with random-effects models.

Results.—Two randomized trials and four retrospective cohorts involving 1522 patients met inclusion criteria. Across studies, mean age ranged from 65 to 76 years, and the majority of patients were male (64%-83%); mean follow-up ranged from 18 to 37 months. Most interventions were in the femoropopliteal segment, and overall, 68% of patients had stents placed. Pooled estimates demonstrated that the addition of cilostazol was associated with decreased restenosis (relative risk [RR], 0.71; 95% confidence interval [CI], 0.60-0.84; $P < .001$), improved amputation-free survival (HR, 0.63; 95% CI, 0.47-0.85; $P = .002$), improved limb salvage (HR, 0.42; 95% CI, 0.27-0.66; $P < .001$), and improved freedom from target lesion revascularization (RR, 1.36; 95% CI, 1.14-1.61; $P < .001$). There was no significant reduction in mortality among those receiving cilostazol (RR, 0.73; 95% CI, 0.45-1.19; $P = .21$).

Conclusions.—The addition of cilostazol to antiplatelet therapy after peripheral vascular interventions is associated with a reduced risk of restenosis, amputation, and target lesion revascularization in our meta-analysis of six studies. Consideration of cilostazol as a medical adjunct after peripheral vascular interventions is warranted, presuming these findings are broadly generalizable.

▶ The authors have performed a meta-analysis of the literature to answer the question of whether cilostazol improves outcomes after peripheral vascular interventions, as suggested by the coronary literature. The authors identified 6 articles that fulfilled their inclusion criteria after an extension review of the literature. These articles (2 randomized controlled trials, 4 retrospective reviews) were deemed to be acceptable quality in terms of methodology and risk of bias based on their assessment tools. However, all of the studies were performed in Japan (the home of the pharmaceutical company that markets the product), and the majority of the procedures were performed for femoropopliteal lesions. The authors reported that cilostazol was associated with decreased restenosis (relative risk [RR] 0.71, confidence interval [CI] 0.60—0.84) and improved freedom from target vessel revascularization (RR 1.36, CI 1.14—1.61) in addition to improved amputation-free survival and limb salvage, although the former 2 outcome measures seem most relevant to the peripheral interventions, particularly among claudicants, because the risk of amputation should be negligible. Cilostazol had no impact on mortality, and there was no increased risk of bleeding complications with only minimal drug-related complications. The mechanism by which cilostazol improves outcomes remains unclear given its pluripotent effects. These findings suggest that the addition of cilostazol should at least be considered at the time of peripheral interventions although the study does not address drug-related cost and/or patient compliance. We have not used cilostazol in our practice but are certainly intrigued by the application and have some preliminary laboratory data that it reduces intimal hyperplasia in a vein graft model.

T. S. Huber, MD, PhD

Access

The Venous Window Needle Guide, a hemodialysis cannulation device for salvage of uncannulatable arteriovenous fistulas

Jennings WC, Galt SW, Shenoy S, et al (Univ of Oklahoma, Tulsa; Mountian Med Vascular Specialists, Salt Lake City, UT; Washington Univ School of Medicine, St Louis, MO; et al)

J Vasc Surg 60:1024-1032, 2014

Background.—Arteriovenous fistulas (AVFs) are recommended for hemodialysis access when possible. A noncannulatable but otherwise well functioning AVF leads to prolonged catheter dependency and frustration for the patient and the renal health care provider team. Difficult cannulation patients include obese individuals in whom cannulation sites are too deep, and others with vein segments that are short, tortuous, or otherwise difficult to palpate. The Venous Window Needle Guide for Salvage of AV Fistulae (SAVE) trial was designed to evaluate the efficacy and safety of the Venous Window Needle Guide (VWING; Vital Access Corp, Salt Lake City, Utah) device for salvage of such noncannulatable AVFs that are otherwise functional.

Methods.—The SAVE study included patients with an established and otherwise mature AVF, in whom an additional procedure would otherwise be necessary to establish reliable cannulation. The VWING is a single-piece titanium device that allows repeated access of an AVF through a single puncture site (buttonhole technique). Inclusion criteria included mature AVFs 6.0 to 15.0 mm in depth with multiple failed attempts at cannulation or where the access could not be palpated. The devices were implanted subcutaneously and sutured to the anterior wall of the mature fistula. Study end points were reliable and successful cannulation and avoidance of adverse events during the 6-month follow-up, implant technical success, and clinical cannulation success.

Results.—Enrollment included 54 patients at 11 trial sites with implantation of 82 VWING devices. Body mass index was 26 to 50 (median, 36), 40 (74%) patients were female, and age was 17 to 84 (median, 59) years. Forty (74%) individuals were diabetic. Thirty-three (61%) patients were white, 16 (30%) black, and 10 (18%) patients were Hispanic, Pacific Islander, or Native American. Three patients were excluded from data analysis for reasons unrelated to the device. Successful AVF access was achieved using the VWING in 49 (96%) of the 51 patients evaluated. The rate of device-related serious adverse events was 0.31 per patient-year; each event was resolved leaving the AVF functional. The rates of sepsis and study-related interventions were 0.04 and 0.65 per patient-year, respectively. There were no study-related deaths. One device was removed because of infection. The AVF survival rate at 6 months was 100%. The total number of study days was 9497 and the estimated number of device cannulations was 4238.

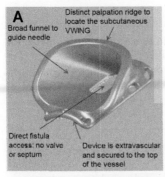
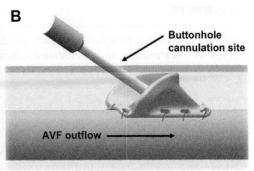

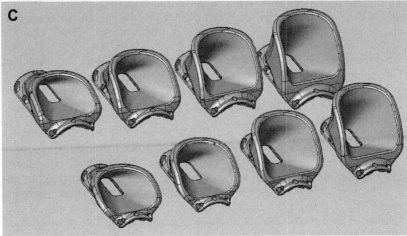

FIGURE 1.—a, The Venous Window Needle Guide (VWING; Vital Access Corp, Salt Lake City, Utah). The cannulation device is comprised of a single piece of titanium that allows repeated access of an arteriovenous fistula (AVF) through a single puncture site (buttonhole technique). b, The schematic image shows the VWING sutured to the anterior AVF wall using the eight suture slots. Cannulation is allowed using the buttonhole technique 3 weeks after implantation. c, Each VWING device is 17.7 mm in length and available in 7 and 9 mm widths for variation in vessel diameter. AVF depth variation is accommodated by available 4-, 6-, 8-, and 10-mm heights. All images were provided by and reproduced with permission of Vital Access Corporation. (Reprinted from the Journal of Vascular Surgery. Jennings WC, Galt SW, Shenoy S, et al. The Venous Window Needle Guide, a hemodialysis cannulation device for salvage of uncannulatable arteriovenous fistulas. *J Vasc Surg.* 2014;60:1024-1032, Copyright 2014, with permission from The Society for Vascular Surgery.)

Conclusions.—The VWING was safe and effective in facilitating AVF cannulation for patients with an otherwise mature but noncannulatable fistula. Successful AVF access was achieved using the VWING in 49 (96%) of the 51 patients evaluated. The AVF survival rate at 6 months was 100% (Fig 1).

▶ The authors report the results of the Venous Window Needle Guide for Salvage of AV Fistulae (SAVE) trial using the Venous Window Needle Guide (VWING), a prospective multicenter trial designed to evaluate the utility of the device ($N = 54$ patients, 82 devices) for patients with autogenous arteriovenous access (AVF) that were deemed unable to be cannulated. The VWING device (Fig 1) is single piece of titanium that is shaped like a funnel and designed to facilitate the buttonhole cannulation technique in "mature" AVFs that are too deep (study inclusion criteria 6—15 mm) or otherwise unsuitable (eg, too tortuous) for cannulation. The device(s) is implanted underneath the skin and sutured to the AVF with the majority of the procedures being performed under local anesthesia in the outpatient setting (median surgical time: single implant, 38 min [range 21—65]; double implant, 78 min [range 37—120]). The authors reported that the technical success rate for implantation was 100% and 95% of the devices could be cannulated at 3 months after implantation. Eighty-six percent of the devices were in use at 6 months, and device-related serious adverse event (SA), AVF intervention, and site infection rates were 0.31 per patient-year, 0.43 per device-year, and 0.08 per device-year, respectively. Overall, the results are quite impressive given that the AVFs were deemed unusable and would have required another surgical procedure to facilitate cannulation, typically some type of "elevation" procedure to reduce the distance of the AVF from the surface of the skin. I am not certain where this device will ultimately fit into our overall armamentarium for establishing permanent hemodialysis access, but it is somewhat intriguing given the epidemic of obesity in our country. Furthermore, it may have a role in the scenario in which patients have a limited segment for cannulation for whatever reason (eg, short AVF, aneurysmal degeneration). The results must be interpreted with some caution given that the follow-up was relatively brief (primary endpoint at 6 months) albeit the total number of implant days (14 172) and estimated device cannulations (4238) were impressive. Furthermore, the study was sponsored by the device manufacturer and conducted at centers of excellence in terms of hemodialysis access, and thus it is not clear that the results are applicable outside of a clinical trial and/or at all centers. Lastly, the use of the buttonhole technique has been somewhat controversial and may be associated with an increased rate of infectious complications.

T. S. Huber, MD, PhD

Randomized Clinical Trial of Cutting Balloon Angioplasty versus High-Pressure Balloon Angioplasty in Hemodialysis Arteriovenous Fistula Stenoses Resistant to Conventional Balloon Angioplasty

Aftab SA, Tay KH, Irani FG, et al (Duke-Natl Univ of Singapore Graduate Med School)

J Vasc Interv Radiol 25:190-198, 2014

Purpose.—To compare the efficacy and safety of cutting balloon angioplasty (CBA) versus high-pressure balloon angioplasty (HPBA) for the treatment of hemodialysis autogenous fistula stenoses resistant to conventional percutaneous transluminal angioplasty (PTA).

Materials and Methods.—In a prospective, randomized clinical trial involving patients with dysfunctional, stenotic hemodialysis arteriovenous fistulas (AVFs), patients were randomized to receive CBA or HPBA if conventional PTA had suboptimal results (ie, residual stenosis > 30%). A total of 516 patients consented to participate in the study from October 2008 to September 2011, 85% of whom (n = 439) had technically successful conventional PTA. The remaining 71 patients (mean age, 60 y; 49 men) with suboptimal PTA results were eventually randomized: 36 to the CBA arm and 35 to the HPBA arm. Primary and secondary target lesion patencies were determined by Kaplan–Meier analysis.

Results.—Clinical success rates were 100% in both arms. Primary target lesion patency rates at 6 months were 66.4% and 39.9% for CBA and HPBA, respectively (*P* =.01). Secondary target lesion patency rates at 6 months were 96.5% for CBA and 80.0% for HPBA (*P* =.03). There was a single major complication of venous perforation following CBA. The 30-day mortality rate was 1.4%, with one non-procedure-related death in the HPBA group.

Conclusions.—Primary and secondary target lesion patency rates of CBA were statistically superior to those of HPBA following suboptimal conventional PTA. For AVF stenoses resistant to conventional PTA, CBA may be a better second-line treatment given its superior patency rates.

▶ The authors have performed a randomized controlled trial to determine whether cutting or high-pressure balloons are more effective for resistant stenoses in "failing" autogenous arteriovenous accesses (AVFs). In their study design, patients were randomized to either cutting or high-pressure balloons only after they failed standard balloon angioplasty (ie, an appropriately sized balloon, insufflation burst pressure, at least 2 insufflations for 1 min). Notably, 516 patients agreed to participate in the study, but the standard balloon angioplasty was successful in 85% of the cases, leaving only 71 patients for randomization. The authors reported that both the primary (6 month—66% vs 40%) and secondary (6 months—97% vs 80%) target lesion patency rates were better for the cutting balloon technique by Kaplan-Meier technique. These findings are helpful and define the optimal treatment for the sclerotic, intimal hyperplastic lesion in autogenous accesses that is refractory to conventional therapy, a problem that seems far more common than the 15% incidence identified in the study. In our own practice, we have used both high-pressure and cutting balloons but have not had sufficient experience in this setting to determine the optimal choice. These findings can likely be extrapolated to other similar clinical scenarios with refractory lesions such as vein graft stenoses or venous outflow stenoses within a prosthetic arteriovenous access (AVG). Notably, the authors had initially planned on enrolling both autogenous and prosthetic accesses, but the enrollment in the latter group was insufficient. The authors emphasized that the high-pressure balloons were twice as expensive as conventional angioplasty balloons in their institution, whereas the cutting balloons were 4 times as expensive. They conceded that the improved patency rates may offset the additional costs for both approaches, but a formal cost analysis was not performed. It is notable that there was only a single complication from a cutting balloon, which was treated with balloon tamponade using a prolonged insufflation. The results should be interpreted with some caution given several limitations of the technique and study. First, the overall primary target lesion patency rates were only fair, even for the cutting-balloon group, and the study participants' follow-up with the mandatory 6-month fistulagram was likewise only fair (18 of 71). Second, it would have been helpful to look at primary assisted patency as well because the procedures were initially performed on "failing" rather than thrombosed accesses. Lastly, the study was halted before optimal enrollment was achieved based on the power analysis, although the sample size was sufficient to achieve statistical significance. Despite these limitations, I would echo the authors' conclusions that conventional balloon angioplasty is sufficient for most stenotic lesions within autogenous accesses and that cutting balloons are superior to high-pressure balloons for refractory lesion.

T. S. Huber, MD, PhD

12 General Thoracic Surgery

Pre- and Postoperative Management

Urokinase Versus VATS for Treatment of Empyema: A Randomized Multicenter Clinical Trial
Marhuenda C, Barceló C, Fuentes I, et al (Universitat Autònoma de Barcelona, Spain; Hosp 12 de Octubre, Madrid, Spain; et al)
Pediatrics 134:e1301-e1307, 2014

Background and Objective.—Parapneumonic empyema (PPE) is a frequent complication of acute bacterial pneumonia in children. There is limited evidence regarding the optimal treatment of this condition. The aim of this study was to compare the efficacy of drainage plus urokinase versus video-assisted thoracoscopic surgery in the treatment of PPE in childhood.

Methods.—This prospective, randomized, multicenter clinical trial enrolled patients aged <15 years and hospitalized with septated PPE. Study patients were randomized to receive urokinase or thoracoscopy. The main outcome variable was the length of hospital stay after treatment. The secondary outcomes were total length of hospital stay, number of days with the chest drain, number of days with fever, and treatment failures. The trial was approved by the ethics committees of all the participating hospitals.

Results.—A total of 103 patients were randomized to treatment and analyzed; 53 were treated with thoracoscopy and 50 with urokinase. There were no differences in demographic characteristics or in the main baseline characteristics between the 2 groups. No statistically significant differences were found between thoracoscopy and urokinase in the median postoperative stay (10 vs 9 days), median hospital stay (14 vs 13 days), or days febrile after treatment (4 vs 6 days). A second intervention was required in 15% of children in the thoracoscopy group versus 10% in the urokinase group ($P = .47$).

Conclusions.—Drainage plus urokinase instillation is as effective as video-assisted thoracoscopic surgery as first-line treatment of septated PPE in children.

▶ Empyema is the most frequent suppurative complication of bacterial pneumonia in childhood and is classical classified into 3 stages of progression: exudative, fibrinopurulent, and organizational. As much as 2% of pneumonia cases in children are complicated by empyema, but there has been a considerable worldwide increase in incidence of empyema with rates reaching 28—53% of all patients hospitalized for pneumonia. The basic treatments remain antibiotics and drainage of the pleural space with a chest tube. Additional interventions including a fibrin lytic agent and video-assisted thoracoscopic surgery (VATS) may be required. In both options, the goal is to break the septa and extract any fluid, fibrin, or debris allowing normal expansion and function of the lung and pleural reabsorption of the fluid as quickly as possible. The authors were able to include 103 patients, including 53 in the VATS group and 50 in the urokinase group. The median length of stay was 10 days in those receiving VATS and 9 days in those receiving urokinase installation.

This trial was important in that there were discrepancies in opinion regarding which treatments are best in clinical practice for children with peripneumonic empyema, with some still favoring the VATS approach and others favoring the intrapleural fibrinolytic agents. This study is one of the few randomized clinical trials on this subject in children and the first multicenter trial. It included children with septated empyema exclusively and ultimately demonstrated that thoracoscopy and fibrinolysis with urokinase was equally effective in this trial. The only word of caution I would add is that, as surgeons, we must scrutinize the imaging studies to see if there are obvious predictors to suggest that one or the other treatment would be better suited to the patient. However, in the middle ground of cases that could be managed either way, I believe this review gives us confidence to proceed with either treatment course.

C. T. Klodell, Jr, MD

How early should VATS be performed for retained haemothorax in blunt chest trauma?

Lin H-L, Huang W-Y, Yang C, et al (Kaohsiung Med Univ, Taiwan; Natl Chiao Tung Univ-Taipei, Taiwan; et al)
Injury 45:1359-1364, 2014

Background.—Blunt chest injury is not uncommon in trauma patients. Haemothorax and pneumothorax may occur in these patients, and some of them will develop retained pleural collections. Video-assisted thoracoscopic surgery (VATS) has become an appropriate method for treating these complications, but the optimal timing for performing the surgery and its effects on outcome are not clearly understood.

Materials and Methods.—In this study, a total of 136 patients who received VATS for the management of retained haemothorax from January 2003 to December 2011 were retrospectively enrolled. All patients had blunt chest injuries and 90% had associated injuries in more than two sites. The time from trauma to operation was recorded and the patients were divided into three groups: 2—3 days (Group 1), 4—6 days (Group 2), and 7 or more days (Group 3). Clinical outcomes such as the length of stay (LOS) at the hospital and intensive care unit (ICU), and duration of ventilator and chest tube use were all recorded and compared between groups.

Results.—The mean duration from trauma to operation was 5.9 days. All demographic characteristics showed no statistical differences between groups. Compared with other groups, Group 3 had higher rates of positive microbial cultures in pleural collections and sputum, longer duration of chest tube insertion and ventilator use. Lengths of hospital and ICU stay in Groups 1 and 2 showed no statistical difference, but were longer in Group 3. The frequency of repeated VATS was lower in Group 1 but without statistically significant difference.

Discussion.—This study indicated that an early VATS intervention would decrease chest infection. It also reduced the duration of ventilator dependency. The clinical outcomes were significantly better for patients receiving VATS within 3 days under intensive care. In this study, we suggested that VATS might be delayed by associated injuries, but should not exceed 6 days after trauma.

▶ In this study, the authors retrospectively reviewed a prospectively maintained trauma database over an 8-year period to identify blunt trauma patients with retained fluid collections in their chests. They attempted to identify any differences in outcomes by timing of intervention. They looked at clinical outcomes such as length of stay at the hospital, intensive care units, and duration of ventilator and chest tube use. In their series, the mean duration from trauma to operation was 5.9 days. They concluded that their study is further justification of early video-assisted thoracoscopic surgery (VATS) intervention to try to decrease potential chest infection from retained hemothorax and possibly also reduce the duration of ventilator dependency; they felt the clinical outcomes were significantly better for patients receiving VATS within 3 days of event.

Blunt injury is the leading cause of chest trauma, and pneumothorax and hemothorax cause severe chest trauma. Approximately 85% of patients with pneumothorax or hemothorax can be successfully treated with just pain control and simple tube thoracostomy. However, the remaining 15% of patients will develop retained pleural fluid collections and may be better managed by further interventions to prevent further complications such as empyema or fibrothorax. VATS is only slightly more invasive than a standard chest tube and allows excellent visualization of the intrathoracic structures as well as evacuation of fluid collections. Although many have advocated for early VATS, the optimal timing for this surgery, and the effect on outcomes, is not yet fully elucidated. Numerous recent studies do state that earlier interventions on injured chest wall with fluid collections lead to better prognosis for patients. However, the exact recommendations for the timing in those operations vary across those studies. It is hoped the earlier the intervention can take place, the more it can help mitigate the most common reasons for prolonged hospitalization of trauma patients, which are infection and respiratory failure.

The authors' trauma service is fairly standard in that all patients received a CT scan at the time of presentation and then a delayed repeat CT scan if the x-ray shows progression of any intrathoracic density. Their indications for performing VATS included a retained volume estimated to exceed 300 cc or the formation of a para-pneumonic effusion, which appeared on CT as a separate loculated pleural collections. All procedures were performed by a thoracic surgeon in a fairly standard fashion through a 2-port approach. One port was utilized as a camera port and the other was used as a working port, ultimately leaving two 36-Fr chest tubes in place at the conclusion of the procedure.

They divided the groups that received their intervention at 2–3 days, 4–6 days, or more than 6 days. Not surprisingly, the shorter lengths of stay were shown in the patients who received earlier interventions. Interestingly, patients with positive cultures were noted to be the ones who had a longer mean period of time to VATS. There is a heavy selection bias in this study, with the longer group having a much higher head injury score and Glasgow Coma Scores that were lower at the time of presentation, which may account for the delay in VATS.

The VATS technique is relatively simple and can be widely applied in the diagnosis and treatment of chest-injured patients. In addition to providing excellent visualization of the pleural cavity, it is a relatively simple way to evacuate pleural collections and ensure excellent expansion of the lung, while being only slightly more invasive than a chest tube. I believe this study further supports the general idea that earlier intervention for retained fluid collection is beneficial for patients; however, I think their timing recommendations are based more on the severity of the injury of the patients and the bias that it brings. The best conclusion that we all can draw from this study and continue to carry forth in our practices is that evacuation of retained chest collections should be performed as early as is safe and feasible for the patient and relatively convenient for the care team. In many patients, it may be appropriate on day 1 or day 2 to proceed with VATS, whereas in others, the associated injuries may mandate a delay that, although not optimal for the intrathoracic process, may be the appropriate choice for the overall care of the patient.

C. T. Klodell, Jr, MD

Management of a pneumopericardium due to penetrating trauma
Nicol AJ, Navsaria PH, Hommes M, et al (Univ of Cape Town, South Africa)
Injury 45:1368-1372, 2014

Introduction.—A pneumopericardium presenting after penetrating chest trauma is a rare event. The surgical management of this clinical problem has not been clearly defined. The aim of this study was to document the mode of presentation and to suggest a protocol for management.

Patient and Methods.—A review of a prospectively collected cardiac database of patients presenting to Groote Schuur Hospital Trauma Centre between October 2001 and February 2009 with a pneumopericardium on chest X-ray after penetrating trauma.

Results.—There were 27 patients with a pneumopericardium (mean age 25 years, range 17—36). The mechanism of injury was a stab wound to the chest in 26 patients and a single patient with multiple low velocity gunshot wounds. Six patients (22%) were unstable and required emergency surgery. One of these patients presented with a tension pneumopericardium. Twenty-one patients were initially stable. Two of these (10%) patients later developed a tension pneumopericardium within 24-h and were taken to theatre. The remaining 19 patients were managed with a subxiphoid pericardial window (SPW) at between 24 and 48 h post admission. Ten of these 19 patients (52%) were positive for a haemopericardium. Only 4 of the 19 underwent a sternotomy and only two of these had cardiac injuries that had sealed. There were no deaths in this series.

Conclusion.—Patients with a penetrating chest injury with a pneumopericardium who are unstable require emergency surgery. A delayed tension pneumopericardium developed in 10% of patients who were initially stable. It is our recommendation that all stable patients with a pneumopericardium after penetrating chest trauma should undergo a SPW. A sternotomy is not required in stable patients.

▶ Pneumopericardium presenting after a penetrating trauma is extremely rare event. However, guidelines concerning its treatment are few. The authors present a 7-year retrospective review of a prospectively maintained database in which they identified 27 patients with pneumopericardium following wounds to the chest. In 26 patients, this was the result of a stab wound, and in 1 patient, it was multiple low-velocity gunshot wounds. They conclude that patients presenting with penetrating chest injury with a pneumopericardium who were unstable require emergency surgery. They further conclude that delayed tension pneumopericardium may develop in 10% of patients who were initially stable. They recommend that all stable patients with a pneumopericardium after penetrating chest trauma should undergo a subxiphoid pericardial window in placement of a drain, but that sternotomy is not required in stable patients.

A pneumopericardium is the collection of air in the pericardial sac. It is most commonly encountered in neonates on positive pressure ventilation or in patients sustaining blunt chest trauma. A pneumopericardium associated with penetrating chest trauma is a rare event. The surgical management of pneumopericardium varies from some that believe that mandatory exploration is required, irrespective of the clinical status of the patient to verify the presence or absence of an underlying cardiac injury, to those who advocate for conservative management in a carefully group of colect patients

The authors aimed to study the clinical presentation of penetrating chest trauma and suggest a treatment protocol based on their 7-year experience. They identified patients with the radiologic appearance of a pneumopericardium on chest x-ray following penetrating trauma and included them in their study. In their protocol, patients that presented either stable or in shock but were easily resuscitated with less than 2 L of crystalloid were investigated with an ultrasound of the heart or a CT scan. All stable patients were observed in a high care unit until a subxiphoid pericardial window of the heart was performed within 24 hours of admission. If at any point the patient became unstable during the period of observation, they were taken immediately to surgery for a subxiphoid pericardial window. Immediate sternotomy was performed in addition to the window only if there was evidence of active bleeding from the heart at time of the window.

It is interesting to note that 3 of their 27 patients at the time of admission were noted to have a small pericardial effusion on echocardiography and were followed with serial echocardiography. Only 1 of these patients progressed to become unstable and require urgent surgery.

Patients with pneumopericardium may have the classic clinical sign of a mill-wheel murmur that was originally described in 1844. Patients may also present with a tension pneumopericardium, which will clinically act as a cardiac tamponade. Chest x-ray will show the heart partially or completely surrounded by air with the pericardium sharply outlined. They may also have an air fluid level in pericardial sac. The diagnosis of pneumopericardium can be made on chest x-ray, ultrasound of the pericardial sac, or CT scan of the chest. In the differential diagnosis, it is always important to consider a pneumothorax or a pneumomediastinum, which may appear radiographically similar but usually the air will extend above the pericardial reflection of the aortic arch, distinguishing it from pneumopericardium. The authors advocate for subxiphoid pericardial window even in stable patients because of the fear of development of a tension pneumopericardial window, which can progress rapidly due to the small confines of the pericardium. I congratulate the authors on this interesting review and support their conclusions that a stable patient does not need a sternotomy after penetrating injury but does require very close observation.

C. T. Klodell, Jr, MD

The Incidence and Management of Postoperative Chylothorax After Pulmonary Resection and Thoracic Mediastinal Lymph Node Dissection

Bryant AS, Minnich DJ, Wei B, et al (Univ of Alabama at Birmingham)
Ann Thorac Surg 98:232-237, 2014

Background.—Our objective was to determine the incidence and optimal management of chylothorax after pulmonary resection with complete thoracic mediastinal lymph node dissection (MLND).

Methods.—This is a retrospective review of patients who underwent pulmonary resection with MLND.

Results.—Between January 2000 and December 2012, 2,838 patients underwent pulmonary resection with MLND by one surgeon (RJC). Forty-one (1.4%) of these patients experienced a chylothorax. Univariate analysis showed that lobectomy ($p < 0.001$), a robotic approach ($p = 0.03$), right-sided operations ($p < 0.001$), and pathologic N2 disease ($p = 0.007$) were significantly associated with the development of chylothorax. Multivariate analysis showed that lobectomy ($p = 0.011$), a robotic approach ($p = 0.032$), and pathologic N2 disease ($p = 0.027$) remained predictors. All patients were initially treated with cessation of oral intake and 200 μg subcutaneous somatostatin every 8 hours. If after 48 hours the chest tube output was less than 450 mL/day and the effluent was clear, patients was given a medium-chain triglyceride (MCT) diet and were observed for 48 hours in the hospital. If the chest tube output remained below 450 mL/day, the chest tube was removed, they were discharged home with directions to continue the MCT diet and to return in 2 weeks. Patients were instructed to consume a high-fat meal 24 hours before their clinic appointment. If the patient's chest roentgenogram was clear at that time, they were considered "treated." This approach was successful in 37 (90%) patients. The 4 patients in whom the initial treatment was unsuccessful underwent reoperation with pleurodesis and duct ligation.

Conclusions.—Chylothorax after pulmonary resection and MLND occurred in 1.4% of patients. Its incidence was higher in those with pathologic N2 disease and those who underwent robotic resection. Nonoperative therapy is almost always effective.

▶ The authors present a high-volume series over a 12-year period of 2838 patients operated on by a single surgeon. In their series, they report a 1.4% incidence of chylothorax that was noted to be statistically significantly associated with lobectomy, robotic operation, or right-sided operation, and pathologic N2 disease by univariate analysis. By multivariate analysis, lobectomy, robotic approach, and pathologic N2 disease were significant.

The treatment of chylothorax was initially with cessation of oral intake and subcutaneous somatostatin and observation of the output. If it falls, they then treat the patient with ongoing medium chain triglyceride diet and discharge to home if the output does not increase.

The authors should be commended on the large series and outstanding outcomes. Chylothorax is an uncommon but potentially serious complication seen after pulmonary resection with complete mediastinal lymph node resection. It is important to remember that the chyle leak seen after pulmonary resection is dramatically different from that seen after esophageal resection. Following esophageal operation, lymph leaks are often related to transection of the thoracic duct, whereas the involved tributary of the thoracic duct is usually a small branch following thoracic lymph node dissection. The authors do note that perhaps the reason the increased incidence is seen after robotic surgery is related to the increased magnification afforded by a robotic approach and perhaps a more complete lymph node dissection. Additionally, they note that when you encounter postoperative chylothorax, it is almost always from the 4R or station 7 lymph nodes, and when they were forced to reoperate, they tried to clip the tributary as well as place a fibrin glue and do a pleurodesis.

This is interesting in that historically many surgeons have felt that high output Chylothorax after pulmonary resection required immediate reexploration, but in fact the authors have importantly demonstrated that conservative management can be effective in a high proportion of these cases. I have included abstracts in previous YEAR BOOKS detailing the use of Midodrine as an oral antilymphatic leak treatment that also showed promise.

The authors of this article note a rather high success rate and routinely used somatostatin, although somatostatin has marginal data in support for its use in chylothorax. Perhaps the optimal therapy may involve other agents such as midodrine or perhaps midodrine in combination with somatostatin and this conservative approach. It is also important to note that in many centers, there is the availability of coil embolization of the thoracic duct, which may be an option for treatment of this condition if this resource is available at your center.

C. T. Klodell, Jr, MD

Postoperative Atrial Fibrillation Prophylaxis After Lung Surgery: Systematic Review and Meta-Analysis

Riber LP, Larsen TB, Christensen TD (Odense Univ Hosp, Denmark; Aalborg Univ Hosp, Denmark; Faculty of Health Aalborg Univ, Denmark)
Ann Thorac Surg 98:1989-1997, 2014

Background.—Atrial fibrillation after thoracic surgery is frequent and increases morbidity and mortality. A number of trials have investigated medical prophylaxis for the prevention of atrial fibrillation after surgery for lung cancer. However, the literature is diverse and hence difficult to review. The aim of this study was to evaluate the safety and efficacy of reducing the risk of postoperative atrial fibrillation by the use of medical prophylaxis in patients undergoing surgery for lung cancer.

Methods.—A systematic review and meta-analysis of randomized, controlled trials investigating prophylactic medical interventions to reduce the risk of postoperative atrial fibrillation was performed.

Results.—A total number of 10 trials were identified. A significant reduction in the risk of postoperative atrial fibrillation was found with a relative risk of 0.53 (95% confidence interval, 0.42 to 0.67) and a number needed-to-treat of 8.5 (95% confidence interval, 6.4 to 13.3). Amiodarone was found to be the most effective prophylactic agent with a relative risk of 0.32 (95% confidence interval, 0.19 to 0.50) and a number needed-to-treat of 4.8 (95% confidence interval, 3.7 to 7.6) and regarded as safe, with no severe adverse events registered. The risk of atrial fibrillation was overall reduced from 25.1% to 13.4% ($p < 0.001$) and for amiodarone as a single therapy from 30.4% to 9.6% ($p < 0.001$).

Conclusions.—Medical prophylaxis with calcium-channel blockers, magnesium sulfate, or amiodarone significantly reduces the risk of developing atrial fibrillation after lung reduction surgery. However, amiodarone and magnesium sulfate were the most effective and safest drugs causing no increased risk of adverse events.

▶ Atrial fibrillation after thoracic surgery is frequent and increases morbidity and mortality. The authors set out to evaluate the safety and efficacy of reducing the risk of atrial fibrillation through the use of medical prophylaxis in patients undergoing surgery for lung cancer. They performed a systematic review and meta-analysis of randomized, controlled trials investigating prophylactic medical interventions and identified 10 total trials. They ultimately conclude that medical prophylaxis with calcium-channel blockers, magnesium sulfate, or amiodarone significantly reduces the risk of developing atrial fibrillation after lung reduction surgery. However, amiodarone and magnesium were the most effective and the safest drugs, causing no adverse events.

Multiple studies have confirmed that supraventricular arrhythmias, and particularly atrial fibrillation, are common after thoracic surgery. They may occur as frequently as 46% of the time after pneumonectomy and in as many as one-third of patients following lobectomy. The ideology involves a combination of hyperadrenergic activity and atrial dilatation, as well as changes in vagal tone, inflammation, pulmonary hypertension, and dilatation of the right ventricle. It most commonly occurs on the second or third postoperative day but can occur later in the postoperative course. Although originally thought to be a relatively benign event, we now know that patients who have atrial fibrillation may have as much as a 2-fold increased chance of hypotension, heart failure, and embolism. They also have a worse short- and long-term prognosis after surgery. Atrial fibrillation may further more increase the length of stay, anxiety, reduce mobilization, and increase medical cost.

The authors should be commended for their comprehensive review initially identifying 157 studies and distilling it down to 10 total studies for systematic review. Of these studies, 3 examined the use of calcium channel blockers, 2 Digoxin, 1 magnesium sulfate, 1 beta-blocker, and 3 prophylactic amiodarone. I believe they have made a solid case that the existing trials support the use of prophylactic magnesium or amiodarone as a safe option to significantly reduce the risk of developing atrial fibrillation after pulmonary resection. The use of 1 of these agents should be strongly considered by all surgeons for incorporation into their perioperative care to minimize the risk of atrial fibrillation postoperatively.

C. T. Klodell, Jr, MD

Early Removal of Urinary Catheter After Surgery Requiring Thoracic Epidural: A Prospective Trial

Hu Y, Craig SJ, Rowlingson JC, et al (Univ of Virginia School of Medicine, Charlottesville)
J Cardiothorac Vasc Anesth 28:1302-1306, 2014

Objectives.—To prevent urinary retention, urinary catheters commonly are removed only after thoracic epidural discontinuation after thoracotomy. However, prolonged catheterization increases the risk of infection. The purpose of this study was to determine the rates of urinary retention and catheter-associated infection after early catheter removal.

Design.—This study described a prospective trial instituting an early urinary catheter removal protocol compared with a historic control group of patients.

Setting.—The protocol was instituted at a single, academic thoracic surgery unit.

Participants.—The study group was comprised of patients undergoing surgery requiring thoracotomy who received an intraoperative epidural for postoperative pain control.

Interventions.—An early urinary catheter removal protocol was instituted prospectively, with all catheters removed on or before postoperative day 2. Urinary retention was determined by bladder ultrasound and treated with recatheterization.

Measurements and Main Results.—The primary outcomes were urinary retention rate, defined as bladder volume >400 mL, and urinary tract infection rate. Results were compared with a retrospective cohort of 210 consecutive patients who underwent surgery before protocol initiation. Among the 101 prospectively enrolled patients, urinary retention rate was higher (26.7% v 12.4%, $p = 0.003$), while urinary tract infection rate improved moderately (1% v 3.8%, $p = 0.280$).

Conclusions.—Early removal of urinary catheters with thoracic epidurals in place is associated with a high incidence of urinary retention. However, an early catheter removal protocol may play a role in a multifaceted approach to reducing the incidence of catheter-associated urinary tract infections.

▶ The purpose of this study was to determine the rates of urinary retention and catheter associated infection after early catheter removal. The authors' intervention was an attempt to remove all catheters on or before postoperative day 2 and compare the results for urinary retention and catheter associated urinary tract infection (CAUTI). They concluded that early removal of the catheters with thoracic epidurals in place was associated with a high incidence of urinary retention. However, an early catheter removal protocol can play a role in a multifaceted approach to reducing CAUTI. The biggest issue surrounding early removal of bladder catheters is postoperative urinary retention. Risk factors for retention include age, male gender, prostatic hypertrophy, type of surgery, and duration of general anesthetic. Thoracic operations are often a little longer and have greater issues with postoperative pain control requiring both epidural and parenteral opioid analgesia when compared with other patients who often use epidural strategies. The incidence of postoperative urinary retention with thoracic epidural in place, whether placed on a continuous infusion or a patient controlled infusion, has received increasing attention as CAUTI has become one of the most common complications following thoracic surgery. Early removal of indwelling urinary catheters may decrease the incidence of CAUTI, but it also may result in increased bladder retention. Additionally, the most common strategy for dealing with postoperative urinary retention is intermittent catheterization, which comes with its own host of complications and patient comfort issues. The Surgical Care Improvement Project (SCIP) has instituted national guidelines for early removal of urinary catheters on or before day 2. However, the impact of this practice on thoracic patients with epidurals is not yet clear.

Therefore, the authors set out to prospectively evaluate the incidence of postoperative urinary retention and CAUTI after adoption of the early removal protocol.

They enrolled consecutive patients undergoing thoracic surgery of the thoracotomy that received an epidural for postoperative pain control and compared them with historical control group from the same institution. Their epidural infusions were a combination of both hydromorphone and bupivacaine, and all indwelling catheters were removed on or before postoperative day 2. Patients were given the opportunity to void, and if they were able to void within 8 hours that was considered a success. If they were unable to void, they were divided into 2 groups, symptomatic or asymptomatic. In the asymptomatic group, bladder residuals greater than 400 cc by ultrasound led to intermittent catheterization, whereas less than 400 cc were reassessed in 4 hours. Symptomatic patients received intermittent catheterization. If they were unable to void within 8 hours, they then received an indwelling catheter again.

The benefits of epidural analgesia after thoracotomy are many and include improved respiratory function and decreased arrhythmias, as well as reduced respiratory infections. However, the incidence of postoperative urinary retention has historically been thought to be exceptionally high with thoracic epidurals in place, particularly when high-dose epidurals using bupivacaine were involved with rates perhaps as high as 33%. Other authors have reported rates as low as 5% with low doses of local anesthetic.

This prospective study demonstrated a urinary retention rate of 26.7%, with a modest improvement in CAUTI. It is reasonable to conclude that a protocol for removing indwelling catheters within 48 hours postoperatively among patients receiving thoracic surgery and epidural analgesia is associated with a relatively high rate of postoperative urinary retention. However, this may be necessary, and an early removal protocol may contribute to a multifaceted approach to reducing the rate of CAUTI.

Certainly, at our center we have experienced attempts at early withdrawal of catheters leading to unacceptable high rates of urinary retention when catheters are removed on postoperative day 1. The authors' strategy of removing them on day 2 and then the algorithmic approach to management may enhance both compliance and satisfaction. This seems a reasonable strategy for many centers to consider now with the emphasis on the SCIP measure for early removal and the intense focus on the reduction of CAUTI.

C. T. Klodell, Jr, MD

Intra-Operative Concerns

Staple Line Coverage After Bullectomy for Primary Spontaneous Pneumothorax: A Randomized Trial

Lee S, Korean Pneumothorax Study Group (Ajou Univ Hosp, Suwon, Korea; et al)
Ann Thorac Surg 98:2005-2011, 2014

Background.—Thoracoscopic wedge resection is generally accepted as a standard surgical procedure for primary spontaneous pneumothorax.

Because of the relatively high recurrence rate after surgery, additional procedures such as mechanical pleurodesis or visceral pleural coverage are usually applied to minimize recurrence, although mechanical pleurodesis has some potential disadvantages. The aim of this study was to clarify whether an additional coverage procedure on the staple line after thoracoscopic bullectomy prevents postoperative recurrence compared with additional pleurodesis.

Methods.—A total of 1,414 patients in 11 hospitals with primary spontaneous pneumothorax undergoing thoracoscopic bullectomy were enrolled. After bullectomy with staplers, patients were randomly assigned to either the coverage group (n = 757) or the pleurodesis group (n = 657). In the coverage group, the staple line was covered with absorbable cellulose mesh and fibrin glue. The pleurodesis group underwent additional mechanical abrasion on the parietal pleura.

Results.—The coverage group and the pleurodesis group showed comparable surgical outcomes. After a median follow-up of 19.5 months, the postoperative 1-year recurrence rate was 9.5% in the coverage group and 10.7% in the pleurodesis group. The 1-year recurrence rate requiring intervention was 5.8% in the coverage group and 7.8% in the pleurodesis group. The coverage group showed better recovery from pain.

Conclusions.—In terms of postoperative recurrence rate, visceral pleural coverage after thoracoscopic bullectomy was not inferior to mechanical pleurodesis. Visceral pleural coverage may potentially replace mechanical pleurodesis, which has potential disadvantages such as disturbed normal pleural physiology.

▶ Primary spontaneous pneumothorax (PSP) is not a serious disease but is troublesome because of its high rate of recurrence. General management strategies include plural drainage, with surgical intervention considered in cases of persistent air leakage or recurrent pneumothorax. The video-assisted thoracoscopic surgery (VATS) probably represents the most commonly applied surgical approach. Some have favored wedge resection alone, although this has been associated with a relatively high postoperative recurrence rate. This has led many surgeons to add additional adjunctive procedures such as mechanical pleurodesis with parietal pleura abrasion or pleurectomy after the wedge resection to minimize the chance of recurrence. However, some have noted concerns with this technique of pleurodesis, including pleural symphysis, which may disturb the normal physiology of the pleura as well as complicate future thoracic procedures. Other groups that have advocated for the use of adjunctive procedures, such as covering the surgical pulmonary margin with an absorbable mesh and fiber glue to reinforce the visceral pleura, report acceptable recurrence rates. Despite several smaller scale studies, no large-scale randomized trial had performed in this area. This led the authors to develop and execute this prospective, randomized, multicenter study aimed at determining the efficacy in preventing postoperative recurrence after thoracoscopic bullectomy with either additional staple line coverage procedure or an additional mechanical pleurodesis after thoracoscopic bullectomy. Over a 4-year period, the authors accrued an impressive 1414 patients who were then randomized at multiple centers but with a common technique that was disseminated by information packets and video clips of the procedure. All blebs were resected with an endoscopic stapling device, and then, after confirmation of no air leak, the patient was randomized to receive either a 3-cm staple line all around the lung, which was covered with absorbable cellulose mesh (Surgicel, Ethicon) and then fibrin glue, or alternatively randomized to mechanical pleurodesis, which was conducted by scrubbing the parietal pleura with sandpaper or gauze until oozing with pleura was confirmed. The results were quite reasonable with the coverage group and the pleurodesis group both demonstrating comparable surgical outcomes. At a median follow-up of 19.5 months, the recurrent rates were essentially the same at 9.5% in the coverage group and 10.7% in the pleurodesis group. Furthermore, the 1-year recurrence rate requiring intervention was only 5.8% in the coverage group and 7.8% in the pleurodesis group.

VATS has showed many advantages, such as reduced operation time, drainage time, and lower complication rates as well as perhaps less inflammatory response, shorter hospital stay, and clearly a more cosmetic outcome. However, with just bleb resection alone, the recurrence rate following VATS is unacceptably high perhaps, because of fewer adhesions after thoracoscopic surgery compared with open procedures of the past. Additional adjunctive procedures such as the authors describe are a reasonable middle ground because mechanical pleurodesis can have some deleterious long-term consequences in terms of pleural function and, perhaps more important, future surgeries in the young patient.

At our center, certainly mechanical pleurodesis is not a contraindication for future surgical interventions, including lung transplantation; however, we do have great concern over chemical pleurodesis. With that said, I think this shows us that perhaps staple-line coverage is a reasonable alternative to mechanical pleurodesis in the treatment of spontaneous pneumothorax, particularly in very young patients.

C. T. Klodell, Jr, MD

A Propensity-Matched Analysis of Wedge Resection and Stereotactic Body Radiotherapy for Early Stage Lung Cancer
Port JL, Parashar B, Osakwe N, et al (Weill Med College of Cornell Univ, NY)
Ann Thorac Surg 98:1152-1159, 2014

Background.—Patients who present with early stage non-small cell lung cancer and are poor candidates for lobar resection may be offered sublobar resection (commonly wedge) or stereotactic body radiotherapy (SBRT). However, comparing the relative effectiveness of these techniques is difficult because of differences in patient selection. We performed a propensity-matched analysis to compare the different treatment modalities. We compared the overall recurrence, overall survival, disease-free survival, and recurrence-free survival between treatment groups.

Methods.—A prospectively collected database was reviewed for patients who underwent a wedge resection, a wedge plus brachytherapy, or SBRT for clinical stage IA non-small cell lung cancer from 2001 to 2012. Patients who underwent SBRT were further assessed to confirm operability. Univariate and Cox regression multivariate analysis were performed for predictors of a composite end point of recurrence and mortality.

Results.—There were 164 patients identified, from which 99 were matched by age, sex, and histology. There were 61 women (62%) and 38 men (38%) with a median age of 73 years. Thirty-eight patients underwent a wedge resection only, 38 patients underwent a wedge with brachytherapy, and 23 patients had SBRT. Median follow-up was 35 months. Overall recurrence (local and distant) was significantly higher after SBRT (wedge, 9%; SBRT, 30%; $p = 0.016$). Although recurrence-free 3-year survival was significantly better after wedge resection (88% versus 72%; $p = 0.001$), there was no difference between the two groups in disease-free 3-year survival (77% versus 59%; $p = 0.066$). Multivariate regression analysis identified male sex and SBRT as significant predictors for mortality and recurrence.

Conclusions.—Patients with clinical stage IA non-small cell lung cancer treated by SBRT appear to have higher overall disease recurrence than those treated by wedge resection. However, there was no significant difference in disease-free survival. A randomized trial is needed to define the role of SBRT in the potentially operable patient.

▶ Patients who present with early stage non-small cell lung cancer but are poor candidates for lobar resection may occasionally be considered for therapeutic options such as sublobar resection or stereotactic body radiotherapy (SBRT). To date, there has not been a good comparative study performed, and the authors undertake a retrospective review of a prospectively collected database comparing these 2 groups of patients. Their findings include an overall recurrence rate that was significantly higher after SBRT and a recurrence-free survival that was significantly better after wedge resection; there was no difference between the groups in disease-free 3-year survival. The authors conclude that patients with clinical stage 1A non-small cell lung cancer should be treated by wedge resection as a first therapy but that SBRT may be appropriate in some circumstances.

This vexing problem confronts surgeons frequently when treating elderly and more medically compromised patients with lung cancer. Although lobar resection remains the standard of care, there are many times that a sublobar resection may be offered as an alternative for a medically compromised patient. The background of this type study comes from the excellent results of SBRT found in medically inoperable patients and, now, the transfer of that thought process to patients who are medically compromised but may still have adequate pulmonary reserve for sublobar resection, albeit borderline.

SBRT cases in this trial were routinely discussed in a multidisciplinary conference with thoracic surgical input. The SBRT patients most commonly fell into 2 groups. The first had adequate cardiopulmonary function but, because of a combination of prior lobar resection and a new central lesion, these patients would have required a completion pneumonectomy. The second group had adequate cardiopulmonary reserve for a limited resection; however, these patients were deemed not candidates because of the centrality of their lesions.

In contrast, the surgery patients who were selected for the sublobar resections were generally from 2 groups. All of the patients had centrally located lesions, but the first group had inadequate pulmonary function with a prior history of lobar resection. The second group had borderline cardiopulmonary reserve precluding lobar resection. Wedge resections were performed with a curative intent with a margin equaling to the diameter of the tumor plus at least 1-cm margin. Wedge resections were performed by both video-assisted thoracoscopy surgery and thoracotomy depending on the tumor depth location, reoperation, and the year of resection. Patients in both groups were followed in routine office visits and underwent routine CT scans every 6 months and, when clinically warranted, a positron emission tomography scan was obtained. Analysis demonstrated equivalent survival and recurrence rates between wedge resection alone and wedge resection with brachytherapy, and therefore, the surgical groups were combined for the remaining comparisons with SBRT. It was noted that the patients treated with SBRT were significantly older than the 2 surgical groups and that tumors in the surgical group were more peripheral in location. Of the patients who underwent surgery, 63% were performed by a VATS approach, and it is important to note that in the surgical groups, lymph nodes were harvested, resulting in a pathologic upstaging in 24% of patients in the surgical arm. There was no mortality in the surgical or SBRT patients at 30 days.

Recurrence occurred after surgery in 9.2% of the patients and after SBRT in 30.4% of the patients. Recurrence-free 3-year survival was higher after wedge resection, although there was no statistically significant difference in disease-free 3-year survival between the wedge resection and the SBRT groups.

Surgery remains the treatment of choice for early-stage lung cancer. Improvements in surgery and perioperative care along with greater adoption of video-assisted thoracoscopic and robotic surgery have reduced surgical mortality to approximately 1% and have led to a decreased length of stay for a majority of the patients. It is thought that up to 25% of early-stage lung cancer patients are not considered candidates for lobar resection because of severe medical comorbidities and previous lung resections. This important propensity-matched study compares patients having treatment that occurs contemporaneously and the outcomes of the surgical groups are consistent with modern standards. I think this reinforces our belief that patients that are candidates for sublobar resection should have surgery as their primary treatment while patients who cannot have sublobar resection because of being medically inoperable should have SBRT offered as a therapeutic intervention. Further studies will have to determine whether SBRT is ever going to be appropriate as a first-line therapy for borderline patients, but currently the data are not yet mature enough to make that conclusion.

C. T. Klodell, Jr, MD

Is Sleeve Lobectomy Comparable in Terms of Short- and Long-Term Results With Pneumonectomy After Induction Therapy? A Multicenter Analysis

Cusumano G, Marra A, Lococo F, et al (Catholic Univ, Rome, Italy; Niels Stensen Clinics, Ostercappeln, Germany; et al)
Ann Thorac Surg 98:975-983, 2014

Background.—Sleeve lobectomy (SL) is considered a valid therapeutic option in untreated, centrally located non-small cell lung cancer (NSCLC) even in patients "fit" for pneumonectomy (PN). Nevertheless, SL feasibility and long-term results after induction therapy (IT) have been only rarely investigated. We herein report the results of a multicenter retrospective study on NSCLC patients who underwent PN or SL after IT for locally advanced NSCLC.

Methods.—From January 1992 to January 2012, 119 consecutive patients (94 males, 25 females) underwent in three tertiary referral centers either SL (bronchial, arterial, or both) or PN for locally advanced NSCLC after IT (chemotherapy alone or combined chemoradiotherapy). The indication for SL was based on technical feasibility. Clinical and pathologic variables were retrospectively reviewed, and treatment results were assessed and compared in both groups. Survival was calculated by Kaplan-Meier method and compared by the log-rank test as well the Cox regression model.

Results.—Sleeve lobectomy was performed in 51 patients and PN, in 68 patients. Thirty-day mortality and morbidity rates were 3.9% and 9.8% for SL and 2.9% and 22.1% for PN, respectively. Five-year survival rates were 53.8% after SL and 43.1% after PN, respectively ($p = 0.28$). Overall recurrence rate was 42.8% after SL and 47.0% after PN ($p = 0.34$); relapse was locoregional in 22.4% of SL cases and 12.1% after PN, respectively ($p = 0.011$). The Cox analysis suggested pN status and right side as independent risk factors for death in the SL group (hazard ratio, 1.96; 95% confidence interval, 1.12 to 3.44; $p = 0.018$; and hazard ratio, 2.96; 95% confidence interval, 1.13 to 8.66; $p = 0.047$, respectively). As well, pN status and right side were a strong predictor of relapse (hazard ratio, 2.33; 95% confidence interval, 1.17 to 4.64; $p = 0.016$; and hazard ratio, 2.96; 95% confidence interval, 1.13 to 8.66; $p = 0.046$, respectively) in SL patients.

Conclusions.—For locally advanced NSCLC, SL represents a safe and effective surgical option when compared with PN even after IT, with substantially comparable early and long-term results. Nevertheless, further investigations on a large cohort of patients are needed.

▶ Pneumonectomy has been considered for many years the gold standard in the treatment of centrally located non-small cell lung cancer. Considering the potential high risk of morbidity, mortality, and reduction of quality of life associated with removal of an entire lung, a lung-sparing strategy of resection has been widely supported with the aims of completeness of tumor resection and at the same time preserving maximal lung function.

Sleeve lobectomy is usually reserved for centrally located lung masses with the tumor located in a lobar bronchus that invades the main stem bronchus. Although this kind of procedure was originally adopted in patients with limited pulmonary function and judged as clinically unfit for pneumonectomy, more recently, consideration has been given that this could be extended whenever technically possible irrespective of the patient's ability to tolerate a pneumonectomy. Although the feasibility and efficacy of the sleeve procedure has been well confirmed, the short- and long-term results after induction therapy are less well studied, especially with concerns about postoperative risks, including radiation-associated anastomotic failure. The aim of the authors' review was to study the experiences in 3 high-volume centers surrounding this clinical issue. For that purpose, they evaluated the postoperative results and particularly anastomotic failure and survival in a patient cohort that had locally advanced non-cell lung cancer treated with either induction therapy followed with either sleeve lobectomy or pneumonectomy. Finally, they paid particular attention to the impact of preoperative radiation therapy on complication rates.

In all, they studied 119 patients, all of whom had an interdisciplinary risk analysis before starting treatment and in planning the induction therapy. The surgery was performed 2 weeks after clinical restaging and a total of 4 to 6 weeks from the last course of chemotherapy and radiation. Access to the thoracic cavity was a muscle-sparing lateral or postlateral thoracotomy. In all cases, sleeve lobectomy was carried out whenever possible and not limited to those patients in which functional reserve contraindicated pneumonectomy. The 30-day mortality rate was similar between the 2 groups with 3.9% in the sleeve lobectomy group and 2.9% in the pneumectomy. Additionally, radiotherapy did not affect the risk of death or postoperative complications.

The authors have reported the outcomes of a large cohort of a non-small cell patients who underwent either a sleeve lobectomy or a pneumonectomy after induction therapy. Their data suggested that sleeve lobectomy continues to represent a valuable procedure as part of a multimodality treatment with an acceptable risk of postoperative morbidity and mortality. Additionally, several studies have now confirmed encouraging results with acceptable postoperative short- and long-term outcomes after pneumonectomy subsequent to induction therapy. The bronchoplastic approach after induction therapy seems to result in a lower morbidity rate when compared with standard pneumonectomy and results in preservation of a greater amount of residual lung.

This and other current data continue to support extending the indication of sleeve lobectomy for non-small cell lung cancer after induction therapy whenever technically possible. Considering the relatively low morbidity and mortality rate and the preservation of the appropriate surgical outcomes, it would seem appropriate to consider this as the standard of care first-line approach, irrespective of the pulmonary function test ability to tolerate a complete pneumonectomy.

C. T. Klodell, Jr, MD

Lobectomy, Sublobar Resection, and Stereotactic Ablative Radiotherapy for Early-Stage Non-Small Cell Lung Cancers in the Elderly

Shirvani SM, Jiang J, Chang JY, et al (The Univ of Texas MD Anderson Cancer Ctr, Houston)

JAMA Surg 149:1244-1253, 2014

Importance.—The incidence of early-stage non–small cell lung cancer (NSCLC) among the elderly is expected to rise dramatically owing to demographic trends and increased computed tomographic screening. However, to our knowledge, no modern trials have compared the most common treatments for NSCLC.

Objective.—To determine clinical characteristics and survival outcomes associated with the 3 most commonly used definitive therapies for early-stage NSCLC in the elderly.

Design, Setting, and Participants.—The Surveillance, Epidemiology, and End Results database linked to Medicare was used to determine the baseline characteristics and outcomes of 9093 patients with early-stage, node-negative NSCLC who underwent definitive treatment consisting of lobectomy, sublobar resection, or stereotactic ablative radiotherapy (SABR) from January 1, 2003, through December 31, 2009.

Main Outcomes and Measures.—Overall and lung cancer-specific survival were compared using Medicare claims through December 31, 2012. We used proportional hazards regression and propensity score matching to adjust outcomes for key patient, tumor, and practice environment factors.

Results.—The median age was 75 years, and treatment distribution was 79.3% for lobectomy, 16.5% for sublobar resection, and 4.2% for SABR. Unadjusted 90-day mortality was highest for lobectomy (4.0%) followed by sublobar resection (3.7%; *P* =.79) and SABR (1.3%; *P* =.008). At 3 years, unadjusted mortality was lowest for lobectomy (25.0%), followed by sublobar resection (35.3%; *P* < .001) and SABR (45.1%; *P* < .001). Proportional hazards regression demonstrated that sublobar resection was associated with worse overall survival (adjusted hazard ratio [AHR], 1.32 [95% CI, 1.20-1.44]; *P* < .001) and lung cancer–specific survival (AHR, 1.50 [95% CI, 1.29-1.75]; *P* < .001) compared with lobectomy. Propensity score–matching analysis reiterated these findings for overall survival (AHR, 1.36 [95% CI, 1.17-1.58]; *P* < .001) and lung cancer–specific survival (AHR, 1.46 [95% CI, 1.13-1.90]; *P* =.004). In proportional hazards regression, SABR was associated with better overall survival than lobectomy in the first 6 months after diagnosis (AHR, 0.45 [95% CI, 0.27-0.75]; *P* < .001) but worse survival thereafter (AHR, 1.66 [95% CI, 1.39-1.99]; *P* < .001). Propensity score–matching analysis of well-matched SABR and lobectomy cohorts demonstrated similar overall survival in both groups (AHR, 1.01 [95% CI, 0.74-1.38]; *P* =.94).

Conclusions and Relevance.—Lobectomy was associated with better outcomes than sublobar resection in elderly patients with early-stage

NSCLC. Propensity score matching suggests that SABR may be a good option among patients with very advanced age and multiple comorbidities.

▶ In the coming years, 2 public health developments are expected to affect the incidence of early-stage non-small cell lung cancer (NSCLC) in the United States. The first is the recent recommendations in favor of CT screening for lung cancer among long-term smokers. This is in response to the National Lung Cancer Screening Trial, which demonstrated a reduction in lung cancer mortality among patients undergoing appropriate screening. Secondarily, the advancing age of the population estimates that by 2030 the incidence of non-small cell lung cancer among adults older than 65 years is expected to rise to 271 000 cases annually. These 2 factors will additively place pressure on the health care system to provide effective and cost-conscious care. However, no recent randomized trials have compared contemporary treatment strategies for elderly patients. In fact, the most recent trial on which most of our recommendations are based is the Lung Cancer Study Group (LCSG) 821 trial, which suggested lobectomy resulted in fewer failures and improved survival compared to sublobar resections for non-small cell lung cancer. However, this trial was completed more than 20 years ago.

Several new trials have been opened in an attempt to further elucidate this issue. However, they have been stalled by poor enrollment, and several have been closed. The authors reviewed 9093 patients treated definitively for early-stage non-small cell lung cancer over a 6-year period in contemporary times. The median age was 75, and 54% were female. Seventy-nine percent (79%) underwent lobectomy, 16% sublobar resection, and 4.2% stereotactic ablative radiotherapy. As expected, the surgical patients were younger and had fewer comorbidities than those who were treated with radiation therapy. When comparing lobectomy with sublobar resection, the lobectomy again proved superior in terms of overall survival and lung cancer-free survival.

The adoption of widespread CT screening for lung cancer will increase the number of patients identified with non-small cell lung cancer and the number of patients seen by surgeons for evaluation. Overall, this will be an outstanding benefit for patient care because a mortality benefit will accrue from the timely identification of malignant lung nodules. However, the strain on the US health care system will be significant. This will be especially true as more elderly patients with more comorbidities, such as chronic obstructive pulmonary disease, coronary artery disease, and other concerns are diagnosed as having non-small cell lung cancer. The findings of this trial are essentially concordant with those of the LCSG 821 trial, suggesting that lobectomy should be the standard of care for all patients who can tolerate it irrespective of their chronologic age. The findings in this trial also support the efficacy of stereotactic ablative radiotherapy in frail patients with advanced age, and this technology appears promising and may offer a lower rate of periprocedural mortality with encouraging long-term survival results that are deemed to be marginal candidates for surgery.

C. T. Klodell, Jr, MD

Staging of Non-small Cell Lung Cancer

Cost-Effectiveness of Initial Diagnostic Strategies for Pulmonary Nodules Presenting to Thoracic Surgeons

Deppen SA, Davis WT, Green EA, et al (Vanderbilt Univ Med Ctr, TN)
Ann Thorac Surg 98:1214-1222, 2014

Background.—Patients presenting to thoracic surgeons with pulmonary nodules suggestive of lung cancer have varied diagnostic options including navigation bronchoscopy (NB), computed tomography-guided fineneedle aspiration (CT-FNA), ^{18}F-fluoro-deoxyglucose positron emission tomography (FDG-PET) and video-assisted thoracoscopic surgery (VATS). We studied the relative cost-effective initial diagnostic strategy for a 1.5- to 2-cm nodule suggestive of cancer.

Methods.—A decision analysis model was developed to assess the costs and outcomes of four initial diagnostic strategies for diagnosis of a 1.5- to 2-cm nodule with either a 50% or 65% pretest probability of cancer. Medicare reimbursement rates were used for costs. Quality-adjusted life years were estimated using patient survival based on pathologic staging and utilities derived from the literature.

Results.—When cancer prevalence was 65%, tissue acquisition strategies of NB and CT-FNA had higher quality-adjusted life years compared with either FDG-PET or VATS, and VATS was the most costly strategy. In sensitivity analyses, NB and CT-FNA were more cost-effective than FDG-PET when FDG-PET specificity was less than 72%. When cancer prevalence was 50%, NB, CT-FNA, and FDG-PET had similar cost-effectiveness.

Conclusions.—Both NB and CT-FNA diagnostic strategies are more cost-effective than either VATS biopsy or FDG-PET scan to diagnose lung cancer in moderate- to high-risk nodules and resulted in fewer non-therapeutic operations when FDG-PET specificity was less than 72%. An FDG-PET scan for diagnosis of lung cancer may not be cost-effective in regions of the country where specificity is low.

▶ The authors review the varied diagnostic options, including navigation bronchoscopy (NB), CT-guided fine needle aspiration (CT-FNA), and fludeoxyglucose positron emission tomography (FDG-PET) as well as video-assisted thoracoscopy surgery (VATS). They conclude that both NB and CT-FNA are more cost-effective than either VATS biopsy or FDG-PET to diagnose lung cancer in moderate to high-risk nodules and resulted in fewer nontherapeutic operations when FDG-PET specificity was less than 72%. An FDG-PET scan for the diagnosis of lung cancer may not be cost-effective in regions of the country where specificity is low. This is an interesting twist on a diagnostic decision that surgeons face frequently in that it encompasses the cost-effectiveness of the various strategies.

The management of pulmonary nodules suggestive of lung cancer is a combination of both art and science and most recently the U.S. Preventive Services

Task Force has recommended low-dose CT screening for healthy individuals at high risk for lung cancer. It is predicted that this may lead to the discovery of as many as 1 to 2 million more suspicious nodules annually, given the current clinical screening recommendations. Patients with these suspicious nodules will require additional test for diagnosis, and many will be evaluated by a surgeon. Currently, FDG-PET is suggested for noninvasive diagnosis of nodules greater than 0.8 cm with a clinical probability of lung cancer between 5% and 65%. CT-guided FNA is an alternative diagnostic technique with diagnostic accuracy of approximately 77% in peripheral nodes that are amenable to needle biopsy. However, it is known that approximately 41% of CT-FNAs biopsies are non-diagnostic. Alternative strategies include the computer-assisted NB, the virtual bronchoscopy, and radial endobronchial ultrasound to help clinicians navigate beyond the hilum and biopsy suspicious lesions in the peripheral lung fields with increased diagnostic yield.

Their test case for their analysis is a 60-year-old man with a 15-pack-a-year history, no prior history of lung cancer, and a 1.5- to 2-cm nodule in an upper lobe incidentally observed on a CT scan. The nodule is either spiculated or has grown at 15% in diameter on serial radiographs, but not both. The individual is deemed a good operative candidate and would tolerate lobectomy. Based on clinical risks lung cancer scoring lists, this patient would have an approximately 65% prediction of lung cancer. In their analysis, the FDG-PET had the lowest expected cost for diagnosing patients at $10 410; compared with FGD-PET, patients' diagnoses with by NB incurred an expected incremental cost of only $191, making it also a very cost-effective strategy.

In clinical practice, we are frequently asked to see patients with suspicious lesions, and the first step should be an estimation of the likelihood of cancer made by a combination of some clinical model for cancer risk prediction combined with clinical judgment and acumen. Patients with a probability of cancer ranging between 5% and 65% need a diagnostic workup such as FDG-PET or NB. Patients with a greater than 65% chance of cancer may be recommended to go directly to VATS biopsy. However, in the authors' analysis, the use of VATS biopsy for the diagnosis was not preferred over the other diagnostic methods unless the prevalence of malignancy was thought to be greater than 85%.

The authors should be congratulated on taking the guidelines and placing some cost-effectiveness data alongside them to help guide us. If the lung screening program truly does yield 1 to 2 million additional nodules needing workup each year, this data will be invaluable in helping surgeons select the appropriate diagnostic methods based on a combination of clinical risk scoring models and their clinical expertise.

C. T. Klodell, Jr, MD

Tumor Biology and Prognostic Variables

Optimal timing of pulmonary metastasectomy — Is a delayed operation beneficial or counterproductive?

Krüger M, Schmitto JD, Wiegmann B, et al (Hannover Med School, Germany; Brigham and Women's Hosp and Harvard Med School, Boston, MA)
Eur J Surg Oncol 40:1049-1055, 2014

Introduction.—Pulmonary metastasectomy represents an established approach in the treatment of lung metastases related to several solid malignant tumors, promising the chance of long term survival. Regarding the proper timing of metastasectomy both operation promptly after diagnosis and delayed operation after an interval of 3 months are common practice.

Materials and Methods.—A systematic Medline search addressing the optimal timing of metastasectomy was performed. Since the search query "timing of metastasectomy" yields only a limited number of articles, the Medline search was expanded to include the main arguments for prompt metastasectomy ("metastases of metastasis", "growth rate of pulmonary metastases") and for delayed metastasectomy.

Results.—Based on the data available to date, there is no necessity to expedite the timing of the operation. On the other hand, there is no evidence that a delayed operation, for example after re-staging following an interval of 3 months, provides a benefit.

Conclusion.—Therefore the timing of metastasectomy should only depend on the patient's requirements, such as general state of health and oncologic considerations, such as promising multimodal therapy concepts, extrathoracal tumor manifestations or oncologic type of the primary tumor. A delayed operation seems justified if the indication for resection is questionable due to a high risk of early multilocal recurrence.

▶ Pulmonary metastasectomy remains an established approach in the treatment of lung metastases related to several solid organ malignant tumors. The authors review the available literature, systematically addressing to determine if there is any guidance as to whether immediate metastasectomy should be performed or whether there is an advantage to the commonly applied 3-month interval delay to allow further elucidation of the patient disease. They conclude that the timing of metastasectomy should depend only on the patient requirements, such as general state of health and oncologic considerations promising multimodal therapy concepts and extrathoracic tumor manifestations. They further concluded that a delayed operation seems justified if the indication for resection is questionable or high risk due to early multilocal recurrence.

In general, local control of solid malignant tumors is nearly always achievable; however, it is the malignant metastatic diseases that often prove life limiting. The lung is often the first filter for hematogenous metastases of many solid malignant tumors. Therefore, pulmonary metastases are frequent and have increasingly become a focus for surgical procedures. Several retrospective publications have thoroughly demonstrated significantly increased long-term survival after pulmonary metastasectomy. However, key questions such as the timing of said metastasectomy remain to be more fully elucidated. It is common that some surgeons have recommended operating as soon as the patients' clinical situation allows it, often based on the fear that metastases could generate new metastases or concern for rapid local tumor progression. Yet others have preferred a diagnostic interval of 3 months after the initial diagnosis of pulmonary metastases either routinely or in selected patients to allow full characterization of their metastatic disease burden.

Although there are some animal data suggesting that metastases can give off further metastases, there is complete absence of such evidence in humans. In general, it seems most would agree that metastatic foci are not at risk for generating additional metastases after the primary tumor has been removed.

Pulmonary metastasectomy is a widely accepted therapeutic option for metastases of various solid organ tumors; however, because of the lack of randomized data, there are certainly distinct variability among the practice of different thoracic surgeons regarding the approach and timing. Interestingly, about 15%–20% of patients with pulmonary metastases will demonstrate mediastinal hilar lymph node involvement. The majority of series lymph node involvement is seen as an adverse prognostic factor. Furthermore, although repeated metastasectomies are not per se a negative predictor for overall survival, it certainly does have consequences for the patient physically. It should be noted that the majority of data evaluated in the review these authors have undertaken is based on metastasectomies from metastases of colorectal cancer, soft-tissue sarcoma, and renal cell carcinoma. It is unclear whether the results can be extrapolated to other solid tissue tumors.

In summary, the timing of metastasectomy should depend only on patients' condition such as general state of health, and on oncologic considerations, promising multimodal therapy concepts, extrathoracic tumor manifestations, and oncologic type of the primary tumor. As the authors have pointed out, it is justified to perform a delayed operation if the indication for resection is questionable because of a high risk of early multilocal relapse. However, I do think it is prudent to approach each patient individually because some patients have already had a period of observation before being evaluated by a thoracic surgeon, and the tumor doubling time can be roughly estimated by the intervals on the scans. In these cases, there may be exceptions in which it is prudent to watch for a short period of time to allow what is noted as small nodules to grow to a palpable size to ensure therapeutic resection and "clearing of the chest."

C. T. Klodell, Jr, MD

Unexpected Lymph Node Disease in Resections for Pulmonary Metastases
Seebacher G, Decker S, Fischer JR, et al (Klinik Löwenstein, Germany; Missionsärztliche Klinik, Würzburg, Germany; Saarland Univ Med Ctr, Homburg/Saar, Germany)
Ann Thorac Surg 99:231-237, 2015

Background.—Pulmonary metastasectomy is widely accepted for different malignant diseases. The role of mediastinal lymph node (LN) dissection in these procedures is discussed controversially. We evaluated our results of LN removal at the time of pulmonary metastasectomy with respect to the frequency of unexpected LN disease.

Methods.—This was a retrospective analysis of 313 resections performed in 209 patients. Operations were performed in curative intention. Patients with known thoracic LN involvement and those without lymphadenectomy (n = 43) were excluded. Patients were analyzed according to the type of LN dissection. Subgroups of different primary cancers were evaluated separately.

Results.—Sublobar resections were performed in 256 procedures with lymphadenectomy, and 14 patients underwent lobectomy. Patients underwent radical lymphadenectomy (n = 158) or LN sampling (n = 112). The overall incidence of unexpected tumor in LN was 17% (radical lymphadenectomy, 15.8%; sampling, 18.8%). Unexpected LN involvement was found in 17 patients (35.5%) with breast cancer, in 120 (9.2%) with colorectal cancer, and in 53 (20.8%) with renal cell carcinoma. The 5-year survival was 30.2% if LN were tumor negative and 25% if positive ($p = 0.19$). LN sampling vs radical removal had no significant effect on 5-year survival (23.6% vs 30.9%; $p = 0.29$).

Conclusions.—Dissection of mediastinal LN in resection of lung metastases will reveal unexpected LN involvement in a relevant proportion of patients, in particular in breast and renal cancer. Routine LN dissection appears necessary and may become important for further therapeutic decisions. On the basis of our data, LN sampling seems to be sufficient.

▶ Depending on the histology of the primary tumor, resection of pulmonary metastases is widely accepted and supported by various studies. The role of lymph node dissection during surgery for metastatic lung nodules is certainly a controversial topic. Whereas some groups perform no lymph node dissection, others prefer sampling, and yet others prefer a radical regional lymphadenectomy. The decision for lymph node dissection is frequently based on preoperative imaging such as the CT or positron emission tomography scans. The authors attempted to analyze the incidence of unexpected metastatic disease at the time of mediastinal lymph node dissection during pulmonary metastasectomy for different extrapulmonary tumor entities. The lymph node sampling versus systematic dissection was also investigated. The authors included 110 men and 99 women in their retrospective review, including the 3 most frequent tumor entities of colorectal carcinoma, renal carcinoma, and breast cancer. In the 270 procedures with lymph node resection, the incidence of unsuspected tumor involvement of the lymph nodes was 17%. The incidence of colorectal carcinoma having positive mediastinal lymph nodes was 9.2%; it was higher in breast cancer patients at 35% and in renal cell carcinoma patients at nearly 21%. The number of resected metastatic foci appeared to be a prognostic factor for the development of unexpected lymph node disease. Not surprisingly, survival at 5 years was noted to be higher in patients that did not have unexpected lymph node metastasis.

The dissection of mediastinal lymph nodes during the resection of lung metastasis should be considered a standard portion of the operation. The lymph nodes will be noted to reveal unexpected lymph node involvement with metastatic tumor in a not insignificant percentage of patients, particularly in kidney and breast cancer patients. This may not only offer additional therapeutic treatment options as part of study protocols but also offers important prognostic information to the patient. This may represent a departure from how many of us were classically trained in just performing a wedge resection for metastatic foci without lymph node dissection. I believe that anyone participating in routine metastatsectomies should perform lymph node resection as part of the procedure.

C. T. Klodell, Jr, MD

Intermediate-term oncologic outcomes after video-assisted thoracoscopic thymectomy for early-stage thymoma
Sakamaki Y, Oda T, Kanazawa G, et al (Osaka Police Hosp, Japan; et al)
J Thorac Cardiovasc Surg 148:1230-1237, 2014

Objective.—To evaluate the impact on patient survival of video-assisted thoracoscopic surgery (VATS) thymectomy for the treatment of early-stage thymoma, by comparing the intermediate-term oncologic outcomes with outcomes after open thymectomy.

Methods.—Eighty-two patients who underwent complete resection of a Masaoka stage I or II thymoma between November 1998 and December 2011 were reviewed.

Results.—The patients included 32 men and 50 women (median age, 57 years; range, 20-90 years), of whom 44 had stage I thymoma and 38 had stage II thymoma. Seventy-one patients underwent VATS, of whom 4 (5.6%) underwent conversion to open thymectomy; the remaining 11 patients underwent planned open thymectomy. Thirty-six patients underwent total thymectomy and 46 underwent partial thymectomy. Operative mortality was nil. The tumor stage, tumor size, and proportion of patients who underwent total thymectomy were not significantly different between the open and VATS thymectomy groups. The median follow-up period was 49 months (VATS, 48 months; open, 52 months). There was a significant difference between the 2 groups for the estimated 5-year overall survival (VATS, 97.0%; open, 79.5%; P =.041) but not in the estimated 5-year recurrence-free survival.

Conclusions.—Our findings indicate that the intermediate-term oncologic outcomes after VATS thymectomy for early-stage thymoma are as favorable as outcomes after open thymectomy. Further follow-up is still required to evaluate the long-term outcomes after VATS thymectomy.

▶ The authors set out to evaluate the impact on patient survival of video-assisted thoracoscopic surgery (VATS) thymectomy for the treatment of early-stage thymoma and compared the intermediate-term oncologic outcomes with outcomes after open thymectomy. They ultimately conclude that the intermediate-term oncological outcomes are favorable for VATS thymectomy for early-stage thymoma and that it remains a viable alternative.

Complete resection is the most important predictor of long-term survival in patients with stage I or II thymoma. In stage I or II thymoma, a thymectomy usually achieves complete resection, resulting in favorable long-term outcomes. Although many reports have suggested that VATS thymectomy for early stage-thymoma is technically feasible and safe, long-term follow-up studies have not yet become available in great number.

This article presents the single-center experience of treatment of early-stage thymoma over a 13 year period using VATS as the most common surgical approach. Interestingly, in their data set, partial thymectomy was performed more commonly than total thymectomy for stage I and stage II thymoma. During the study period, the surgical approach selected was VATS thymectomy as the default choice if the planned tumor characteristics on computed tomography and/or magnetic resonance imaging were noninvasive, and then open thymectomy if there appeared to be tumor invasion of the great vessels or the pericardium was either suggested or could not be excluded.

There were no statistically significant differences between open and VATS thymectomy in terms of age, male-to-female ratio, proportions that underwent total thymectomy, adjuvant radiotherapy, or with improvement in myasthenia gravis after surgery. Patients who underwent VATS thymectomy tended to have smaller thymomas and a higher likelihood of stage I disease. Clearly, the patients who had open thymectomy had a higher incidence of resection of adjacent structures including pericardium, left innominate vein, phrenic nerve, and peripheral lung tissue.

There were no statistically significant differences in the operating times between patients who underwent open total thymectomy and those who underwent VATS total thymectomy or between those who underwent partial thymectomy either open or via VATS. Their conversion rate was 5.6% and usually resulted from either adhesions between the tumor and the innominate vein or was due to uncontrollable bleeding.

Most previous studies for thoracoscopic thymectomy for thymoma have reported favorable short-term surgical outcomes but have not highlighted the oncological outcomes. However, some other studies have reported survival and recurrence data up to 10 years after VATS thymectomy. These authors 13-year experience continues to support the role of VATS for treatment of stage I and stage II thymoma and to demonstrate favorable intermediate-term oncological outcomes compared with open surgery.

It is critical for the surgeon to consider the radiographic findings in the likelihood of invasion of adjacent structures when selecting VATS vs open thymectomy. Additionally, although there is no absolute size cutoff for VATS thymectomy, it is thought to be technically feasible for thymoma measuring up to 5 cm in diameter. This study is somewhat limited by the retrospective, nonrandomized design and the obvious selection bias by how they decided on either VATS or open approach. However, their findings of favorable intermediate-term oncological outcomes after VATS thymectomy for treatment of early-stage thymoma are reassuring to many of us who have continued to use this minimally invasive approach for early-stage thymoma. I have personally found the robotic approach using a unilateral right-sided robotic approach to most thymomas to be exceptionally favorable and the enhanced magnification afforded by the robot valuable in ensuring total thymectomy and excellent control of the thymic veins.

C. T. Klodell, Jr, MD

Lung Transplantation

Diverticulitis occurs early after lung transplantation
Larson ES, Khalil HA, Lin AY, et al (UCLA; et al)
J Surg Res 190:667-671, 2014

Background.—Lung transplantation recipients are at an increased risk for developing diverticulitis. However, the incidence and natural history of diverticulitis have not been well characterized. Our objective was to identify patient and transplant-related factors that may be associated with an increased risk of developing diverticulitis in this patient population.

Materials and Methods.—This is a retrospective single institution study. All patients who received a lung transplant between May 2008 and July 2013 were evaluated using an existing lung transplantation database. Patient-related factors, the incidence and timing of diverticulitis, and outcomes of medical and surgical management were measured.

Results.—Of the 314 patients who received a lung transplant, 14 patients (4.5%) developed diverticulitis. All episodes (100%) of diverticulitis occurred within the first 2 y after transplantation. Eight patients (57%) required surgery with a mortality rate of 12.5%. Six patients (43%) were managed medically and did not require surgery with a mean follow-up period of 442 d.

Conclusions.—Diverticulitis is common after lung transplantation and occurs with a higher incidence compared with the general population. Diverticulitis occurs early in the posttransplant period, and the majority of patients require surgery. Patients who respond promptly to medical treatment may not require elective resection. A greater awareness of the risk of diverticulitis in the early posttransplant period may allow for earlier diagnosis and treatment.

▶ Intra-abdominal complications are a major source of postoperative morbidity in patients who have undergone solid organ transplantation. Lung transplantation is particularly troublesome in that it requires some of the highest levels of immunosuppression due to the constant contact with the external environment. This high immunocompromised state predisposes the patient to infectious complications such as diverticulitis. The authors' purpose for their study was to better define the natural history in diverticulitis in the lung transplant population, and they sought to determine patient- or transplant-related factors that may be associated to increased risks for developing diverticulitis. They also evaluated the outcomes of surgery for diverticulitis in lung transplant population and the appropriateness of conservative nonoperative management in elective resection.

They performed a retrospective single institution review of lung transplantation over a 5-year period. In their institution, standard immunosuppression regimen included thymoglobulin for patients aged less than 60 years and basiliximab for patients older than 60 years. Additionally, patients received pulsed dose Solu-Medrol concurrent with transplantation and are maintained on prednisone with a tapering schedule over a 6-week period to a maintenance dose of 10–15 mg daily. Subsequently, they may receive additional pulsed-dose steroids for rejection episodes. In their study, there were 8 surgically managed patients who had abdominal scanned findings that were consistent with a more severe form of diverticulitis, including thickening of the sigmoid colon and pericolonic fat stranding as well as extraluminal gas or free air or an abscess. In contrast, 6 patients were successfully treated with medical therapy that radiographically has less severe disease.

Although few guidelines exist regarding the optimal management of diverticulitis in the lung transplant population, the authors should be congratulated on this review in which they point out that these are high-risk patients because they can mask physical signs and symptoms due to an immunosuppression regimen that is high even compared with other solid organ transplants. Importantly from their study, they identify that diverticulitis typically occurs within the first 2 years after lung transplantation. They additionally identify that lung transplant patients who required surgery for diverticulitis were more likely to have a prior history of diverticulitis and to have CT scan findings consistent with more severe disease population. In this group that underwent surgery, the mortality rate was 12.5%. Conversely, favorable CT scan findings suggested that they would respond to medical treatment and many could be managed conservatively without elective surgical resection. Furthermore, the overall incidence of diverticulitis in this population was 4.5%, which is consistent with other studies and is much higher than the incidence of the general population, which is estimated at 0.5%. The incidence of diverticulitis in their population was higher in the single lung transplant population compared with the bilateral transplant group. However, this is likely because the patients who received the single-lung transplantation were of a more advanced age group. Diverticulitis tends to occur in older recipients and is more common in the early posttransplant period.

This study is exceptionally important in reminding us that infectious complications—in particular, intra-abdominal processes such as diverticulitis—can be quite common after solid organ transplantation, especially when compared with the rates of the general population. An attitude of hypervigilance toward the identification and subsequent treatment of these patients may help reduce the relatively high 12.5% mortality noted in the patients with severe enough disease to require surgical treatment.

C. T. Klodell, Jr, MD

Miscellaneous

Spontaneous Pneumomediastinum: An Extensive Workup Is Not Required
Bakhos CT, Pupovac SS, Ata A, et al (Albany Med College, NY)
J Am Coll Surg 219:713-717, 2014

Background.—Spontaneous pneumomediastinum is a rare entity usually caused by alveolar rupture and air tracking along the tracheobronchial tree. Despite its benign nature, an extensive workup is often undertaken to exclude hollow viscus perforation. We sought to review our experience with this condition and examine the optimal management strategy.

Study Design.—We conducted a retrospective review of all radiographic pneumomediastinum cases at a tertiary hospital between 2006 and 2011. The main outcomes measures included length of hospital stay, mortality, and need for investigative procedures.

Results.—Forty-nine patients with spontaneous pneumomediastinum were identified, including 26 male patients (53%). Mean age was 19 ± 9 years. Chest pain was the most common presenting symptom (65%), followed by dyspnea (51%). Forceful coughing (29%) or vomiting (16%) were the most common eliciting factors, and no precipitating event was identified in 41% of patients. Computed tomography was performed in 38 patients (78%) and showed a pneumomediastinum that was not seen on chest x-ray in 9 patients. Esophagography was performed in 17 patients (35%) and was invariably negative for a leak. Thirty-eight patients (78%) were hospitalized for a mean of 1.8 ± 2.6 days. No mortality was recorded. Compared with patients who presented with pneumomediastinum secondary to esophageal perforation, spontaneous pneumomediastinum patients were younger, had a lower white cell count, and were less likely to have a pleural effusion.

Conclusions.—Spontaneous pneumomediastinum is a benign entity and rarely correlates with true esophageal perforation. Additional investigation with esophagography or other invasive procedures should be performed selectively with the aim of expediting the patient's care. The prognosis is excellent with conservative management and the risk for recurrence is low.

▶ Pneumomediastinum is defined by the presence of free air in the mediastinum and is generally caused by alveolar rupture resulting from a sudden increase in the intrathoracic pressure. This air then escapes from the alveoli to the interstinum and tracks along the tracheobronchial tree as well as along the vasculature. Pneumomediastinum can generally be categorized into 2 types: the spontaneous and secondary types. The secondary type usually reflects a violation of the aerodigestive tract and can be due to trauma, surgery, and other interventions or caused by gas forming mediastinal infections. In contrast, spontaneous pneumomediastinum is a diagnosis of exclusion and usually a benign condition related to intrathoracic pressure such as forceful coughing or a Valsalva maneuver. Besides the basic history and physical examination, many imaging studies and/or invasive procedures are often performed, and patients are often hospitalized to exclude a more serious aerodigestive tract injury or perforation. The authors report one of the largest series in literature performing a retrospective review over a 5-year period and identifying 49 patients. Of the 49 patients, in the group that had no history of intervention, induced vomiting, or trauma 53% were male and the mean age was 19 years. Chest pain was the most common presenting symptom followed by dyspnea and neck pain, and no precipitating event could be identified in 41% of the patients. Esophagography was performed in 35% of the patients and was invariably negative for a leak. Seventy-eight percent (78%) of the patients were admitted to the hospital with a mean length of stay of 1.8 days. Conversely, group 2 included patients who had a higher potential of pneumomediastinum thought to be secondary to esophageal perforation. These patients were older, had higher white cell count at admission, and tended to have a higher body mass index and heart rate. They were also often noted to have a pleural effusion. Obviously, their mortality rate and length of stay were significantly higher when compared with the other group.

The authors present a fairly compelling management algorithm that includes a presentation of pneumomediastinum on chest x-ray and CT scan as the initial diagnostic test, which includes a CT of the chest, upper abdomen, and neck. Then, if the patient is found to have low-risk factors (such as age less than 40 years, a history of cough or upper respiratory infection, and clinical nontoxic appearance), the CT scan findings do not demonstrate pleural effusion or pneumopericardium, and there is no evidence of dyspnea or dysphonia, then these patients can be managed with supportive care. Conversely, if there is any history of dysphagia, then those patients require esophagram. If the esophagram is negative, then they can still be managed with supportive care. Furthermore, patient high-risk factors include age older than 40, history of severe vomiting and retching, elevated white cell count, and abdominal tenderness. In these patients, the CT scan may find pleural effusion, atelectasis, pneumopericardium, or pneumoperitoneum, and an esophagram is next indicated. If no perforation is identified, they may be managed with supportive care. However, if an esophageal perforation is identified, then clearly they need either a stent or an esophageal repair. The important findings in this article are a reminder that pneumomediastinum is an uncommon, benign, and self-limited disease primarily affecting young adults. Chest pain, shortness of breath, and subcutaneous emphysema are the main findings accompanying the pneumomediastinum and CT scan of the chest remains the gold standard initial screening study in establishing the diagnosis. It may also be useful, based on this article, to allow the algorithmic approach to management in order to have a standardized triaging mechanism and more carefully scrutinize who requires hospital admission vs who can be managed at home with supportive care.

C. T. Klodell, Jr, MD

Penetrating cardiac injuries and the evolving management algorithm in the current era

Kong VY, Oosthuizen G, Sartorius B, et al (Univ of KwaZulu Natal, Pietermaritzburg, South Africa; Univ of KwaZulu-Natal, Durban, South Africa)

J Surg Res 193:926-932, 2015

Background.—Penetrating cardiac injuries carry a significant mortality, especially if operative intervention is delayed because of diagnostic difficulties.

Methods and Materials.—We reviewed our experience of 134 consecutive cases over a 6 year period. For the initial 5 years, the diagnosis was based on clinical grounds only. During the final year of study, focused ultrasound focused abdominal sonar for trauma (FAST) and subxiphoid pericardial window were introduced.

Results.—Ninety-six per cent (128/134) were males and the overall mean age was 27 y. Eighty-four per cent (112/134) sustained isolated cardiac injury and the remaining sixteen per cent (22/134) had concurrent injuries elsewhere. A total of 10 FAST's were performed and the sensitivity was 20%. Fifteen subxiphoid pericardial window were performed (8 had diagnostic uncertainty, 2 with double jeopardy, and 5 with delayed tamponade) and had a sensitivity of 100%. The survival rate for the 109 patients from the pre-adjunct period was 83% and 88% for the 25 patients in the post-adjunct period, which was not statistically significant (P value $= 0.765$). There was no significant difference in the complication rate, mean intensive care unit stay, or mean total hospital stay.

Conclusions.—Penetrating cardiac injuries are highly lethal. A high index of suspicion, coupled with early operative intervention remains the key in securing the survival of these patients.

▶ Penetrating cardiac injuries are highly lethal with less than 10% of victims reaching the hospital alive. Of those who do make it to the hospital, rapid diagnosis and surgical intervention may be key to survival. Historically, the diagnostic workup of a suspected penetrating cardiac injury was predominantly clinical; however, a number of new diagnostic and therapeutic modalities are now widely used. The focused abdominal sonar for trauma (FAST) and the subxiphoid pericardial window (SPW) are both mainstays in the management of penetrating cardiac injuries. Although the FAST scan may only offer diagnostic potential, the SPW may be both diagnostic and therapeutic in a defined cohort of patients. The authors review 6 years of data from their trauma registry and identify patients in whom penetrating cardiac wound was suspected. They have only been routinely been performing the FAST scan since 2013, and their general algorithm is that a patient with a positive FAST scan is taken for operative exploration. In an unstable patient with a negative FAST scan, but the clinical suspicion is high, they perform a SPW and proceed accordingly based on the results. In a stable patient with a negative FAST scan but low clinical suspicion, they were comfortable observing the patient and did not perform further imaging. The only additional pearl for the SPW is that they only mention inspecting the pericardial space for fluid contents. I believe it is essential that the pericardial space is irrigated with warm saline and that it is demonstrated that the saline returns to the suction at the subxiphoid space. If repeated attempts at irrigation at the pericardium result in loss of that saline volume, consideration of a large rent in the pericardium into the pleural space should be considered and investigated.

Penetrating cardiac injuries are still commonly encountered and remain highly lethal. The overall mortality from all penetrating thoracic trauma is approximately 30% and in penetrating cardiac injuries, the mortality is approximately 76%. Of those who do survive long enough to reach the hospital, then the early diagnosis and immediate intervention becomes critical to save the patient. The diagnostic approach that the authors outline based on a combination of clinical presentation and FAST scan and the use of SPW is both appropriate and relatively common among our ranks. They do highlight, importantly, that hemodynamic instability even in the setting of a negative FAST scan should provoke further investigation.

C. T. Klodell, Jr, MD

Air Transport of Patients with Pneumothorax: Is Tube Thoracostomy Required Before Flight?

Braude D, Tutera D, Tawil I, et al (Univ of New Mexico Health Science Ctr. Albuquerque)
Air Med J 33:152-156, 2014

Objective.—It is conventionally thought that patients with pneumothorax (PTX) require tube thoracostomy (TT) before air medical transport (AMT), especially in unpressurized rotor-wing (RW) aircraft, to prevent deterioration from expansion of the PTX or development of tension PTX. We hypothesize that patients with PTX transported without TT tolerate RW AMT without serious deterioration, as defined by hypotension, hypoxemia, respiratory distress, intubation, bag valve mask ventilation, needle thoracostomy (NT), or cardiac arrest during transport.

Methods.—We conducted a retrospective review of a case-series of trauma patients transported to a single Level 1 trauma center via RW with confirmed PTX and no TT. Using standardized abstraction forms, we reviewed charts for signs of deterioration. Those patients identified as having clinical deterioration were independently reviewed for the likelihood that the clinical deterioration was a direct consequence of PTX.

Results.—During the study period, 66 patients with confirmed PTX underwent RW AMT with an average altitude gain of 1890 feet, an average barometric pressure 586-600 mm Hg, and average flight duration of 28 minutes. All patients received oxygen therapy; 14/66 patients (21%) were supported with positive pressure ventilation. Eleven of 66 patients (17%) had NT placed before flight and 4/66 (6%) had NT placed during flight. Four of 66 patients (6% CI 0.3-11.7) may have deteriorated during AMT as a result of PTX; all were successfully managed with NT.

Conclusions.—In shit series, 6% of patients with PTX deteriorated as result of AMT without TT, yet all patients were managed successfully with NT. Routine placement of TT in patients with PTX before RW AMT may not be necessary. Further prospective evaluation is warranted.

▶ It is conventionally thought that patients require tube thoracostomy before air transport, particularly in unpressurized aircraft. The authors retrospectively reviewed 66 patients transported with known pneumothorax and no tube thoracostomy in place. Interestingly, in their series, only 6% of patients deteriorated during air medical transport without a tube thoracostomy and required a needle thoracostomy. They conclude that perhaps the routine placement of tube thoracostomy in patients with pneumothorax before air medical transport may not be necessary.

Thoracic trauma is responsible for one-quarter of all trauma deaths and is a frequent component of multisystem trauma. Pneumothorax is observed in 10% to 22% of severe blunt trauma cases. Some experts have held that the presence of an unresolved pneumothorax is an absolute contraindication for air medical transport. However, tube thoracostomy may not be possible in all settings and may be associated with both transport delays and serious complications particularly when being placed by less experienced providers.

This study is performed by retrospectively reviewing a prospectively maintained database over a 6-year period and distilling down only to those patients that were transported with a pneumothorax without a tube thoracostomy. Their patients had an average altitude gain of 1884 feet and a barometric pressure between 586 and 600 mm Hg. The average duration of transport was 28 minutes. Twenty-four percent (24%) of the patients were transported between facilities, and the remainder came directly from the accident scene. Only 7 of the 66 patients (11%) deteriorated during transport. In 3 of these cases, the deterioration was felt to be unrelated to the pneumothorax. In 4 cases (6%), deterioration was thought to be due to the pneumothorax. Each of these patients was successfully managed with needle decompression and did not suffer any apparent morbidity from not having a tube thoracostomy in place before transport.

Air medical transports present a theoretical risk for patients with pneumothorax because of increasing altitude especially in nonpressurized rotary-wing aircraft. Increasing altitude results in decreasing atmospheric pressure and subsequent increases in the volume in a closed system. According to Boyles Law, an increase in 2000 feet of elevation would allow the volume of a closed air space to expand by approximately 10%. With those data in mind, although larger and prospective trails may be helpful in developing more definitive evidence-based clinical based guidelines, it is interesting to consider that perhaps not all patients require tube thoracostomy for pneumothorax prior to transport. One caveat is that the air medical transport in this study does use 3-inch-long catheters for needle decompressions. This should be the standard for any who are considering using this as a treatment algorithm because the shorter catheters may not always reach into the chest space.

In summary, in this small retrospective study only 6% of patients with traumatic pneumothorax deteriorated as a result of unpressurized air medical transport without tube thoracostomy. All of those patients were managed successfully with needle decompression without apparent morbidity or mortality. Therefore, the routine placement of tube thoracostomy prophylactically before air transport may not be necessary. Ultimately, this is a decision that each referring physician or referring center and receiving physician may have to make on an individual basis, but this article does provide some evidence to allow us to consider transporting patients without chest tubes for small, stable pneumothoraces.

C. T. Klodell, Jr, MD

Predictors of outcome and different management of aortobronchial and aortoesophageal fistulas
Mosquera VX, Marini M, Pombo-Felipe F, et al (Complejo Hospitalario Universitario de A Coruña, Spain)
J Thorac Cardiovasc Surg 148:3020-3026, 2014

Objective.—Aortoesophageal and aortobronchial fistulas are uncommon but life-threatening conditions. The present study aimed to identify potential differences in outcomes, depending on the etiology, type, and management of the fistulas, and to determine mortality predictors.

Methods.—We retrospectively reviewed a series of 26 consecutive patients with thoracic aorta fistulas admitted to our institution from 1998 to 2013 (18 aortobronchial, 7 aortoesophageal, and 1 combined fistula).

Results.—The mean age was 61.5 ± 13.4 years, with 22 men. Management was thoracic endovascular aortic repair (TEVAR) in 8, open repair in 7, and conservative in 11. The TEVAR and nonoperative patients were significantly older and presented with more comorbidities. Shock developed in 15 patients and sepsis in 9. The most common radiologic findings were intramural hematoma (65.4%), pseudoaneurysm (53.8%), and bronchial compression (46.20%). Active contrast extravasation (23.1%) and ectopic gas (19.2%) were associated with a worse prognosis. In-hospital mortality was 100% in the conservative group, 37.5% in the TEVAR group, and 14.3% in the open repair group ($P = .04$). Septic shock was the most common cause of death. The risk factors for in-hospital mortality were hemodynamic instability on admission ($P = .02$), sepsis ($P = .04$), and conservative management ($P < .001$). The overall long-term survival in surgical patients at 1 and 5 years was 66% and 58.7%, respectively. Infectious and malignant etiologies resulted in the worst prognosis.

Conclusions.—The outcomes are ultimately conditioned by the etiology of the fistula. Both open and endovascular management of aortic fistulas can prevent death by exsanguination; however, patients remain at high risk of infectious complications. Failure to treat the underlying cause will result in poor midterm outcomes.

▶ Aortoesophageal and aortobronchial fistulas pose one of the most challenging surgical problems to manage. Both types of thoracic aorta fistulas are uncommon but life-threatening if left untreated. Primary aortoesophageal and aortobronchial fistulas are most commonly found in association with aortic aneurysms, ruptured penetrating aortic ulcers, thoracic trauma, ingestion of foreign bodies, and esophageal or bronchogenic malignancies. The classic management of these difficult problems has been open repair; however, in the most contemporary of times, many centers have gone to the primary use of thoracic endovascular aortic repair (TEVAR) and have published their experiences. Both open and endovascular surgical treatment can prevent patient death by controlling the exsanguination; however, irrespective of the approach, patients remain at high risk of infectious complications because neither the bronchus nor the esophagus are sterile cavities. This is of utmost importance when managing aortic fistulas especially when they are either related to or caused by mycotic pseudoaneurysms or malignancy. The aim of the authors' study was to identify the potential differences in early- and long-term results, stratified by the etiology, type, and management of the fistulas and to determine the mortality predictors in this subset of patients. Their cohort of 26 patients over a 15-year period at their center included left bronchial tree to aorta fistula in 18 patients, an aorta to esophageal in 8 patients, and 1 patient with both. In all patients, CT scanning was the most valuable diagnostic test. The patients were managed in both open and TEVAR fashion.

Despite either open or endovascular success managing aortic fistulas, thereby preventing the patients' death by exsanguination, the results of the long-term and midterm outcomes are ultimately dependent on the etiology of the fistula. Therefore, failure to treat the underlying cause will entail a poor midterm outcome. Both open and endovascular management of fistulas can prevent the death, and in that respect, TEVAR seems to be an attractive alternative for most patients even if only used as a bail-out or bridging procedure. At our center, we have moved almost exclusively to the use of TEVAR and endovascular means to control exsanguinating hemorrhage because it is both easier to apply and more rapidly deployable, and it does not involve the coagulopathy and other complications of open surgery. However, the Achilles' heel remains the inability to control the associated infection; prolonged antibiotic therapy and lifelong surveillance is critical and has been our practice paradigm.

C. T. Klodell, Jr, MD

Blunt Cardiac Trauma: A Review of the Current Knowledge and Management
Yousef R, Carr JA (Hurley Med and Level 1 Trauma Ctr, Flint, MI)
Ann Thorac Surg 98:1134-1140, 2014

Blunt cardiac injuries are highly lethal. A review of the world's English literature on the topic reveals a lack of Level 1 Evidence and few cohesive guidelines for the management of these patients. An online database query was performed using the PubMed medical database. All relevant articles from the past 20 years were reviewed. Conclusions are presented with their corresponding Levels of Evidence.

▶ The authors review the world's English literature on the topic of blunt cardiac trauma and attempt to compile some cohesive guidelines to help guide the care of these patients. They felt they reviewed all relevant articles from the past 20 years.

Pathophysiology: Most blunt cardiac trauma injuries occur due to motor vehicle injuries, followed closely by pedestrians being struck by motor vehicles, and then motorcycle crashes. Blunt cardiac trauma is identified in approximately 11.9% of patients sustaining these types of injuries. Seventy to eighty percent of patients who have blunt cardiac injuries have multiple other concurrent injuries, including brain and thoracic aortic injuries as well as lung and hemothorax. The most common lethal cardiac injury is transmural rupture of 1 or more cardiac chambers, as well as tears occurring at the venous-atrial confluence or blunt coronary artery dissection. Owning to its anterior location, the right ventricle is the most commonly injured chamber.

Commotio Cordis: Commotio cordis is a sudden death from a cardiac arrest in a young person often occurring during sports after a blunt chest blow. Unlike motor vehicle accidents or falls, this injury demonstrates no anatomic damage to the heart but is purely a conduction abnormality produced by the trauma. In the United States, there is a commotio cordis registry, which has documented that approximately 50% of these cases are from blunt blows to the chest occurring in competitive sports. Interestingly, the most common sport is baseball, and it is usually triggered when players have been struck in the chest by balls that have either been pitched, batted, or thrown in a variety of circumstances. Other than baseball, commotio cordis is seen in softball, ice hockey, football, and lacrosse. Clearly, most of the blunt trauma victims' blunt cardiac injuries who do survive to the hospital have injuries that are less severe. With the exception of cardiac tamponade from bleeding, the other potentially treatable and reversible cardiac injuries can be divided into 2 groups, which are the structural cardiac lesions, including intramural hematoma and valvular injury, and electrical disturbances, for example.

Intramural Hematoma: Intramural hematoma commonly occurs in the right ventricle and makes up 13% of all patients with blunt cardiac injury. The hematoma can cause premature ventricular contractions, as well as transient bundle branch block, although their clinical course tends to be relatively benign. The knowledge of how to treat intramural hematoma does not come from the trauma literature but rather from the complications that have occurred after surgical and percutaneous coronary interventions resulting in intramural hematomas of the ventricle. With conservative management, virtually all intramural hematomas tend to resolve spontaneously after 4 to 12 weeks.

Valvular Injury: Another common injury pattern from blunt cardiac trauma is papillary muscle rupture leading to acute valvular regurgitation of either the mitral or tricuspid valves. There has also been documentation of blunt aortic valve injury and, very rarely, a blunt pulmonary valve injury. The majority of patients presenting with new atrial-ventricular valve regurgitation will present with a holosystolic murmur and will be diagnosed by echocardiography. Surgical repair is required for these patients and most often will be a valvular replacement. Occasionally, these valves can be reconstructed with repair of the torn papillary muscle and/or chordae.

Coronary artery injury is again most common with direct impact over the left anterior descending coronary artery or the left main coronary artery can also be injured. The apex, septum, or both are the most commonly affected areas of the heart, and often this can be managed with percutaneous techniques, including stenting of the left anterior descending artery. Additionally, traumatic ventricular septal defects can occur and most commonly require surgery and patch closure, although there have been case reports of successful transcatheter closure using a ventricular septal defect occluder device. Finally, in deciding how to screen these patients, one should consider screening by troponin I (TnI) as one of the more accurate mechanisms, as well as electrocardiogram (ECG) for any patient suspected of having a blunt cardiac injury.

Electrical Disturbances: Sinus tachycardia is the most common ECG abnormality among trauma victims. However, atrial fibrillation may also be present as well as supraventricular tachycardia or even paroxysmal ventricular tachycardia. In conclusion, the following list should be considered in any trauma patient with the potential to have a cardiac injury:

- Obtain an initial ECG on all patients in whom blunt cardiac trauma is suspected.
- If the admission ECG does show a new abnormality, the patient should be admitted for continuous monitoring.
- A combination of a fall greater than 20 feet and a sternal fracture should prompt a thorough cardiac evaluation because these patients have a high incidence of blunt cardiac trauma.
- Even a large intramural hematoma in the ventricle can be treated conservatively because most will resolve over time, and usually within 3 months.
- The serum troponin I should be drawn and, when exceeding 1 ng/mL, is abnormal and associated with a true cardiac injury in 60% to 70% of the patients. A formal ECG should be performed in such cases.
- Patients with a suspicion of cardiac injury and then found to have a normal troponin I and a normal ECG can safely be discharged home.
- An interatrial septal hematoma and/or a traumatic tricuspid valve injury can both quickly progress to complete heart block and should be monitored closely with consideration of insertion of transvenous pacemaker prophylactically or at least immediately at the first sign of conduction abnormality.
- Small tears at the venous-atrial confluence may be contained, and the patient may be initially stable; however, diagnosis by echocardiography should lead to prompt surgical restoration of the injury.

C. T. Klodell, Jr, MD

Article Index

Chapter 1: General Considerations

Chapter 2: Trauma

Chapter 3: Burns

Chapter 4: Critical Care

Chapter 5: Transplantation

Chapter 6: Surgical Infections

Chapter 7: Endocrine

Chapter 8: Nutrition

Chapter 9: Gastrointestinal

Chapter 10: Oncology

Chapter 11: Vascular Surgery

Chapter 12: General Thoracic Surgery

Author Index

Printed and bound by CPI Group (UK) Ltd, Croydon, CR0 4YY

08/05/2025

01864679-0005